Anne Marie:
Look forward to
working with you

[signature]

2/16/2016

DESIGNING THE WORLD'S BEST
Children's Hospitals 3

DESIGNING THE WORLD'S BEST Children's Hospitals 3

The future of healing environments

Bruce King Komiske, MHA, FACHE
Editor and Creator

in cooperation with, the National Association of Children's Hospitals and Related Institutions, the Children's Hospital Association, FKP Architects, HDR, HKS Architects, KMD Architects, Stantec, and ZGF Architects LLP

images
Publishing

Published in Australia in 2012 by
The Images Publishing Group Pty Ltd
ABN 89 059 734 431
6 Bastow Place, Mulgrave, Victoria 3170, Australia
Tel: +61 3 9561 5544 Fax: +61 3 9561 4860
books@imagespublishing.com
www.imagespublishing.com

The Images Publishing Group Reference Number: 995

National Library of Australia Cataloguing-in-Publication entry:

Author:	Komiske, Bruce
Title:	Designing the world's best: children's hospital 3
ISBN:	9781864703399 (hbk.)
Subjects:	Children—Hospitals.
	Children—Hospitals—Pictorial works.
	Hospital architecture.
	Hospital architecture—Pictorial works.
	Hospitals—Design and construction.
	Hospitals—Design and construction—Pictorial works.

Dewey Number: 725.57

Edited by Driss Fatih

Designed by The Graphic Image Studio Pty Ltd, Mulgrave, Australia
www.tgis.com.au

Pre-publishing services by Mission Productions Limited, Hong Kong

Printed by Everbest Printing Co. Ltd., in Hong Kong/China on 140gsm GoldEast Matt Art

IMAGES has included on its website a page for special notices in relation to this and our other publications. Please visit www.imagespublishing.com.

Contents

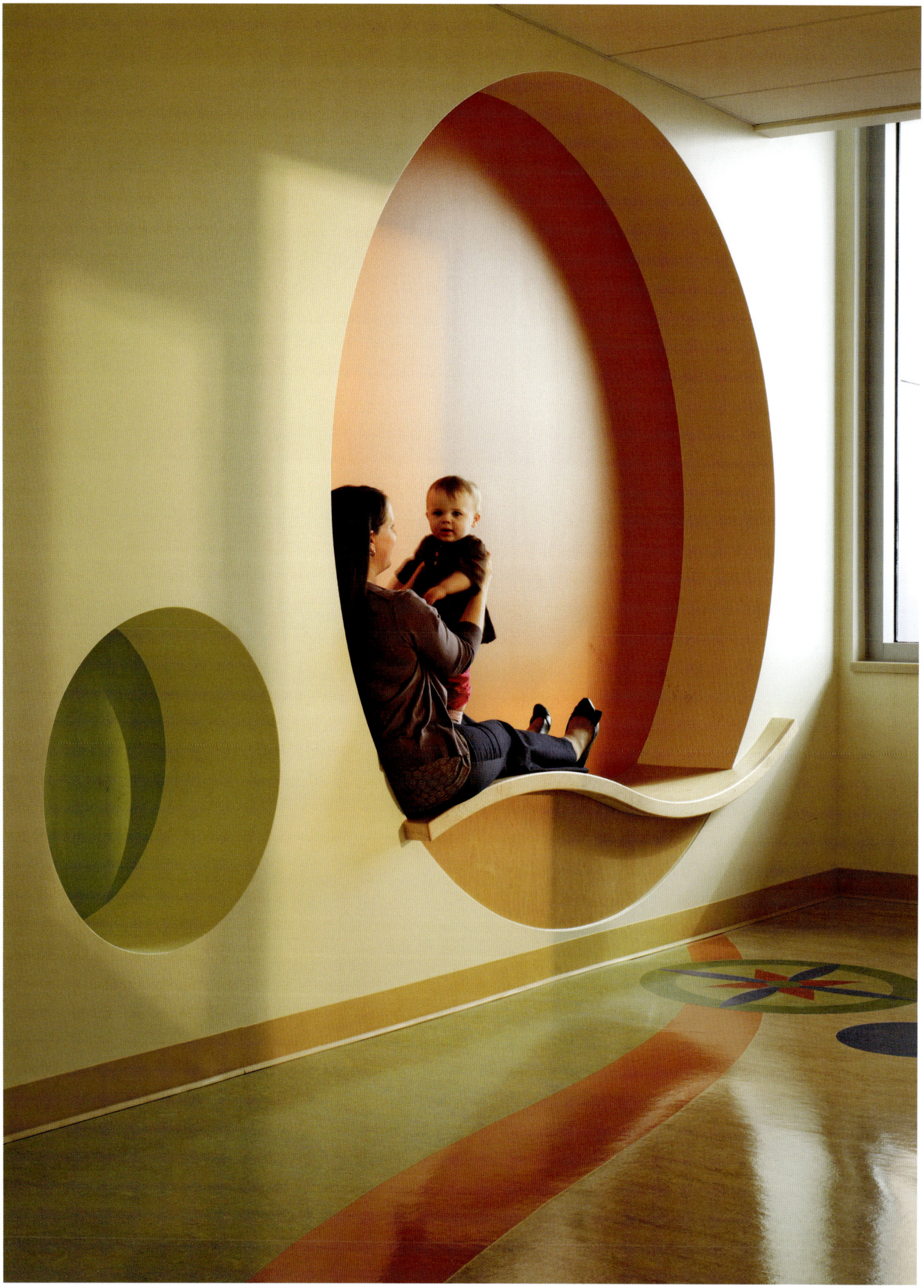

The Purpose

Since the first edition, published by Images in 1999, *Designing the World's Best Children's Hospitals* can be found on the desk of just about anyone interested in starting the long and exciting journey of creating a new children's hospital. Hopefully the book has served as an inspiration to think differently about the look and feel of what is generally thought of as a "very scary place." By sharing photos of the newest and most innovative facilities in the US and around the world, future organizations and their design teams can visualize what resonates or does not resonate within their own culture. This process can also start the planning for site tours, where almost all children's hospitals unselfishly share their experiences. These images can also be the basis of a charrette, which helps the project team to create the vision, design vocabulary, and direction for the project. Through this process, the quality of the healing environments in children's hospitals continues to improve and enhance the healing process, which is the ultimate goal.

This book is also an opportunity to recognize the exciting work of over 70 institutions, their dedicated project teams, and the staff, patients, and families who all had a significant influence on the future of these very special healing environments.

Bruce King Komiske, MHA, FACHE

◀ University of Minnesota Amplatz Children's Hospital, Minneapolis, MN
Photo: Hedrich Blessing Photography, Nick Merrick

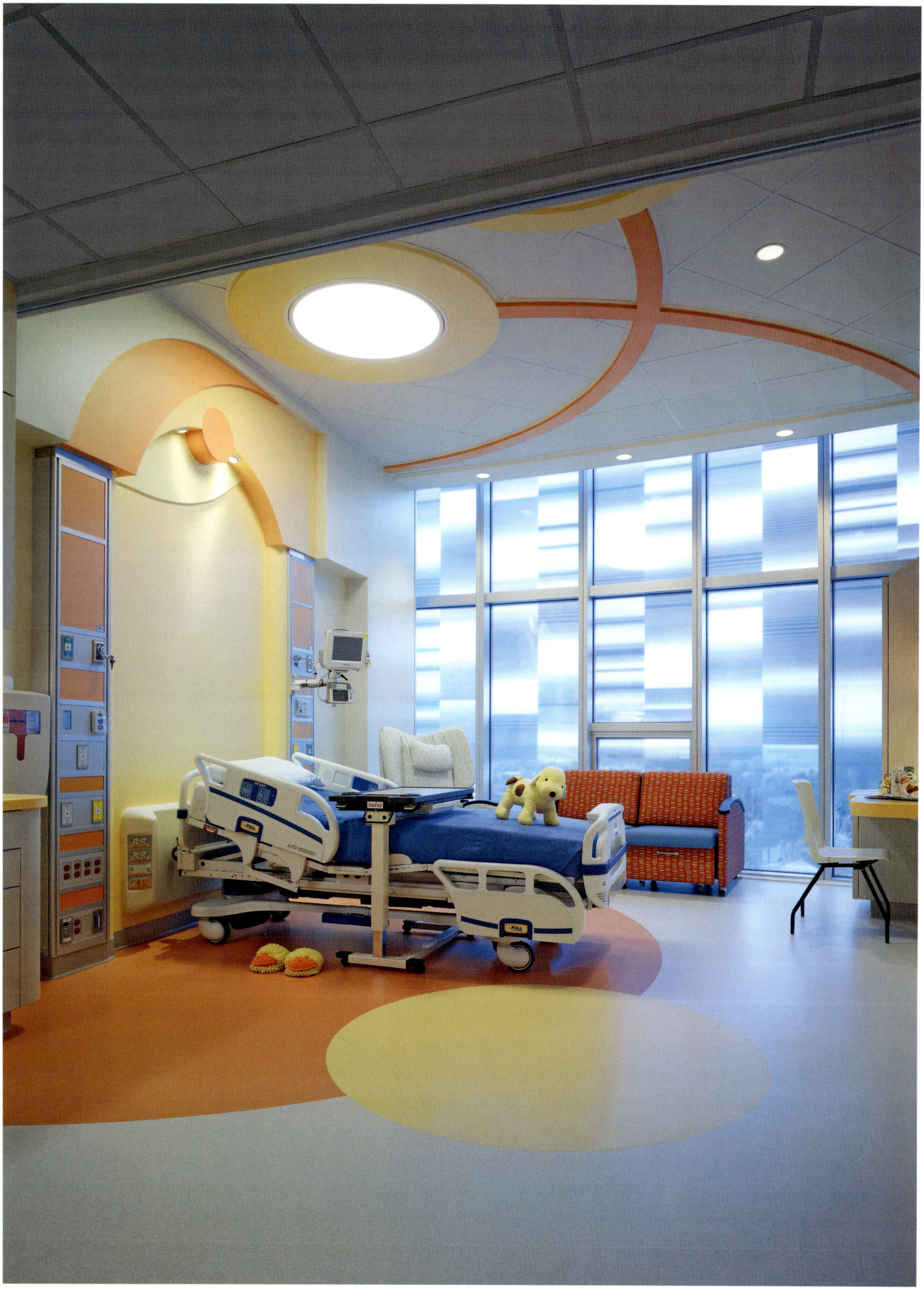

The Challenge

As President and Chief Executive Officer of the National Association of Children's Hospitals and Related Institutions who spent 19 years in office, I have had the opportunity to participate in all three editions of *Designing the World's Best Children's Hospitals*. Each new volume of the book has captured the maturation and sophistication of the roles and functions of children's hospitals. Given that children represent only one quarter of the population and are on the whole healthier than adults, and due to economies of scale and the scarcity of specialized physicians and care givers, children's hospitals have become more and more regional and specialized, and provide care that simply cannot be received elsewhere.

The concentration of children's services into regional centers has permitted and encouraged the design of children's hospitals for the specific needs of children and their families. In addition, with increasing evidence on the impact of design on health and safety, planners and architects have applied their best skills and talents to build features into the facilities that positively impact health and safety. It is tremendously gratifying to see design solutions borne of evidence-based data become the norm. Obviously, with cost remaining a significant consideration in the construction of new children's hospitals, more and more emphasis is being placed on adjacencies and work flow efficiencies to get the most from the investment, as well as the most out of the healing environment.

The essence of this book is to build on what others have learned in the construction of new children's hospitals and to stimulate the imagination through the presentation of beautiful photographic images of richly textured environments, in order to promote a better healing environment for children, a nurturing environment for the children and their families, and a calming environment for children, families, caregivers, and all involved in the healing process. The challenge to you—the next generation of dreamers, planners, architects and staff—is to create ever more pleasing, safe, and cost-effective health care for our children.

Lawrence A. McAndrews
Retired, President and CEO
National Association of Children's Hospitals
and Related Institutions

◀ Helen DeVos Children's Hospital, Grand Rapids, MI
Photo: Hedrich Blessing Photography, Scott McDonald

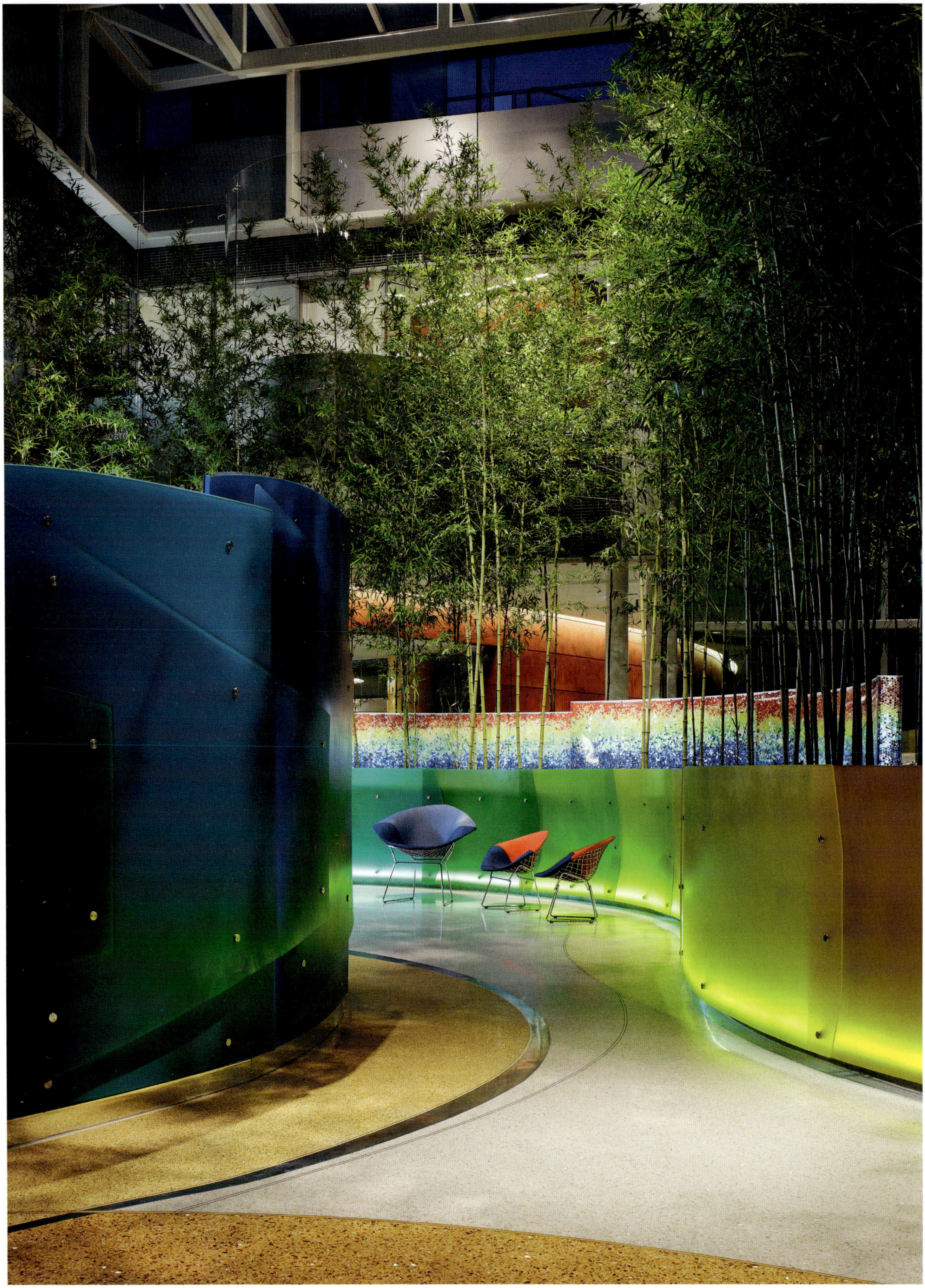

The 10 Guiding Principles of a Successful Project

1 **Vision -** "Make no little plans for they have no magic to stir men's blood"—so wrote Daniel Burnham, responsible for Chicago's Master Plan that more than 100 years later is still used to shape the future of the City.

The size or scope of a project does not matter. If the CEO, project leader, or project team has a grand vision that is supported by the institution and the project strives to accomplish something new through innovation, the chances of a highly successful project significantly improve. Whatever you do—do not simply replace an old building with a new building!

2 **Strategic objectives -** If an institution is committing what might be the largest investment in its history, make sure that at the beginning of the process the team explores the question "If this project was wildly successful, what would it look like and how would you know it?" Be as definitive as possible: for example, market share would increase by 8 percent; patient satisfaction would increase by 15 percent; philanthropy would provide 50 percent of funding, etc. Measure these criteria both before and after construction and also consider completing a Post Occupancy Evaluation (POE) to further modify the building after opening, if necessary. If you do not quantify success, how will you know if you have achieved it?

3 **The team -** The selection of the key members of the team, including the project leader, design and engineering firms, construction management and program management firms, as well as all other consultants, should be based not only on the reputation and experience of the firms, but also on the experience of the actual individuals selected to work on the project, which is of equal importance. Consider narrowing down the key firms and then create opportunities to work closely with each team, in their own environment, before making the final selections. Also make sure that the internal project team comprises the best people that the organization has to offer, with a significant amount of diversity and institutional culture. If at all possible, co-locate the hospital team, designers, engineers, program manager, construction manager, and key consultants at the earliest possible time to foster team building and a team approach to the entire project.

4 **The budget and contract -** Creating a realistic budget is based on both the desired scope of the project and the potential availability of funds.

◀ Ann & Robert H. Lurie Children's Hospital of Chicago, IL
Photo: Hedrich Blessing Photography, Nick Merrick

Spend as much time as necessary to make sure that the project starts with a budget that includes all consultants, owner's work, and all appropriate contingencies. These contingencies must reflect project scope, complexity, and delivery method. Benchmark this draft budget with other similar projects, adjusting for market conditions and regional pricing impacts, and work closely with the construction team for their input. Subject your program and budget to peer reviews by other organizations that have recently completed a similar project.

The next most important document is the contract. Obtain the services of a highly competent expert in healthcare construction contracts to assist in this process. If the budget and contract are fair to all parties, easily understandable, realistic, well-coordinated, and comprehensive, the chances of a successful project are greatly improved.

Finally, the owner must fully understand and accept the risks associated with design and construction and be prepared to deal with changes. Changes come from many sources, and it is necessary to have an effective, time-sensitive, and nimble process to effectively administer the inevitable.

5 **Involvement -** In general, the more engaged staff, faculty, and administrators are in a project, the greater the chances of success. Through ongoing participation in the process, participants become vested in the success of the project. This high level of involvement should extend to the children and families (consider creating a Kid's Advisory Council and a Family Advisory Council), the entire hospital workforce, internal and external committees, as well as interested local community organizations or any other appropriate group. While many groups are advisory in nature, their involvement and participation ultimately provides for a more successful project. Of significant importance, however, is to have a well-defined, efficient, and effective decision-making process that involves the key institutional leaders. This leadership group should be able to take into consideration the feedback and varied opinions of, at times, possibly disparate desires, and keep the focus on the big picture.

6 **Communicate – communicate – communicate -** Communication is one of the most important elements during the life of a project. You can never have too much of it! Consider utilizing every means possible to engage and keep interest at a high level. Use varied communication tools – town hall meetings, email updates, hospital ambassadors, videos, mock-ups, monthly updates at board and staff meetings, community and donor presentations, etc.

7 **Engaging the community -** Each city or community is unique, with its own architecture, art, local culture, geographic features, landmarks, and "bragging rights." Develop a vision and process for incorporating these unique elements into the architecture, art, and landscaping of the building. Make sure that the final building does not look like

a generic hospital that could be located anywhere in the country; rather create a place where patients, families, staff, and community can feel comfortable, heal quickly, and look on it with a deep sense of pride.

8 **Learn from and share with others -** There is a comprehensive body of knowledge that continues to be developed as part of the Evidence Based Design (EBD) initiative started by the Center for Health Design. This base of knowledge provides the project team with a wealth of knowledge that can help make the new facility a safe and healing environment. This knowledge base coalesces from the experience of others and is based on real-world experience and data. Equally important to using this knowledge is the process of sharing your knowledge and the lessons you've learned from your project with others. Consider becoming a "Pebble Project"—a group of facilities around the world that meets twice a year to share their progress and add to the EBD knowledge base. Site visits and mock-ups throughout the life of the project are also critical, and are two of the most cost-effective investments that a team can make. When the project is complete, be generous with your time when other facilities ask for your expertise or wish to tour your site.

9 **Start transition planning early -** Consider starting the transition planning as early as the completion of the programming. By appointing a well-respected member of the organization as the transition team leader, you immediately lend credibility to a critical task that may seem so far away, in terms of time, but requires a significant commitment to be done well. Also consider hiring consultants who have demonstrated a track record of leading many healthcare institutions through the process of successfully relocating and opening their new buildings. Appreciate the fact that if you don't utilize the new building as an opportunity to review and improve upon your basic services, processes, and procedures, you have lost a significant opportunity. Recognize that the cost of transition planning, the actual move, staff training, etc. may be anywhere from 1 to 4 percent of the project budget.

10 **Celebrate –** There are very few times in the life of an institution that have the potential for creating a positive change in the culture of that institution. The planning and construction of a major new addition or an entirely new campus is certainly one of these rare opportunities. Make sure that you take every opportunity to share and enjoy this experience with all constituents. Look for opportunities to celebrate all milestones, for example: groundbreaking, halfway happy hour, topping off, and, most importantly, grand opening events. Provide an opportunity, before receiving patients, to share your new building with the board, the media, the community, the donors, the construction workers, and the families of staff members.

Bruce King Komiske

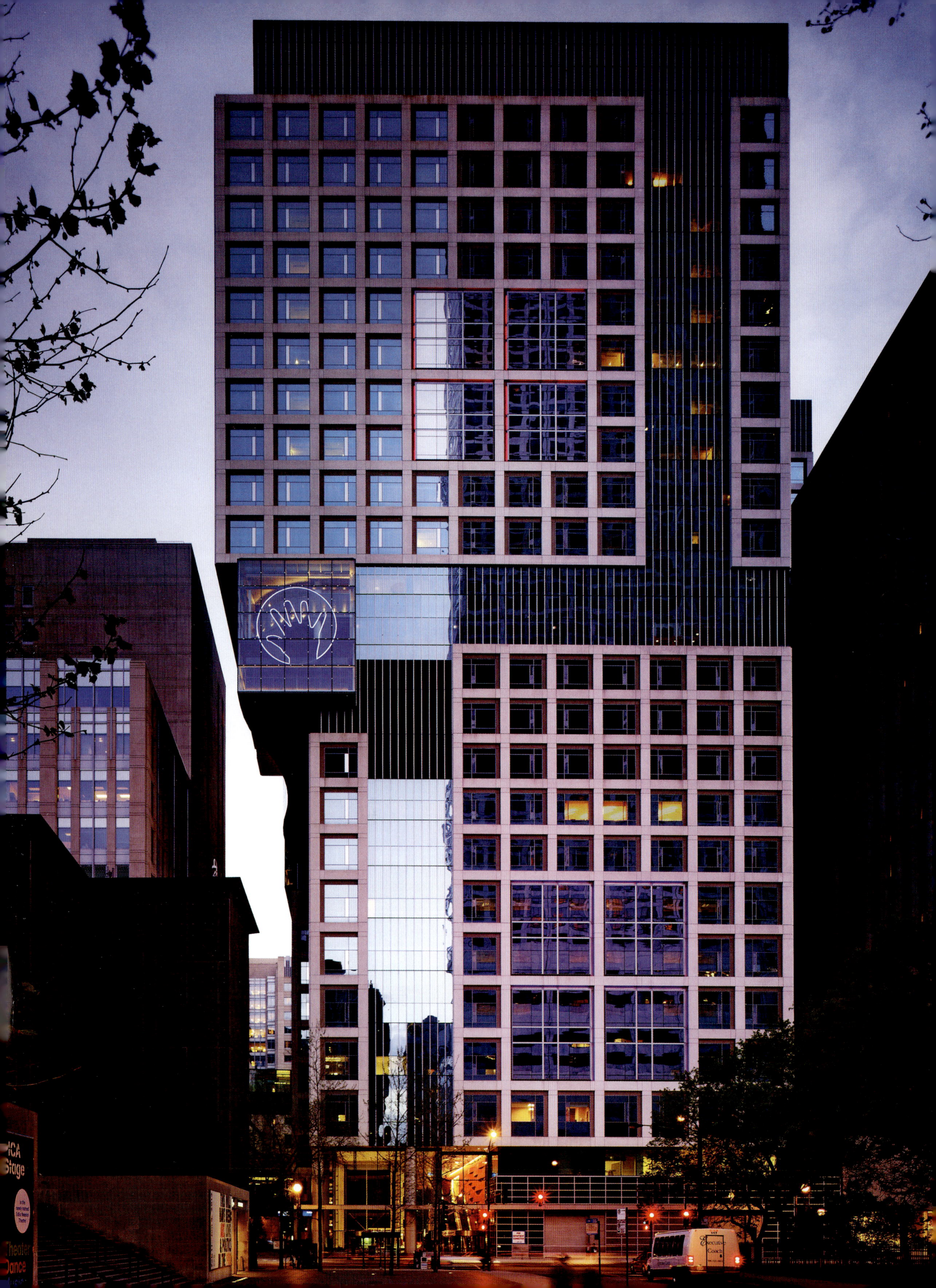
ICA
Stage
Theater
Dance
Executive Coach

Exteriors

The exterior design of the best children's hospitals represents the visual embodiment of the hospital mission, while enhancing the patient and family journey, the brand identity, and the sustainability of the hospital campus.

If a child in pain is transformed through the creative application of form and color, and the stress of loving parents is reduced by creating a place for connectivity, then we have done our part as design professionals.

Creative application of scale, proportion, color, and the relationship of solid and void will strengthen the visual brand identity. A strong brand identity can contribute to the bottom line through enhancing access and market share.

The designers of children's hospitals become the voice for those without a voice, by sculpting the envelope as an outward expression of the critical functions within. With stress reduction as a desired goal, the exterior design of the building should embody experiential transformation with visual elements such as surprise, awe, comfort, safety, and ultimately with the wow factor.

Cues from the surrounding built environment, including materials, scale, orientation, regional, local and micro climate conditions, as well as cultural aspects of the community, influence the design vocabulary, materiality, and systems used to respond sensitively and sustainably to the building's vision. It is our responsibility to integrate innovative ideas that add value to each pediatric facility that we design.

Jeffrey Stouffer, AIA
HKS Architects

◀ Ann & Robert H. Lurie Children's Hospital of Chicago, IL
Photo: Hedrich Blessing Photography, Nick Merrick

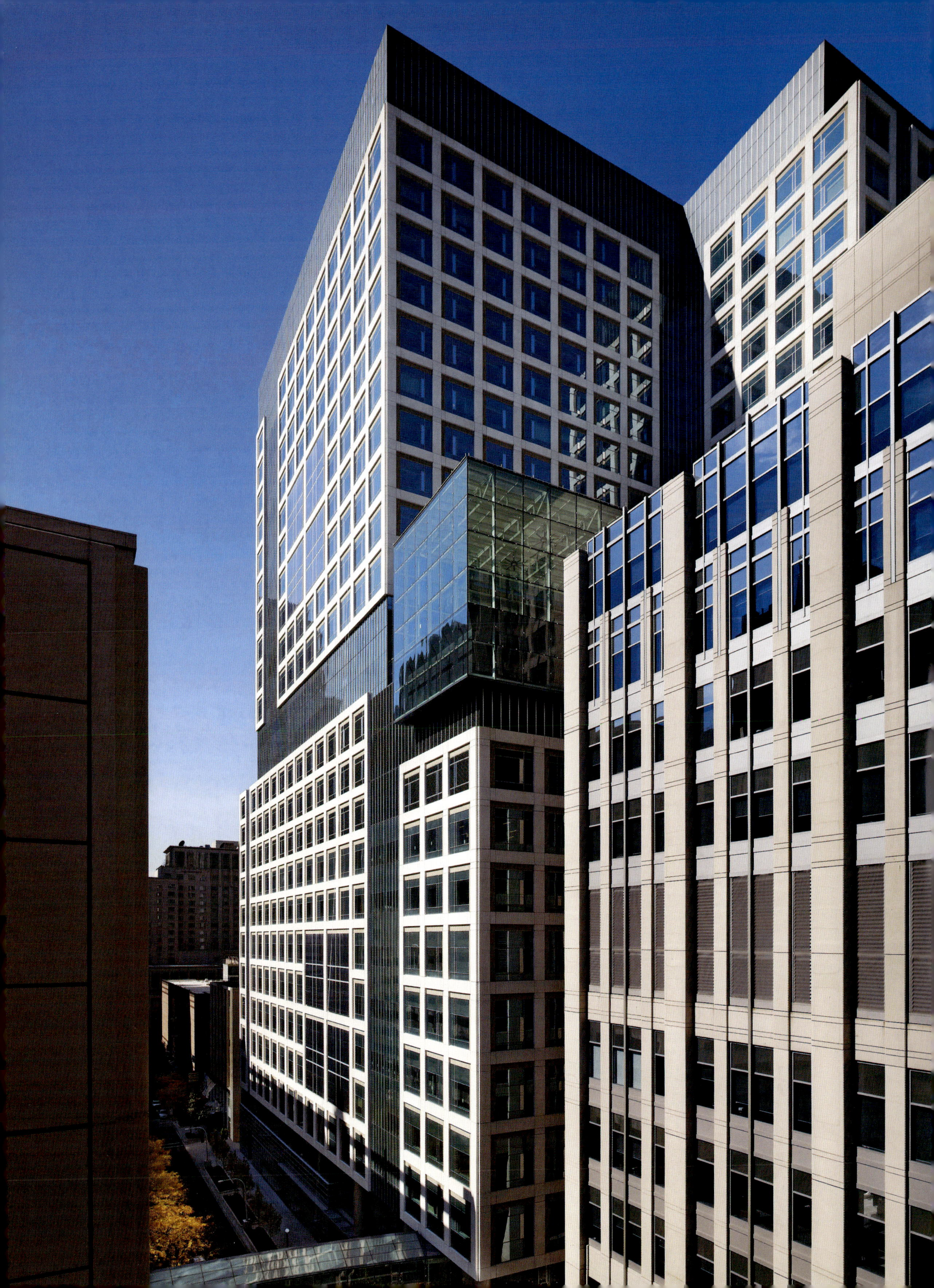

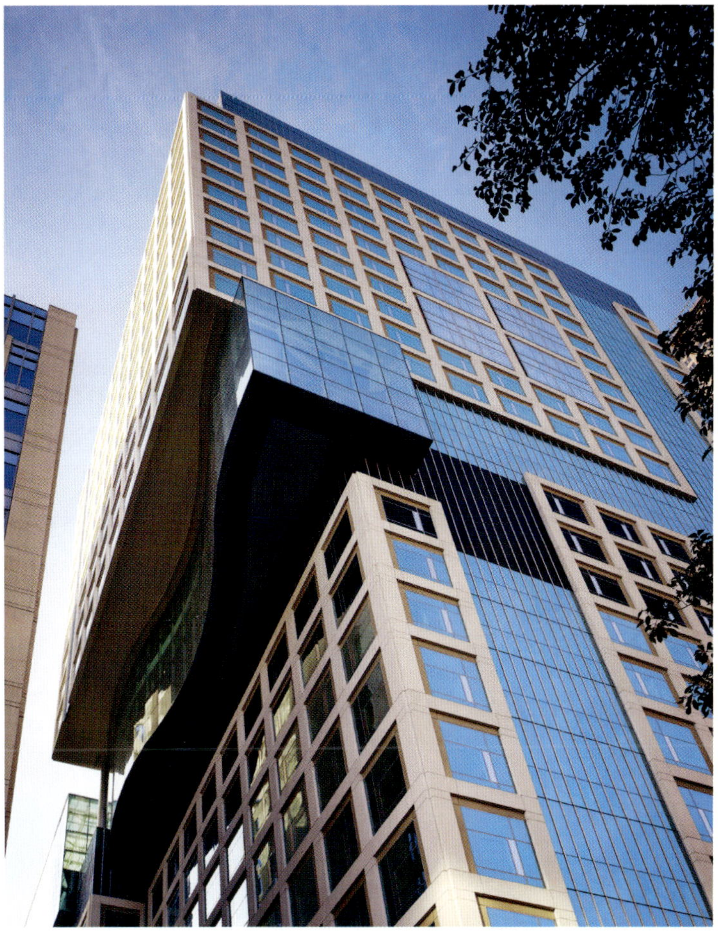

▲ Ann & Robert H. Lurie Children's Hospital of Chicago, IL
◀ *Photos: Hedrich Blessing Photography, Nick Merrick*

▼ Meyer Children's Hospital, Florence, Italy
Photos: Stantec © Alessandro Ciampi and Pietro Savorelli

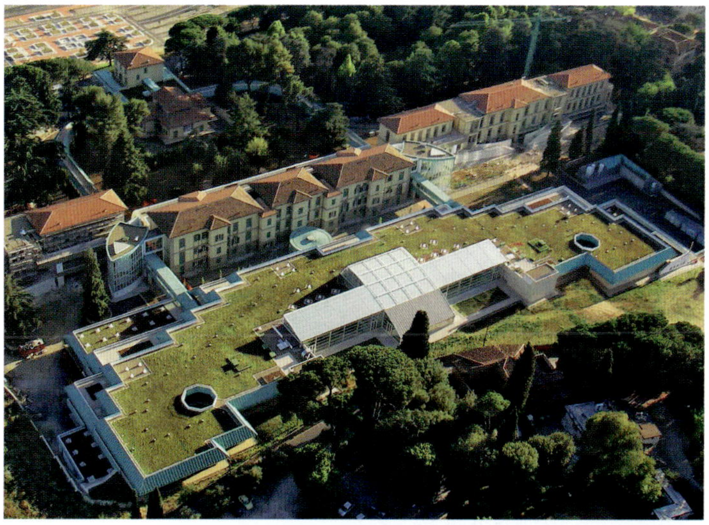

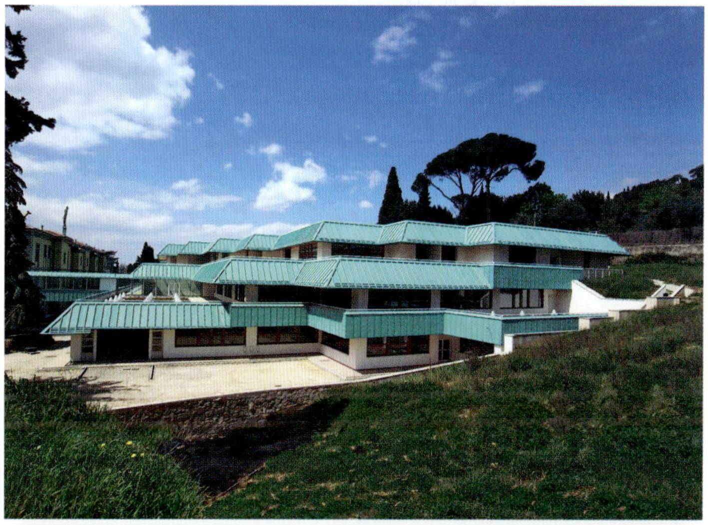

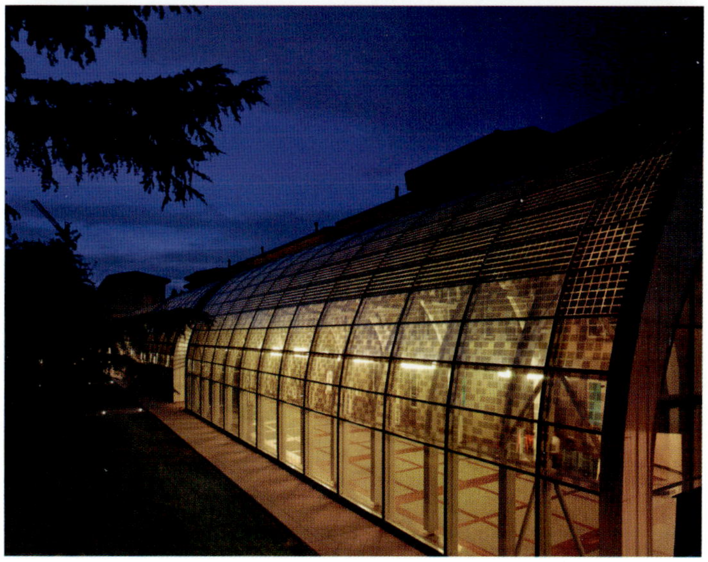

Following pages: Cha Women and Children's Hospital, Seongnam, South Korea
Photo: Jong O Kim

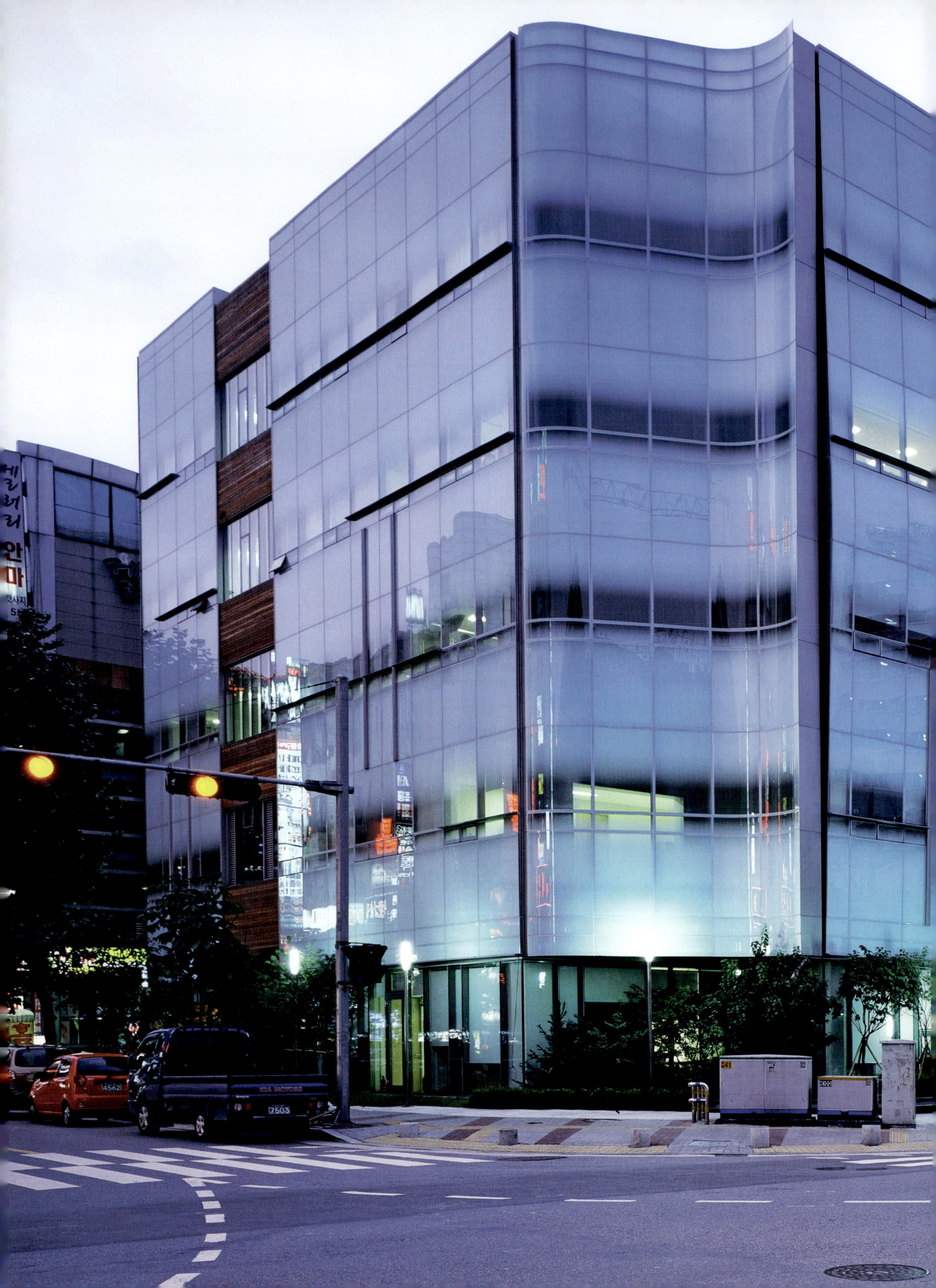

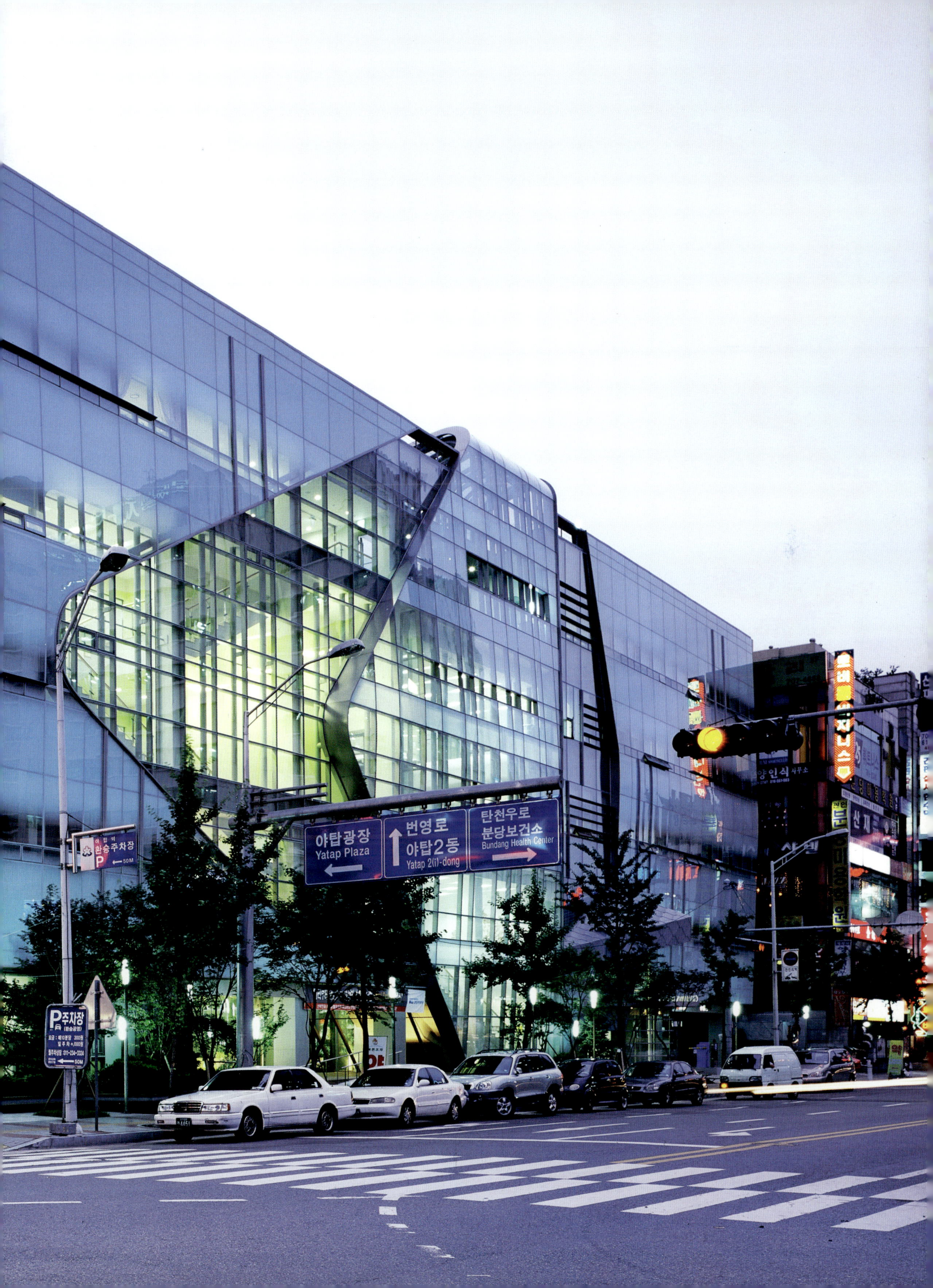
야탑광장
Yatap Plaza
번영로
야탑2동
탄천우로
분당보건소
Bundang Health Center
환승주차장
P주차장

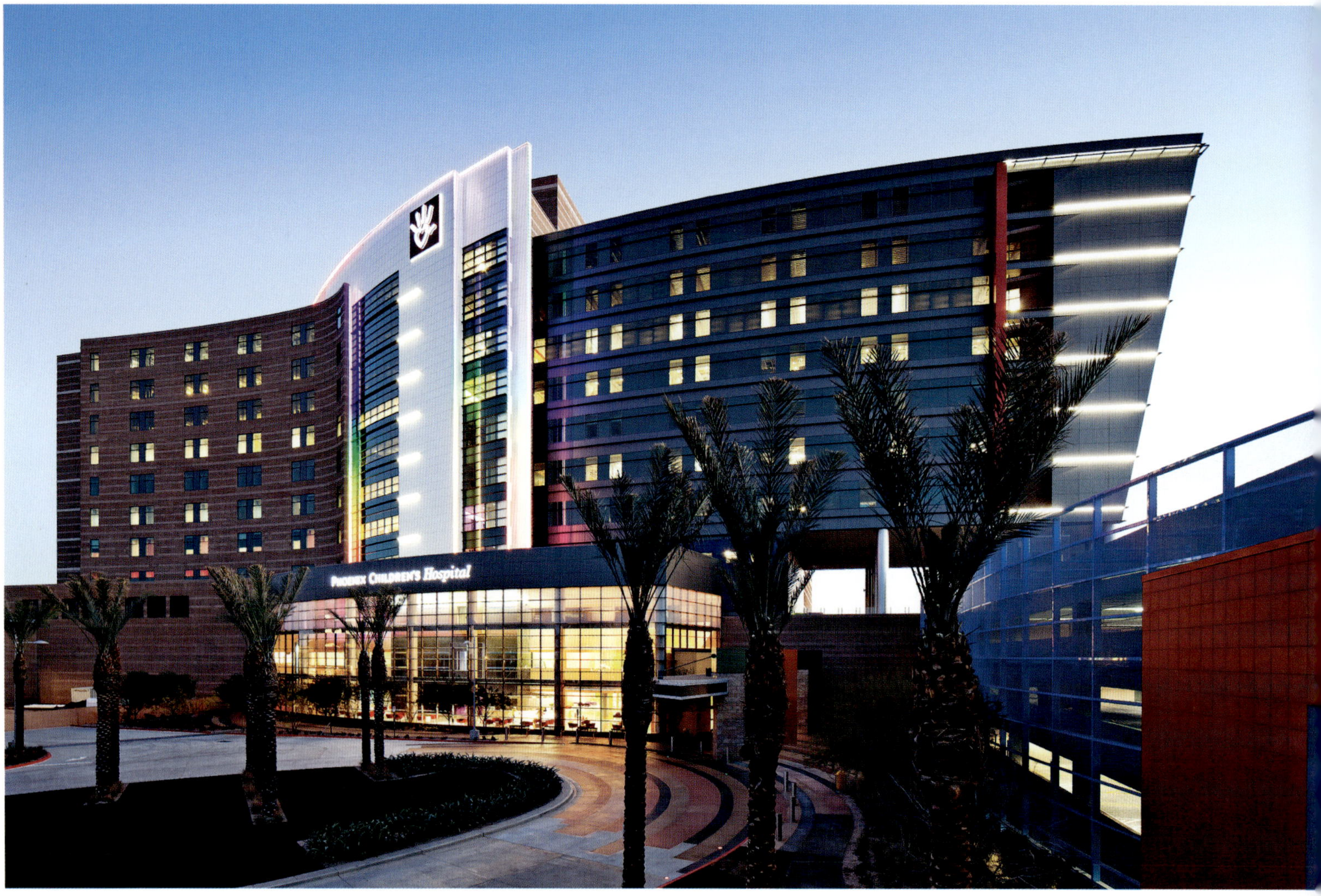

▲ Phoenix Children's Hospital, AZ
Photo: Blake Marvin, HKS

▼ Levine Children's Hospital, Charlotte, NC
Photos: Brad Feinknopf

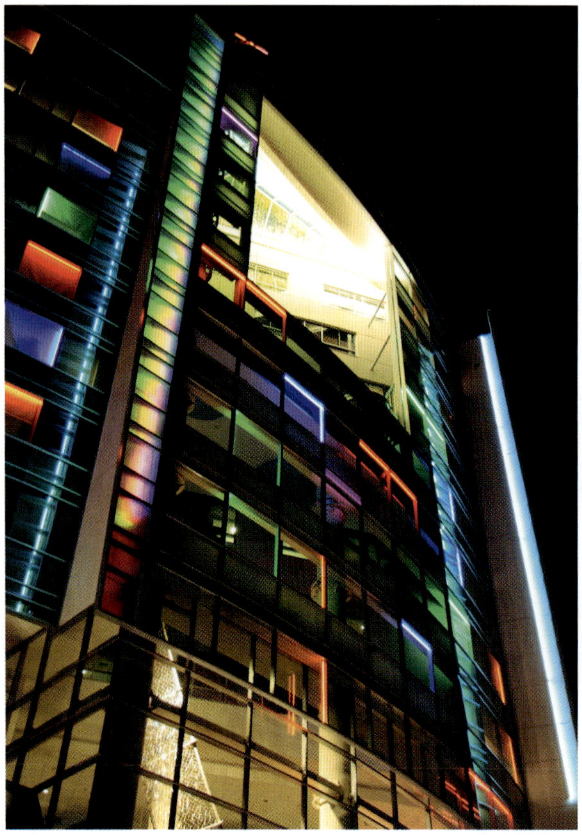

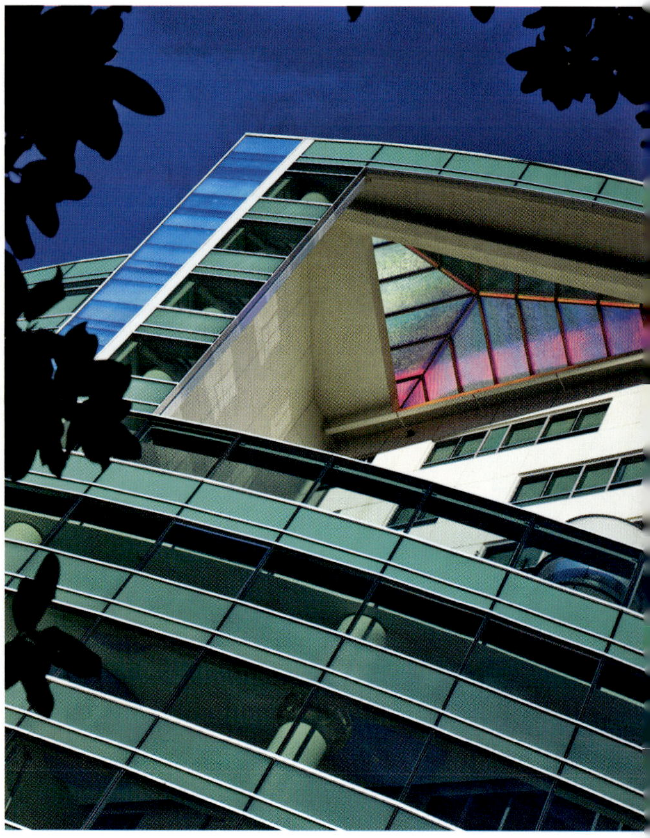

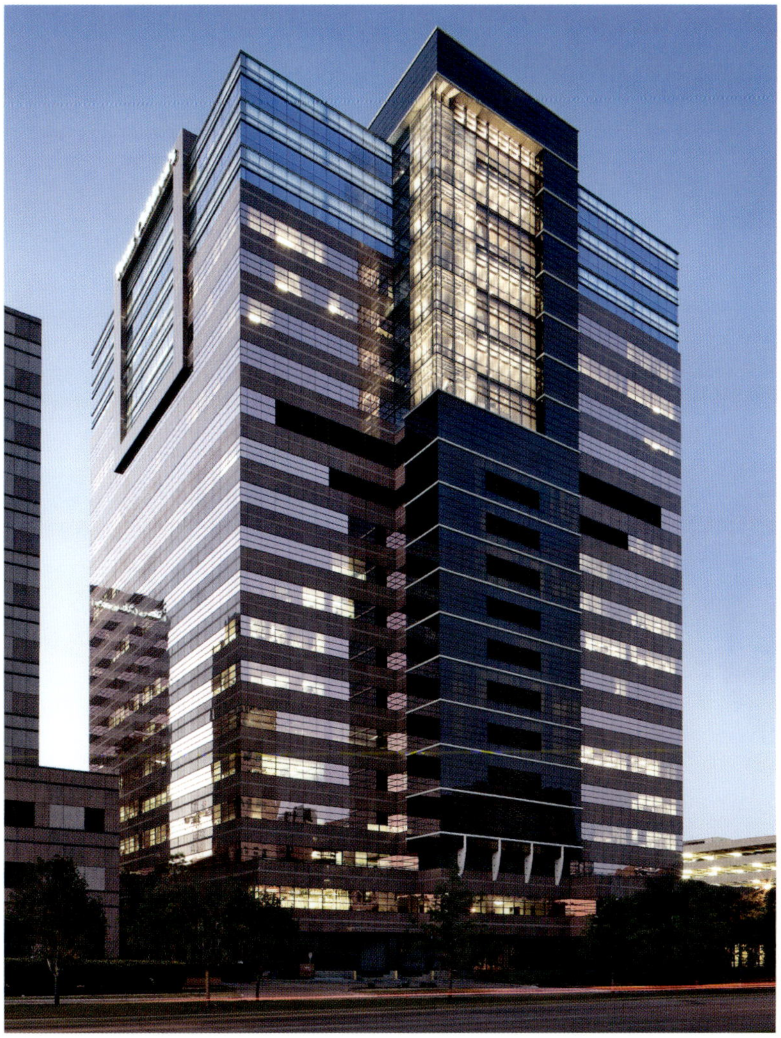

▲ Texas Children's Hospital Feigin Center, Houston, TX
Photo: Aker Imaging

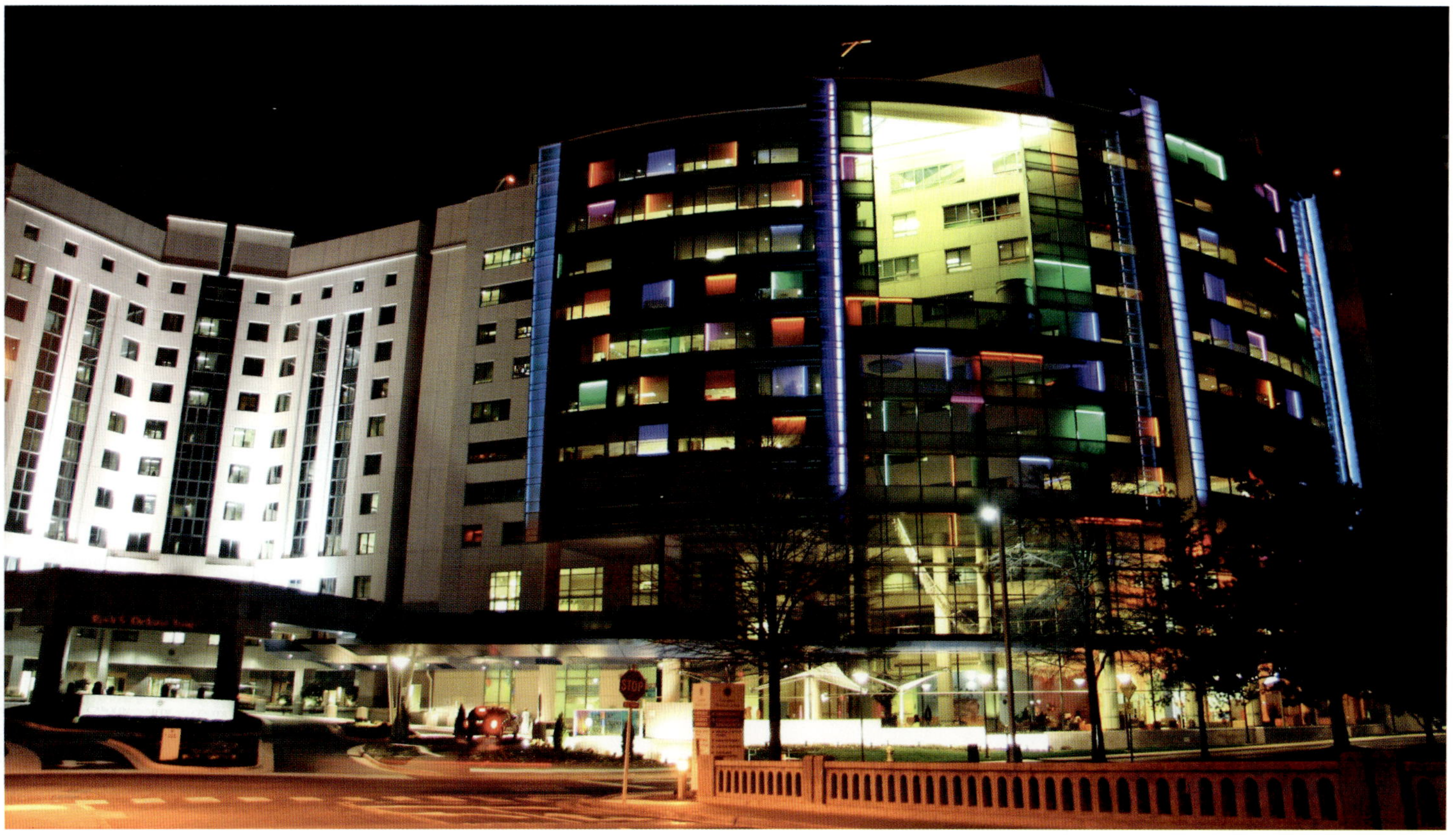

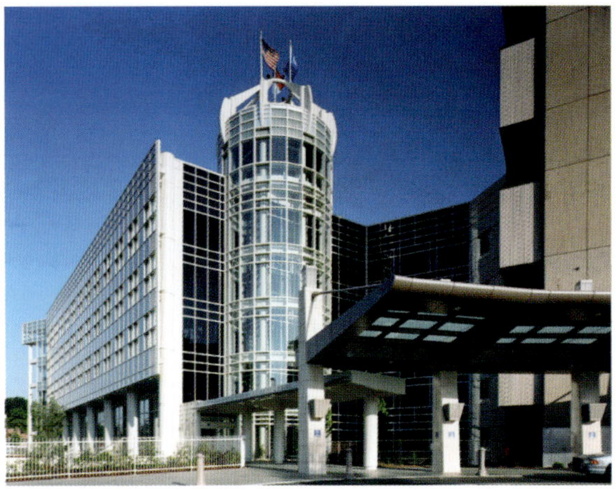

▲ Duke University Children's Hospital, Durham, NC
Photo: Jeff Goldberg/Esto Photography

▼ Children's Hospital of Illinois at OSF Saint Francis Medical Center, Peoria, IL
Photo: James Steinkamp

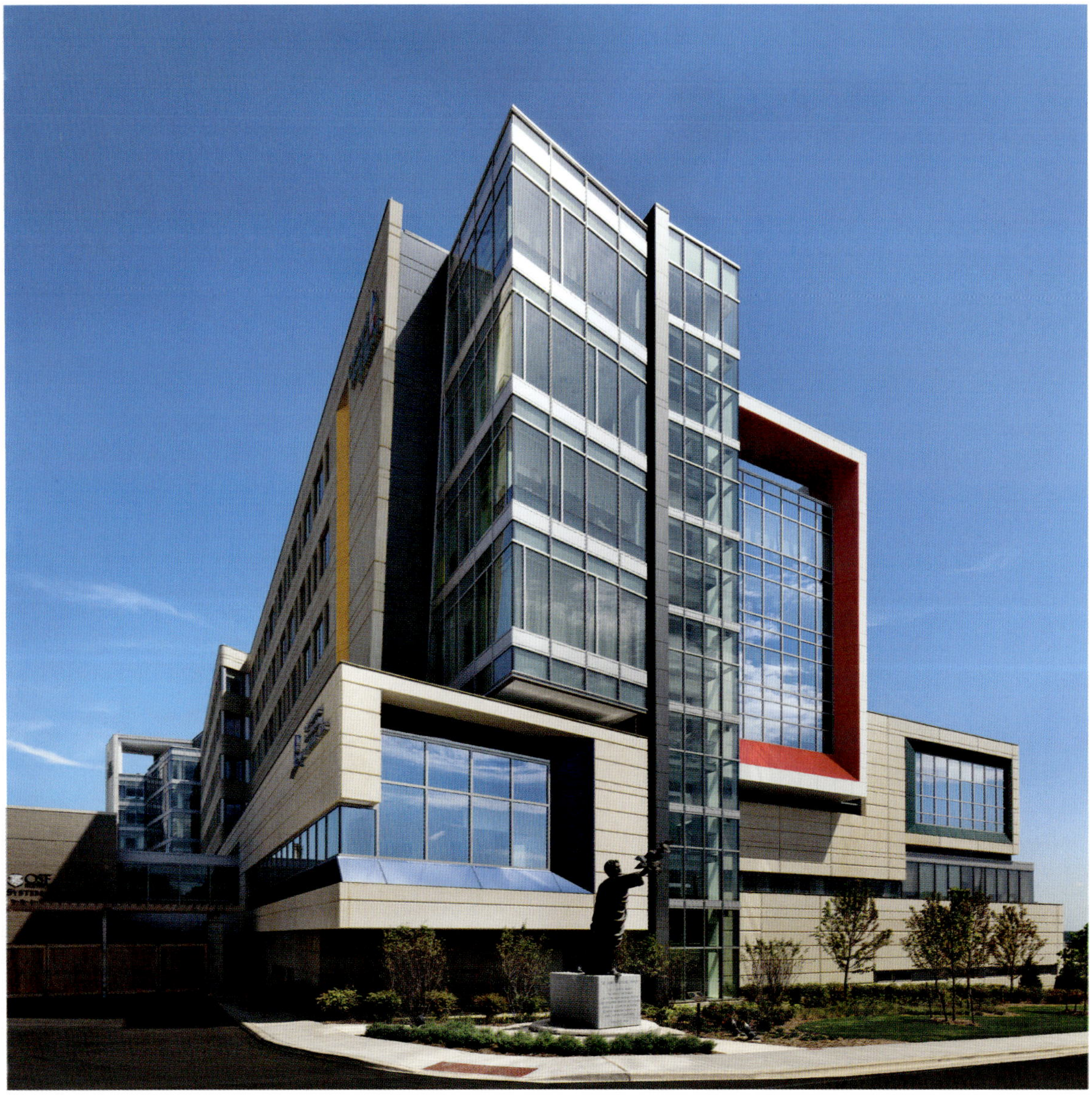

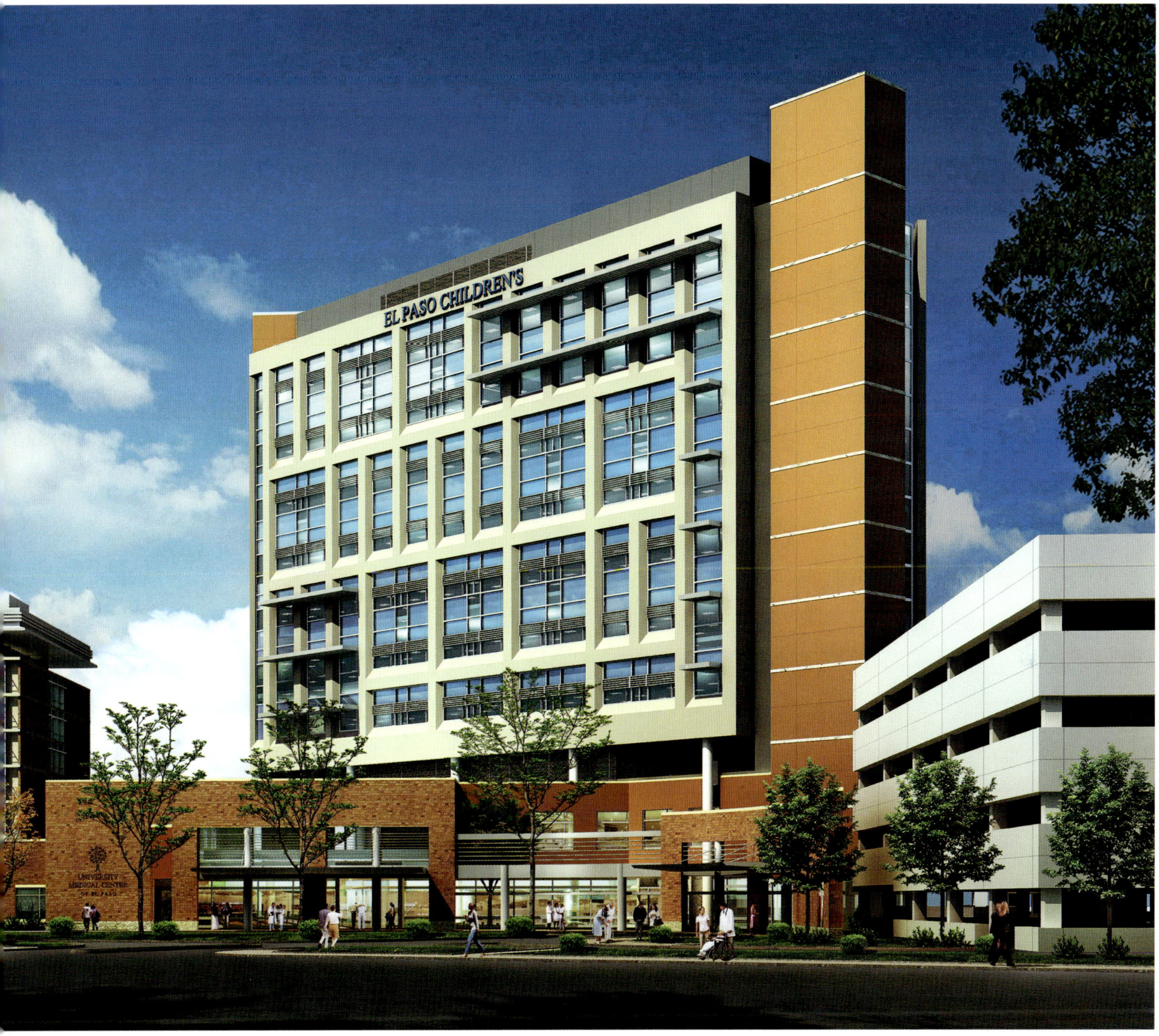

▲ Children's Hospital of El Paso, University Medical Center Expansion, El Paso, TX
Photo: KMD Architects

▼ Helen DeVos Children's Hospital, Grand Rapids, MI

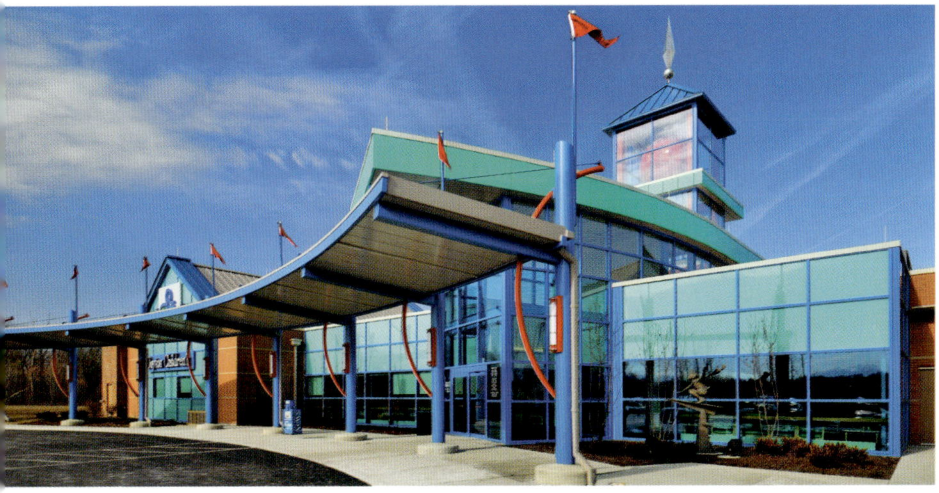

▼ Children's Healthcare of Atlanta, GA
Photo: Blake Marvin, HKS

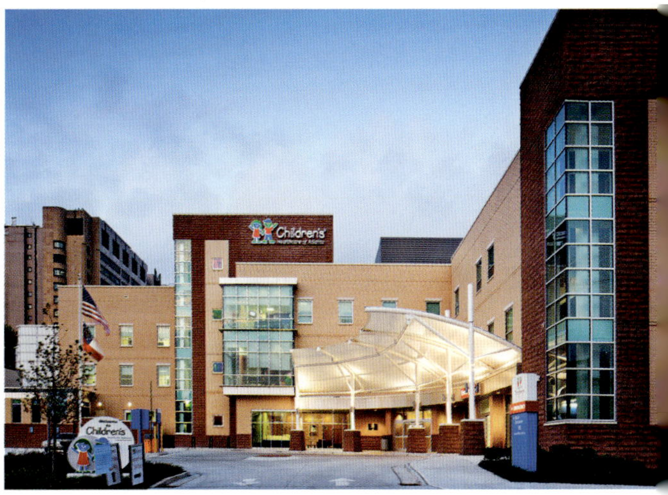

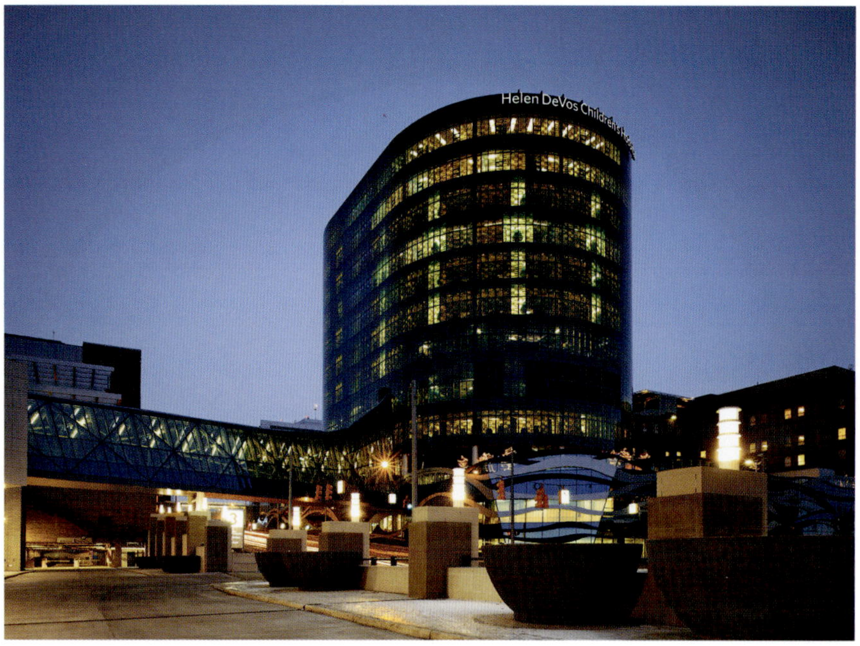

▲ Helen DeVos Children's Hospital, Grand Rapids, MI
▶

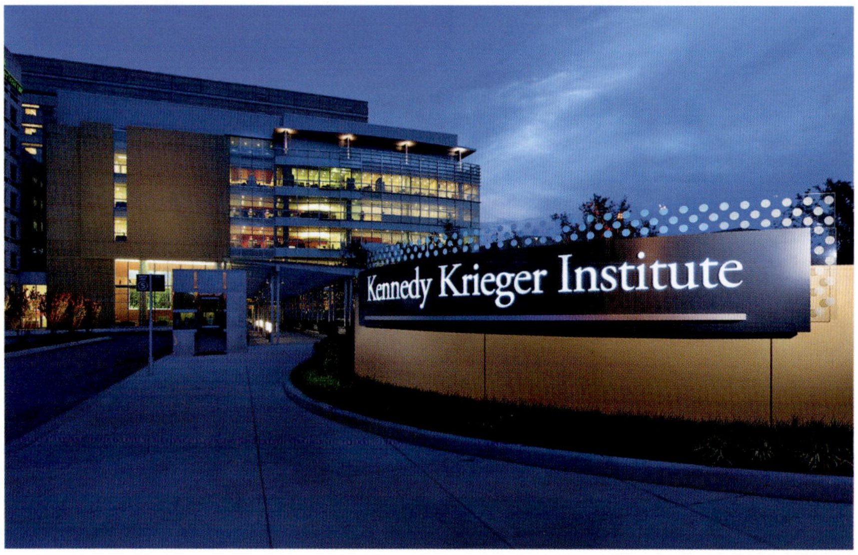

▲ Kennedy Krieger Children's Hospital, Baltimore, MD
Photo: Jim Roof Creative

▼ Sanford Children's Hospital, Sioux Falls, SD

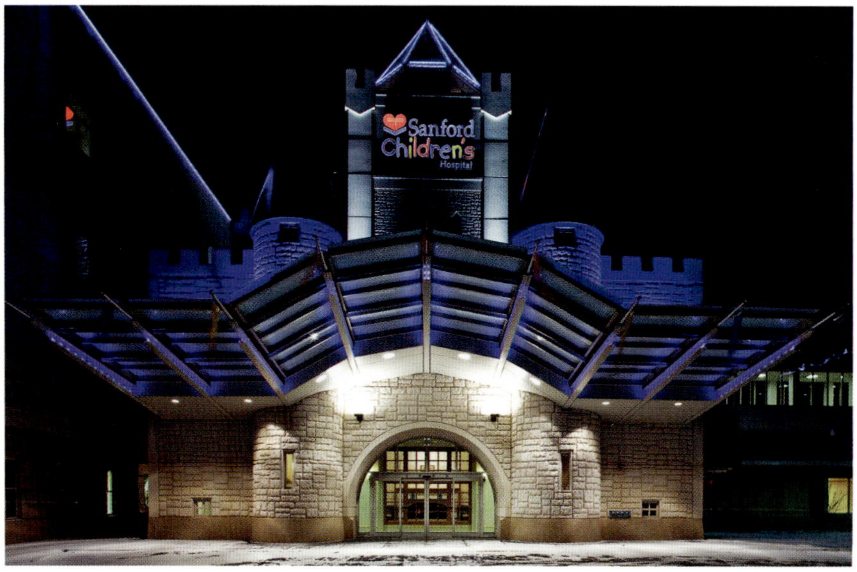

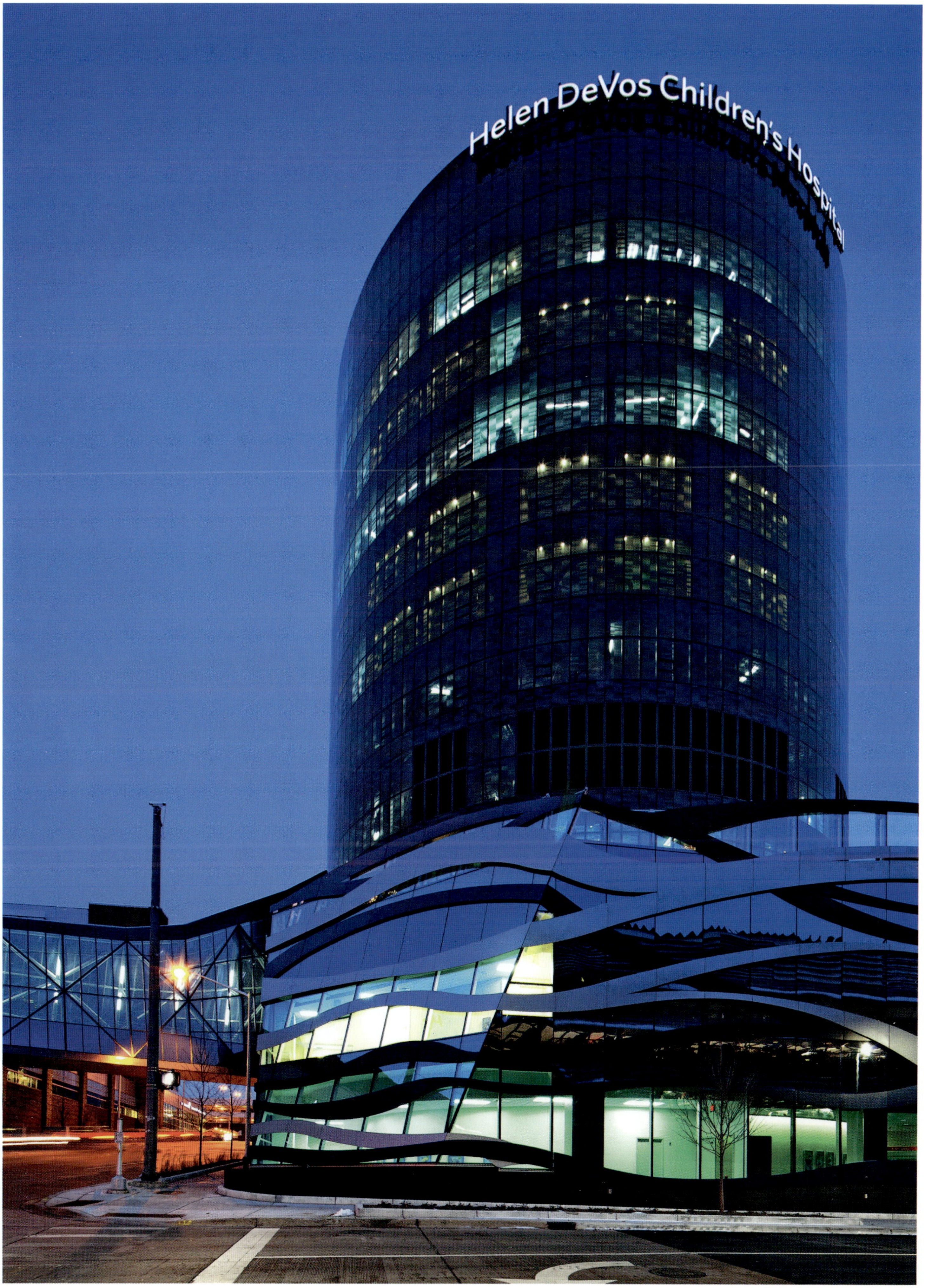
Helen DeVos Children's Hospital

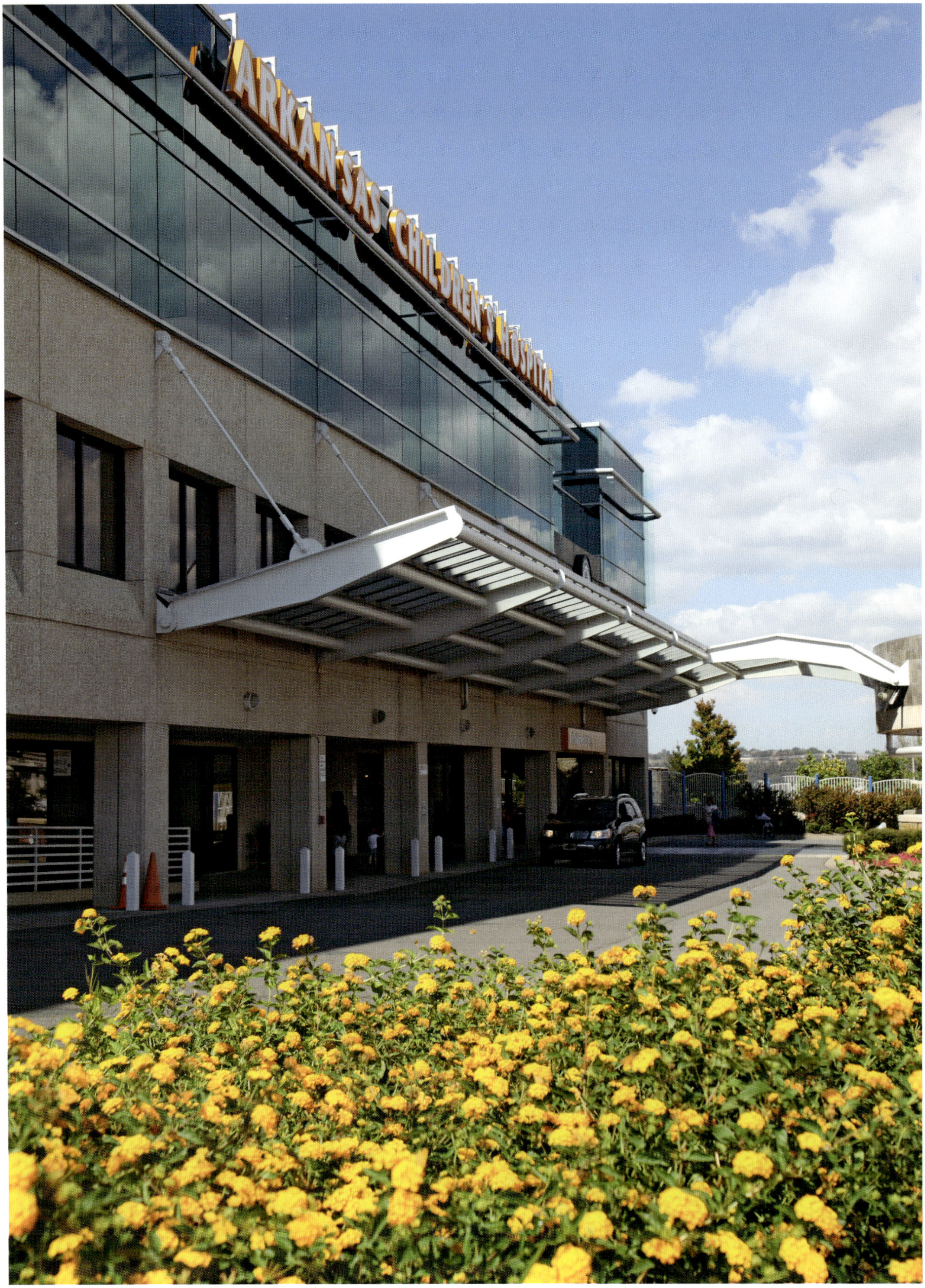
ARKANSAS CHILDREN'S HOSPITAL

◀ Arkansas Children's Hospital, Little Rock, AR
Photo: Kelley Cooper

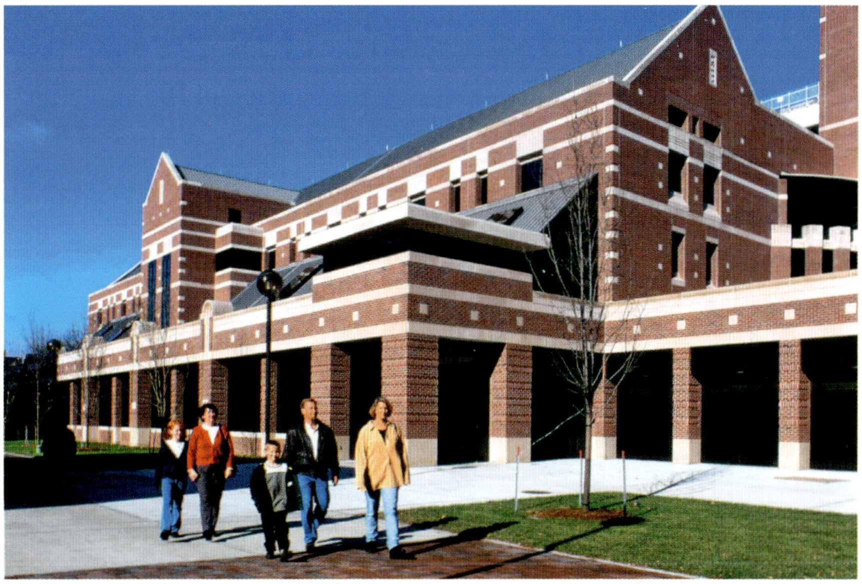

▲ Riley Children's Outpatient Center University of Indiana, Indianapolis, IN
Photo: Michael O'Callahan

▼ Le Bonheur Children's Hospital, Memphis, TN
Photo: Aker Imaging

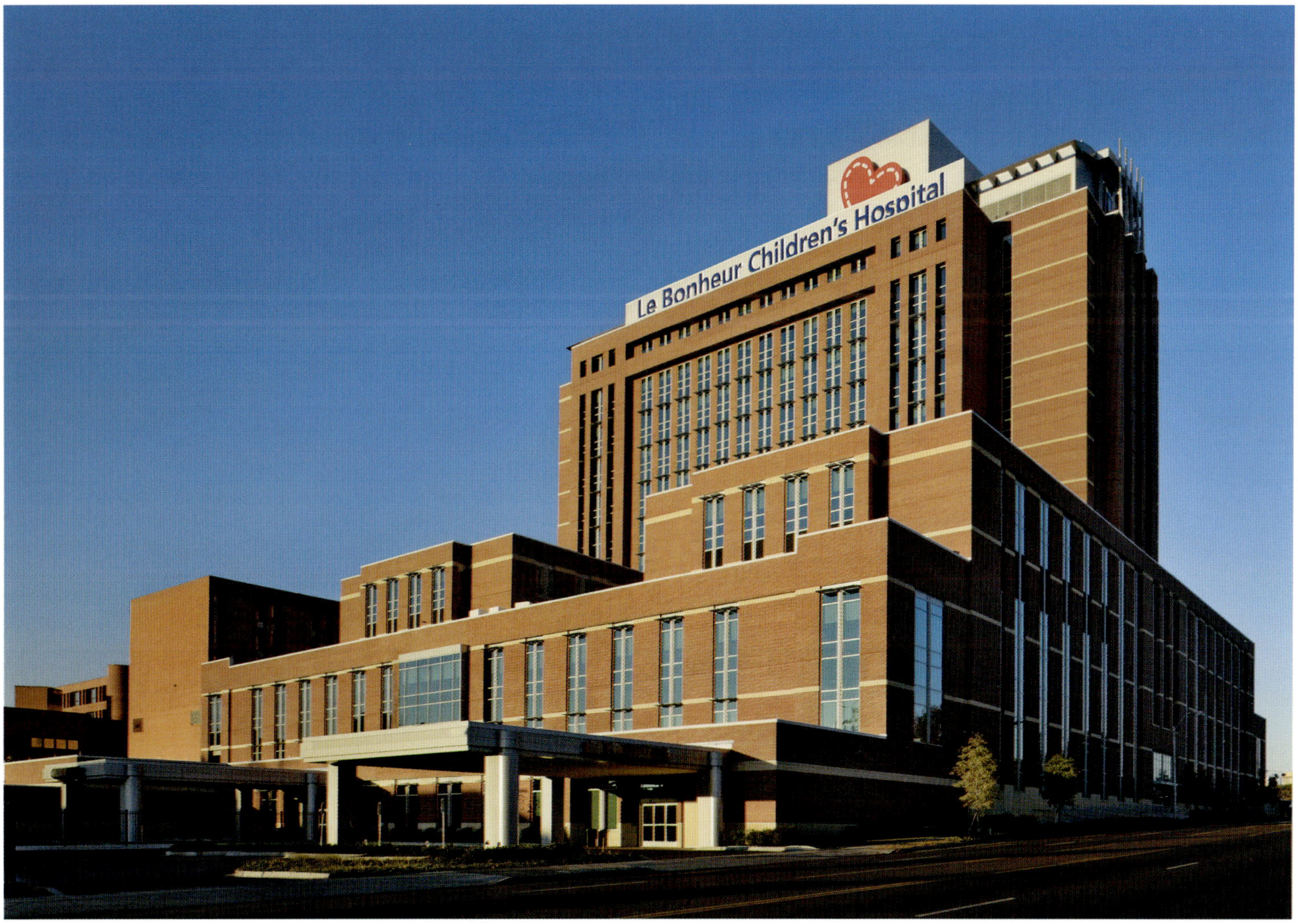

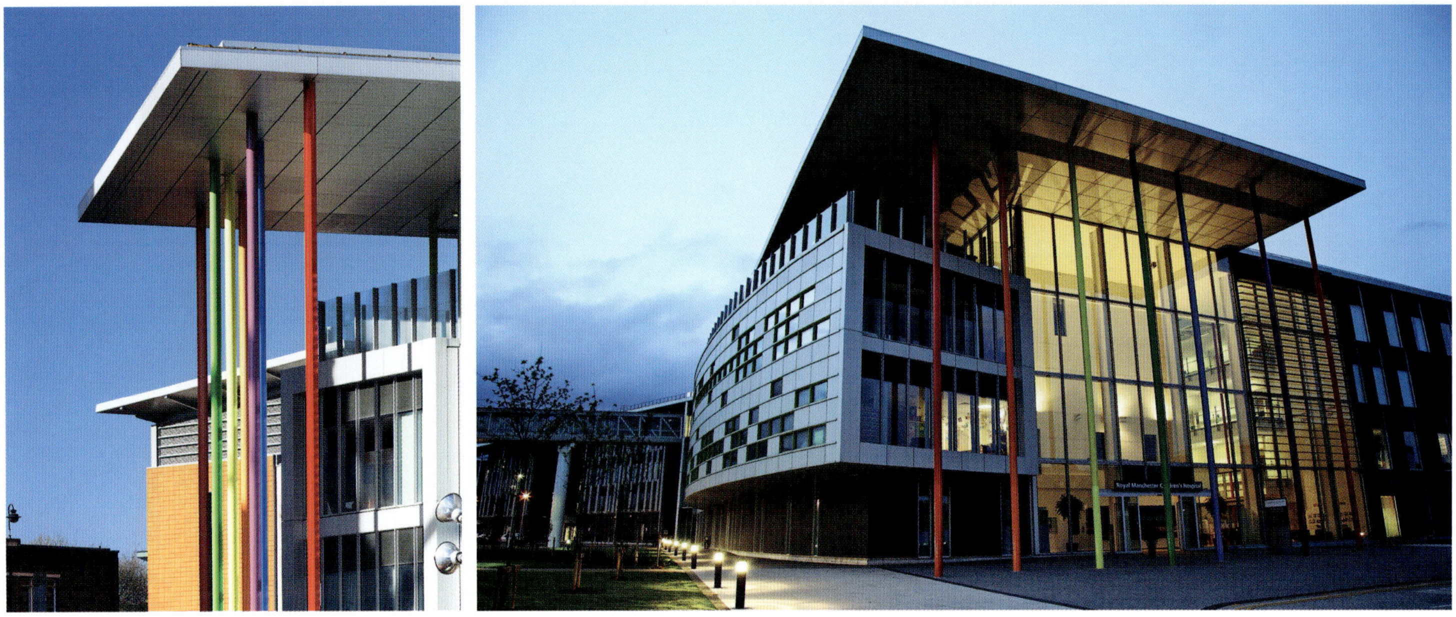

▲ Central Manchester Royal Children's Hospital, Manchester, United Kingdom
Photo: Stantec © Timothy Soar and Greg Harding

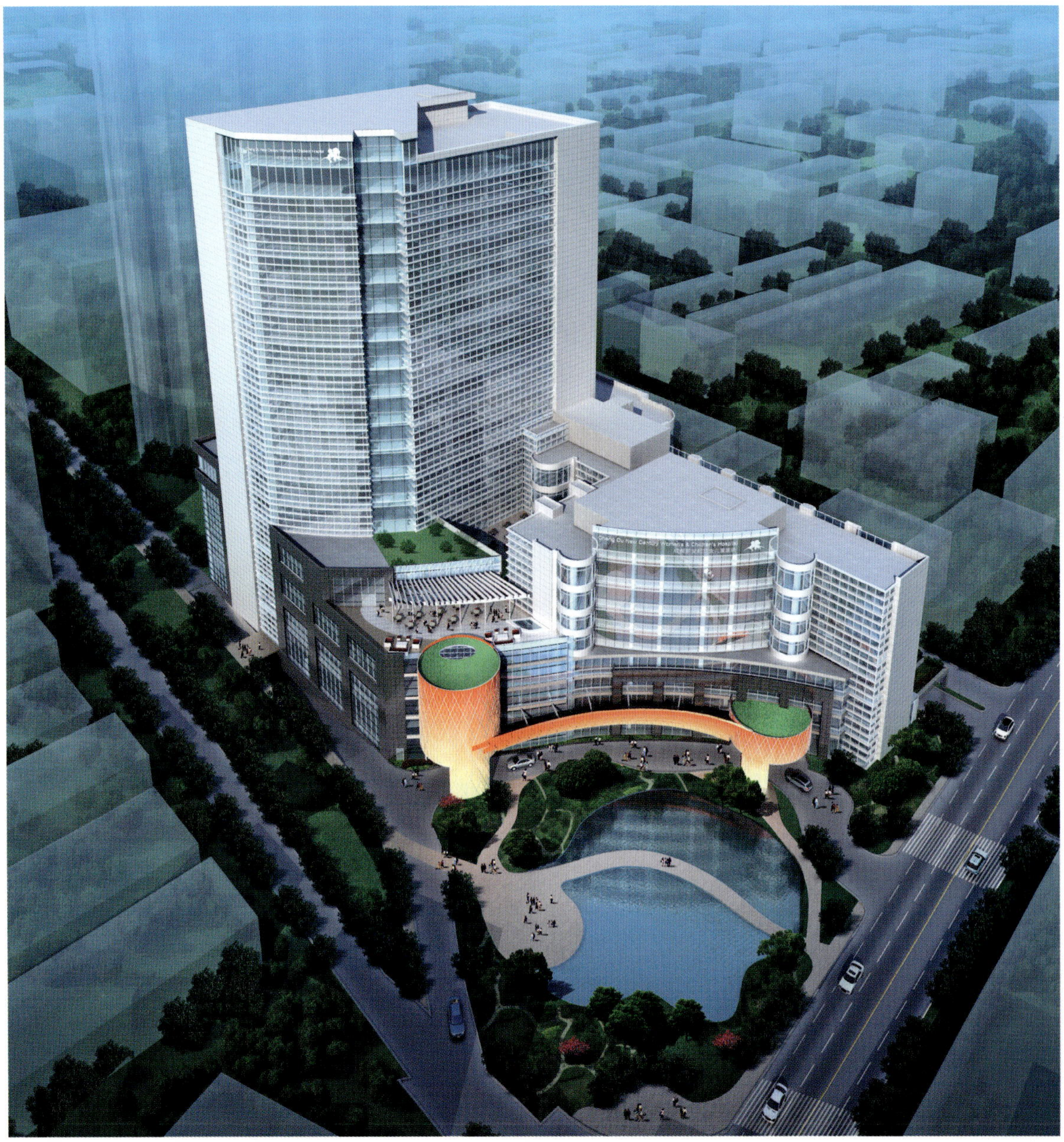

▲ Chengdu New Century Women and Children's Hospital, Chengdu, China
Photo: Provided by FKP Architects

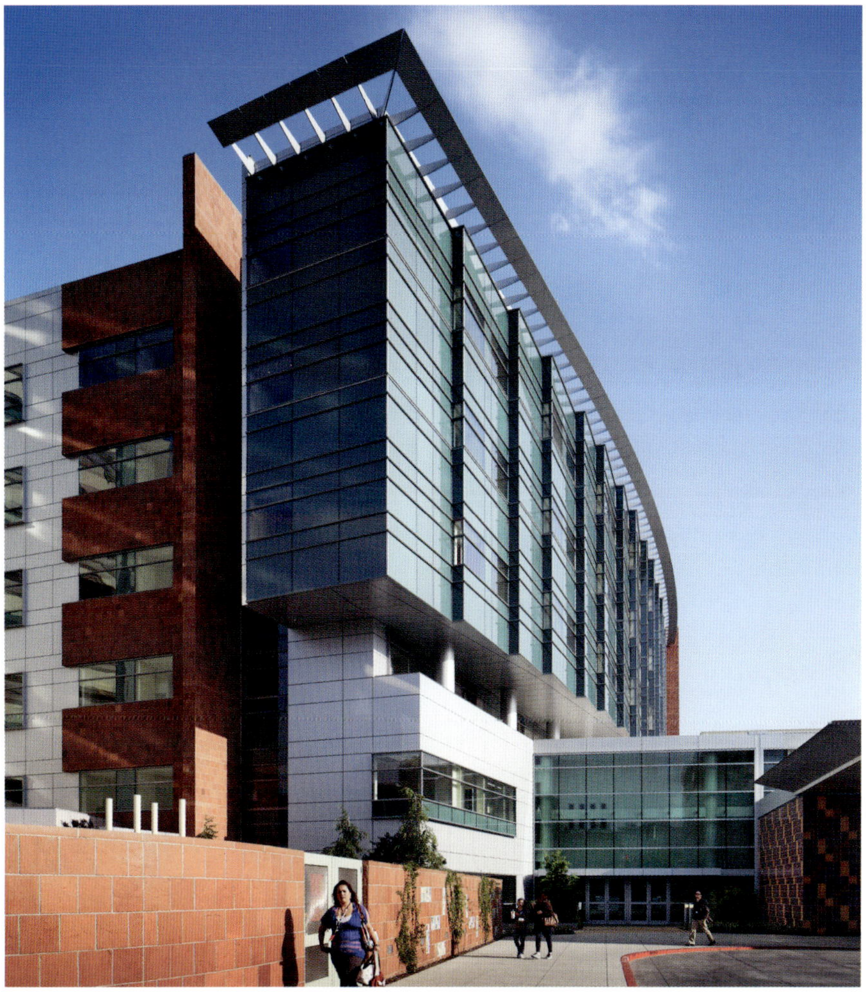

▲ Children's Hospital Los Angeles, CA
▼ ***Photos: Hedrich Blessing Photography, Nick Merrick (above); RMA Photography, Inc. (below)***

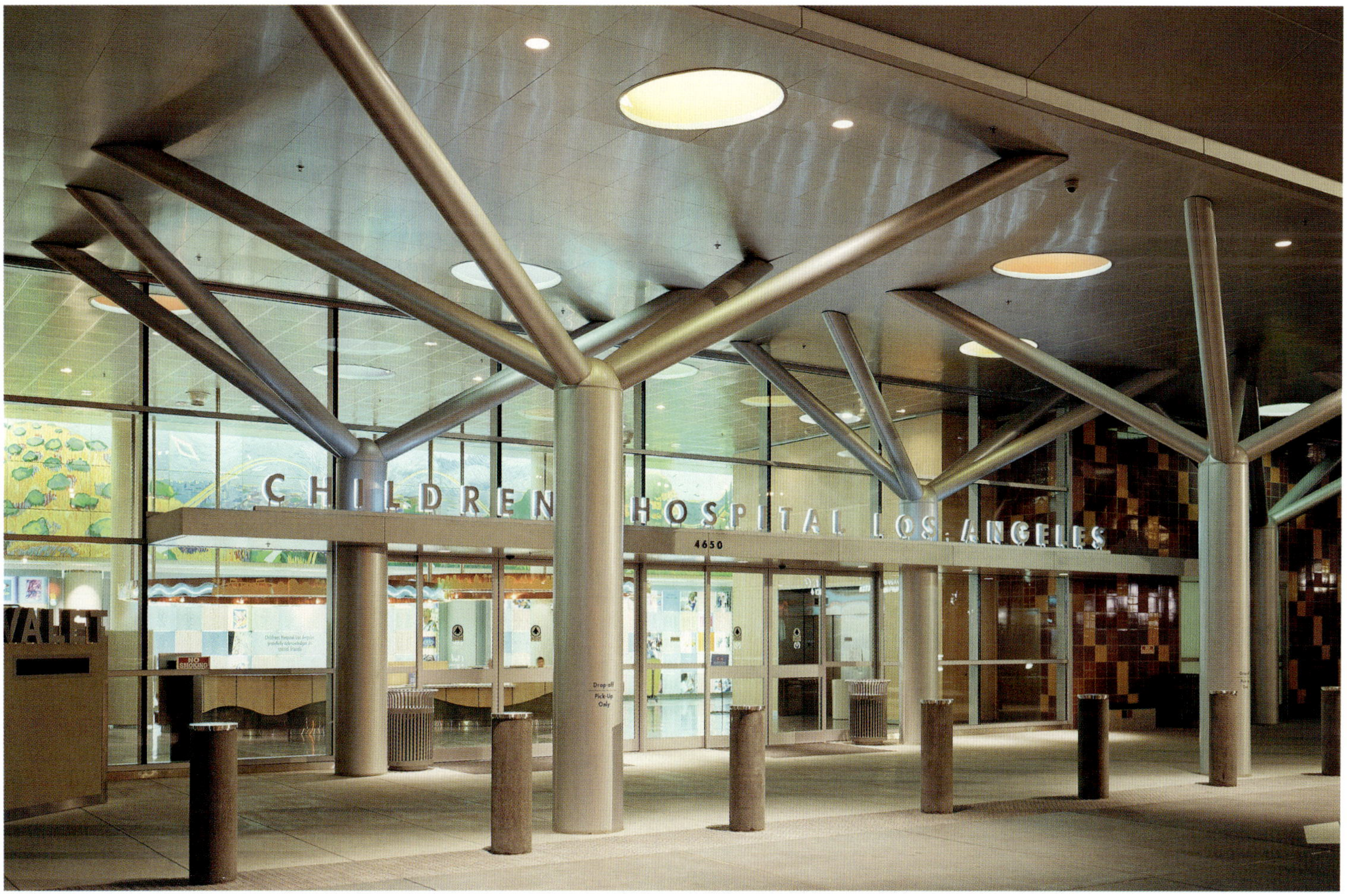

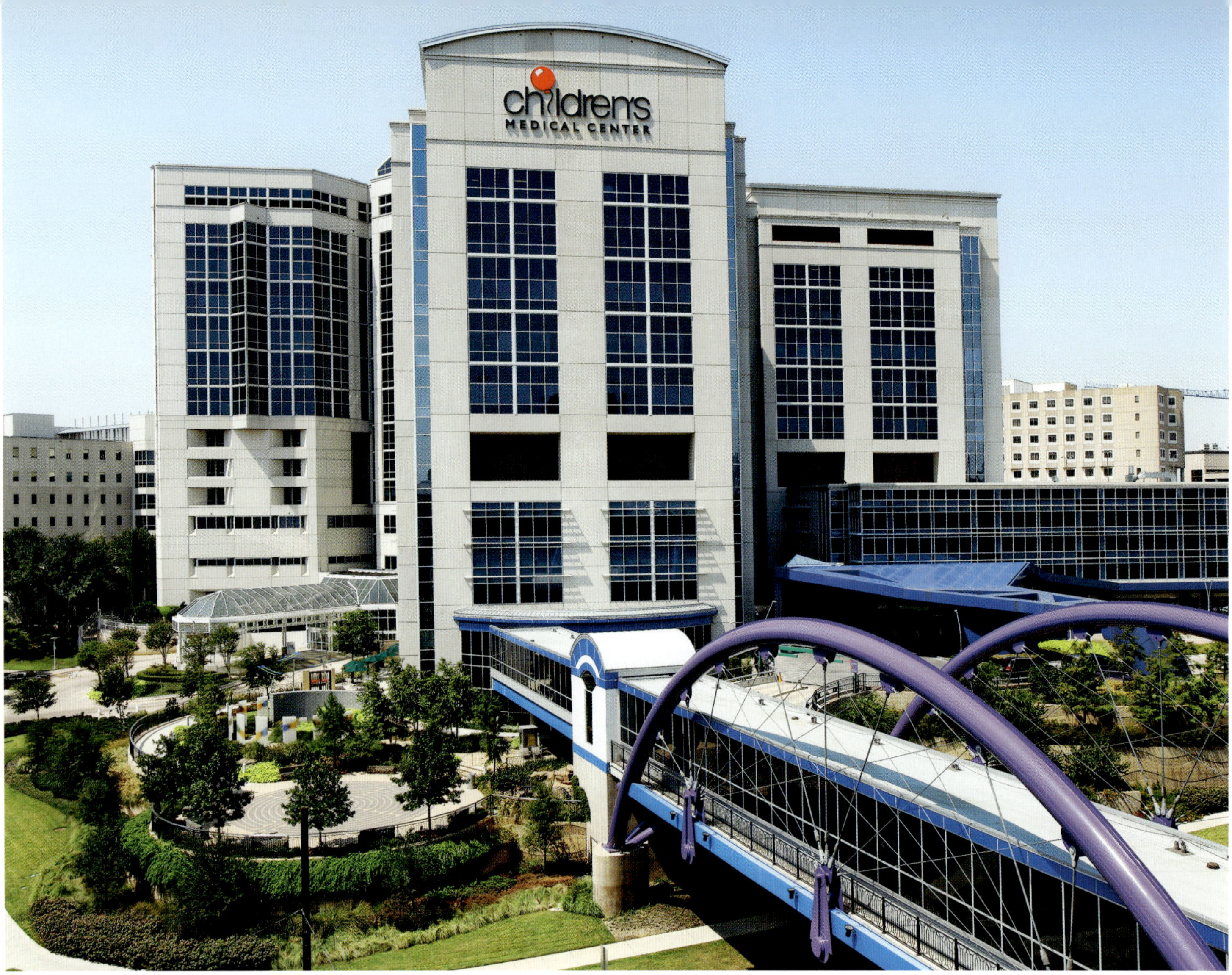

▲ Children's Medical Center, Dallas, TX
Photo: Scott Williams

▼ Arkansas Children's Hospital, Little Rock, AR
Photo: Kelley Cooper

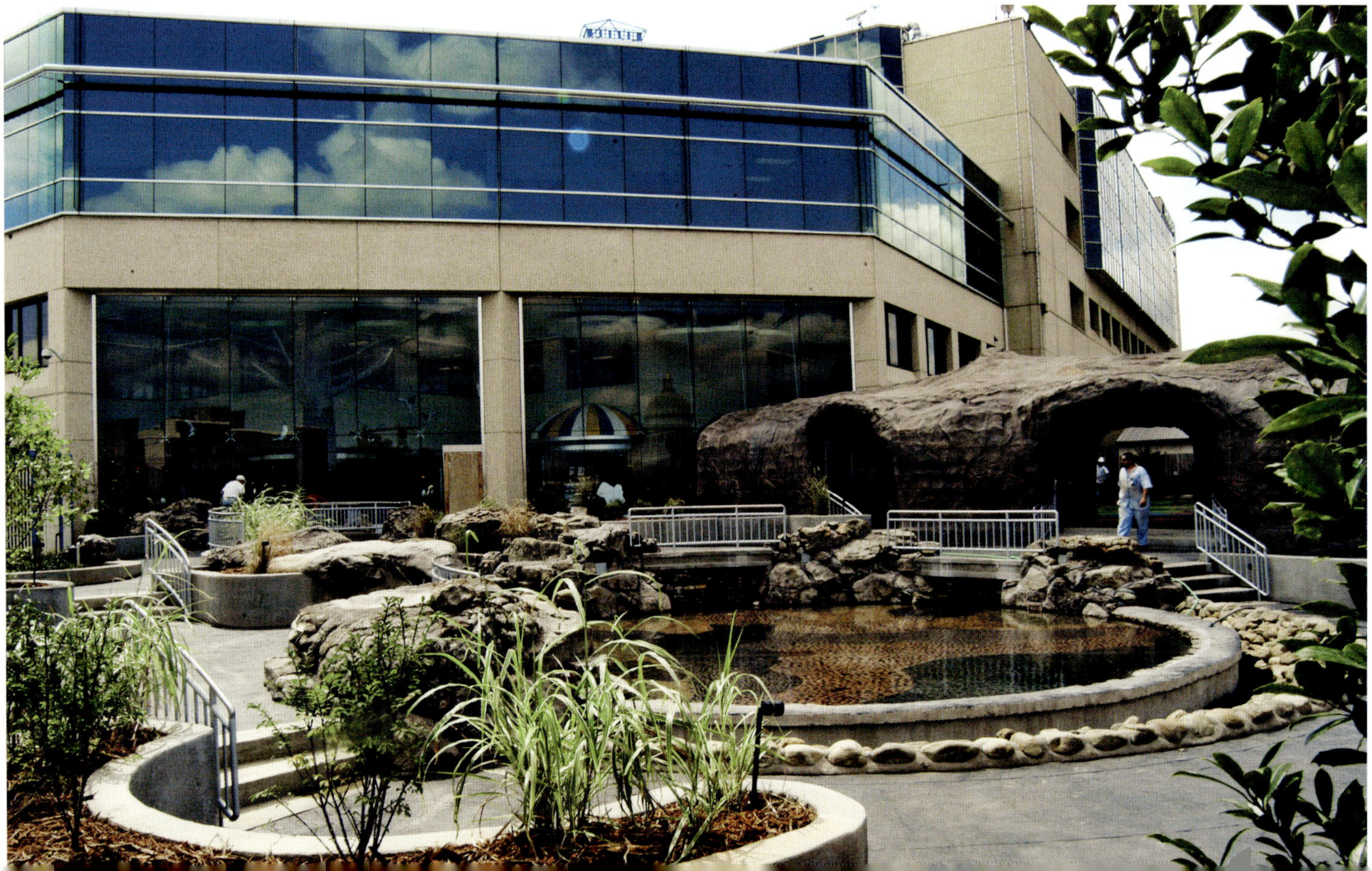

▼ Children's Hospital, Pittsburgh, PA
Photo: Jason Yurkovich

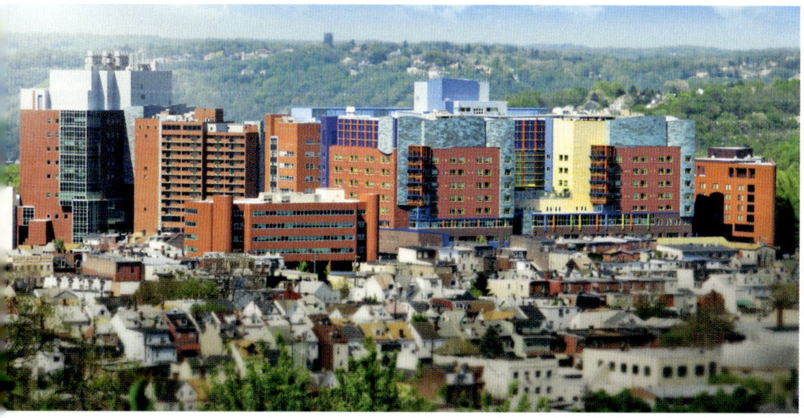

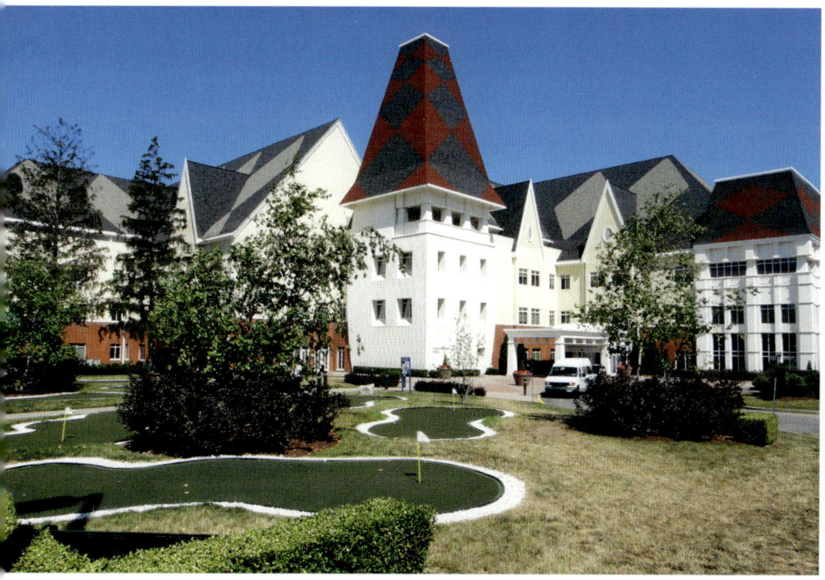

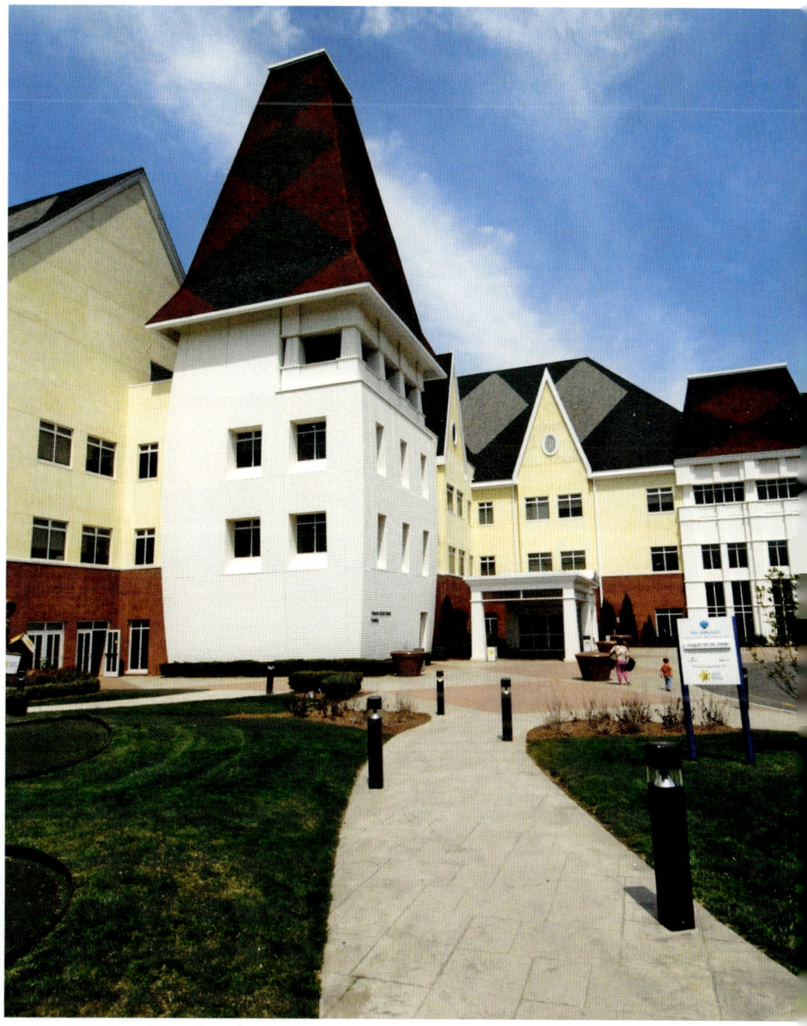

▲ Maria Fareri Children's Hospital, Valhalla, NY
Photos: Westchester Medical Center

Upstate Golisano Children's Hospital, Syracuse, NY
Photos: Susan Kahn

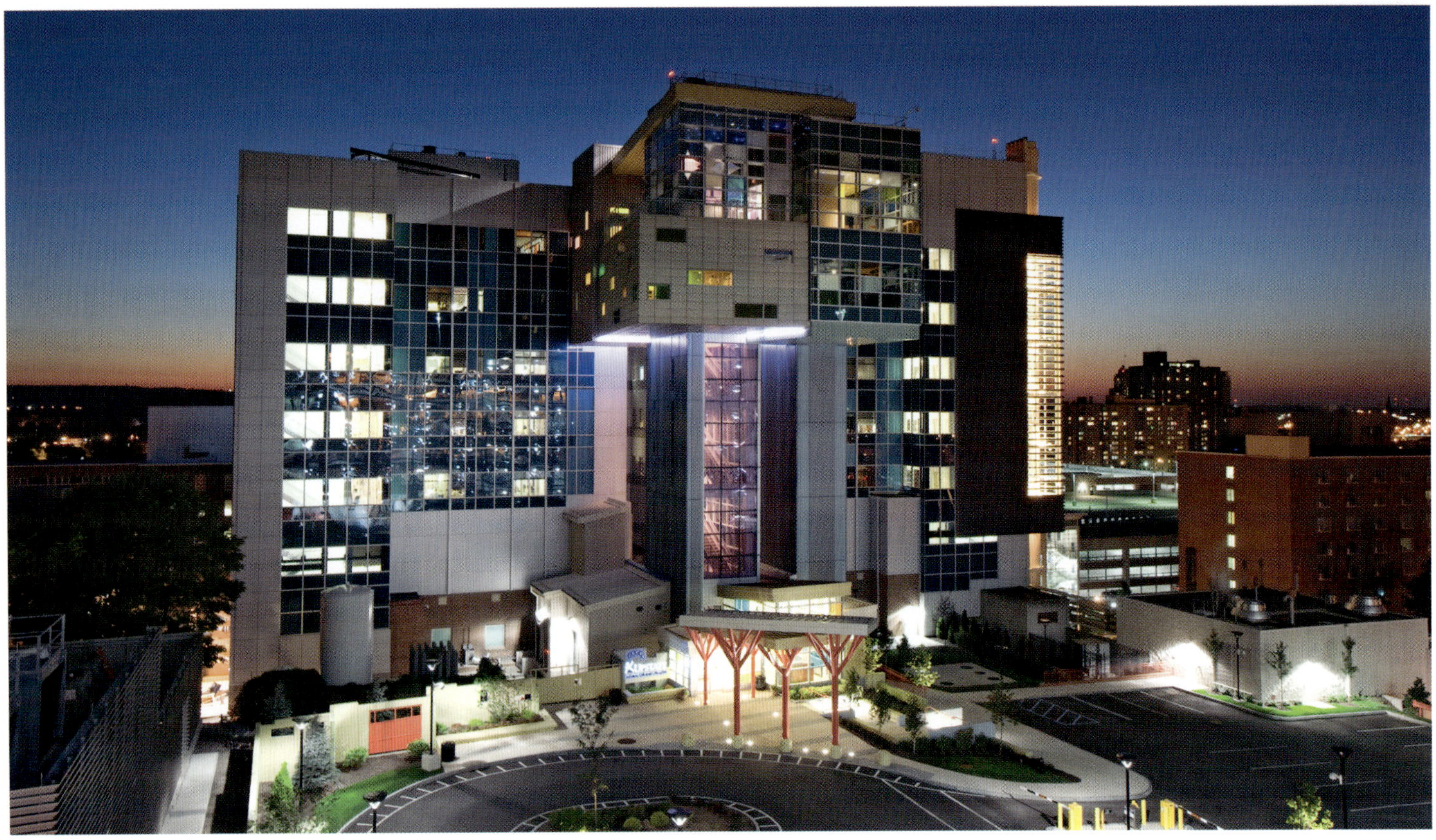

Joseph M. Sanzari Children's Hospital at Hackensack University Medical Center, Hackensack, NJ
Photo: Steve Hockstein, Harvard Studio

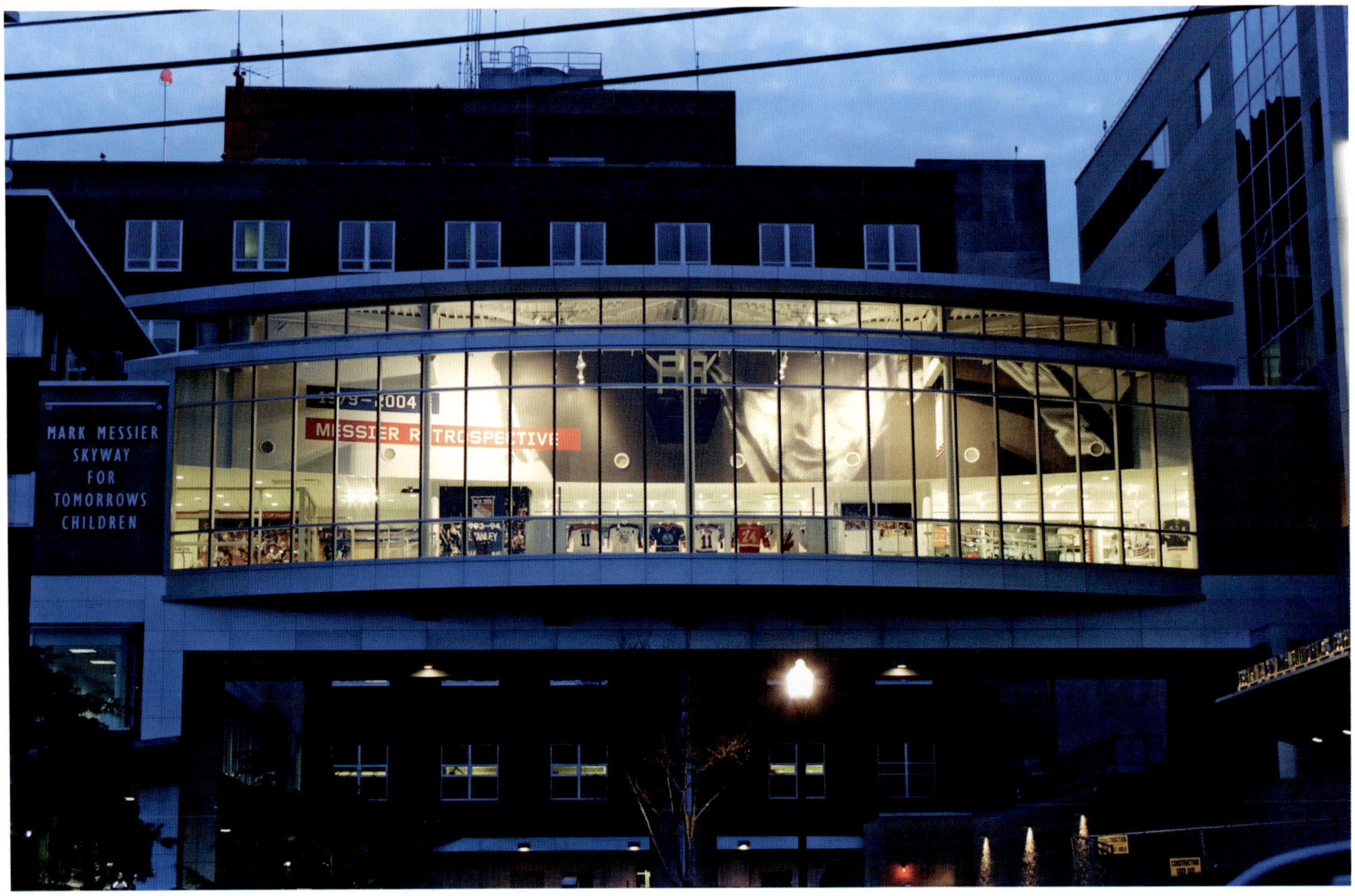

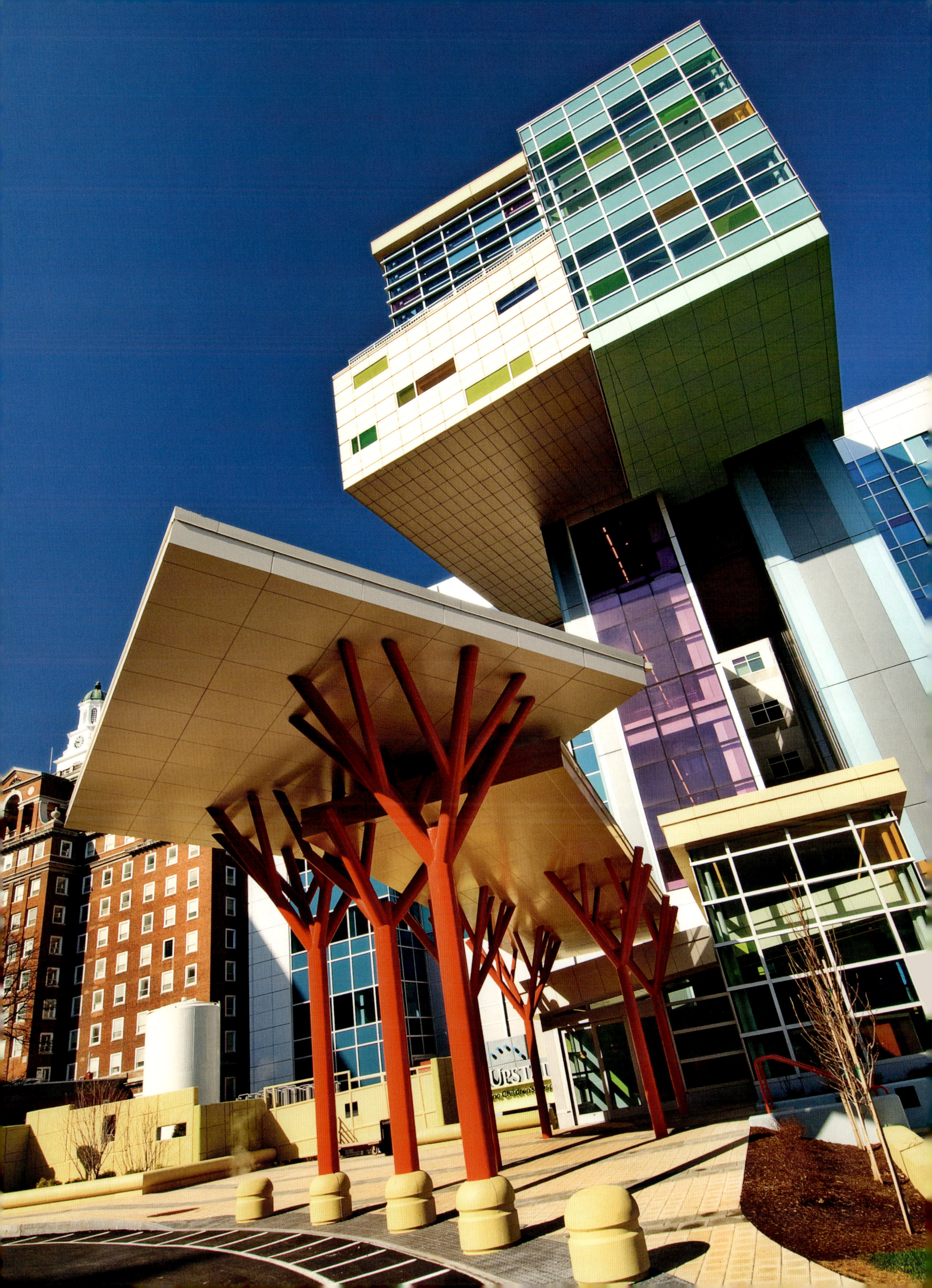

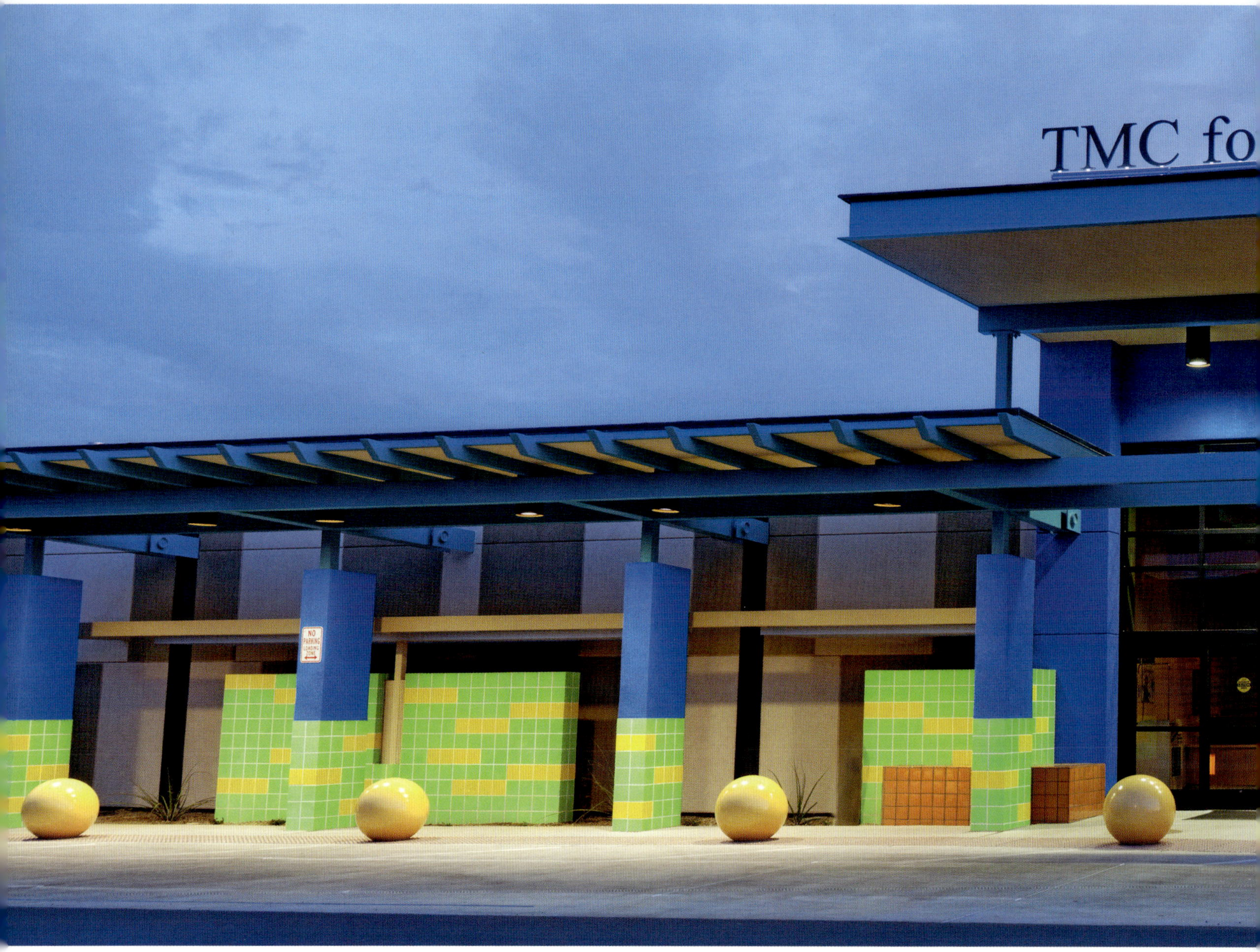

▲ Tucson Medical Center, AZ
Photo: Eric Suhm

▼ University of Minnesota Amplatz Children's Hospital, Minneapolis, MI
Photo: Paul Crosby

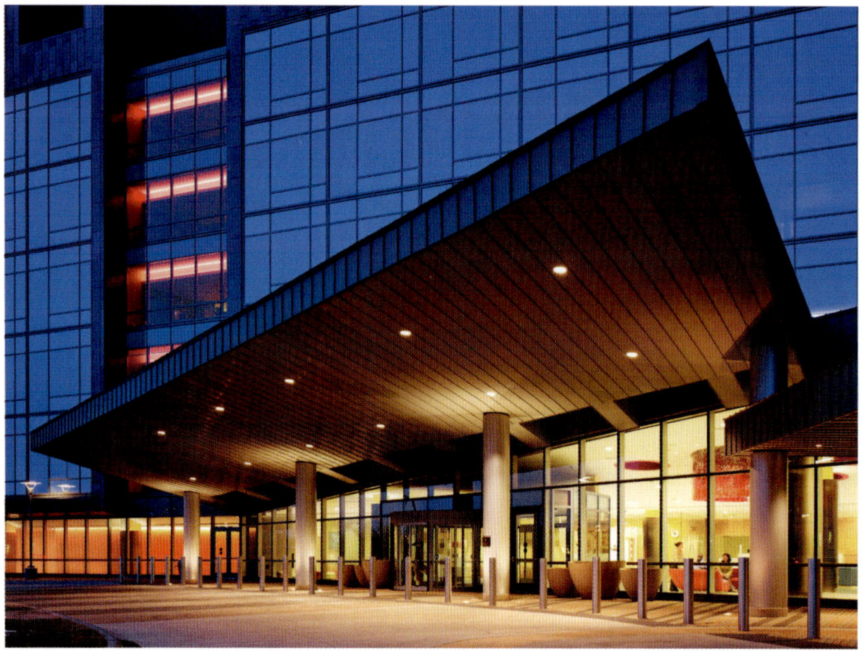

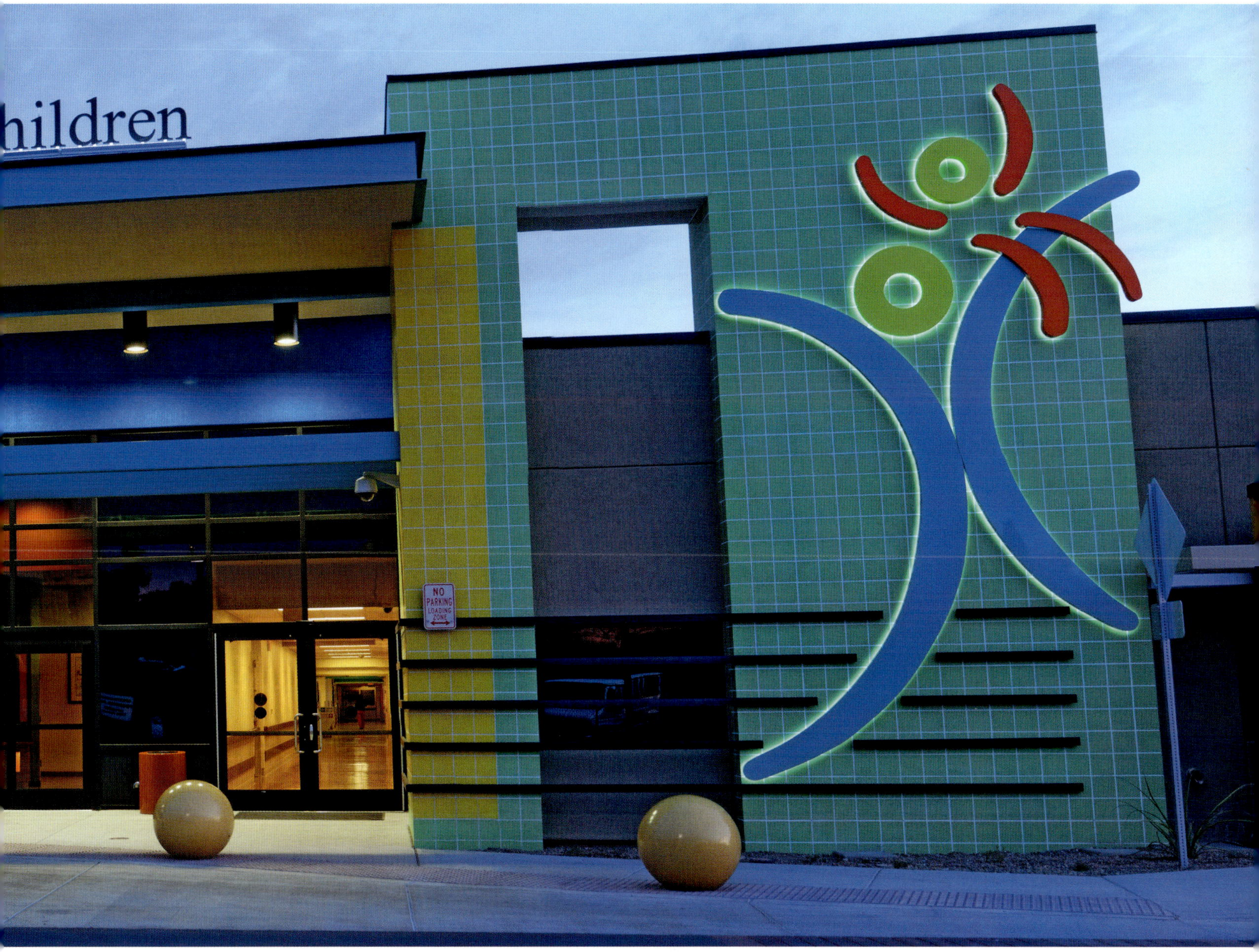

▼ University of Minnesota Amplatz Children's Hospital, Minneapolis, MI
Photo: Paul Crosby

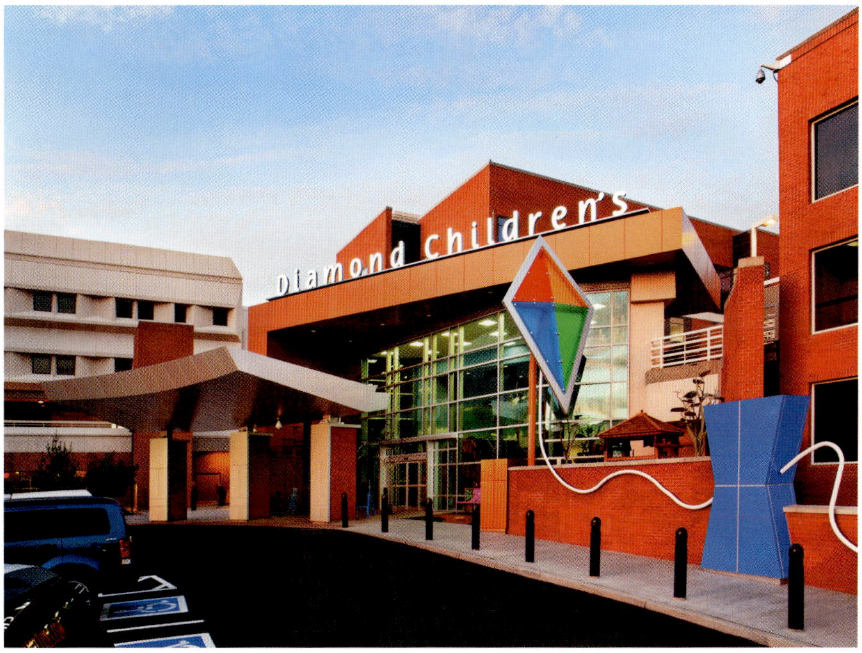

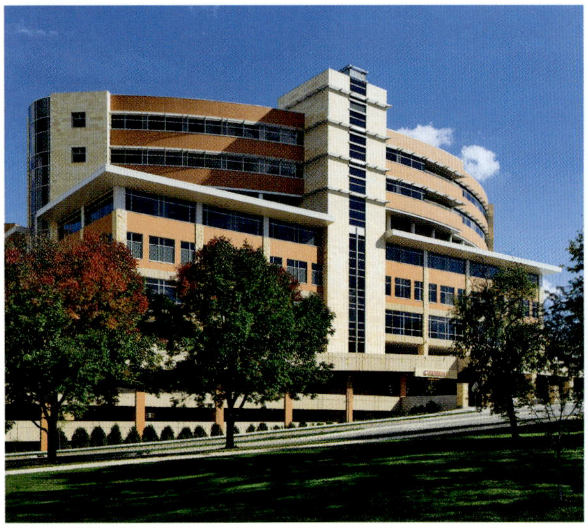

American Family Children's Hospital, Madison, WI ▲

Photos: HDR Architecture, Inc. ▶

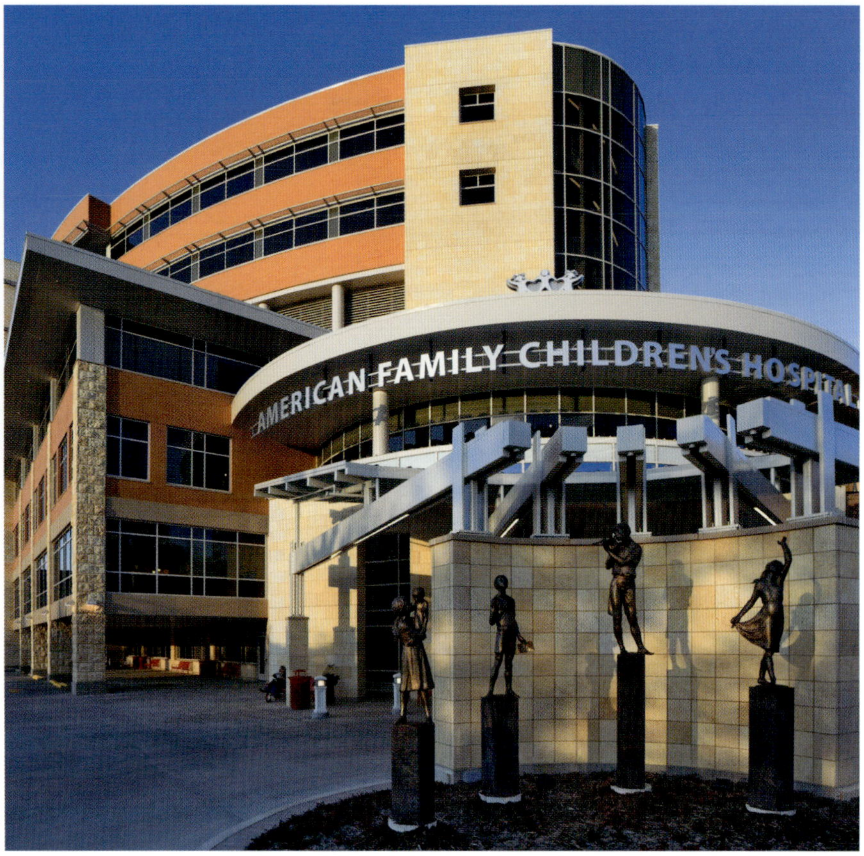

Cardon Children's Centre, Mesa, AZ ▶

Photos: HDR Architecture, Inc. © 2010 Mark Boisclair Photography Inc ▼

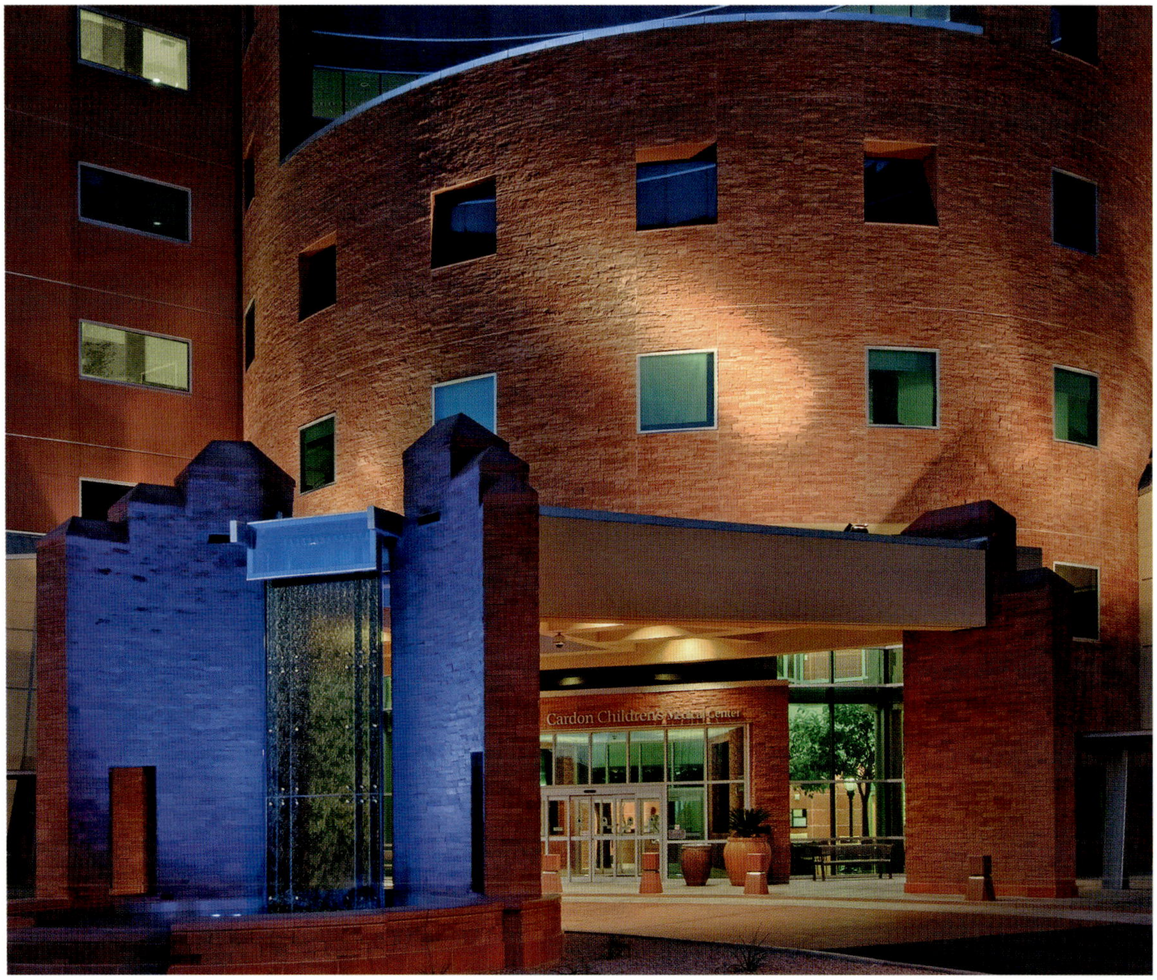

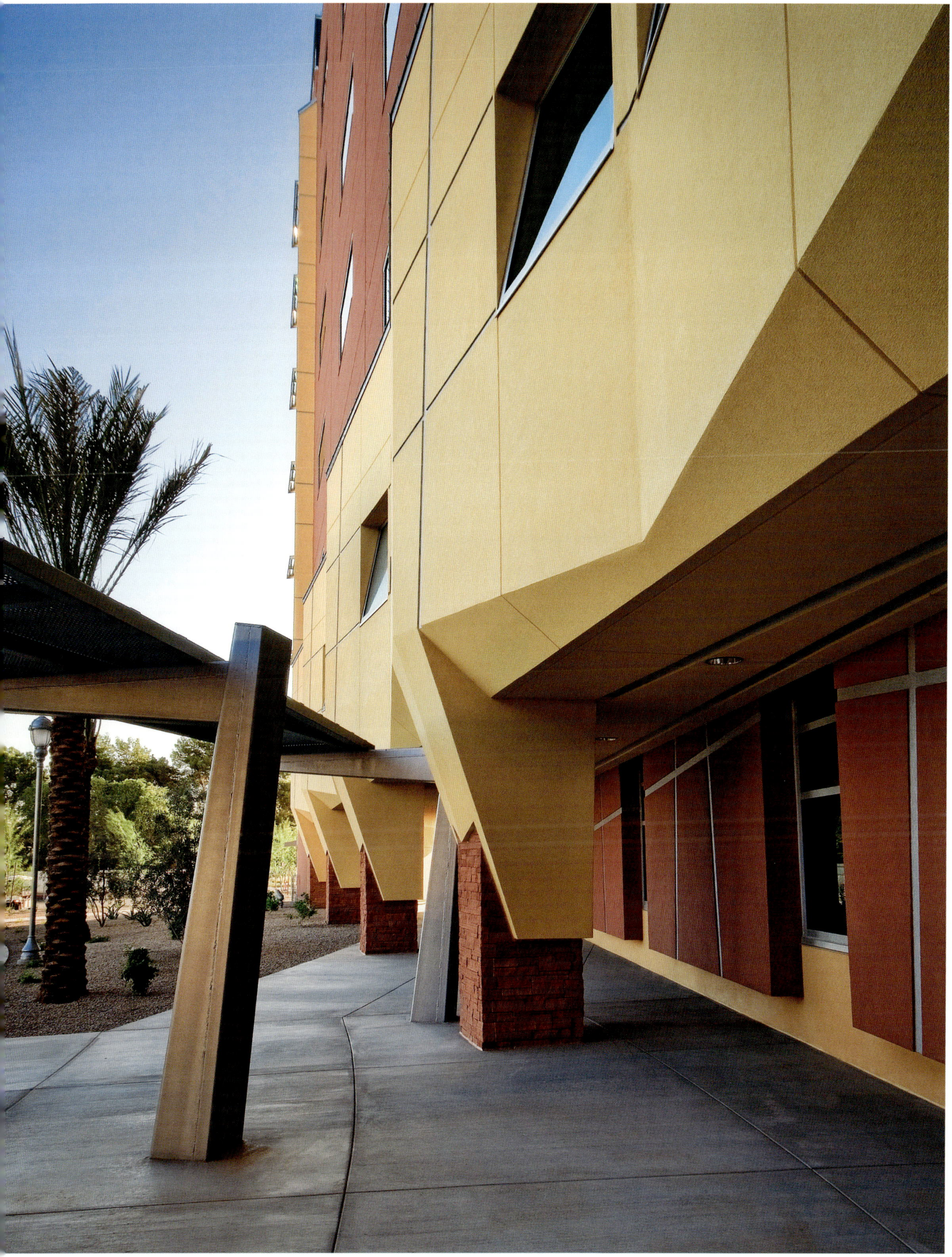

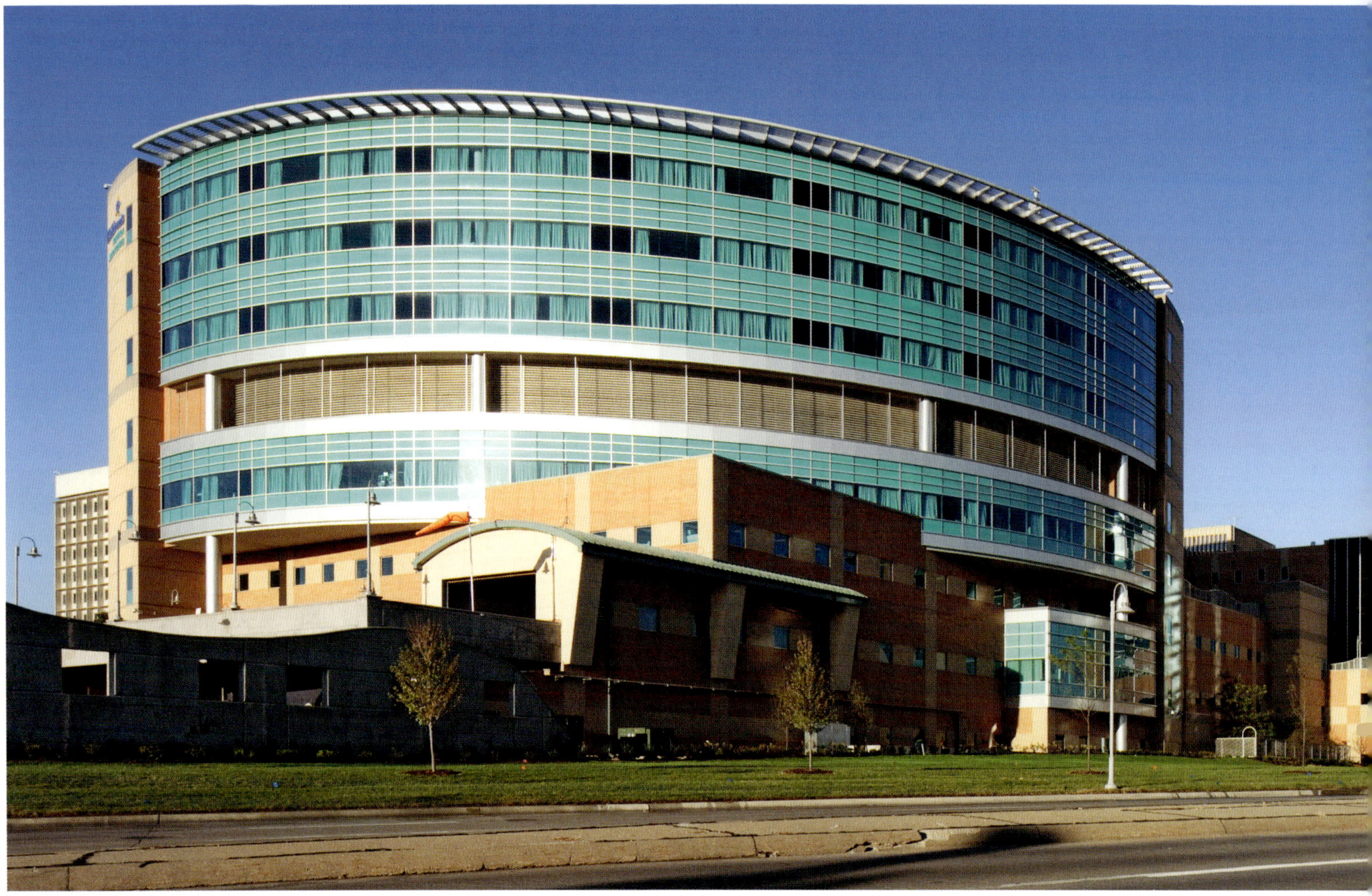

▲ Children's Hospital Omaha, NE
Photo: Matthew Placzek – "Imagine" © 2010 Thomas Grady Photography

▼ Abbott Northwestern Children's Hospital, Minneapolis, MN
Photo: HDR Architecture, Inc.

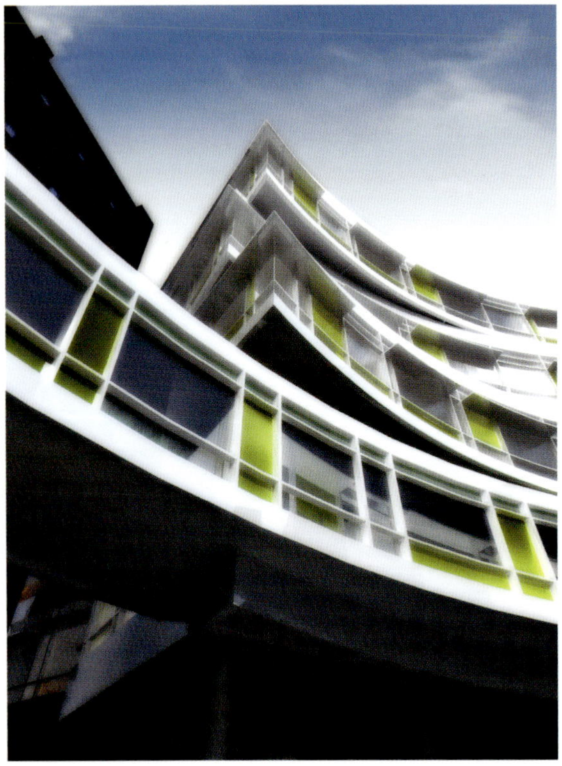

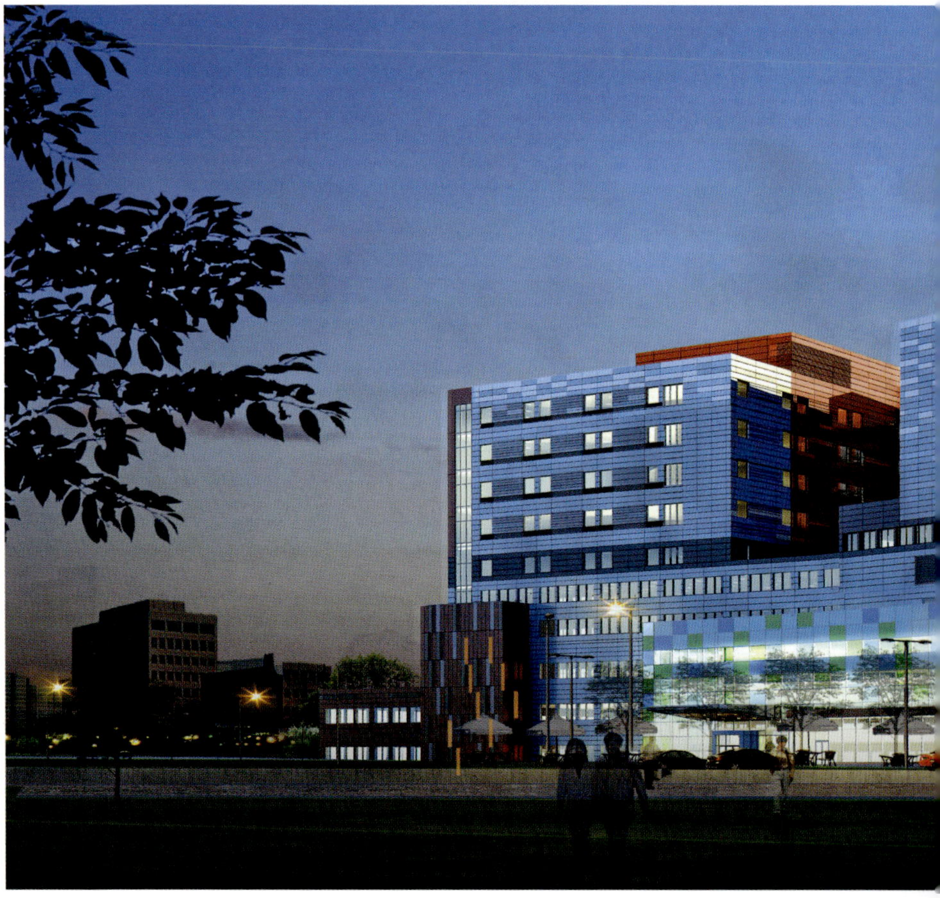

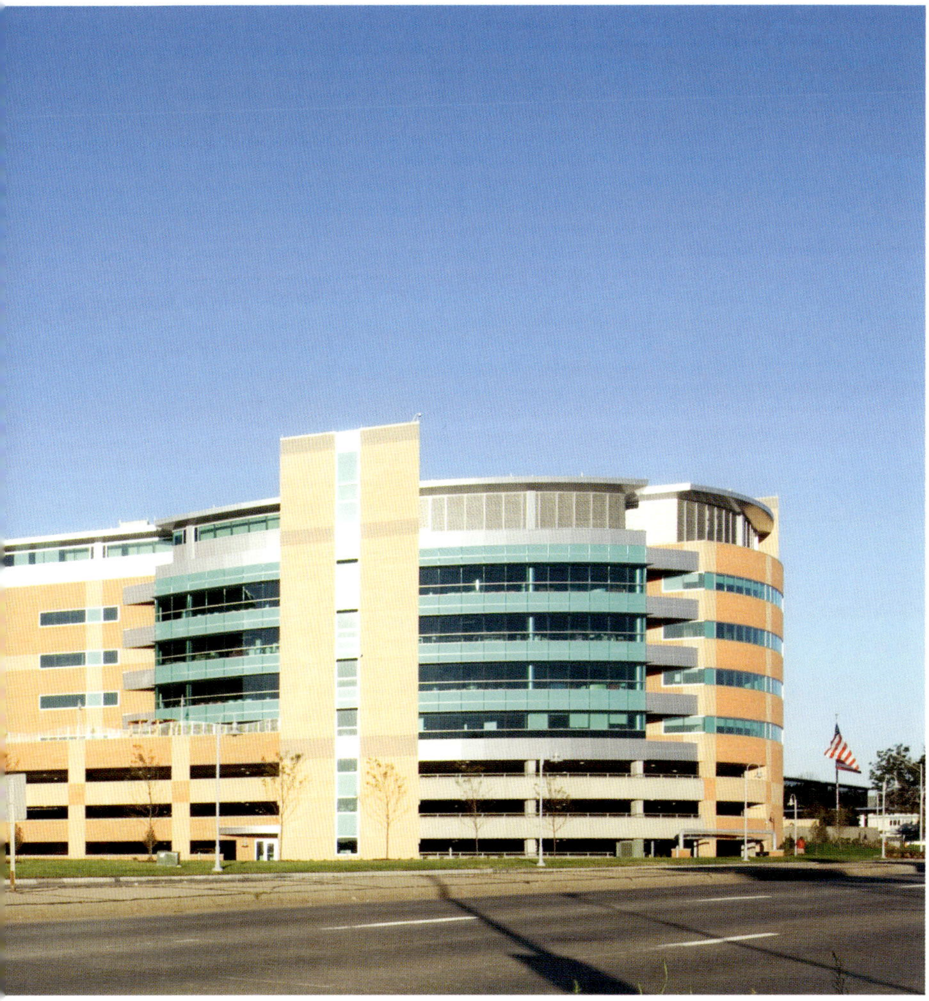

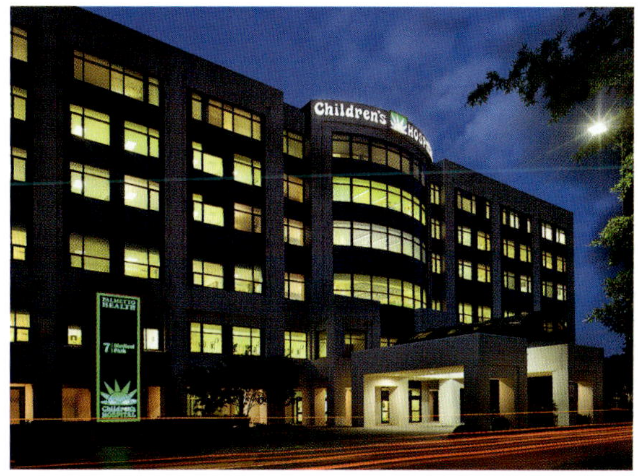

▲ Palmetto Health Children's Hospital, Columbia, SC

▼ Montreal Children's Hospital, McGill, Montreal, Quebec, Canada
Photo: Consortium team: SNC Lavalin, HDR, IBI Group, NFOE Architects and Yelle Maille Architects

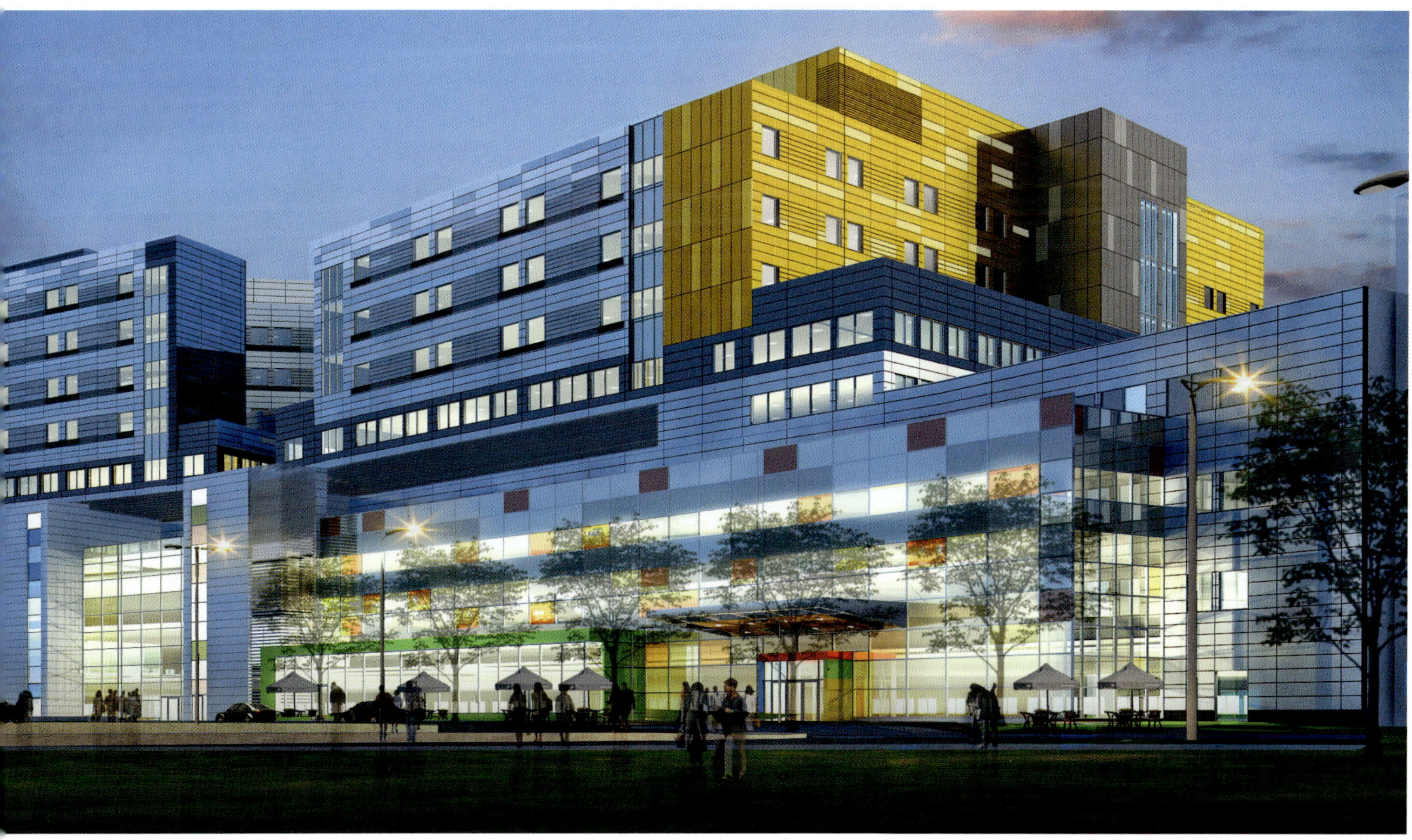

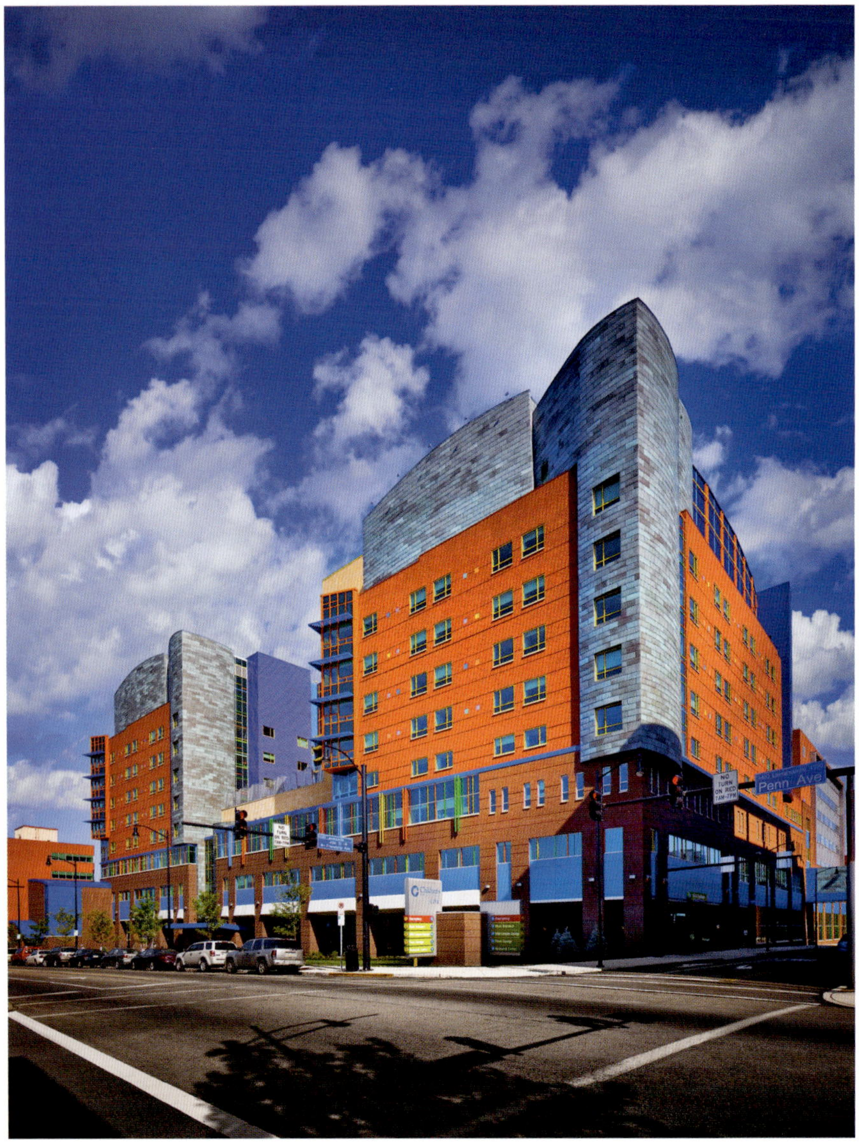

▲ Children's Hospital, Pittsburgh, PA
Photo: Massery Photography, Inc.

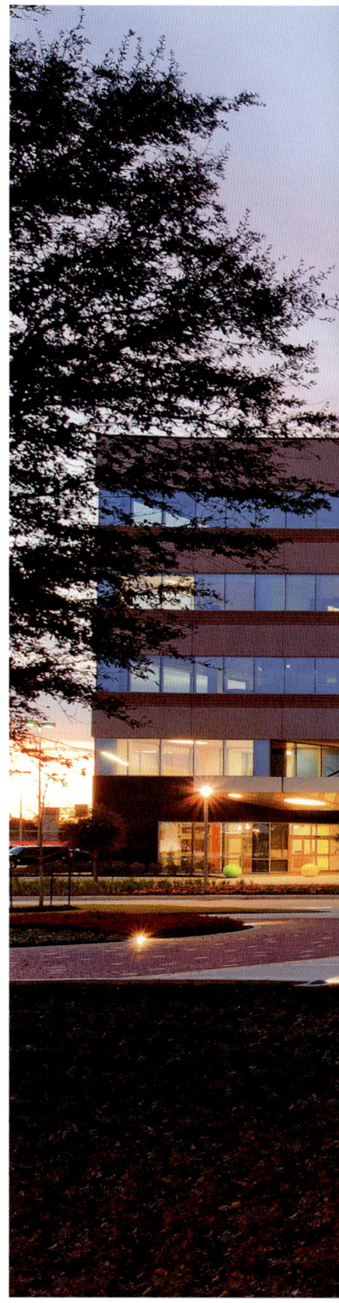

▼ Children's Hospitals and Clinics of Minnesota, Saint Paul, MI
Photo: HDR Architecture, Inc.

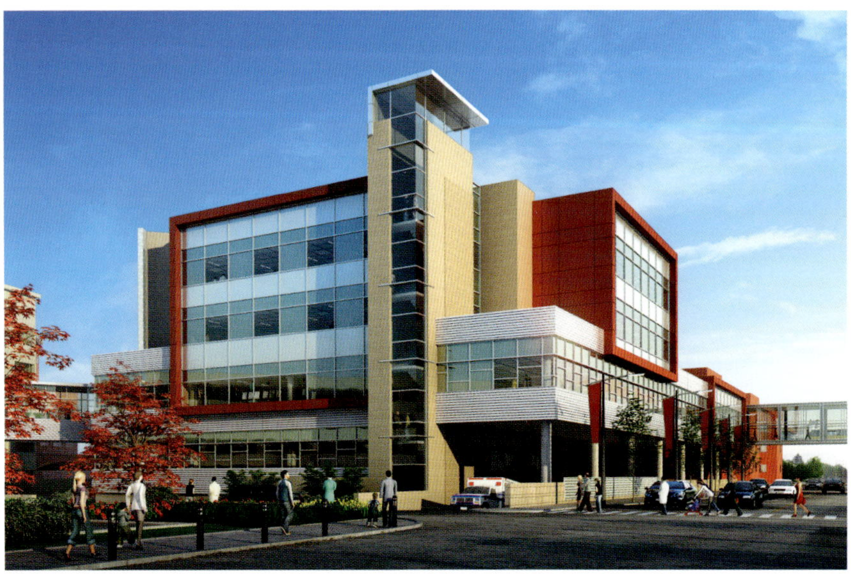

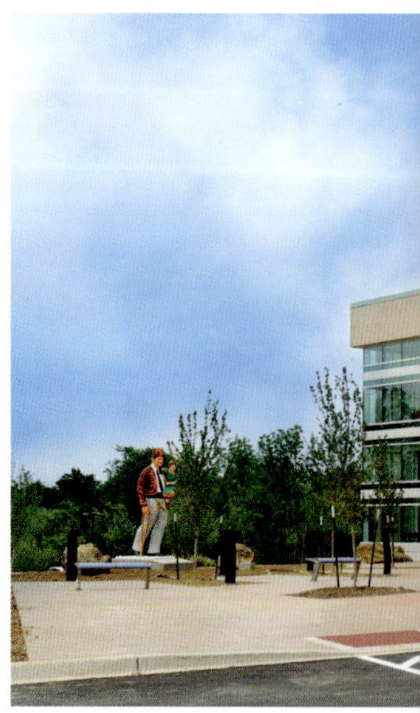

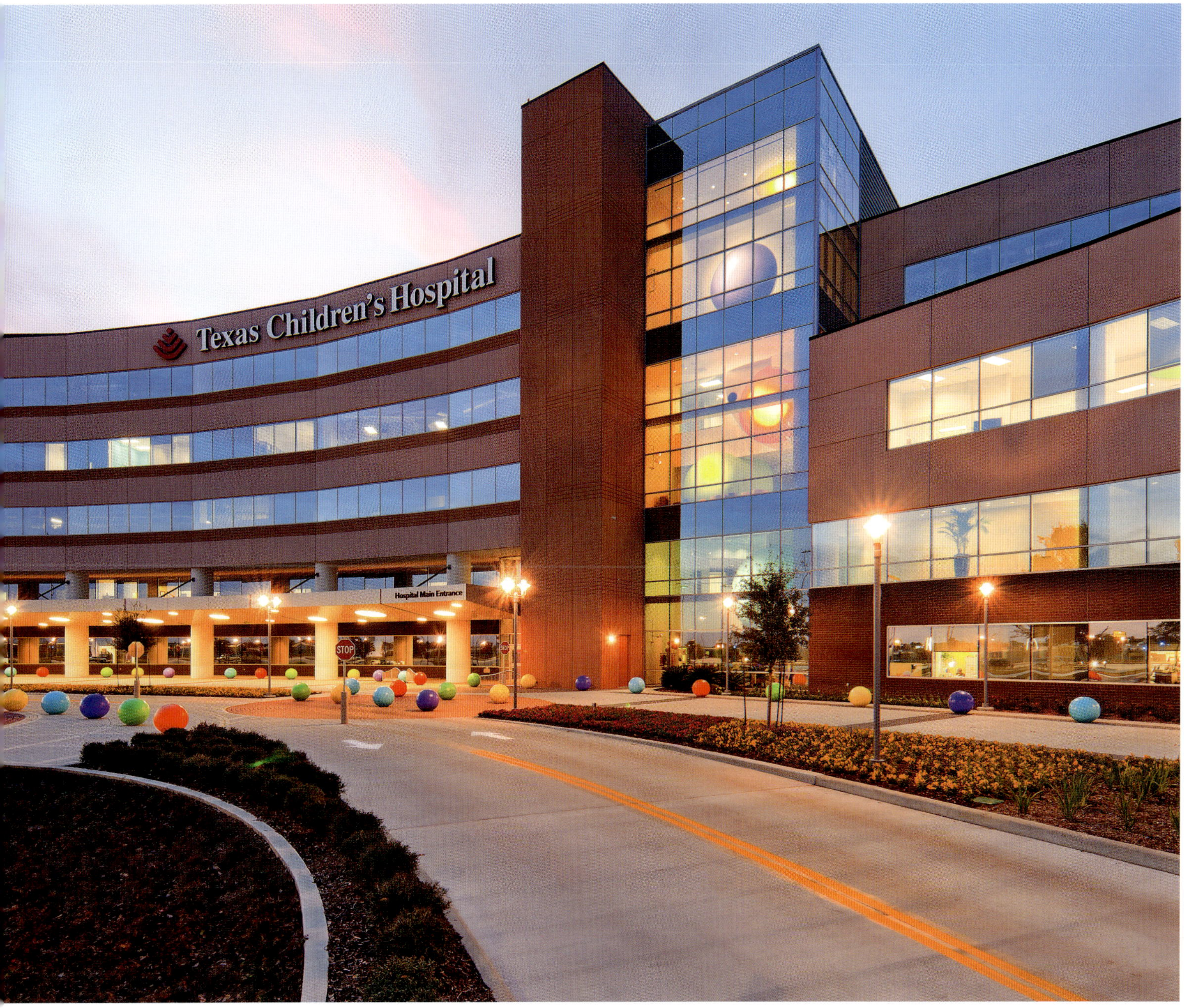

▲ Texas Children's Hospital West Campus, Houston, TX
Photo: Allen Kramer

▼ Kosair Children's Hospital, Louisville, KY

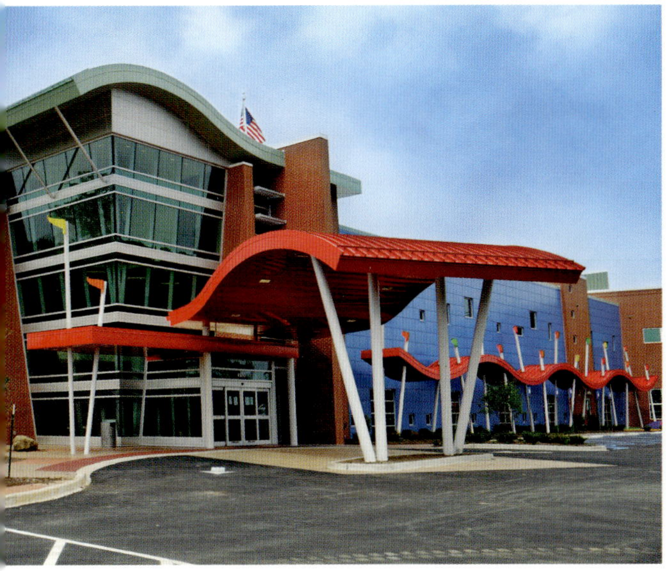

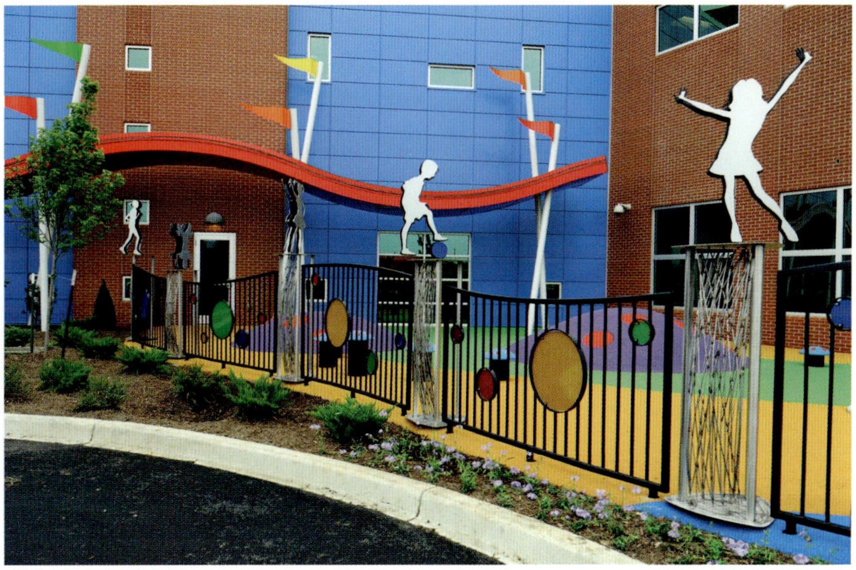

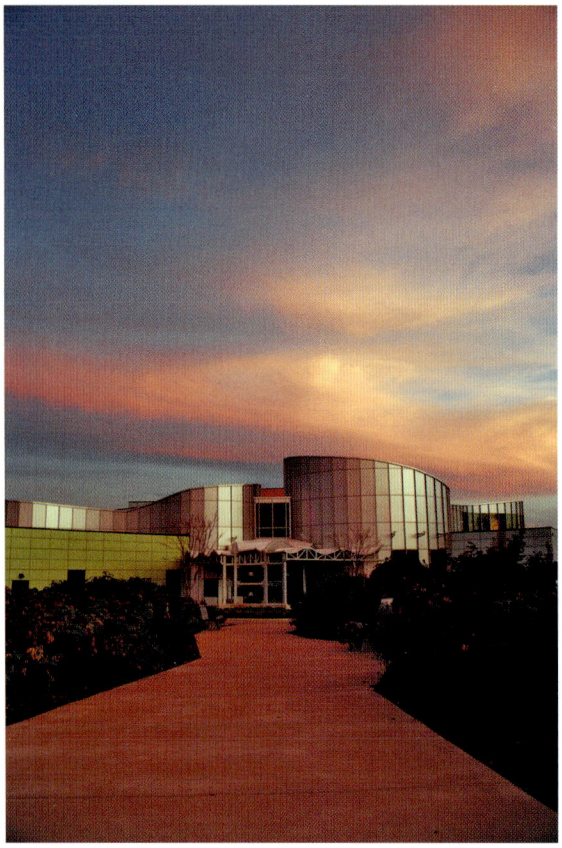

▲ Ranken Jordan - A Pediatric Specialty Hospital, Maryland Heights, MO
Photo: Brian Spurgeon

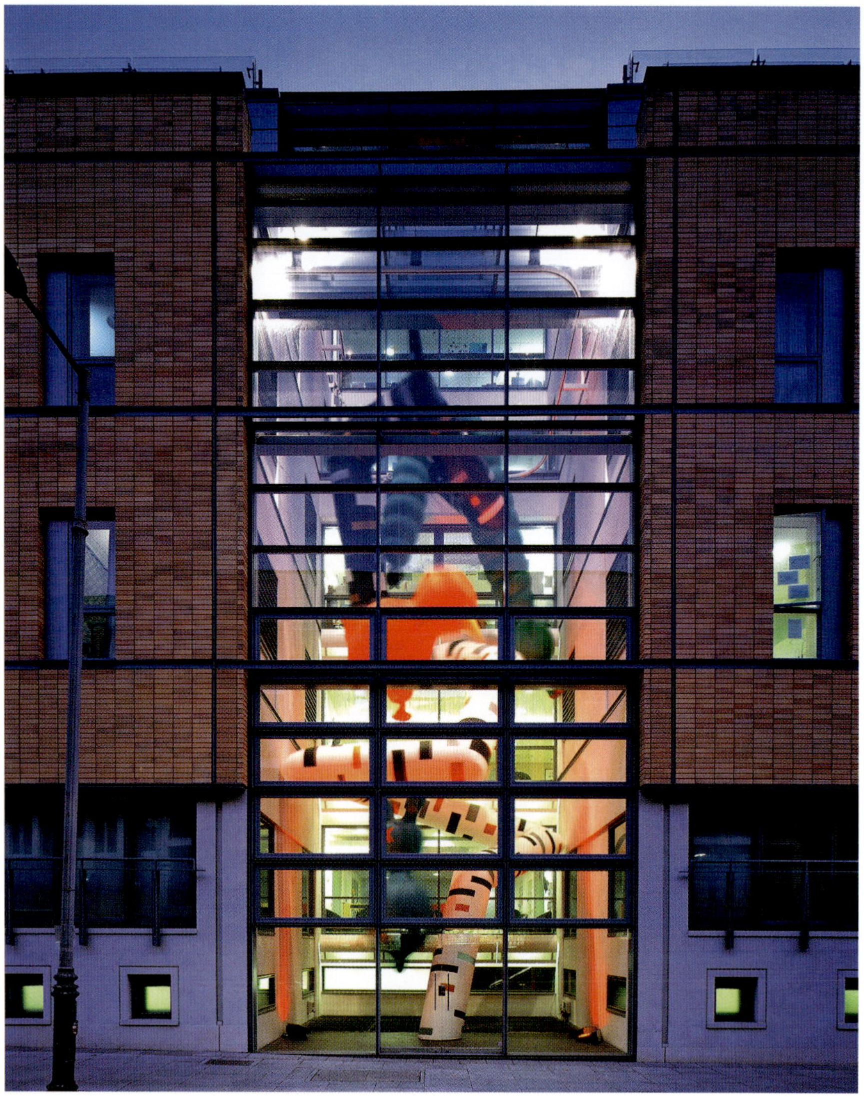

▲ Great Ormond Street Hospital for Children, Octav Botnar Building, London, United Kingdom
Photo: Stantec © Edmund Sumner

▼ Children's Hospital and Medical Center, Omaha, NE
Photos: Thomas Grady

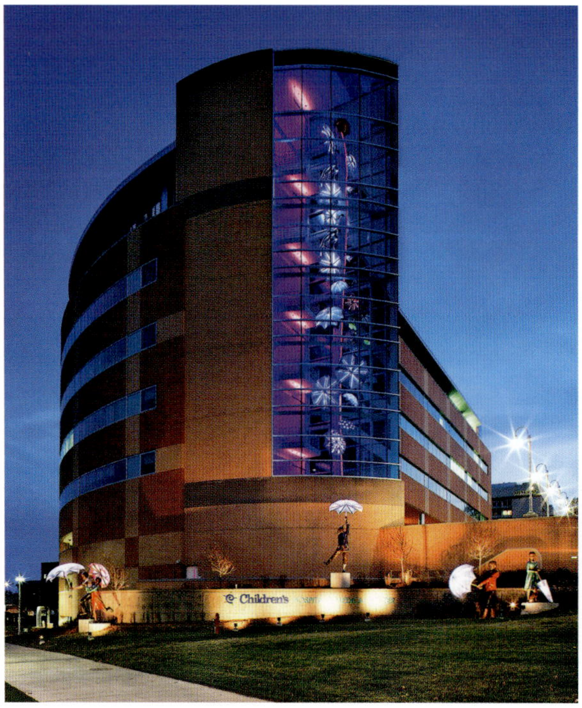

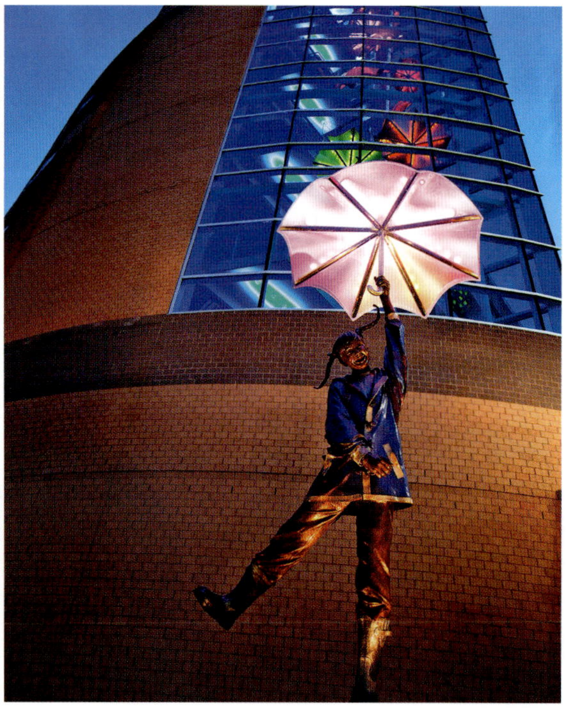

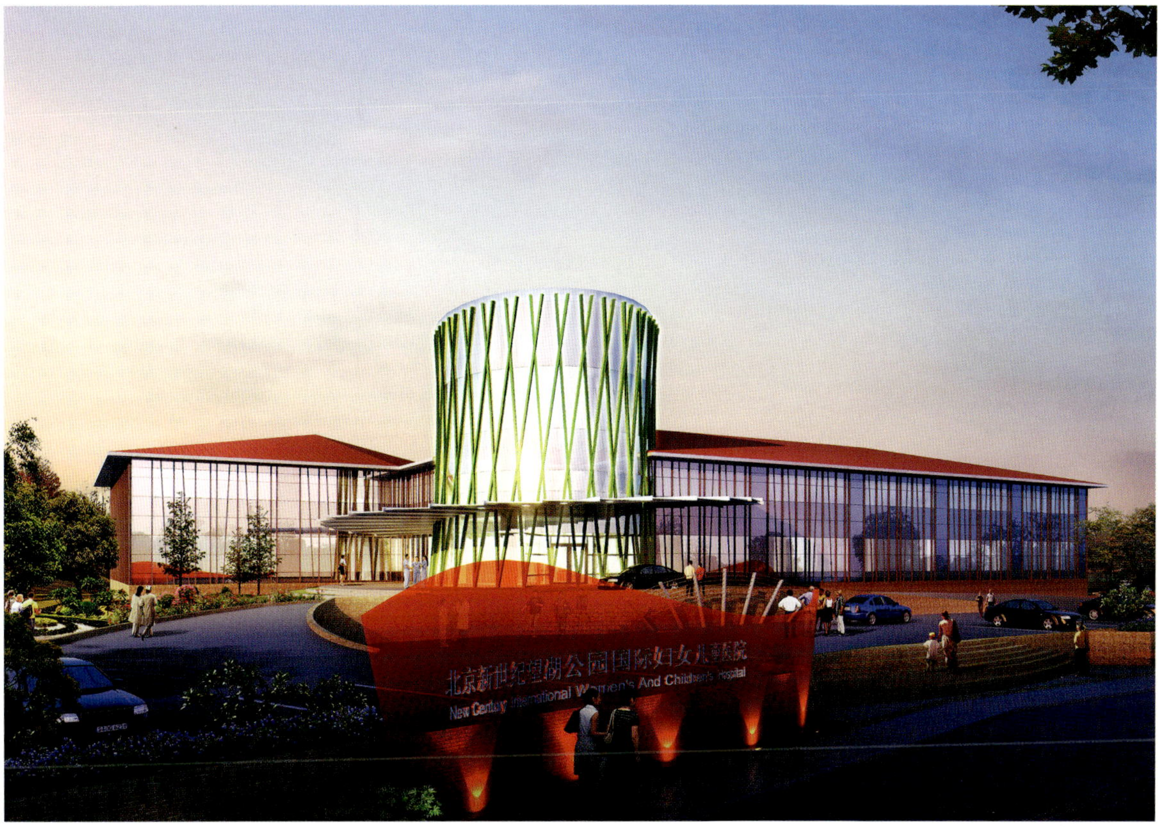

▲ New Century International Women and Children's Hospitals, Beijing, China
Photo: Provided by FKP Architects

▼ Children's Hospital of Philadelphia, PA
Photo: Ed Cunicelli

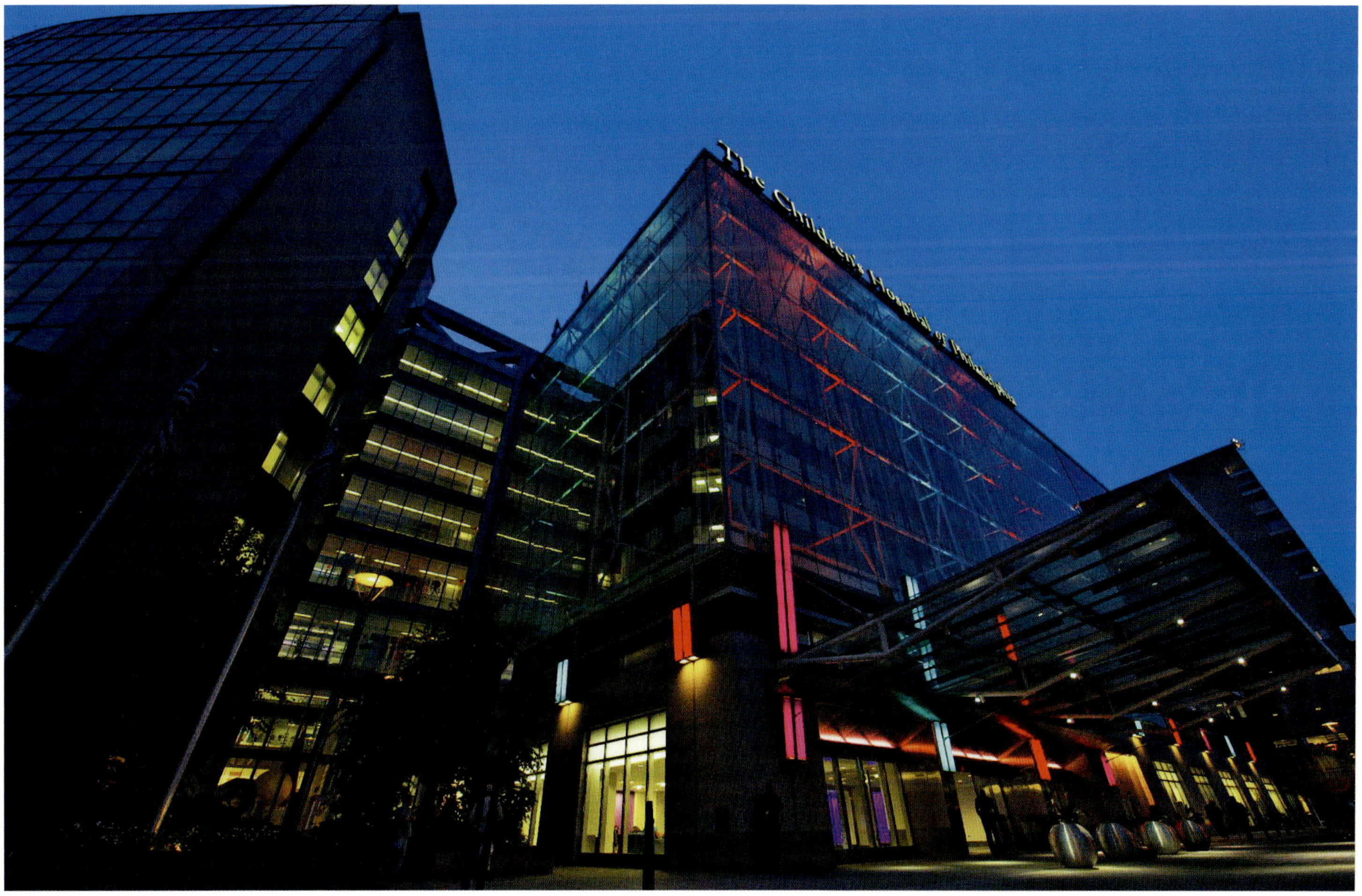

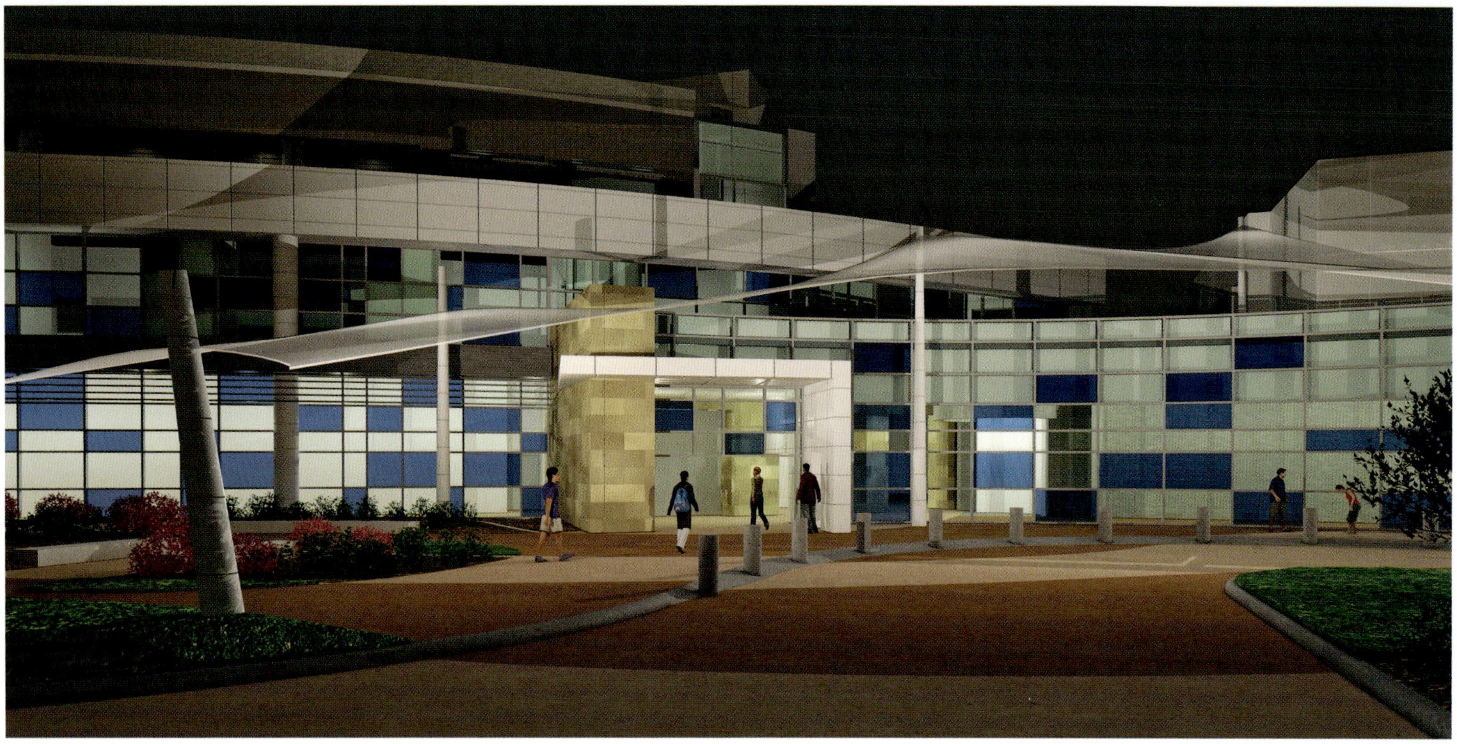

▲ University Health Systems Children's Hospital, Greenville, NC
Photo: HDR Architecture, Inc.

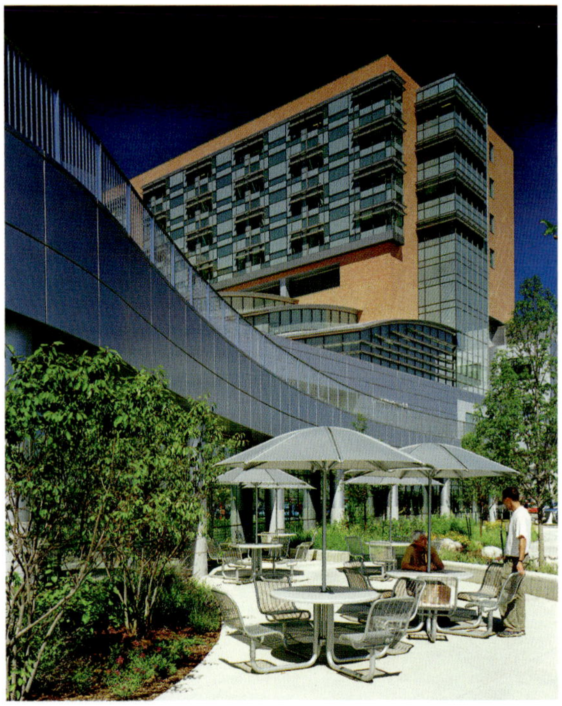

▲ Children's Hospital Colorado, Denver, CO
Photo: Eckert & Eckert

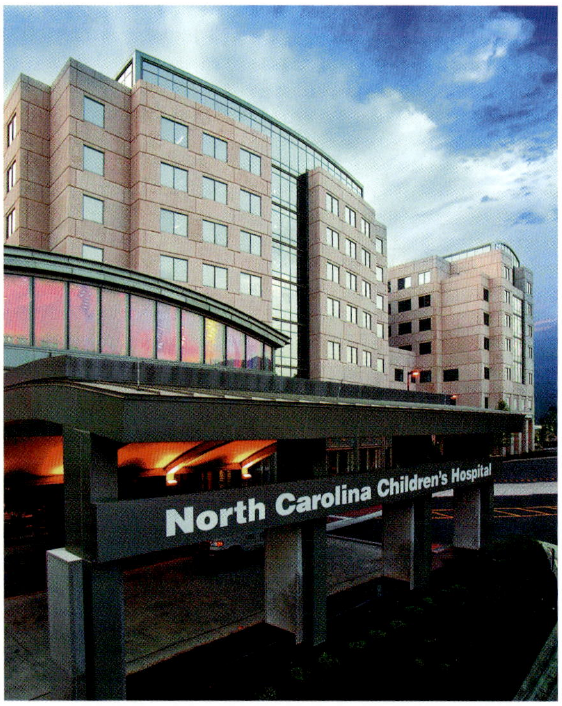

▲ UNC North Carolina Children's Hospital, Chapel Hill, NC
Photo: Brian Strickland

▼ Seattle Children's Hospital, WA

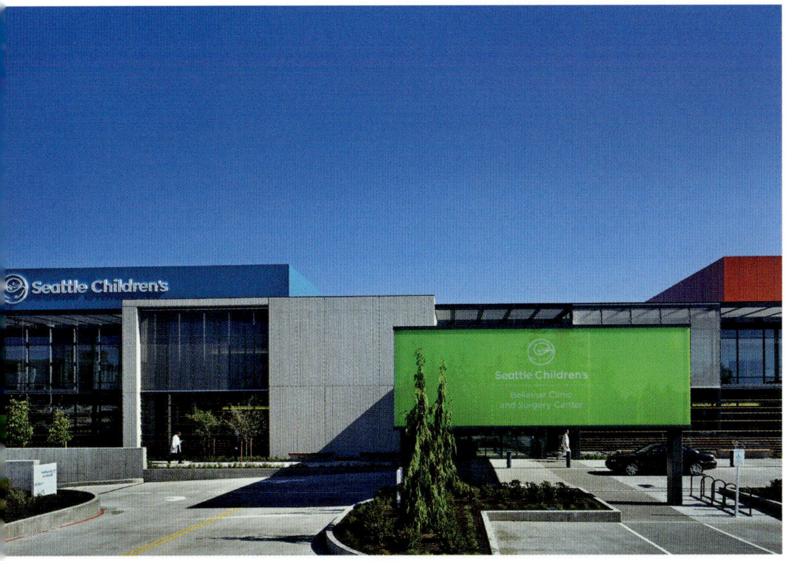

▼ Joseph M. Sanzari Children's Hospital at Hackensack University Medical Center, Hackensack, NJ
Photo: Steve Hockstein, Harvard Studio

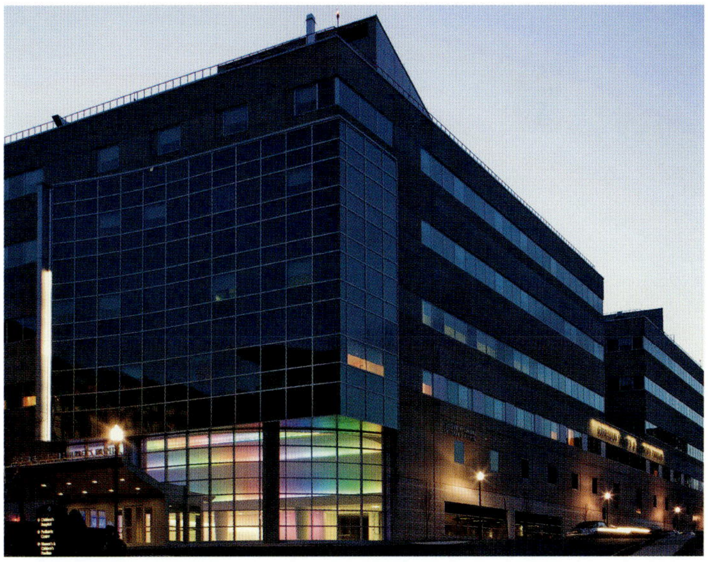

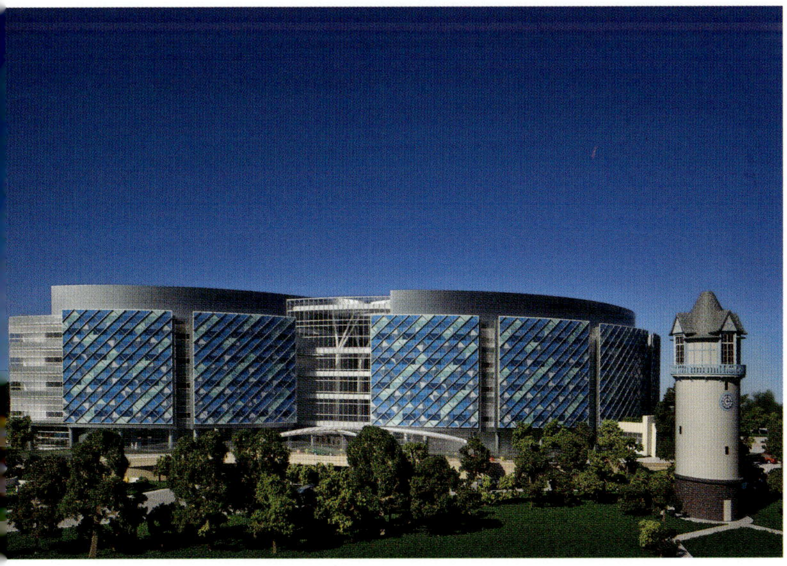

▲ Nemours/AI DuPont Hospital for Children, Wilmington, DE
Photo: Aker Imaging

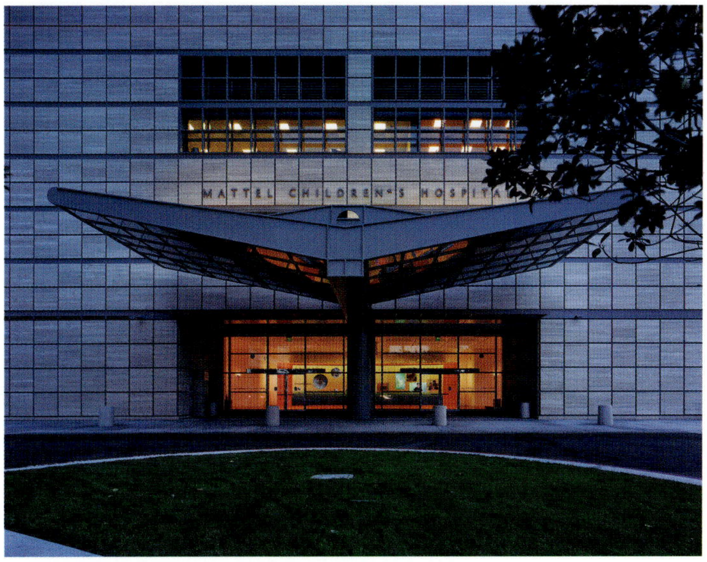

▲ Mattel Children's Hospital UCLA, Los Angeles, CA
Photo: Benny Chan, fotoworks

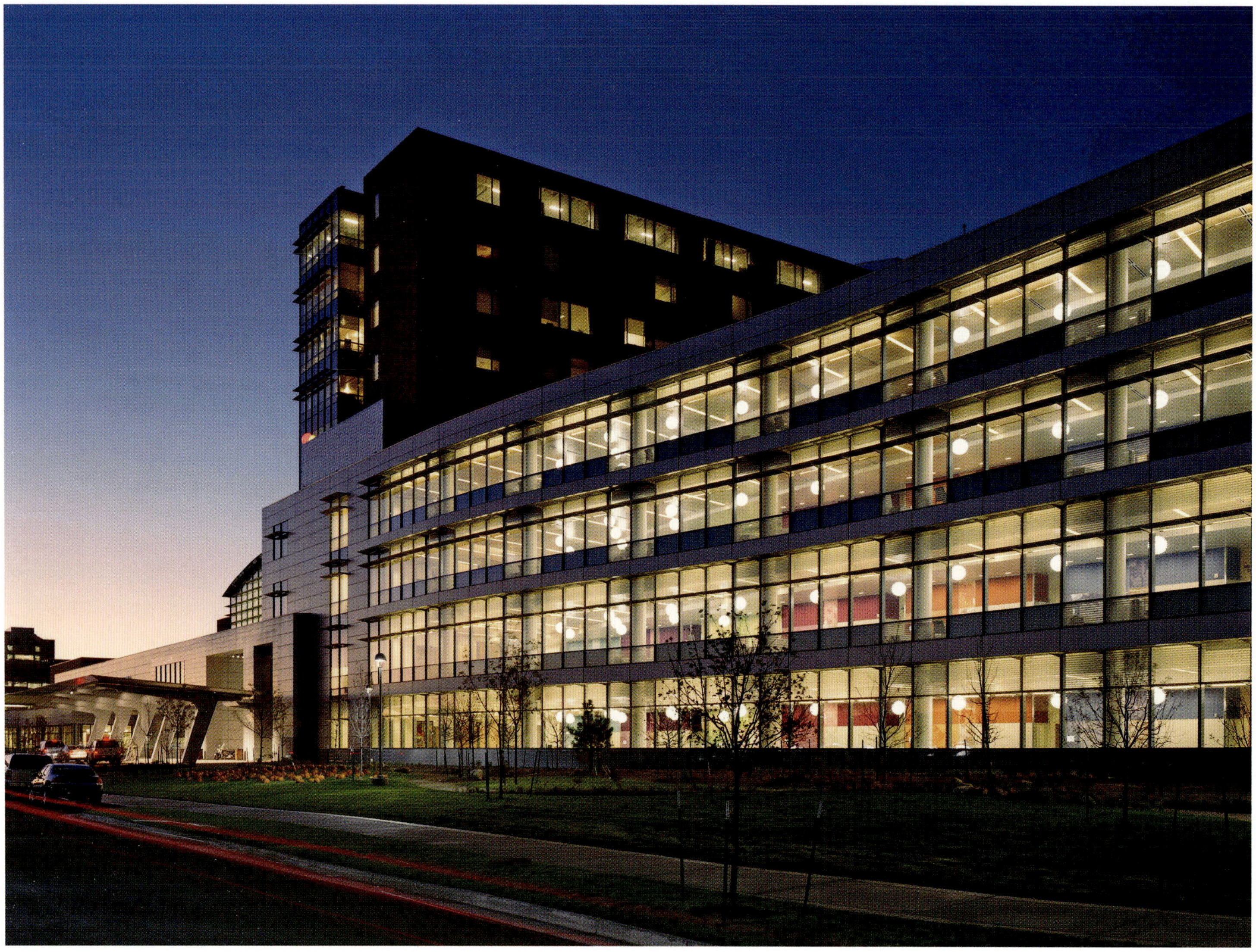

▲ Children's Hospital Colorado, Denver, CO
Photo: Eckert & Eckert

▼ Rady Children's Hospital & Health Center, Acute Care Pavilion, San Diego, CA
Photo: Stantec © RMA Photography

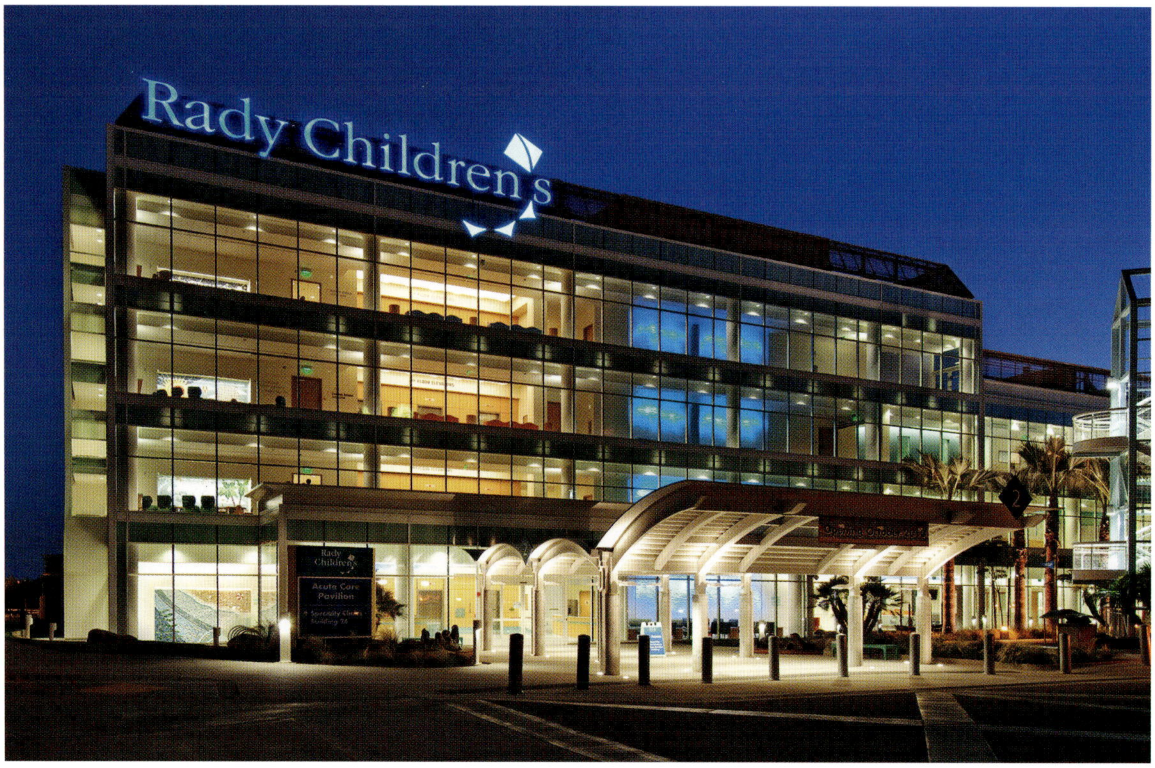

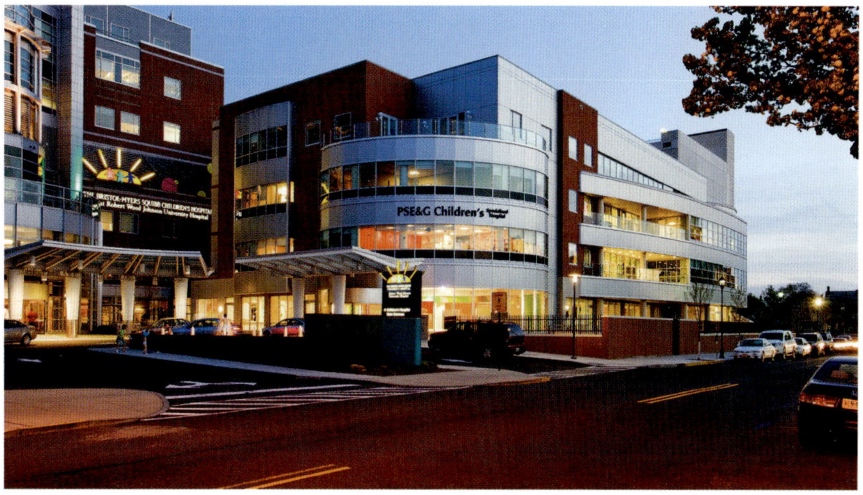

▲ PSE&G Children's Specialized Hospital, Pediatric Rehabilitation Hospital, New Brunswick, NJ
Photo: Blake Marvin, HKS

▼ Texas Children's Hospital Pavilion for Women, Houston, TX
Photo: Craig Dugan Photography

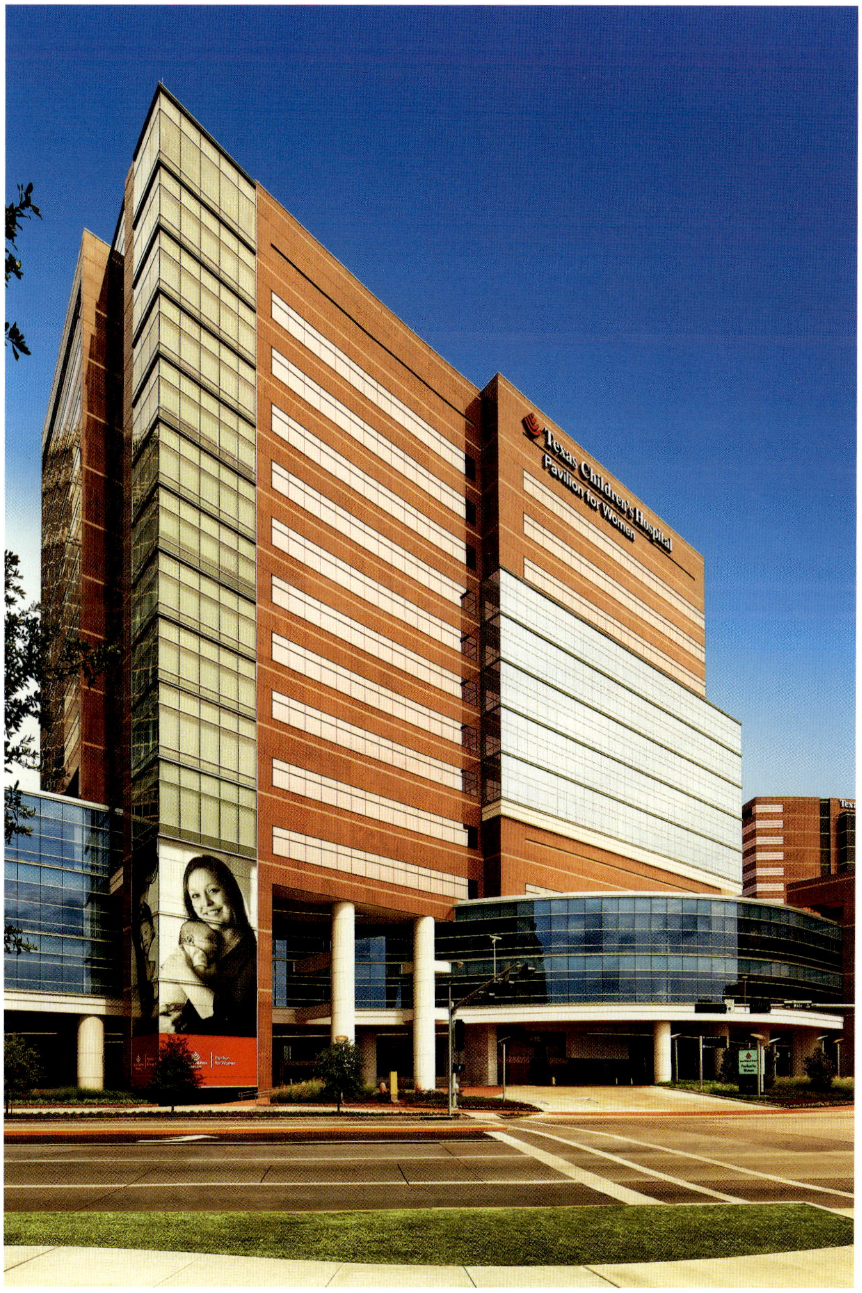

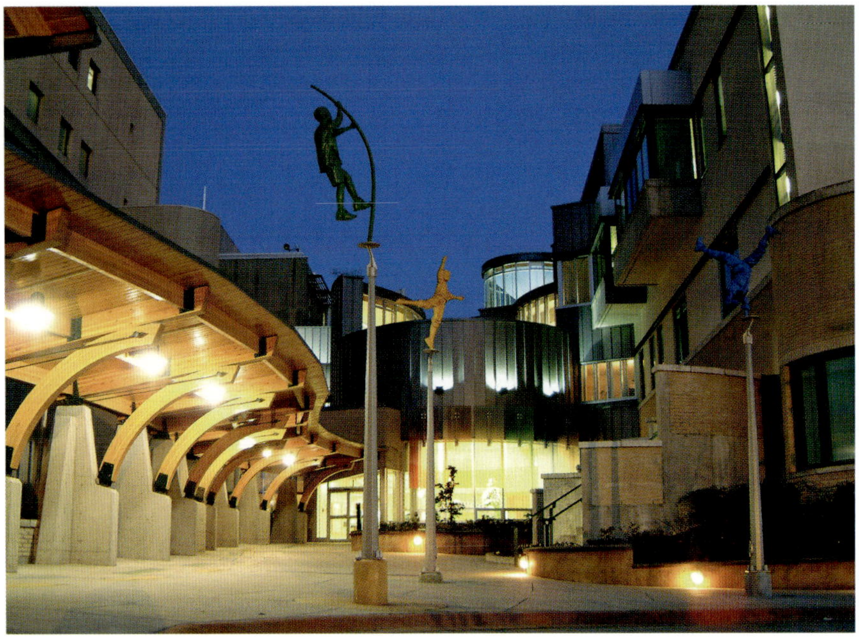

▲ Surrey Memorial Hospital, Children's Health Centre, Surrey, British Columbia, Canada
Photo: Stantec © William Vo

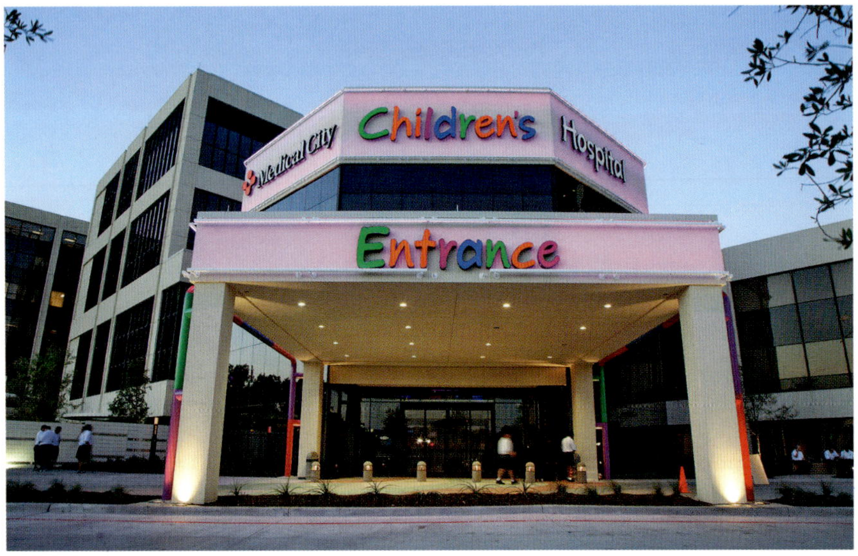

▲ Medical City Children's Hospital, Dallas, TX
Photo: Terry Cockerham

▼ Gillette Children's, Saint Paul, MI
Photo: Terry Mahanna

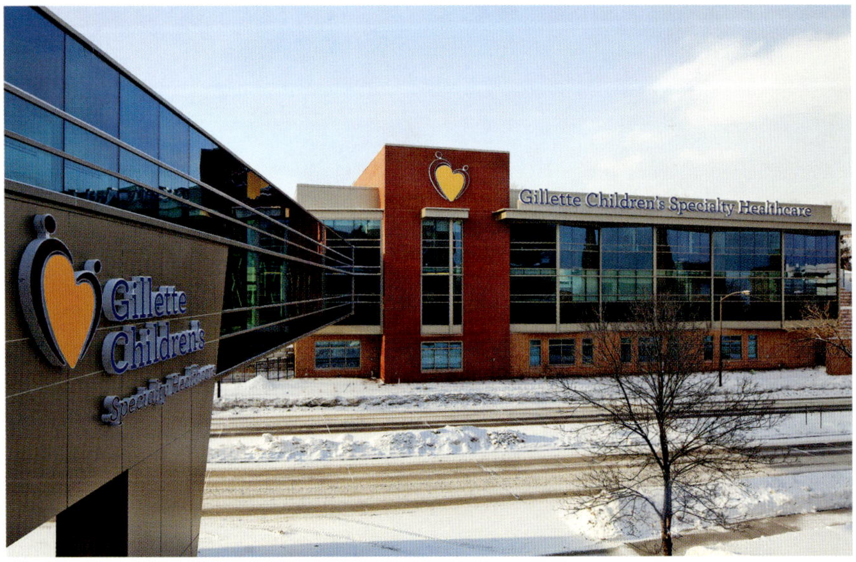

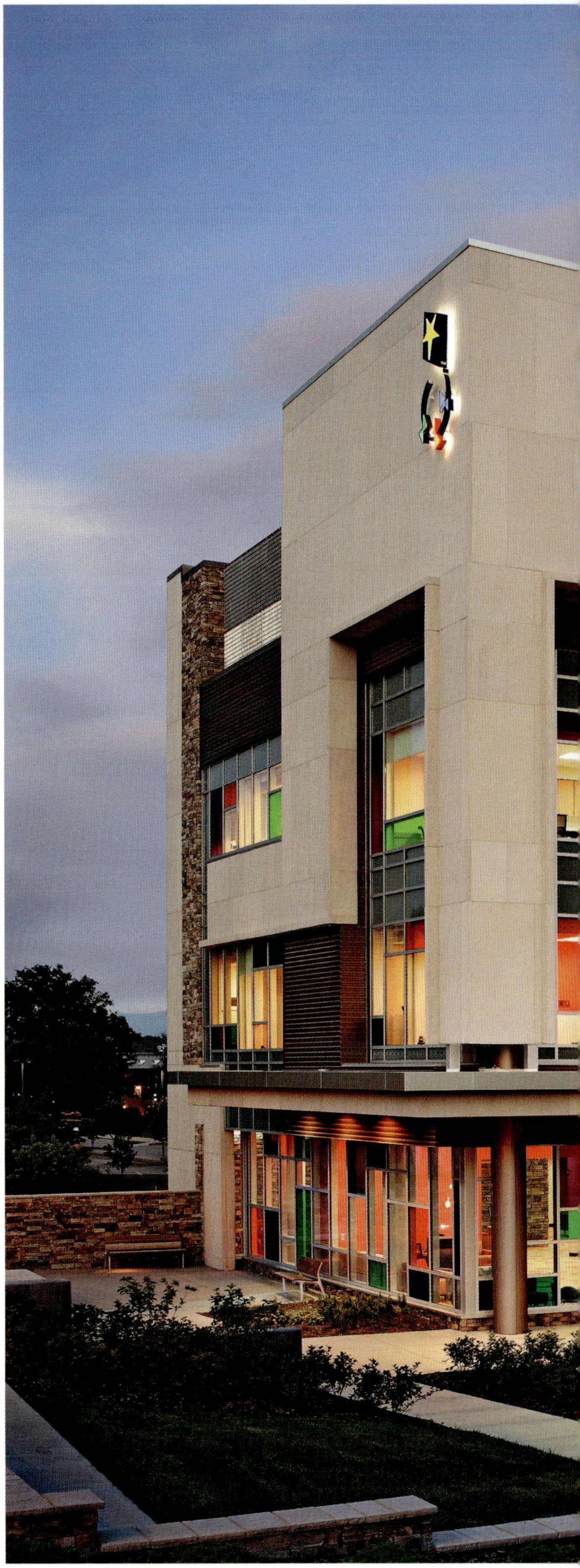

▲ Niswonger Children's Hospital, Johnson City, TN
Photo: Peter Montanti

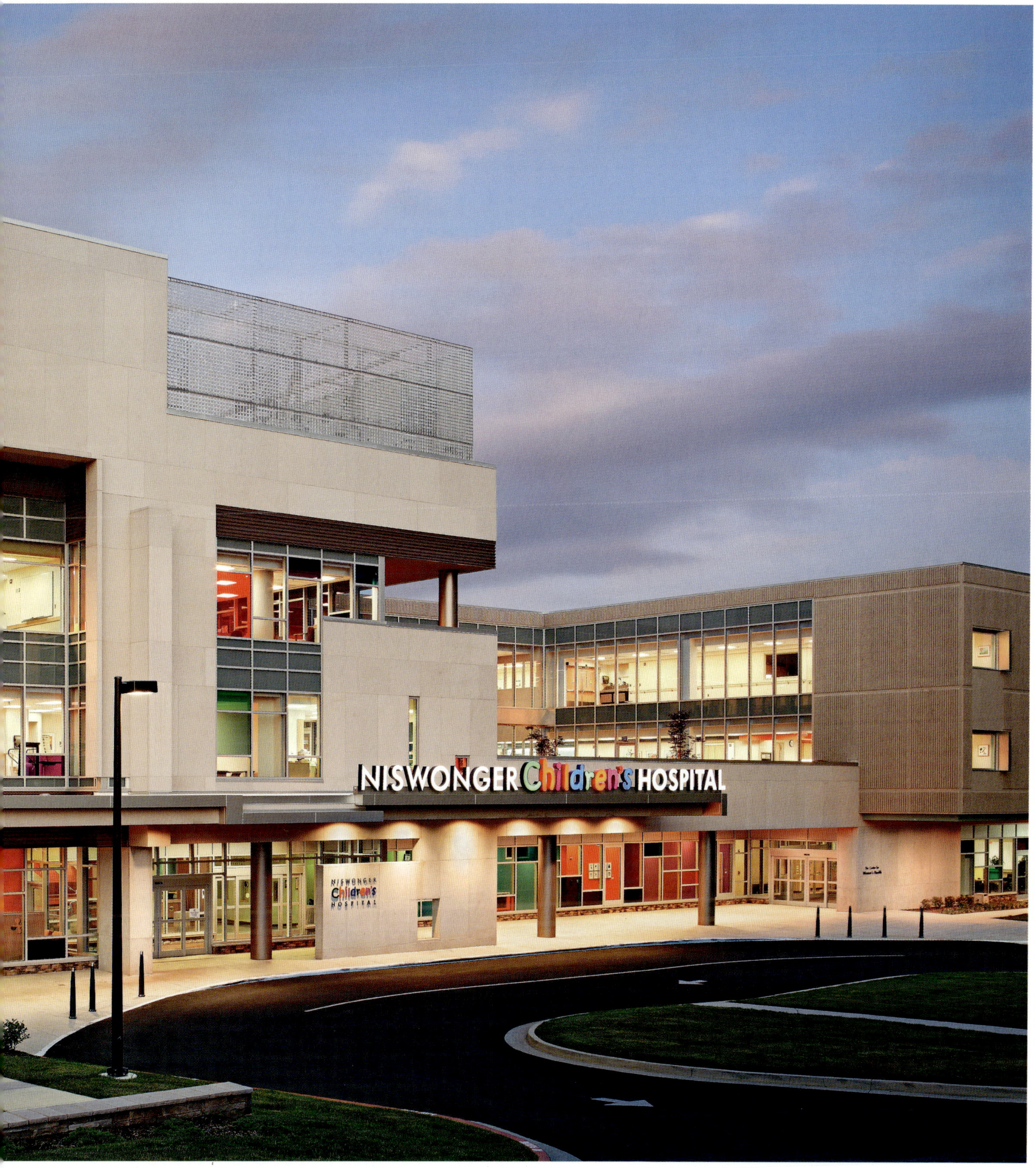
NISWONGER Children's HOSPITAL
NISWONGER Children's HOSPITAL

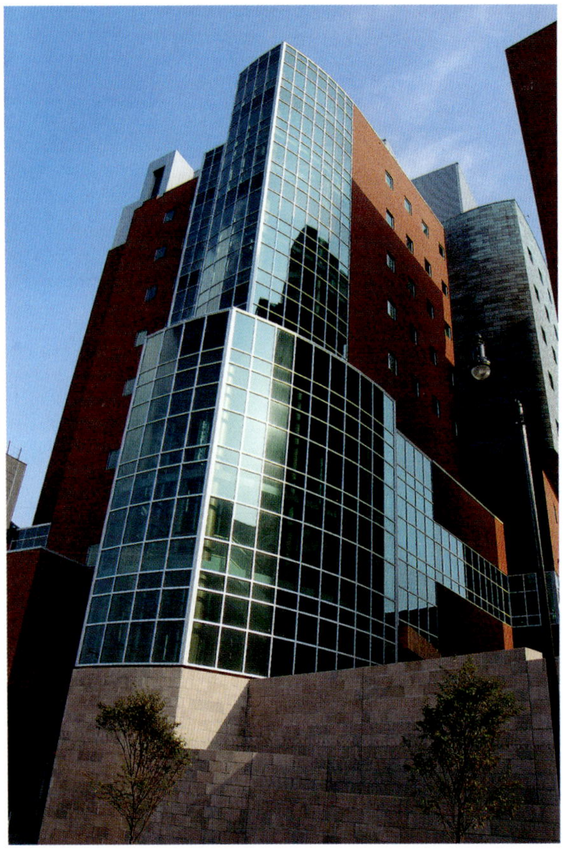

▲ Children's Hospital, Pittsburgh, PA

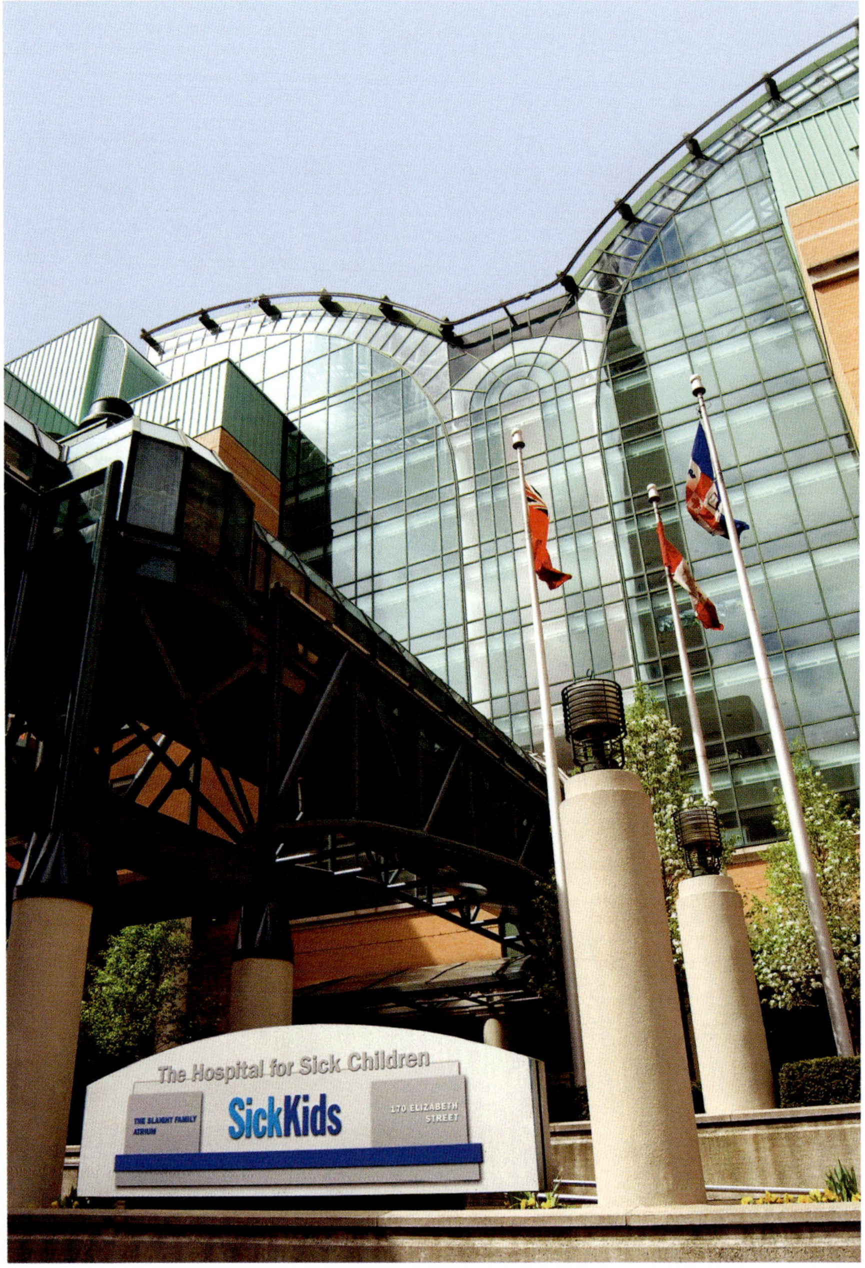

▲ SickKids – The Hospital for Sick Children, Toronto, Ontario, Canada
Photo: Robert Teteruck, SickKids

▼ University of California, San Francisco Medical Center at Mission Bay, Benioff Children's Hospital, San Francisco, CA
Photo: Stantec ©

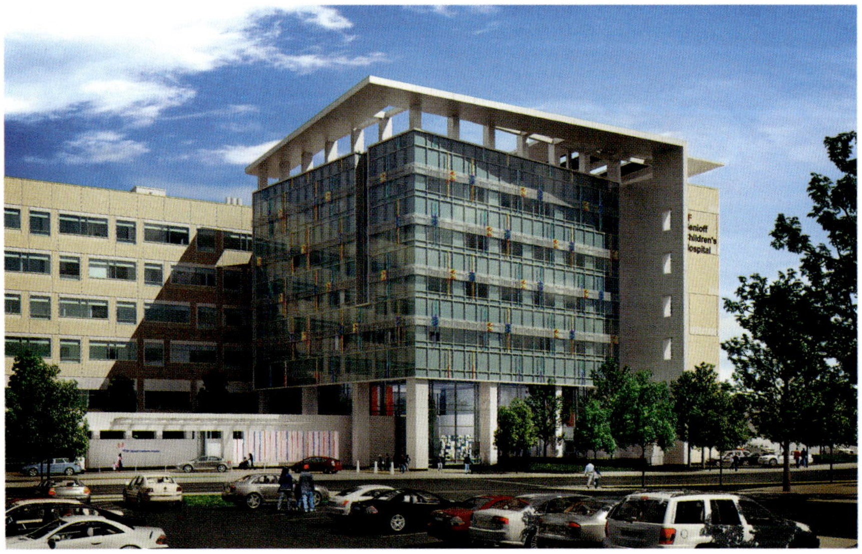

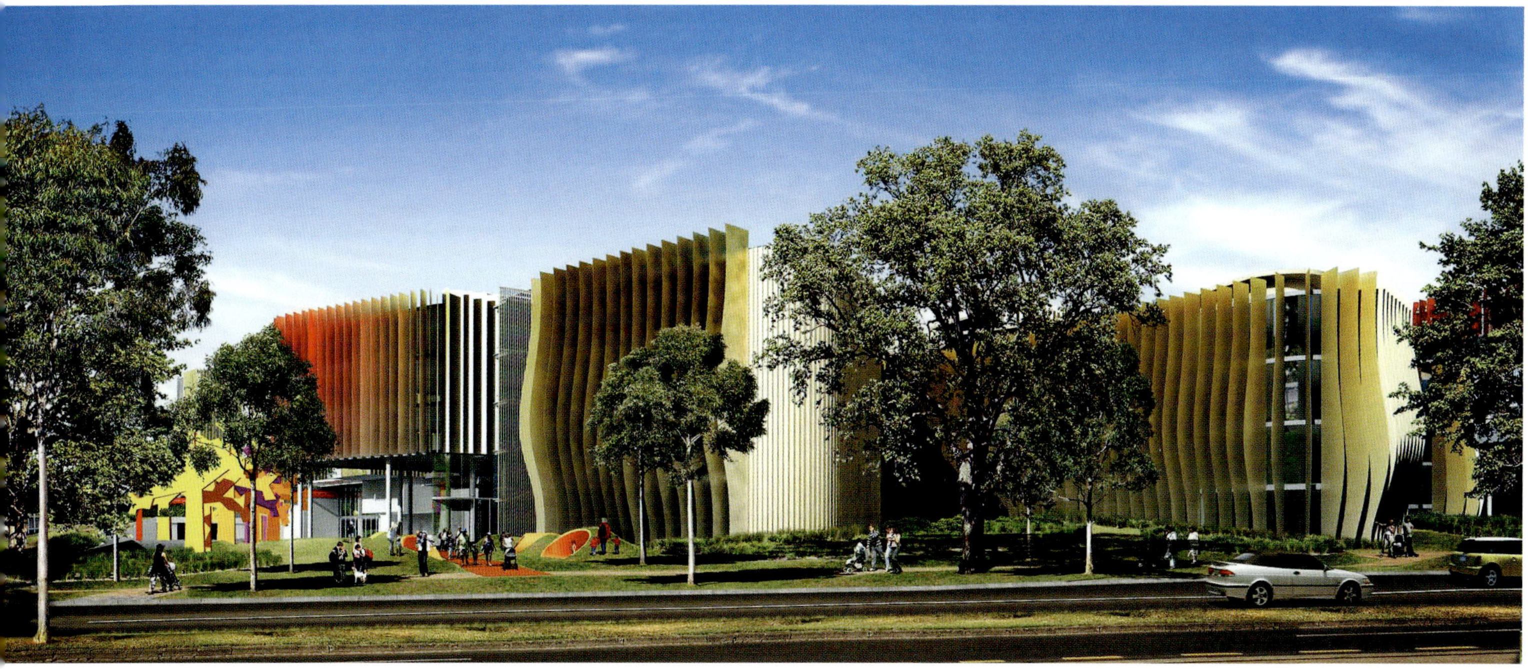

▲ University of Melbourne Hospital, Melbourne, Australia
Photo: Stantec ©

▼ Children's Medical Center at Legacy, Plano, TX
Photo: Robert Canfield

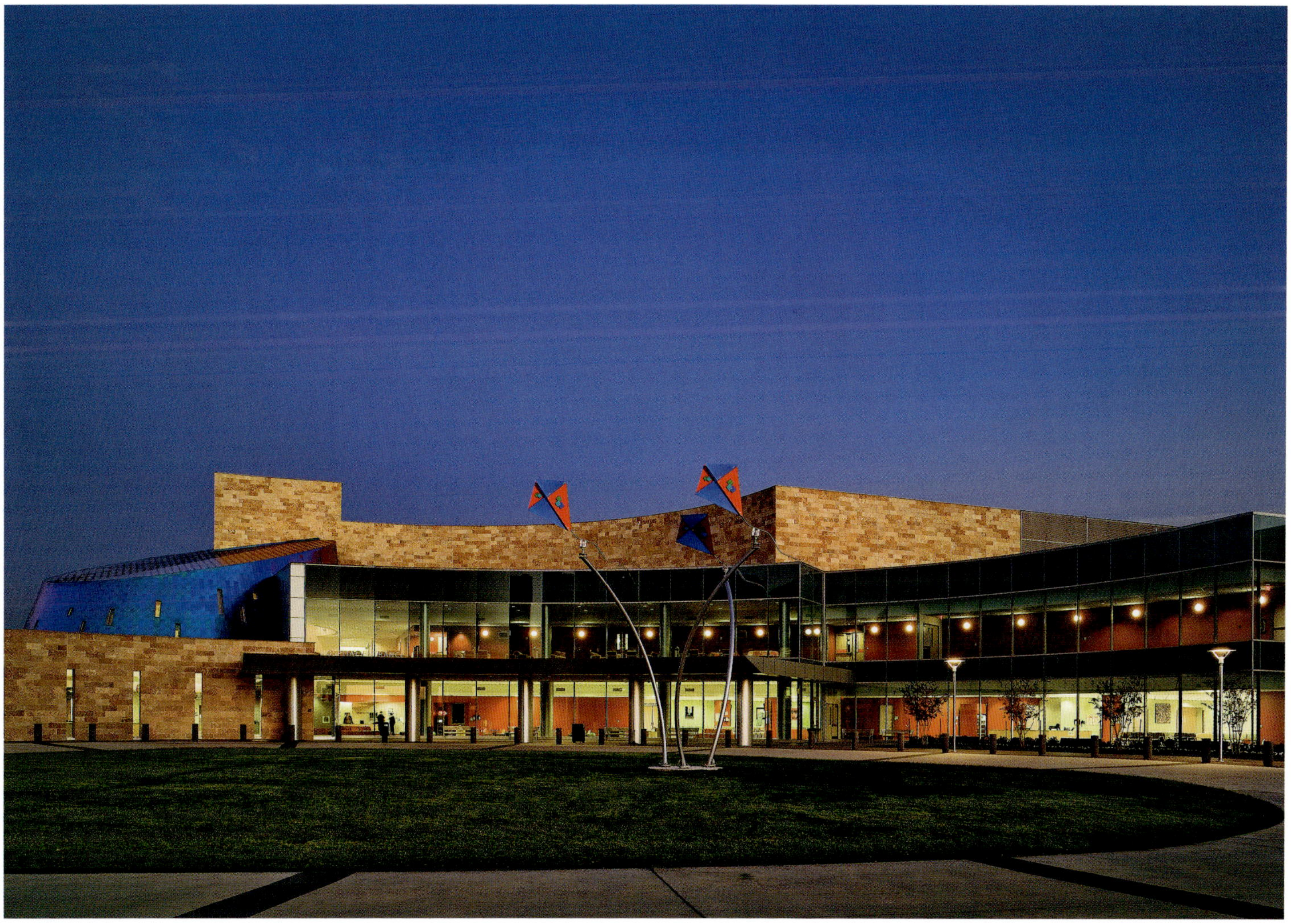

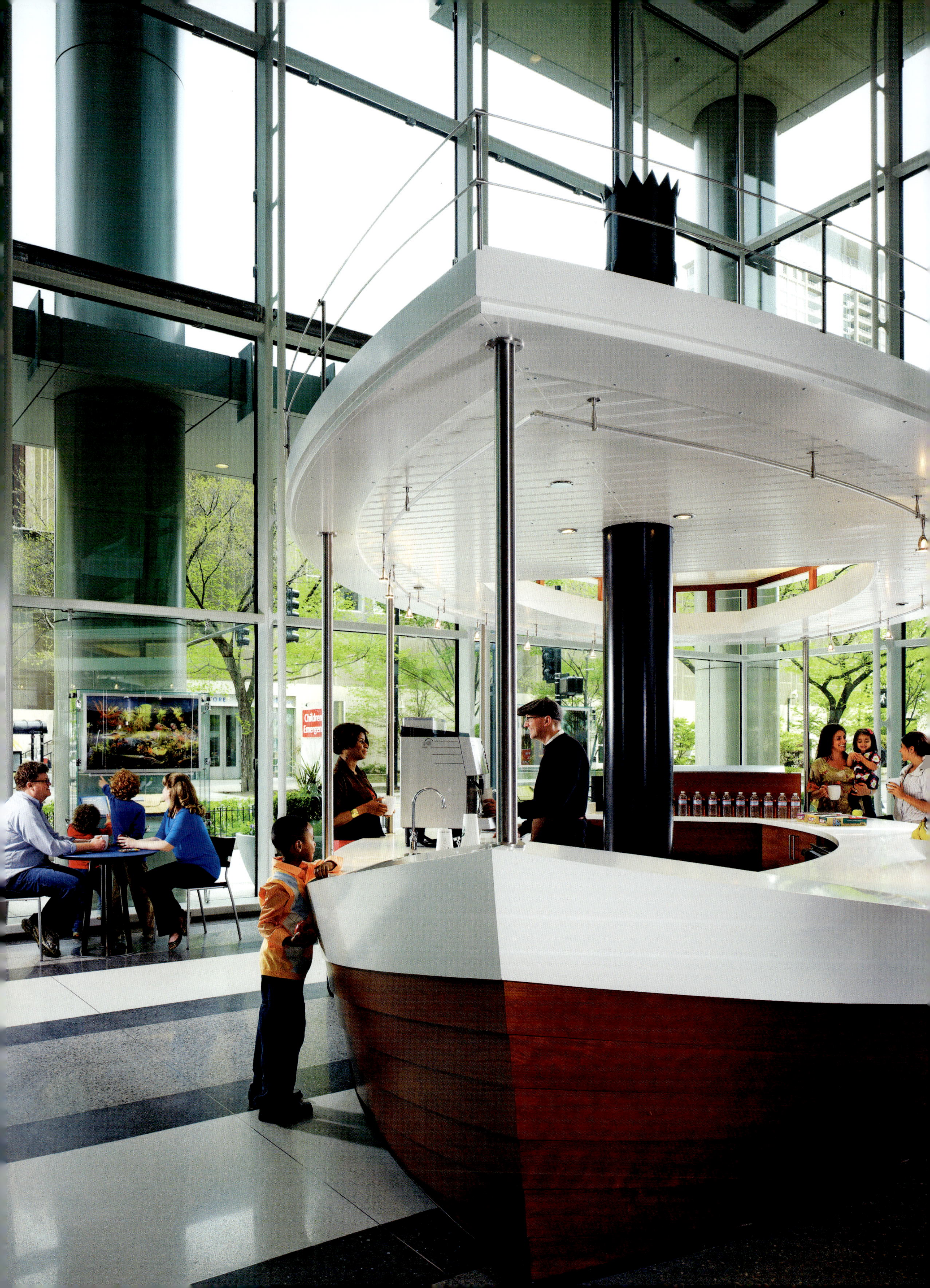

Public Spaces

Public space in a children's hospital is more than just a friendly entrance or a comfortable waiting room. These popular environments provide a unique opportunity for the design team, hospital staff, and patients to create an experience that speaks to each of the institution's stakeholders. More importantly, these common areas offer a way for children's hospitals to distinguish themselves appropriately from their adult counterparts.

Such spaces can be challenging to execute. Too often, the public realm in a children's hospital looks like it was born of a Saturday morning cartoon or a scene out of a fantasy movie. They speak down to the child. Alternatively, they need to be timeless, making sense to all hospital users, whether staff, a mother of a PICU patient, or a teenager who has spent months, if not years, within its walls. Public spaces must also carefully balance a design vision with the medical culture of the hospital. They must be functional in every respect—from efficiently accommodating clinical needs to meeting a hospital's security regulations. To be truly successful, the public spaces of the hospital should create a sense of community, beckon interactivity, and inspire confidence in the patients, families, and staff who use them daily.

Designed the right way, public space in children's hospitals can be a reassuring and captivating place to be.

Jim Diaz, FAIA and Travis Leissner, AIA
KMD Architects

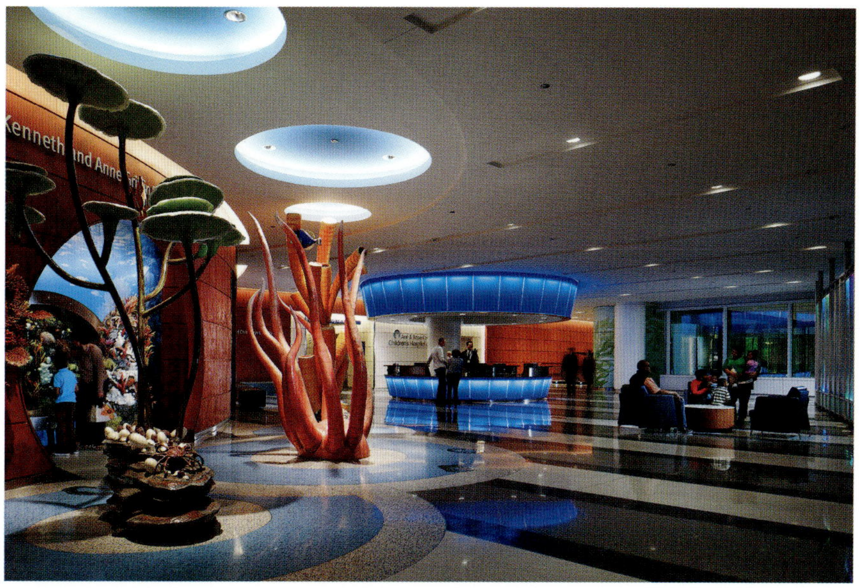

▲ Ann & Robert H. Lurie Children's Hospital of Chicago, IL
◀ ***Photos: Hedrich Blessing Photography, Nick Merrick***

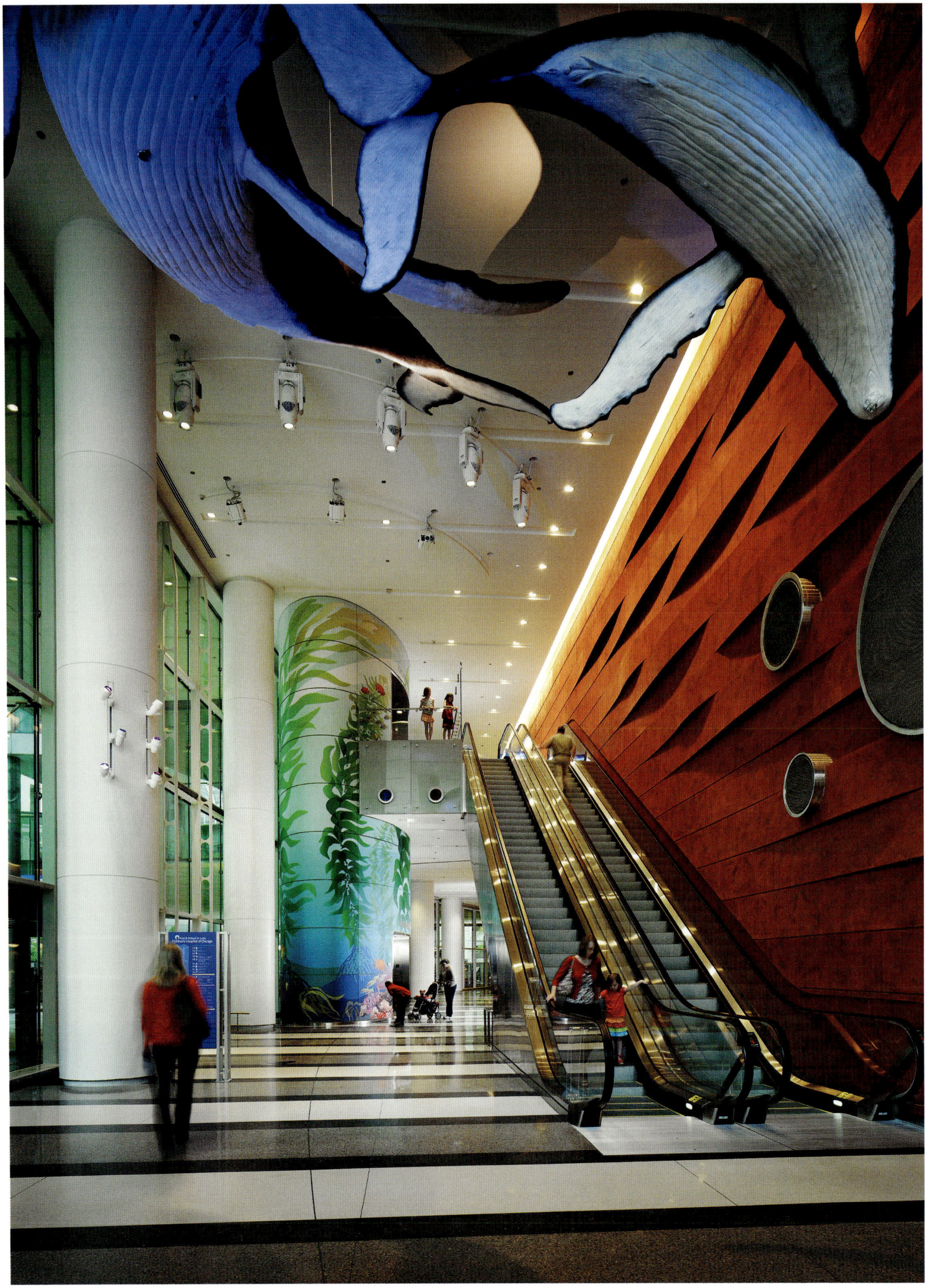

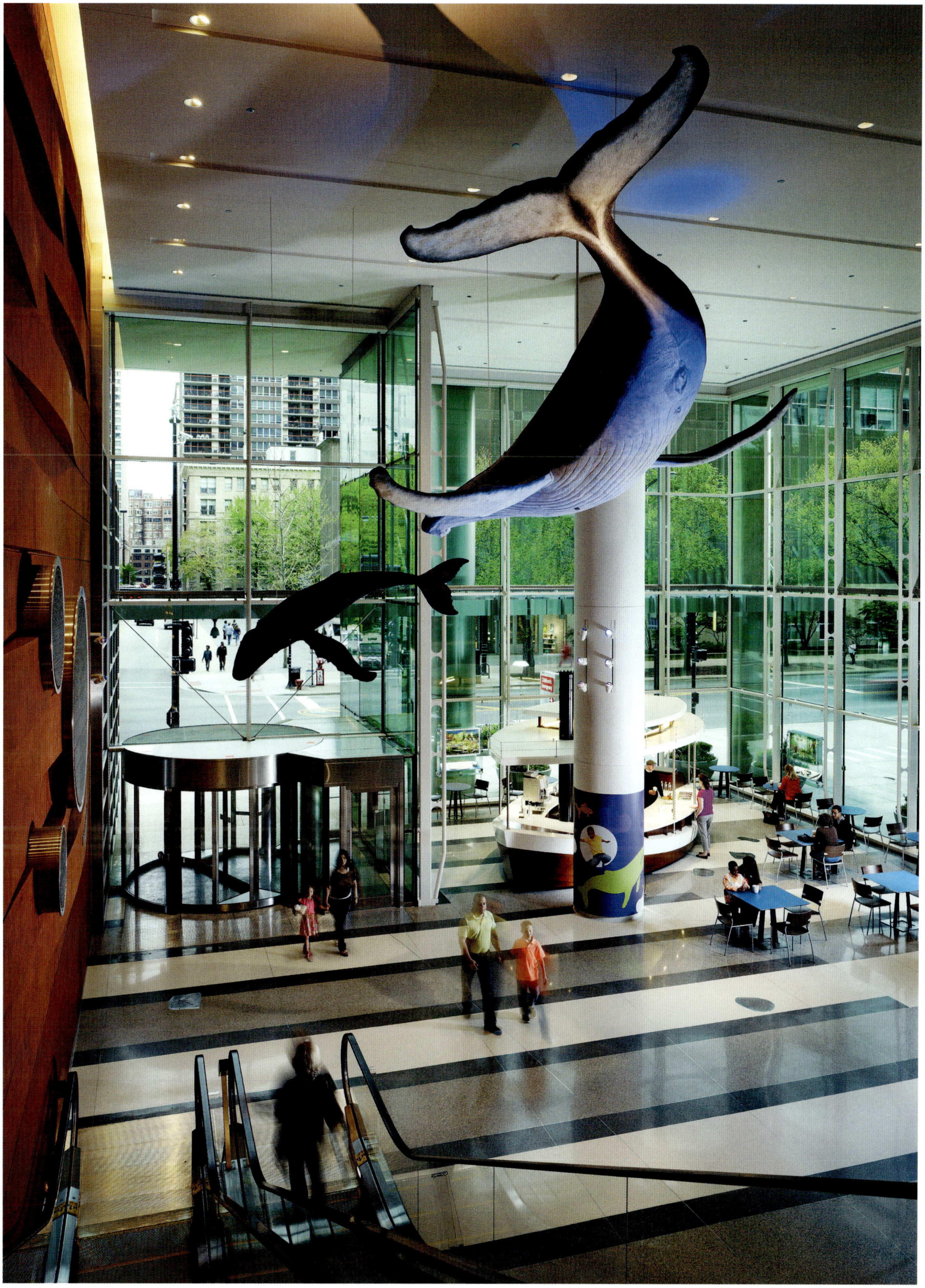

Previous pages: Ann & Robert H. Lurie Children's Hospital of Chicago, IL
Photo: Hedrich Blessing Photography, Nick Merrick

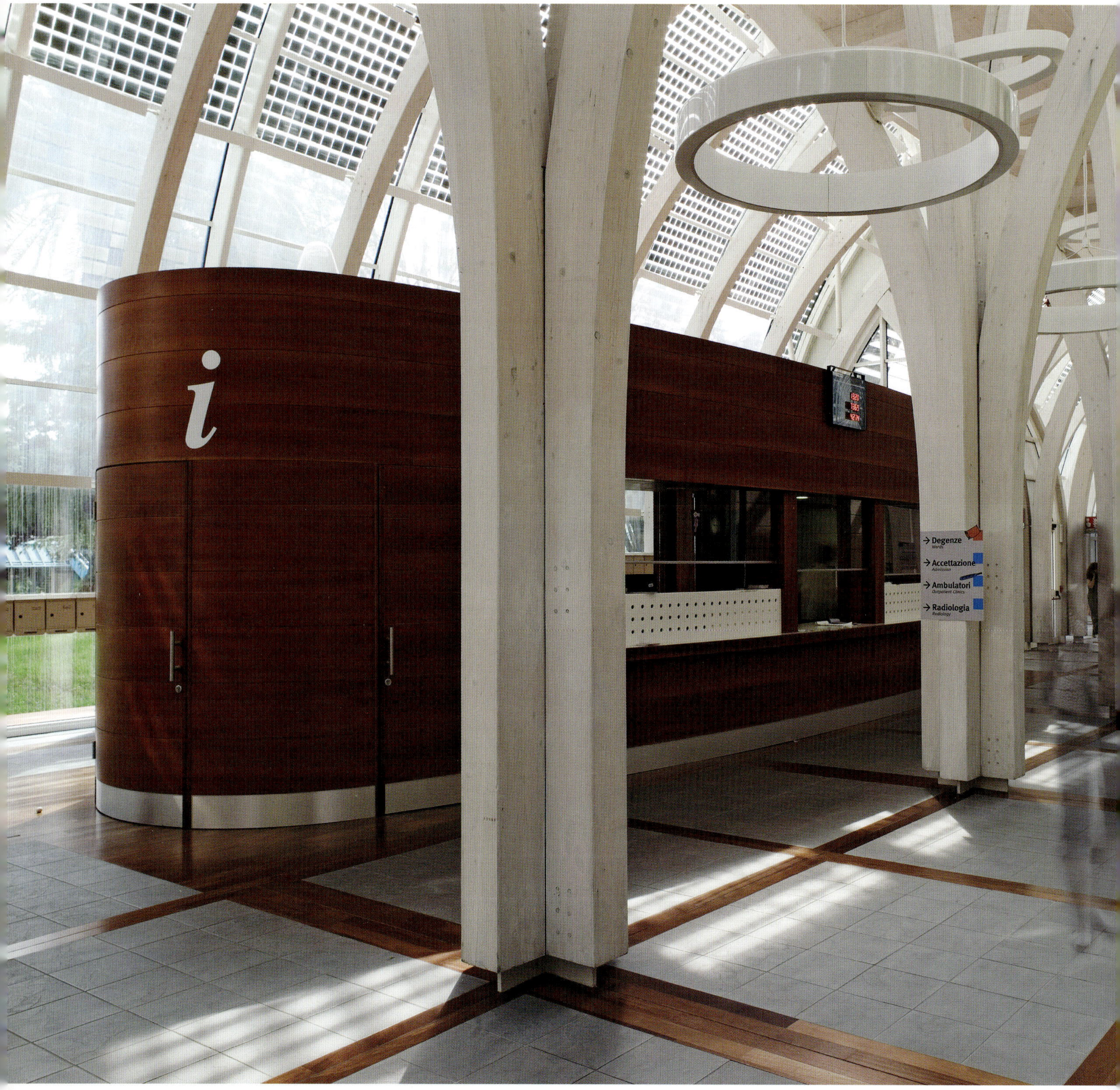

▲ Meyer Children's Hospital, Florence, Italy
Photo: Stantec © Alessandro Ciampo and Pietro Savorelli

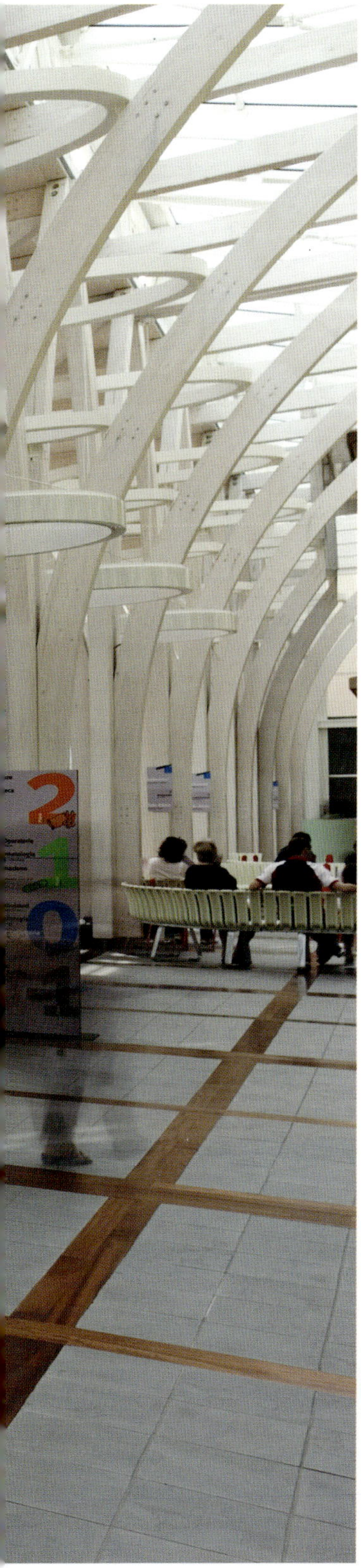

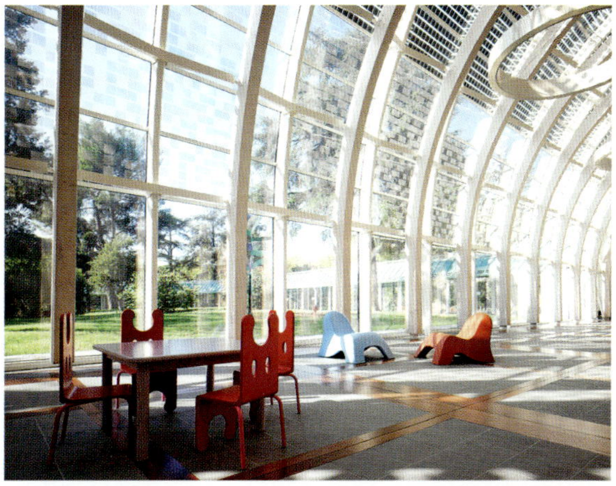

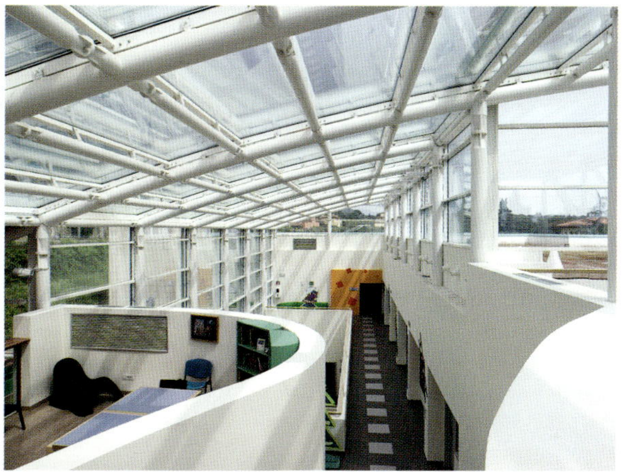

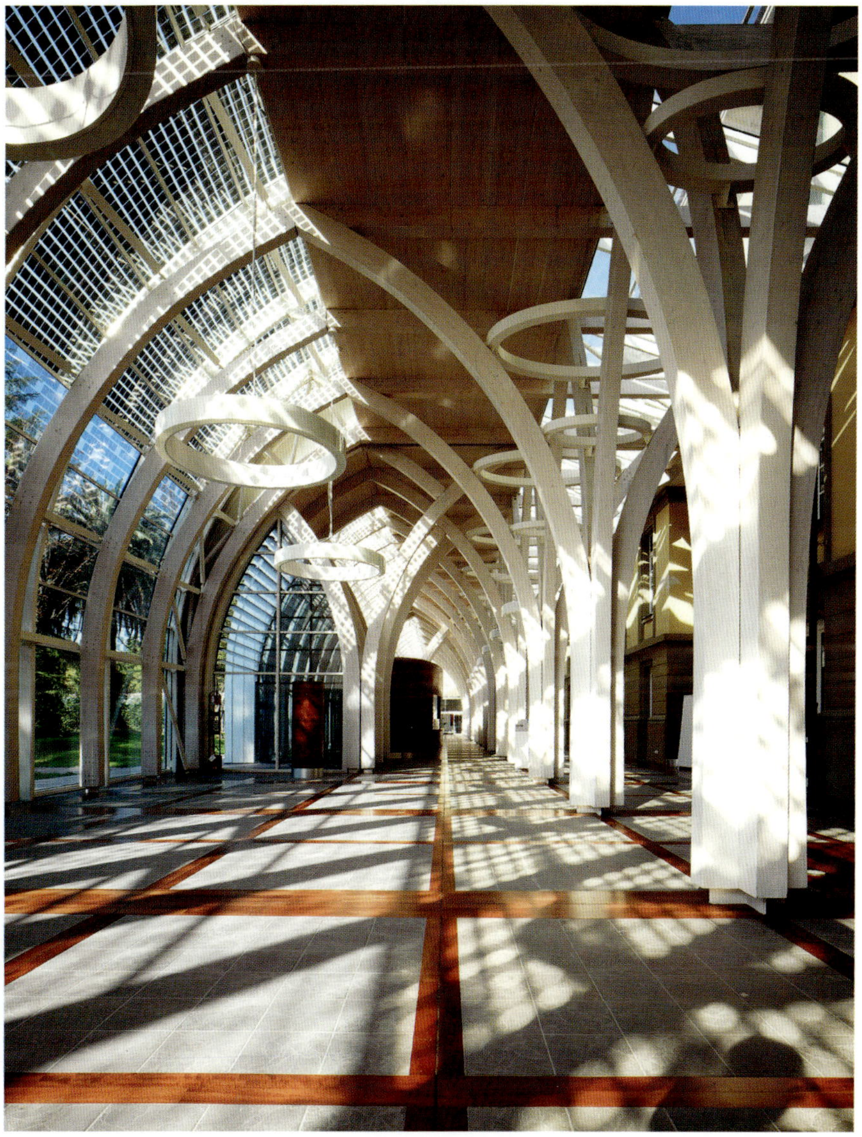

▲ Meyer Children's Hospital, Florence, Italy
Photos: Stantec © Alessandro Ciampo and Pietro Savorelli

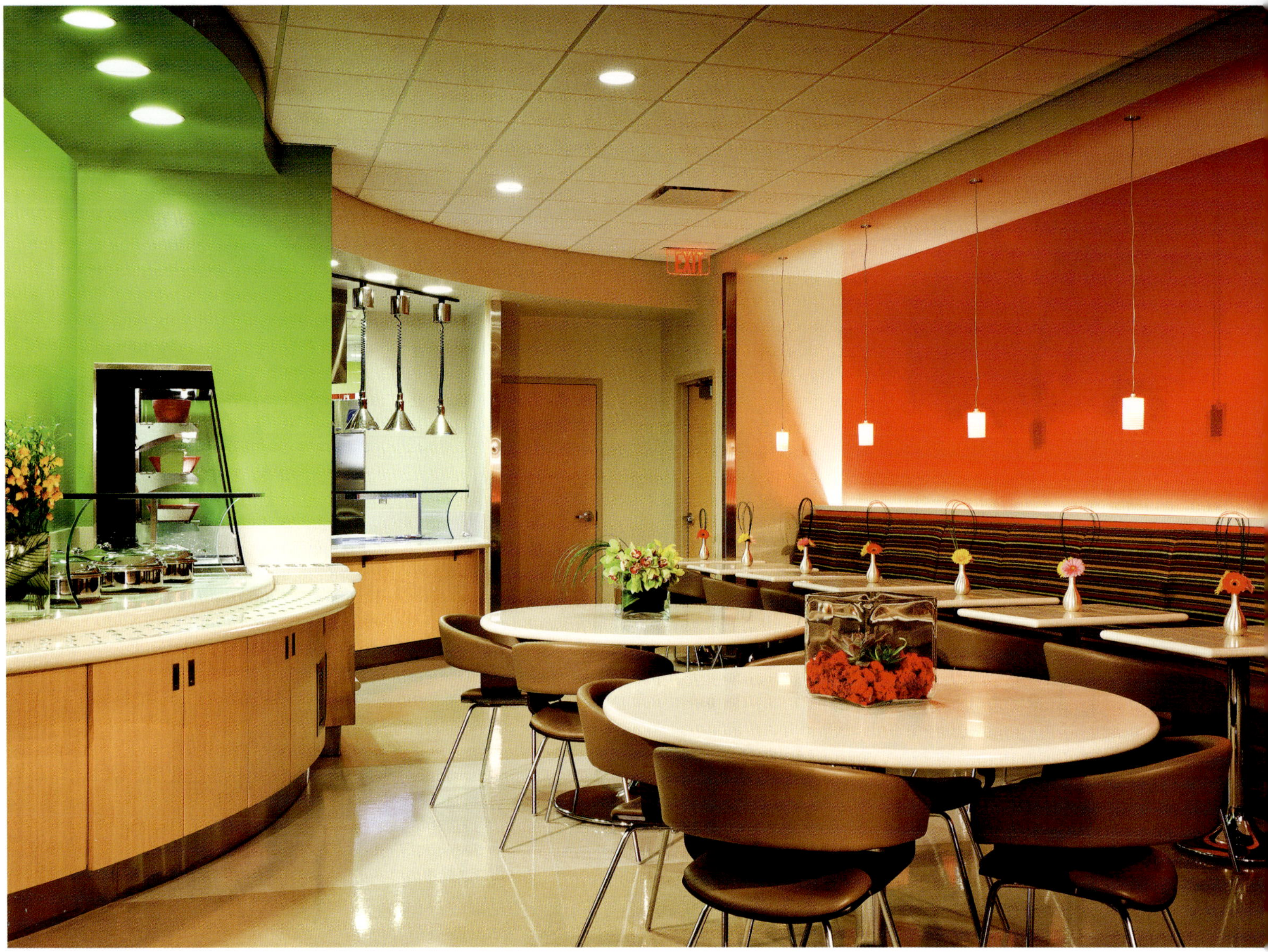

▲ Phoenix Children's Hospital, AZ
Photo: Blake Marvin, HKS

▼ Texas Children's Hospital West Campus, Houston, TX
Photo: Allen Kramer

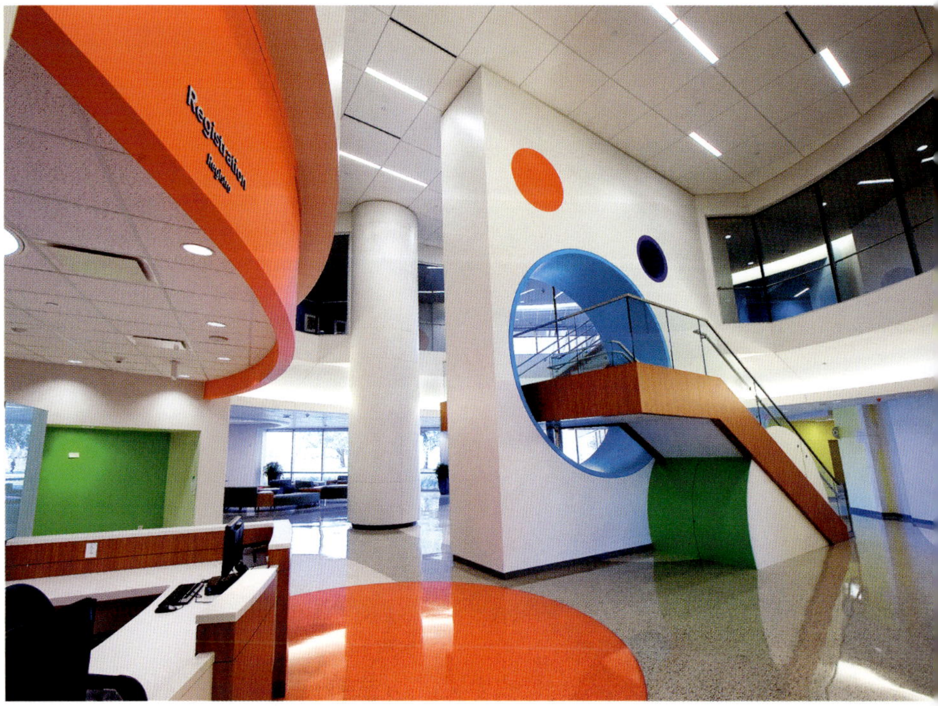

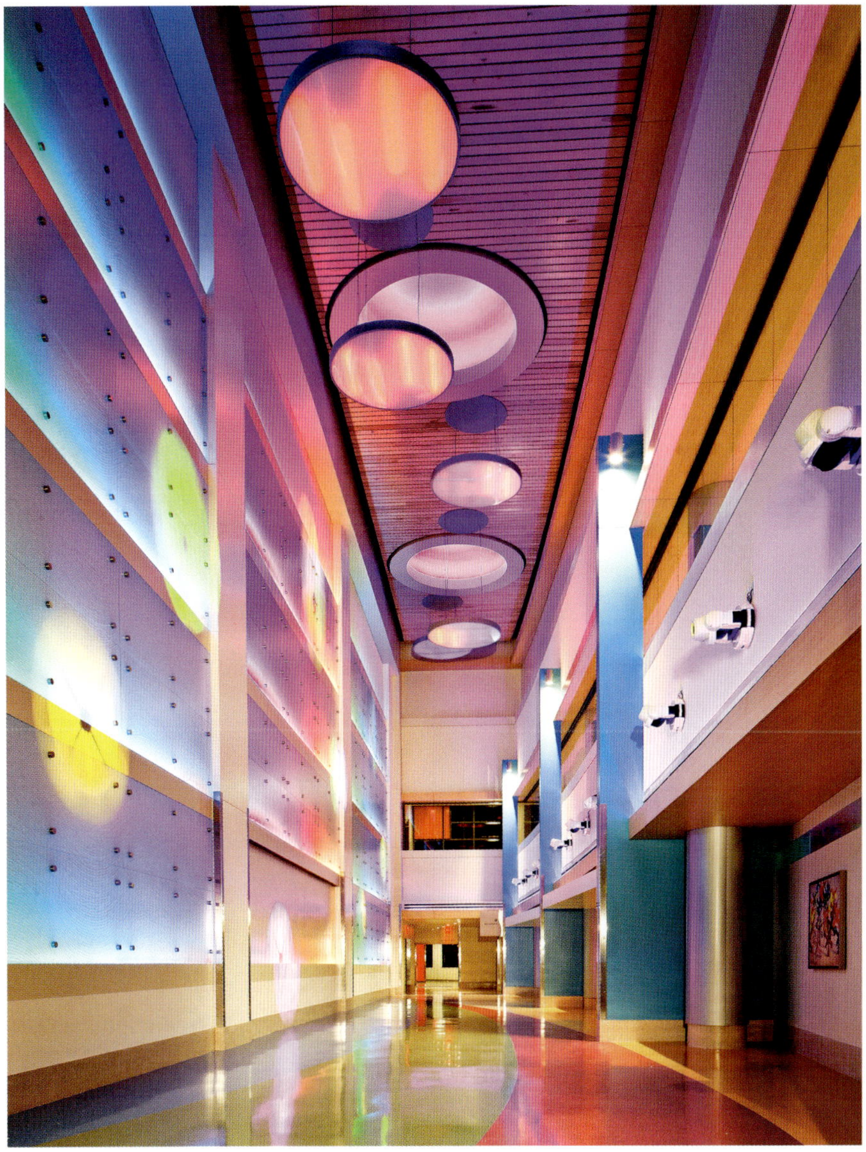

▲ Phoenix Children's Hospital, AZ
Photo: Blake Marvin, HKS

▼ Children's Hospital, Pittsburgh, PA
Photos: Alexander Denmarsh

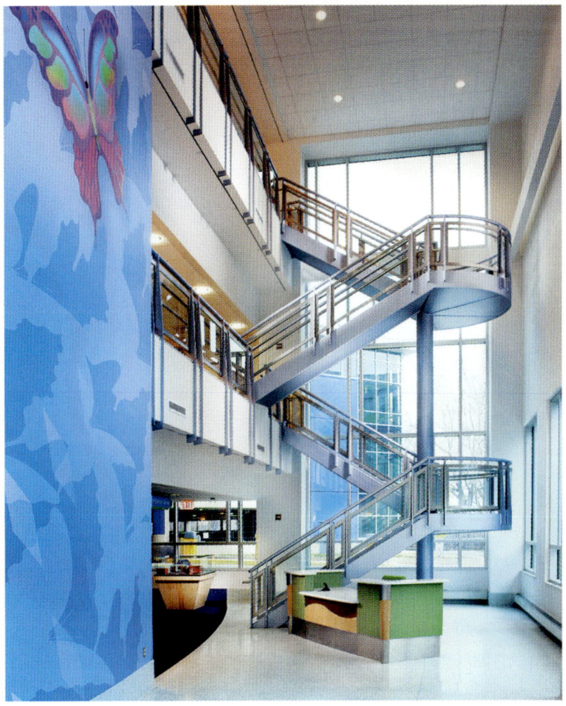

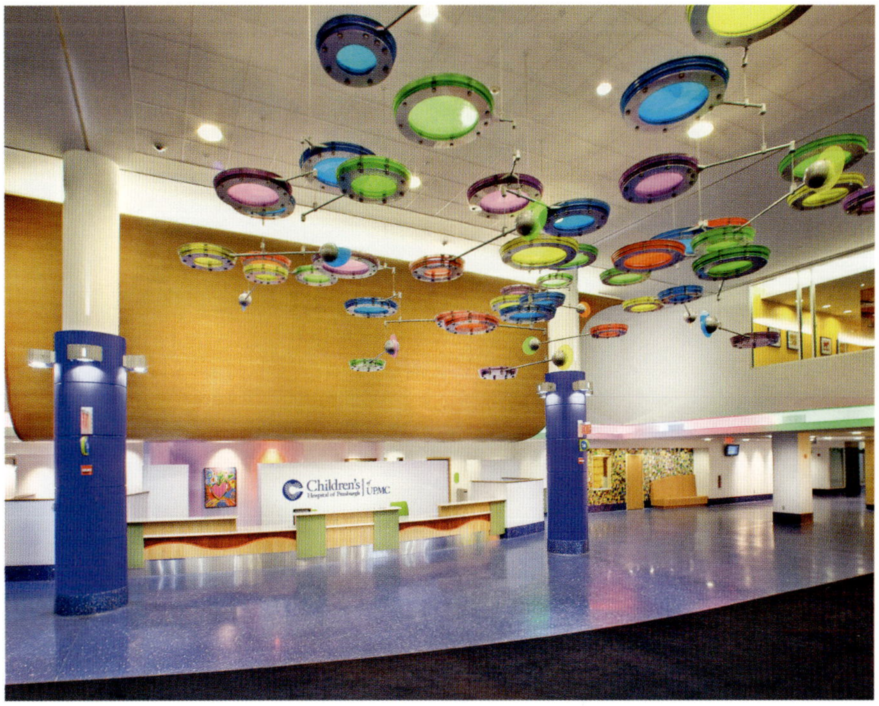

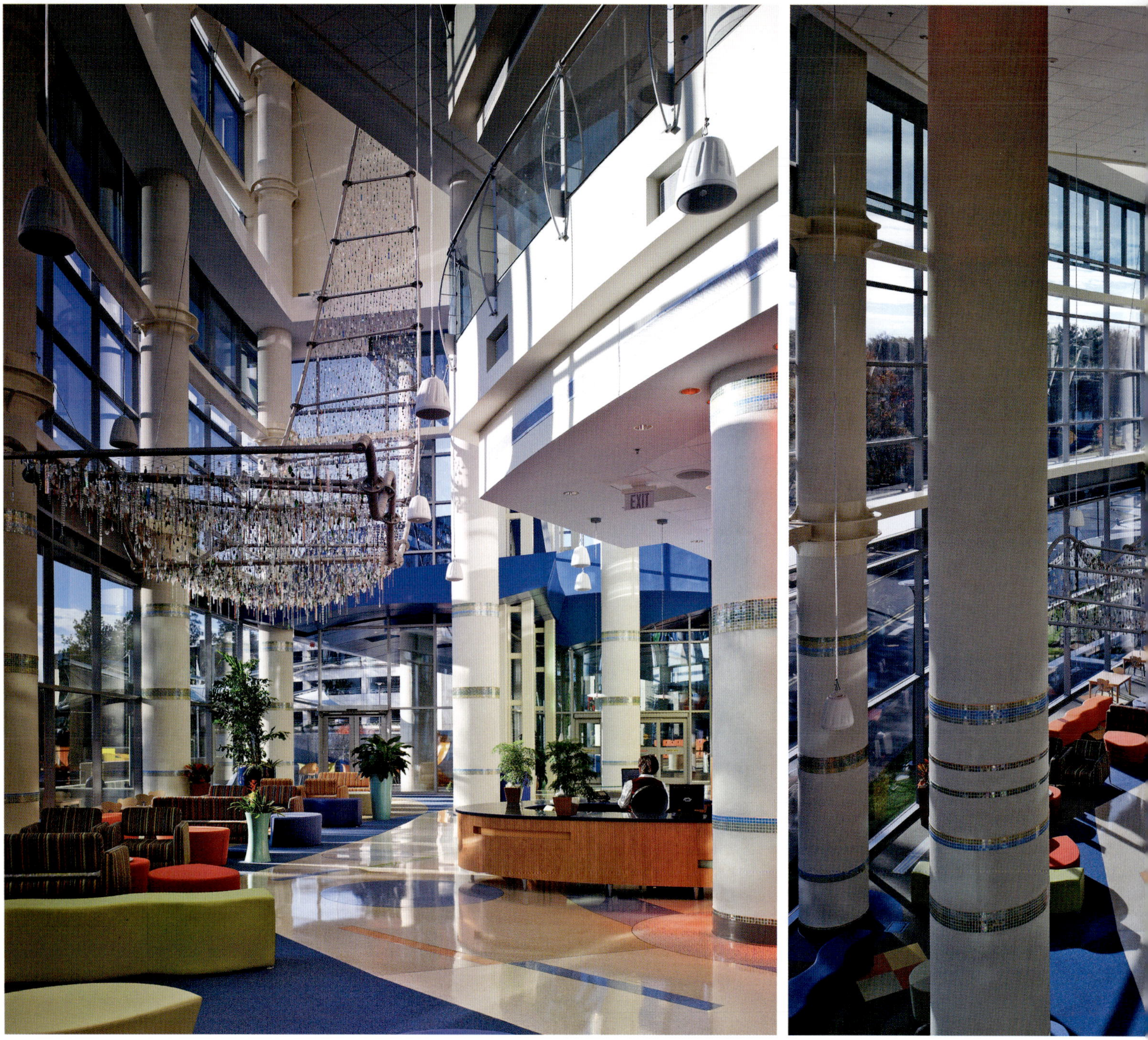

▲ Levine Children's Hospital, Charlotte, NC
Photos: Brad Feinknopf

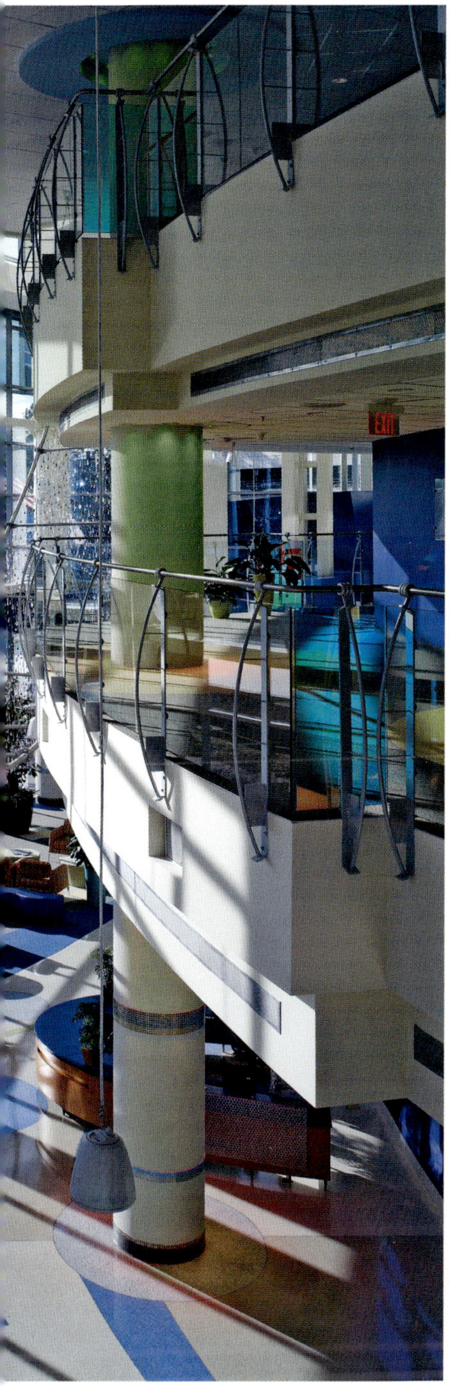

▼ Children's Hospital, Pittsburgh, PA
Photo: Jason Yurkovich

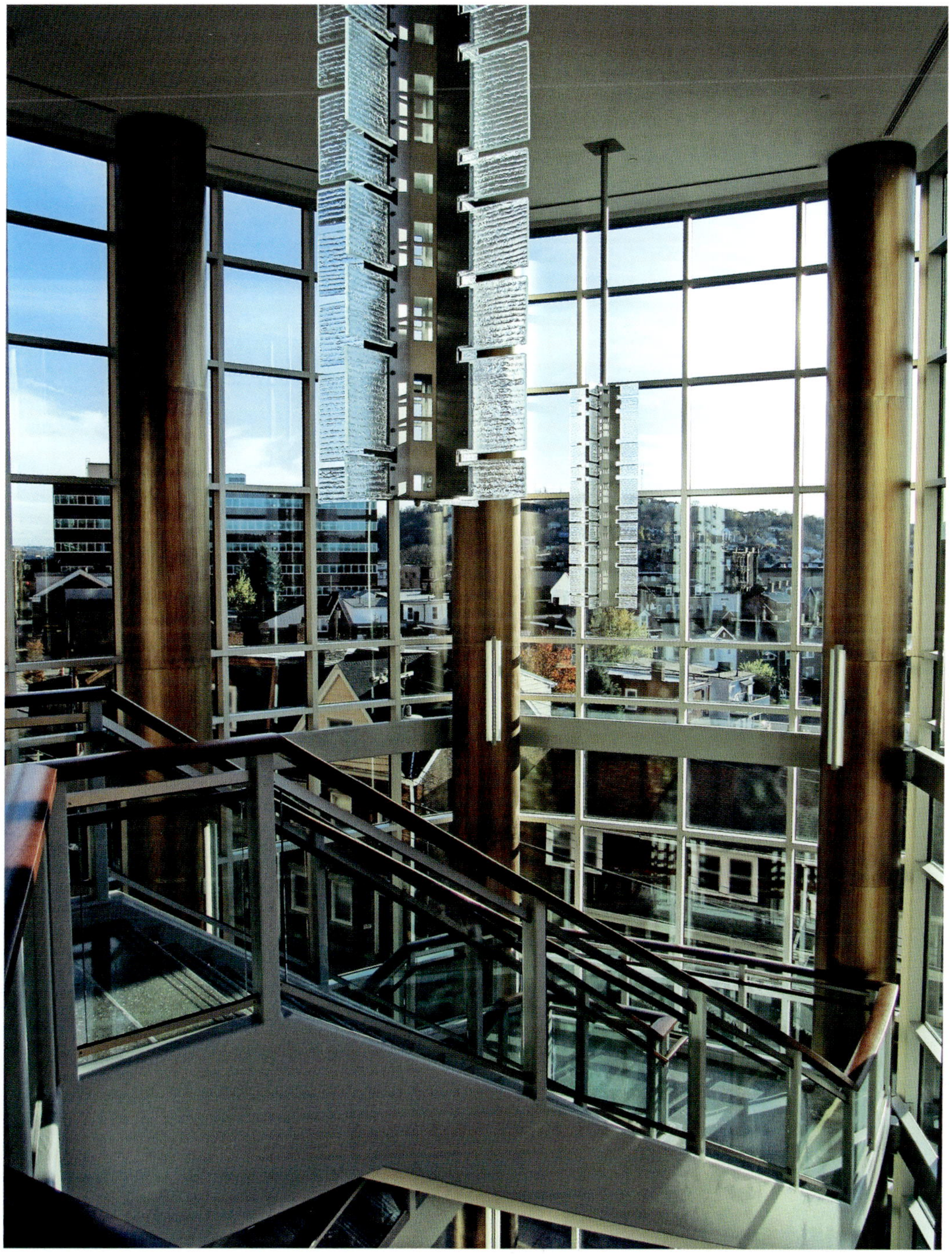

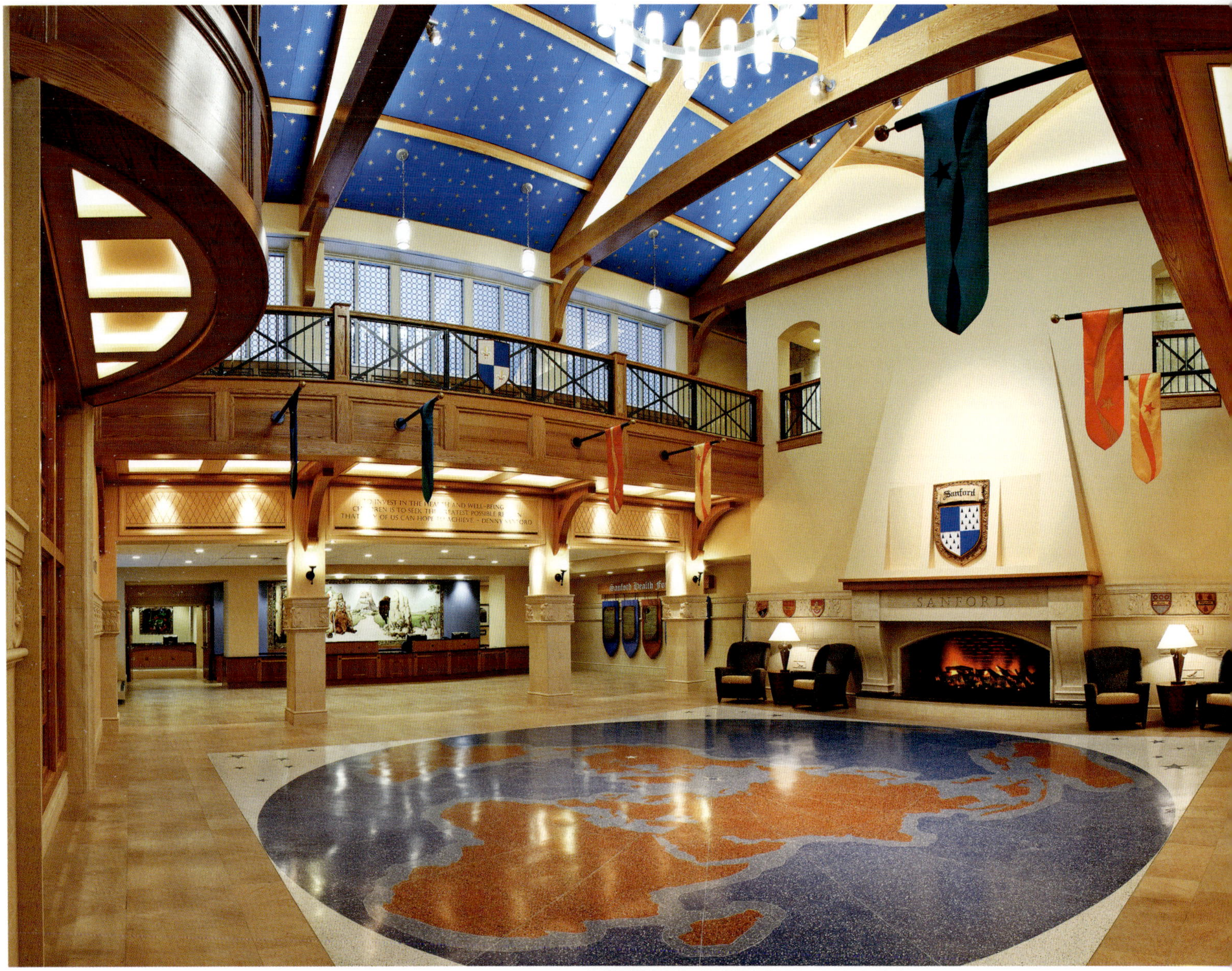

Sanford Children's Hospital, Sioux Falls, MD ▲
▶

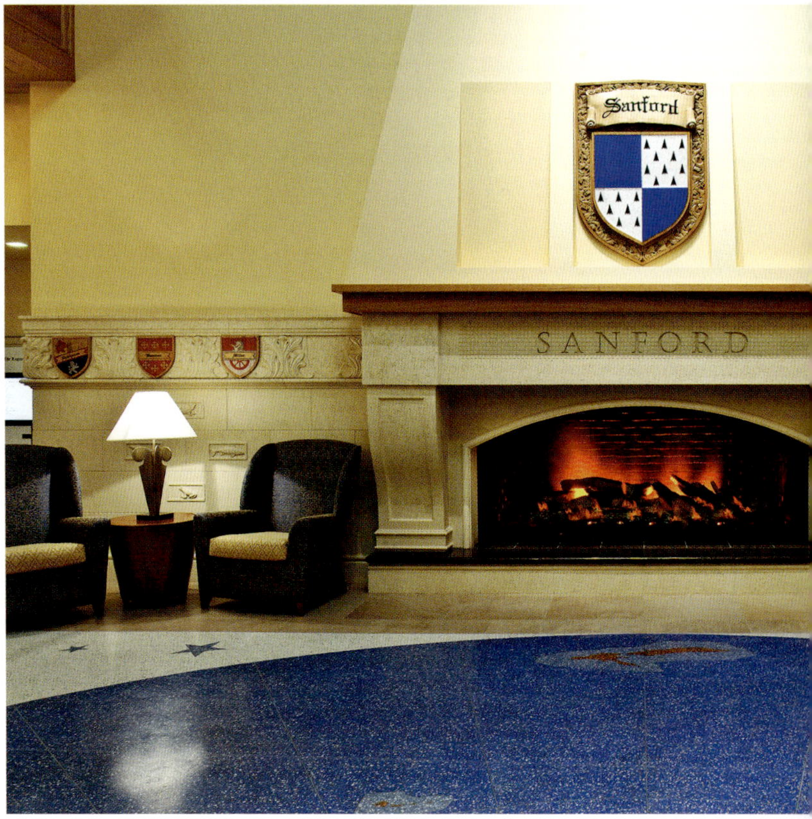

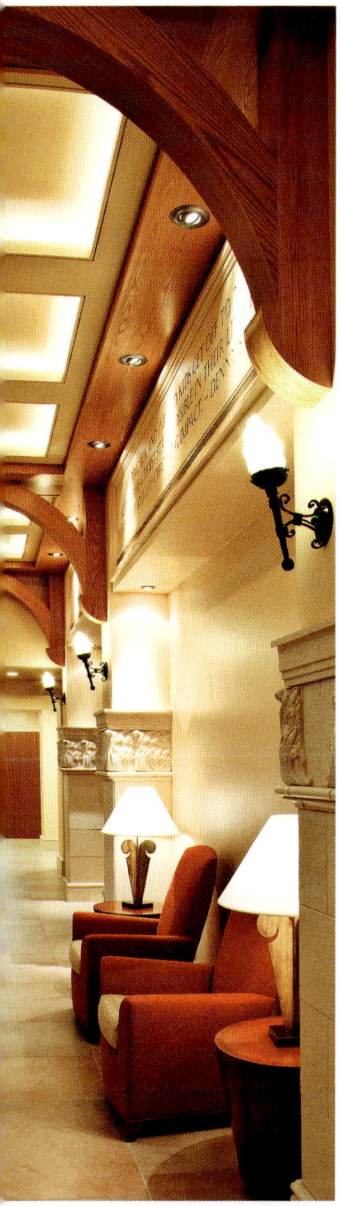

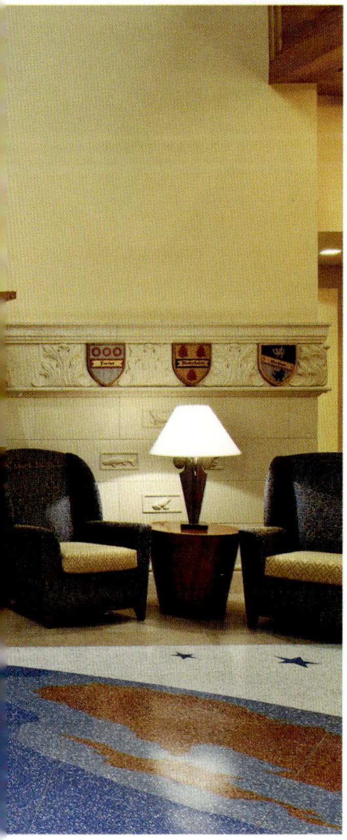

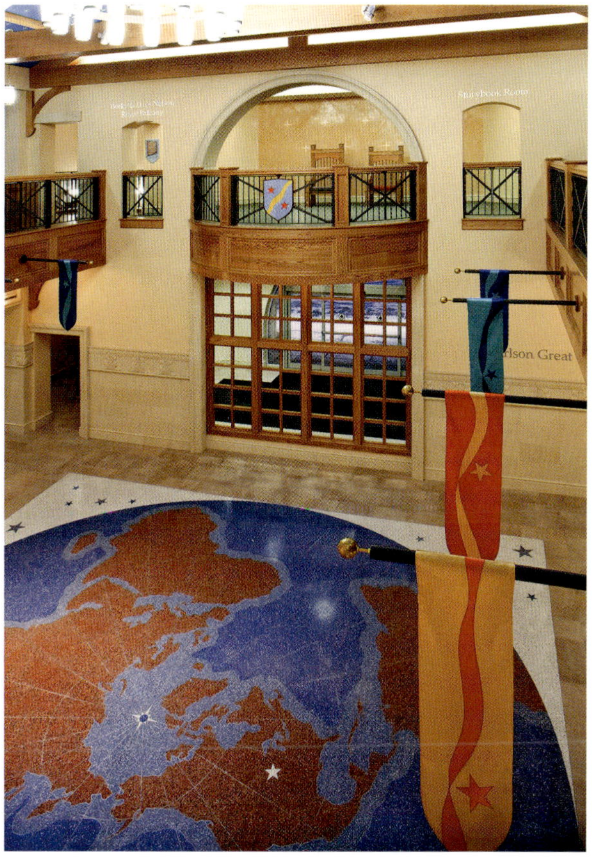

▲ Sanford Children's Hospital, Sioux Falls, MD

▼ Children's Hospital, Pittsburgh, PA
Photo: Alexander Denmarsh

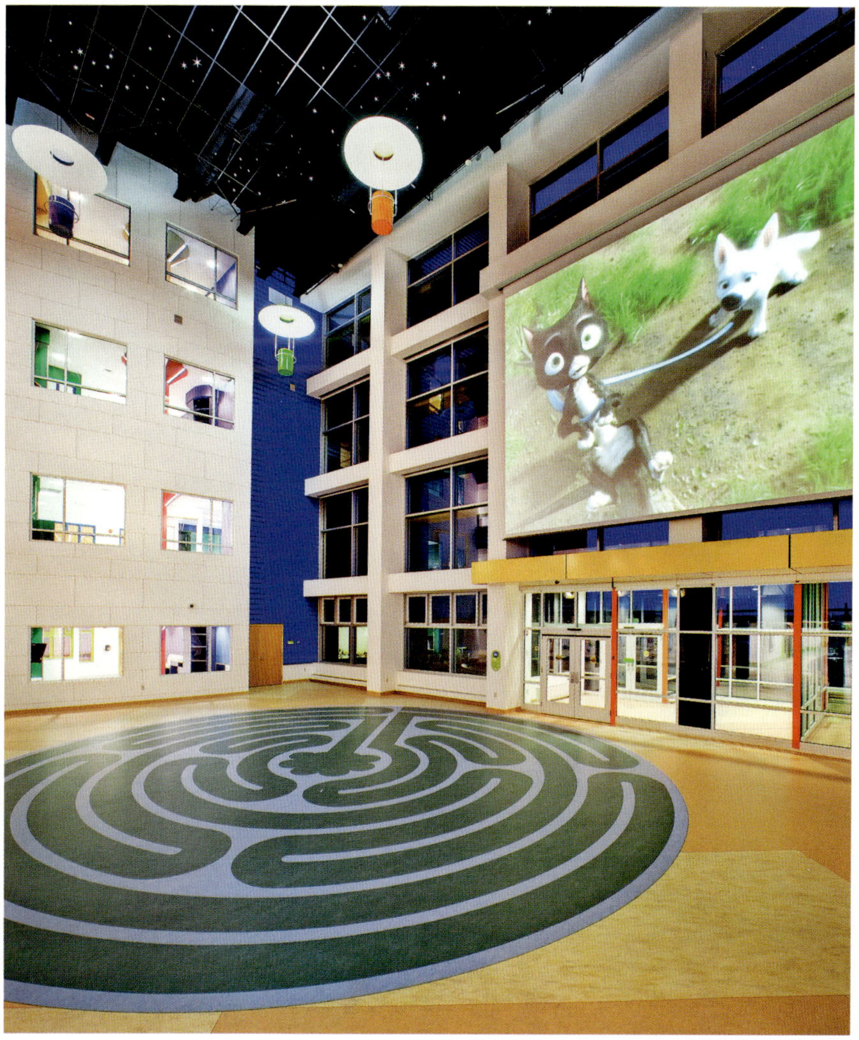

Dayton Children's, OH ▶
Photo: Ken Shory

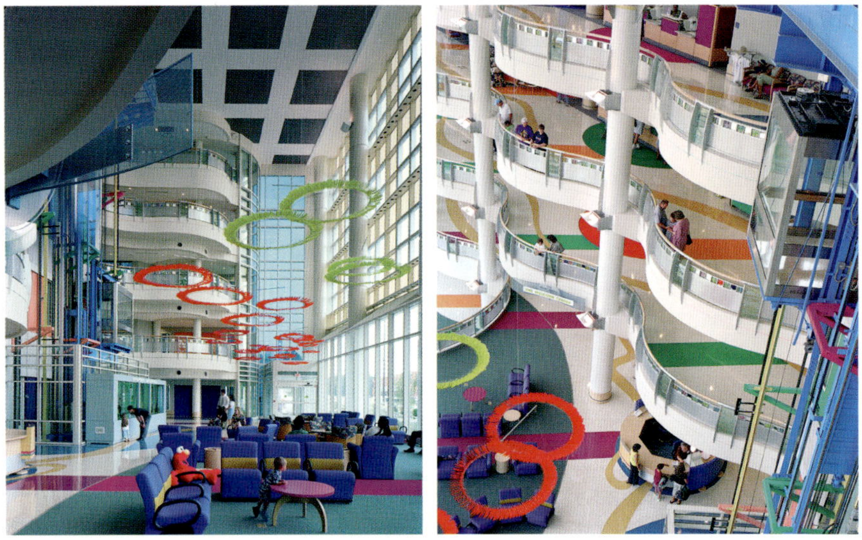

▲ Duke University Children's Hospital, Durham, NC
Photo: Jeff Goldberg/Esto Photography

▼ Central Manchester Royal Children's Hospital, Manchester, United Kingdom
Photo: Timothy Soar

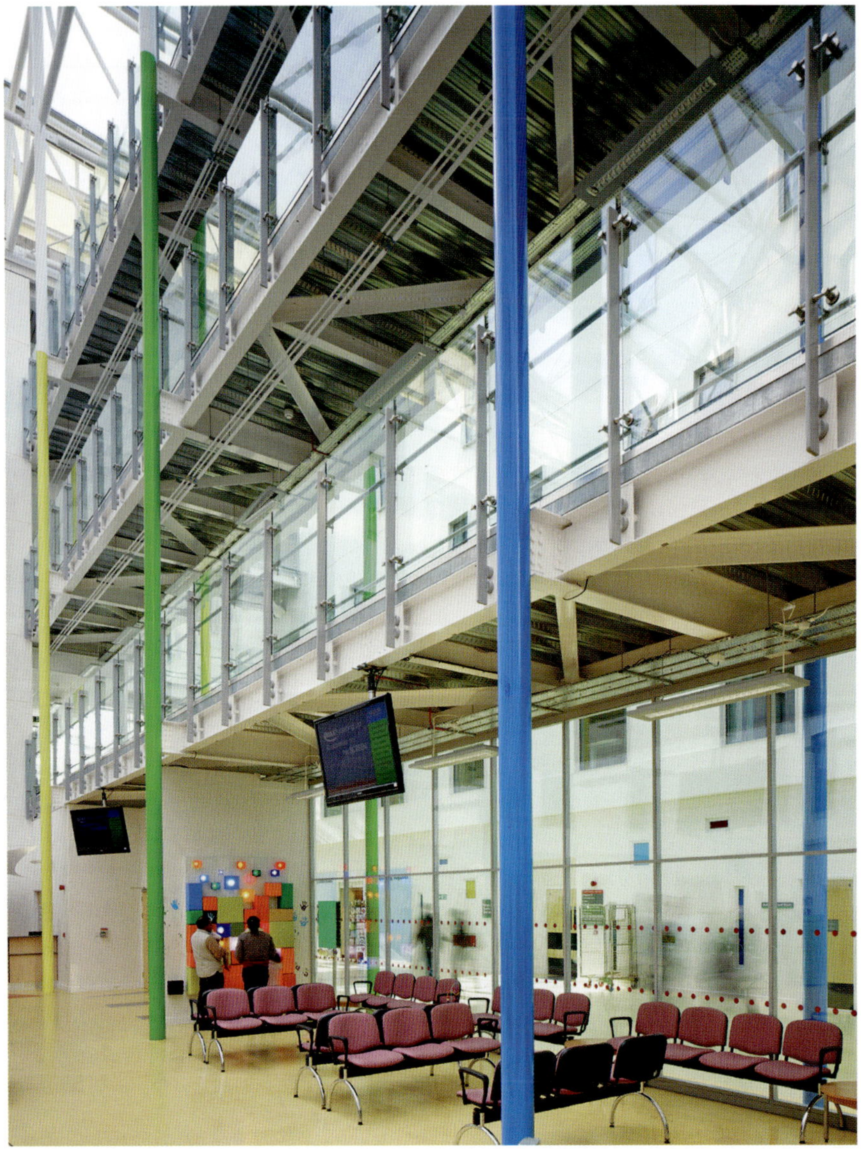

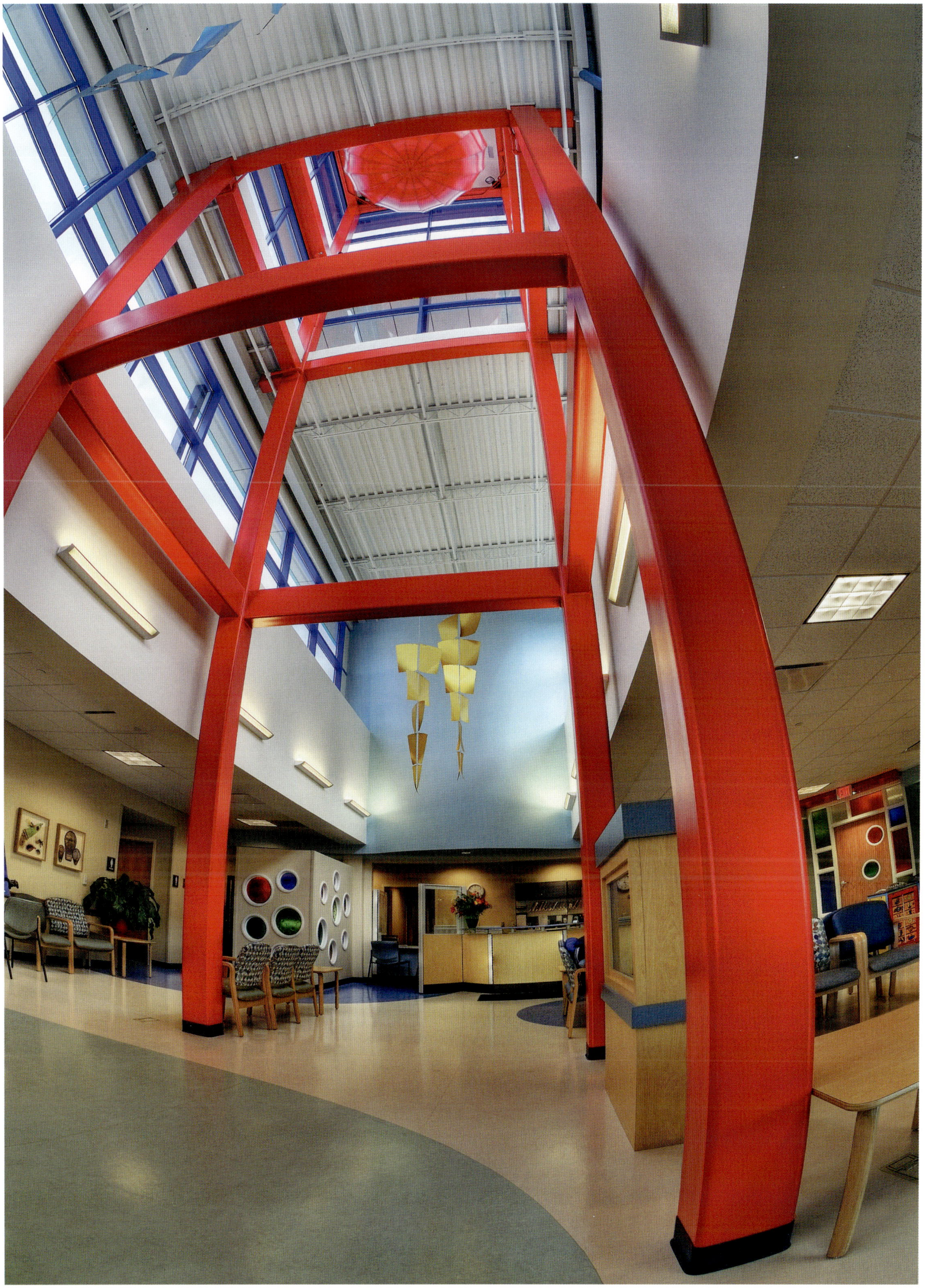

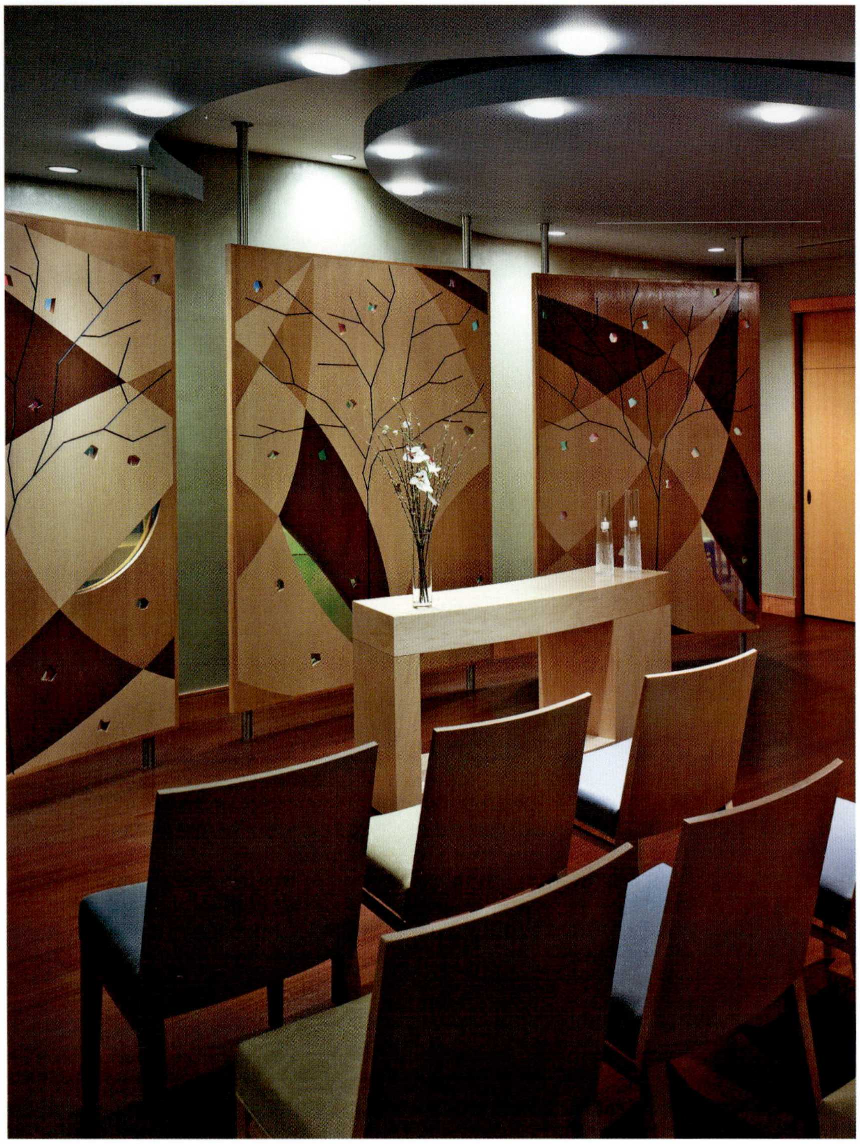

▲ Levine Children's Hospital, Charlotte, NC
Photo: Brad Feinknopf

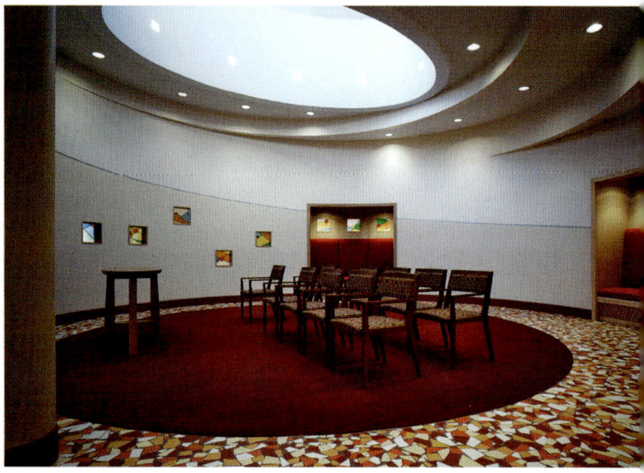

▲ Helen DeVos Children's Hospital, Grand Rapids, MI
Photo: Hedrich Blessing Photography

▼ Children's Hospital Colorado, Denver, CO
Photo: Eckert & Eckert

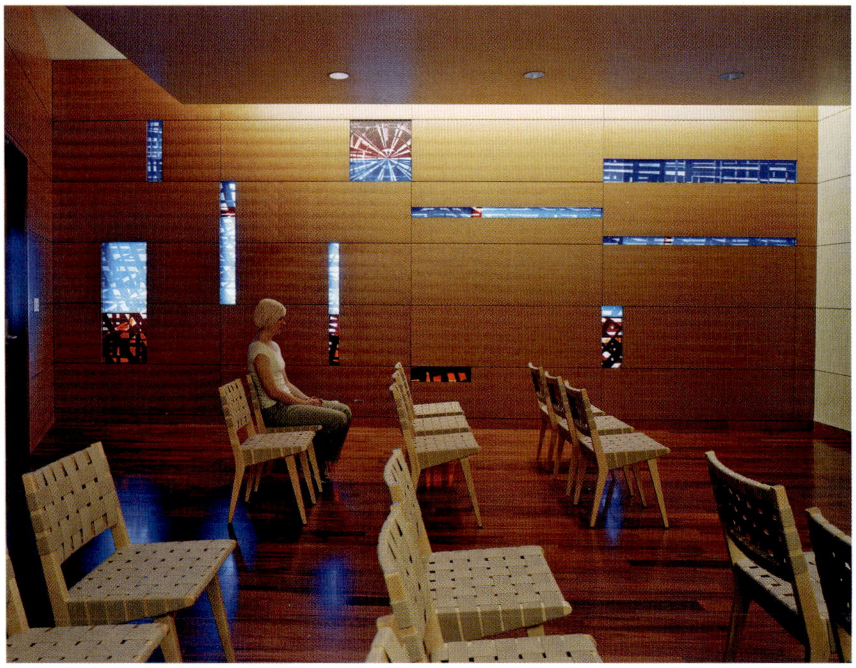

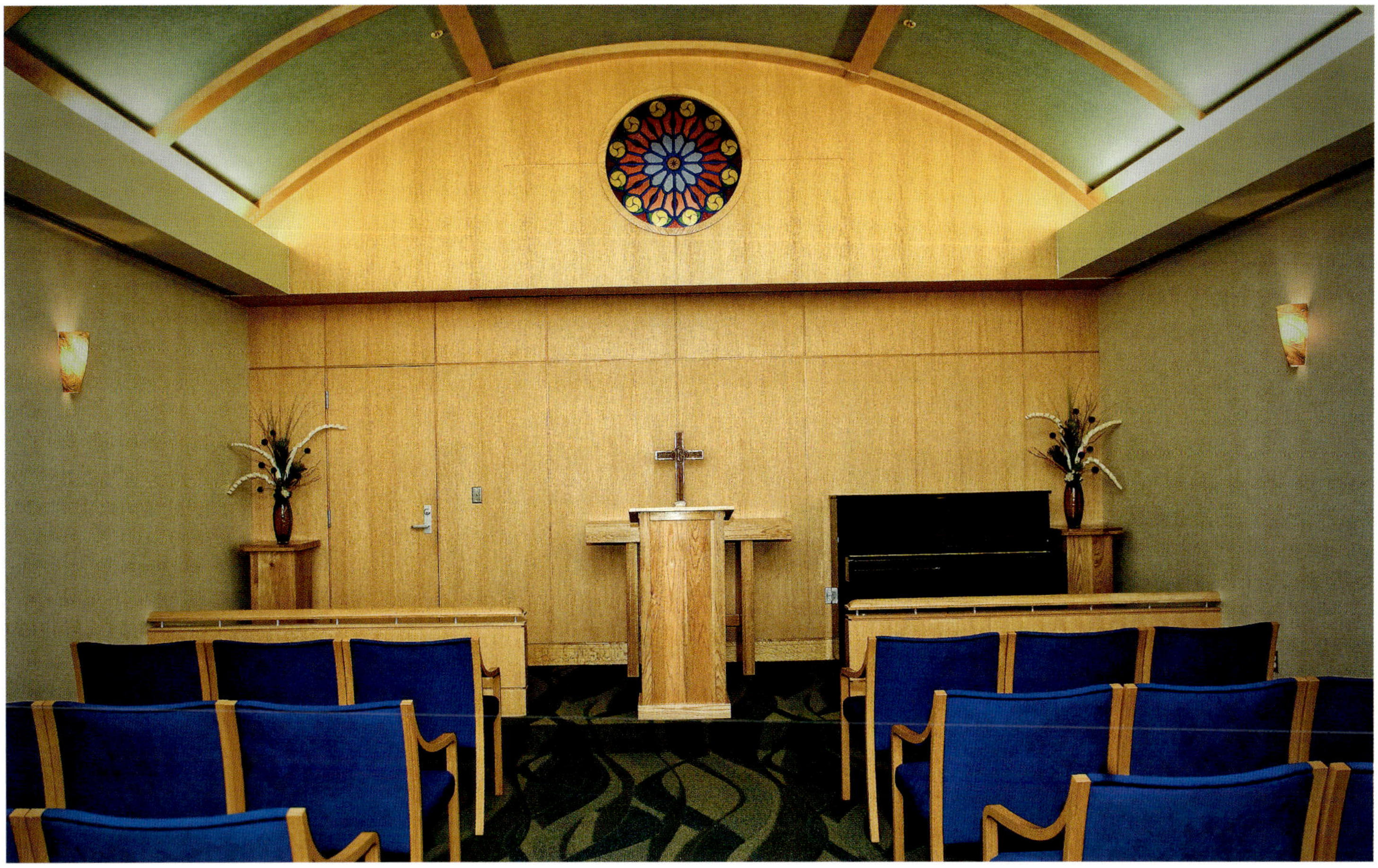

▲ Palmetto Health Children's Hospital, Columbia, SC

▼ Cardon Children's, Mesa, AZ
Photo: Photo courtesy of HDR Architecture, Inc. © 2010 Mark Boisclair Photography Inc.

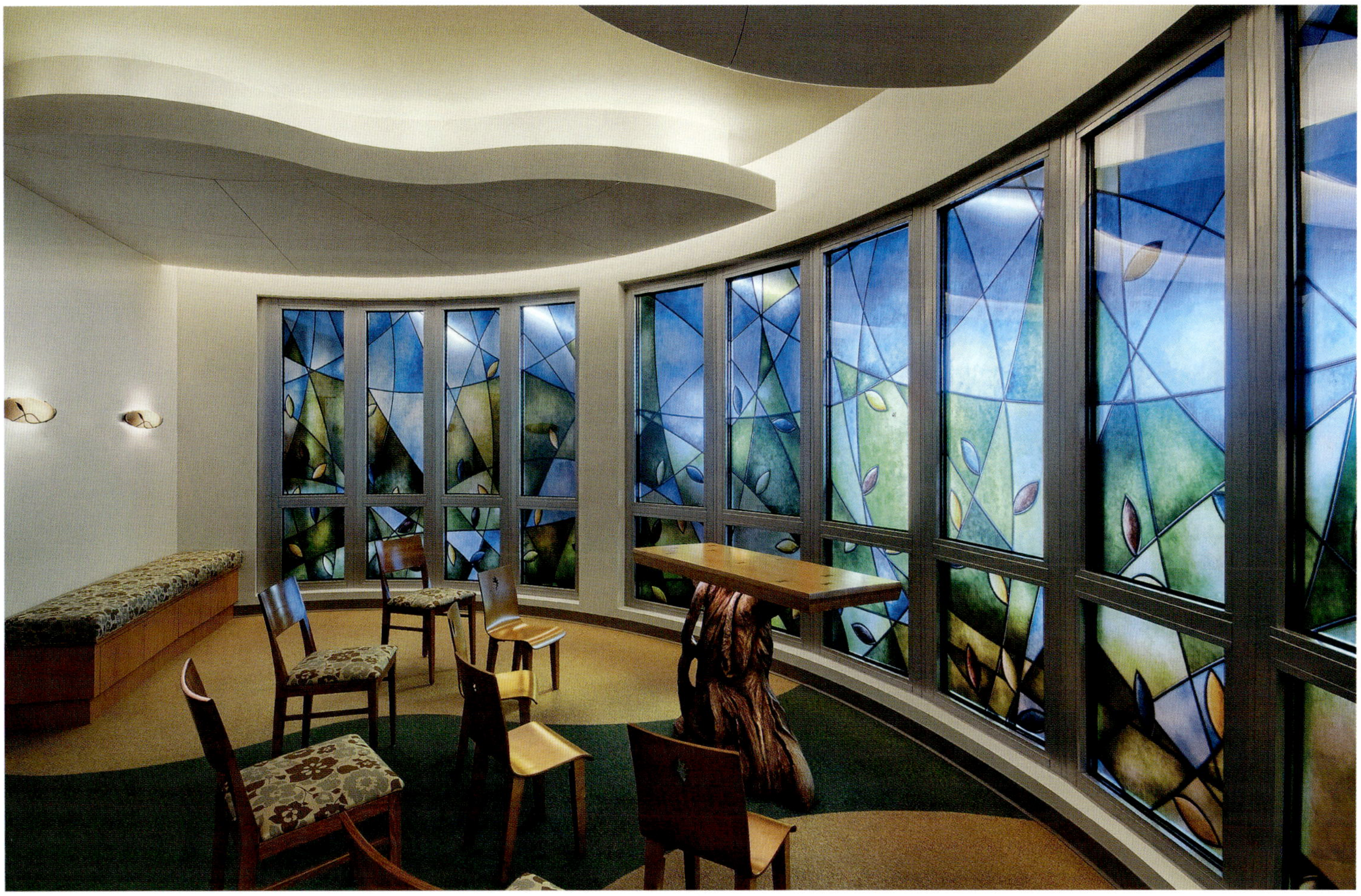

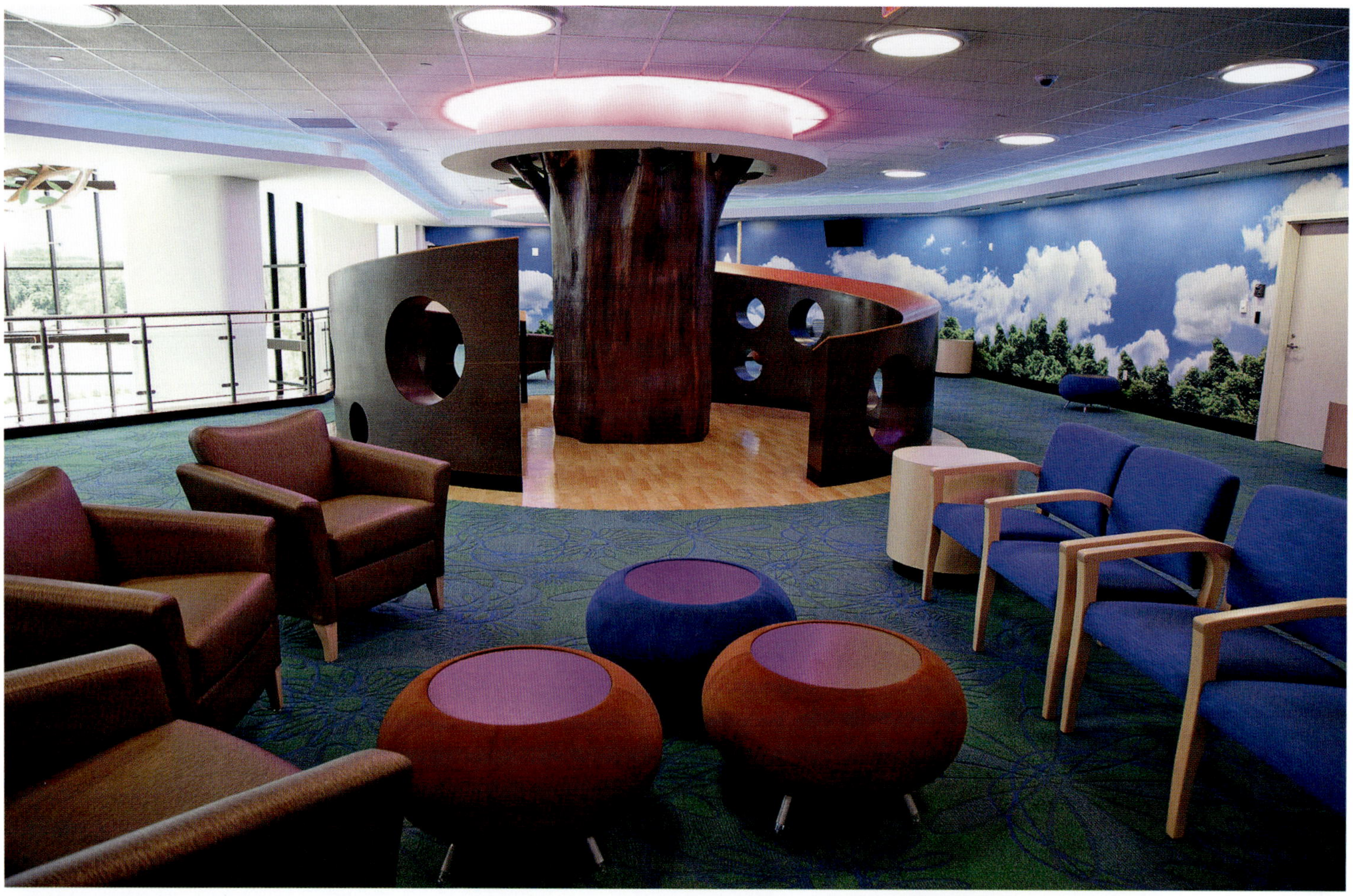

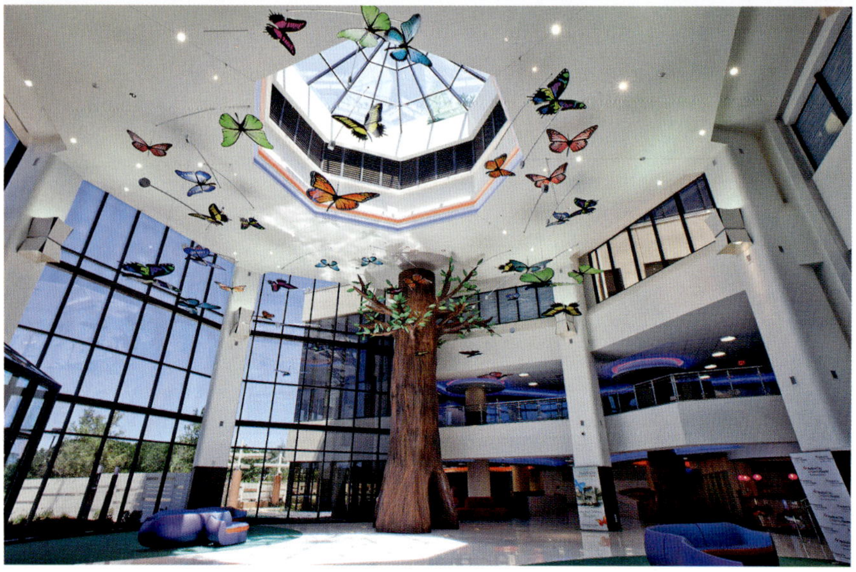

Medical City Children's Hospital, Dallas, TX ▲ ▶
Photos: Terry Cockerham

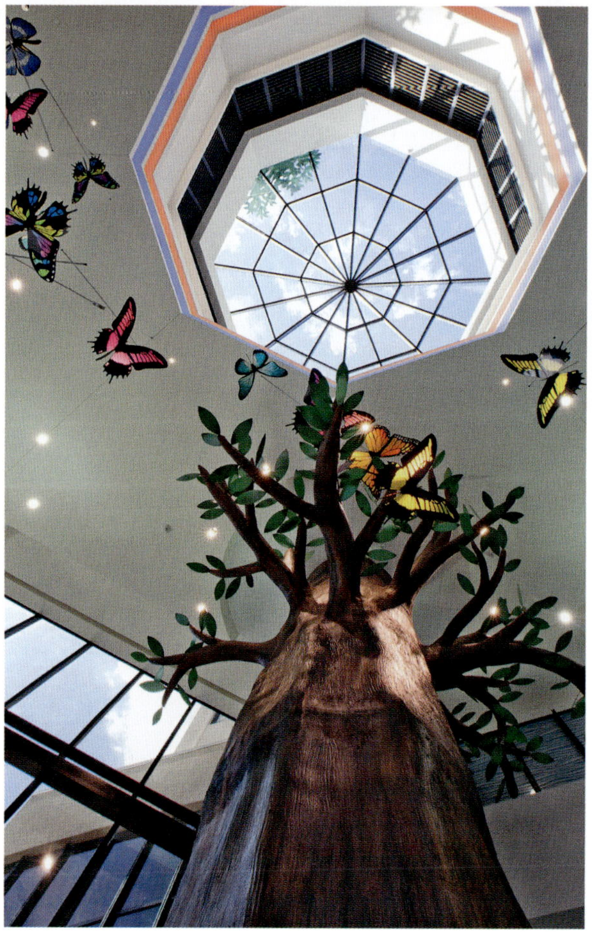

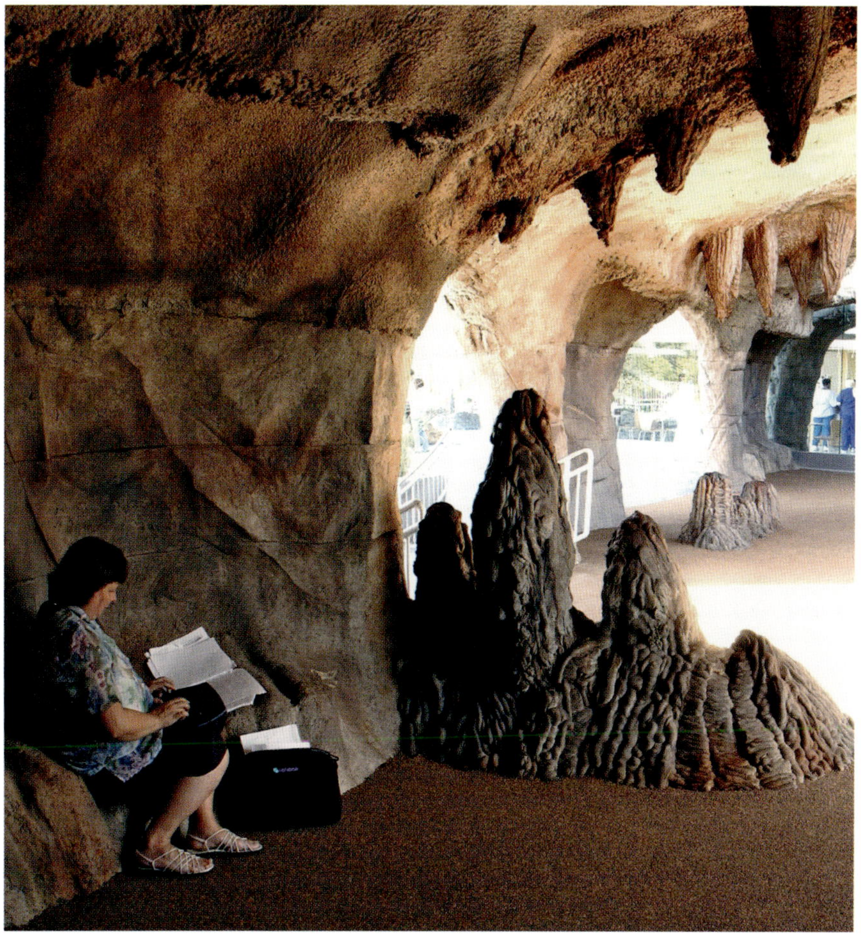

▲ Arkansas Children's Hospital, Little Rock, AR
Photo: Kelley Cooper

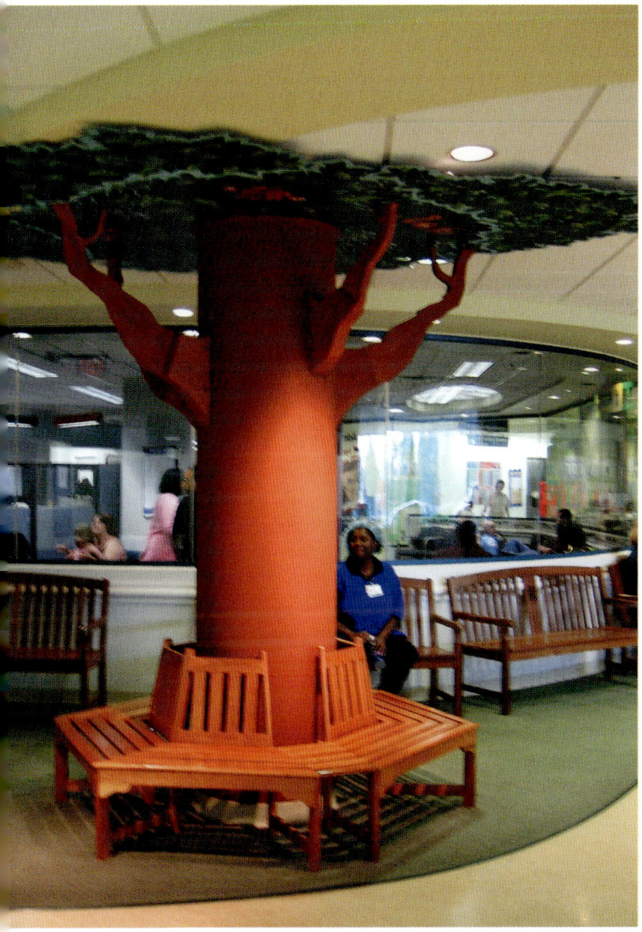

▲ Children's Hospital of Michigan, Detroit, MI

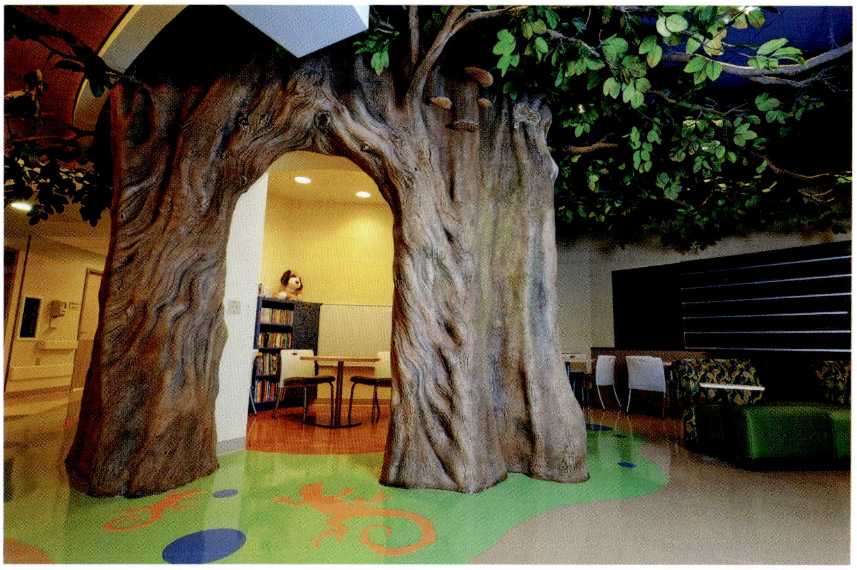

▲ Tucson Medical Center, AZ
Photo: Erik Hinote

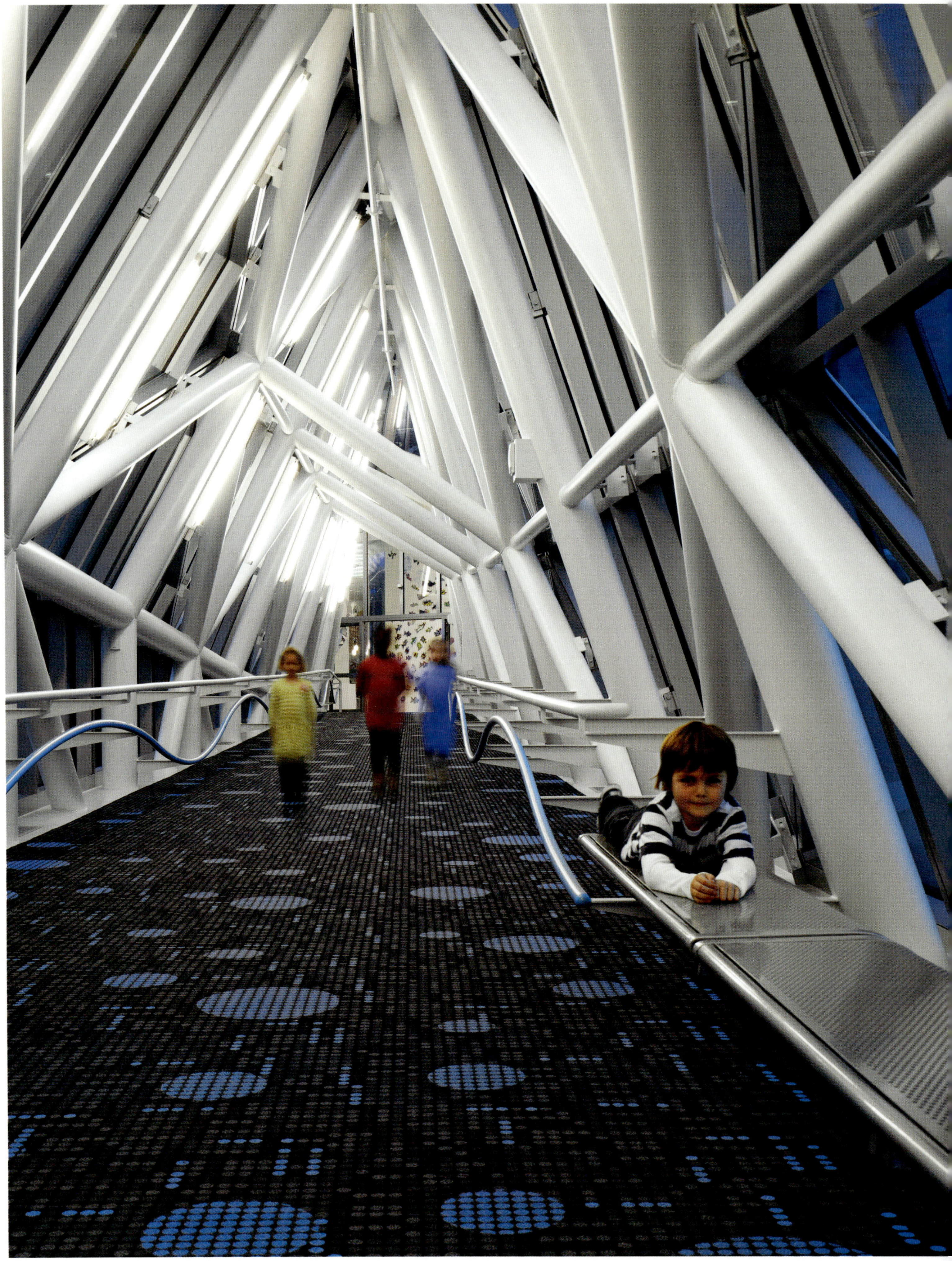

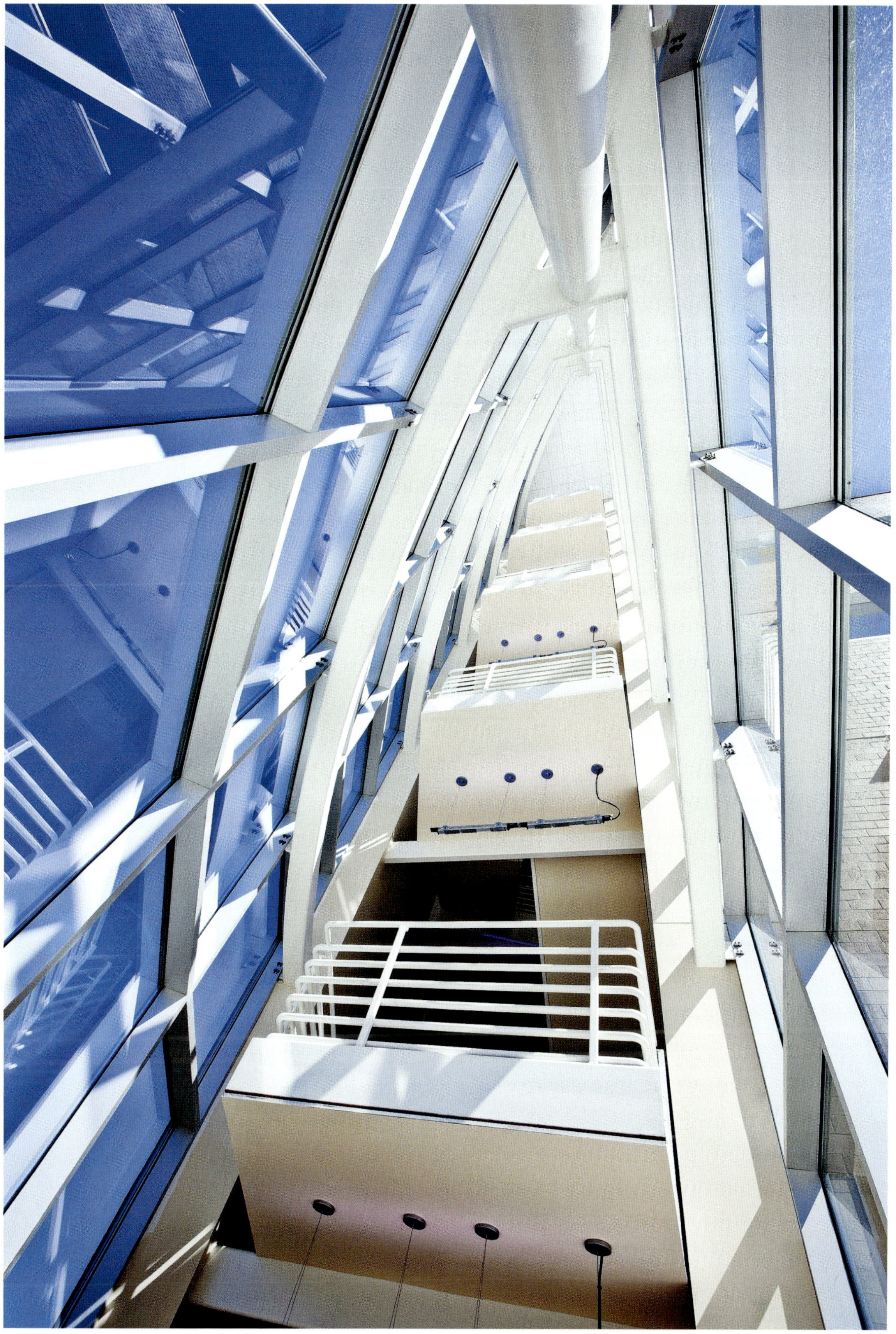

▲ Children's Hospital Omaha, NE
Photo: Matthew Placzek – "Imagine" © 2010 Thomas Grady photography

◀ Helen DeVos Children's Hospital, Grand Rapids, MI
Photo: Hedrich Blessing Photography

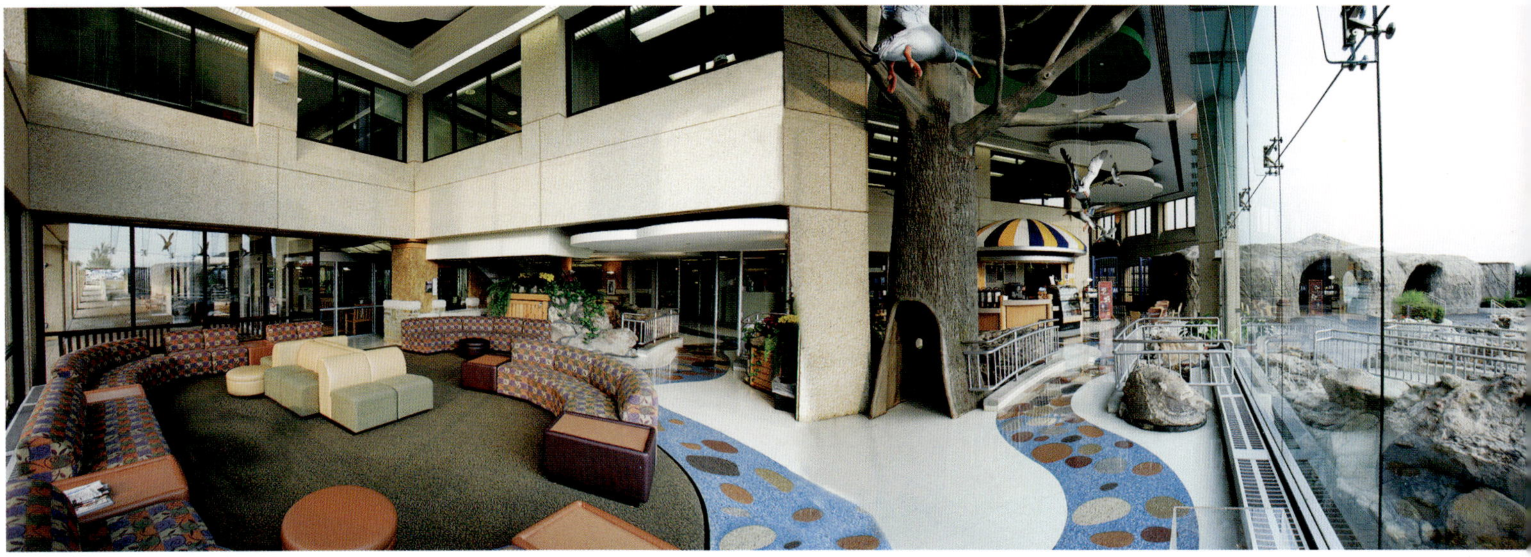

▲ Arkansas Children's Hospital, Little Rock, AR
Photo: Kelley Cooper

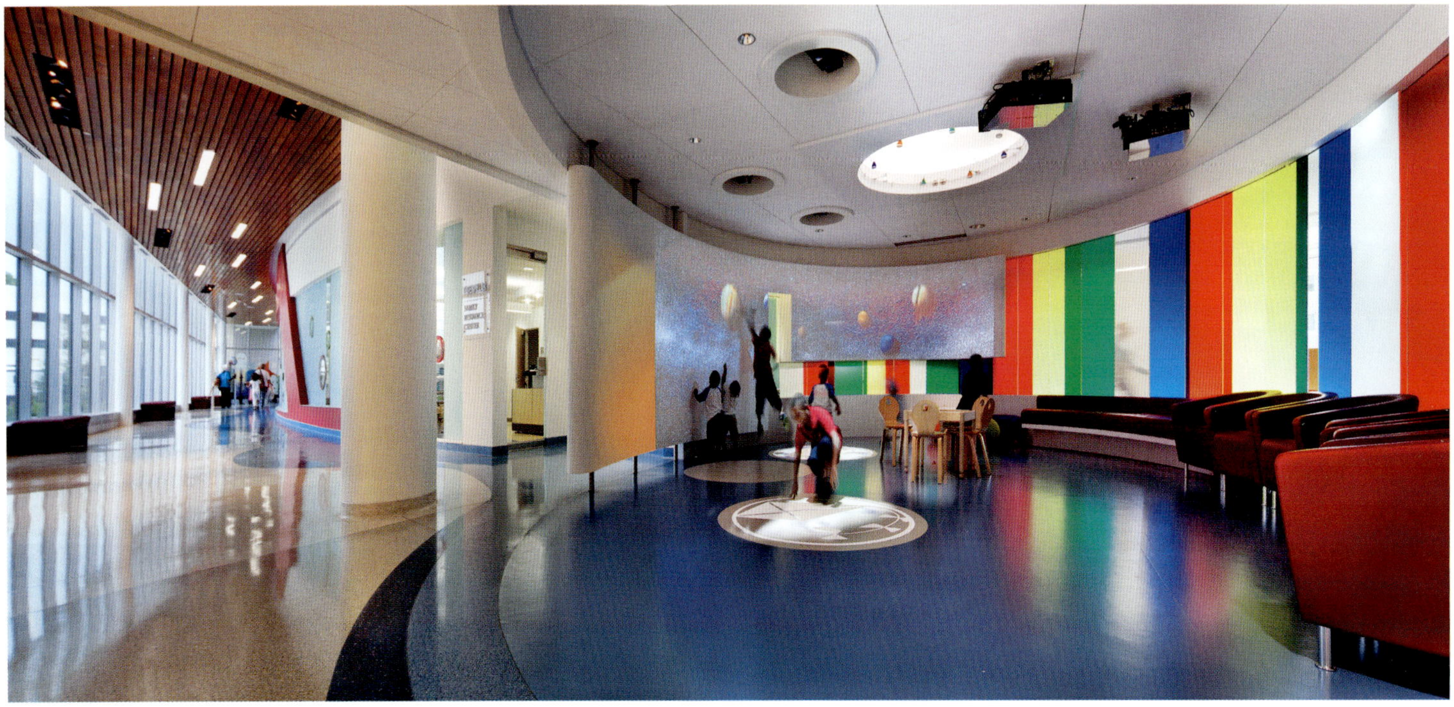

▲ Children's Hospital of Illinois at OSF Saint Francis Medical Center, Peoria, IL
Photo: James Steinkamp

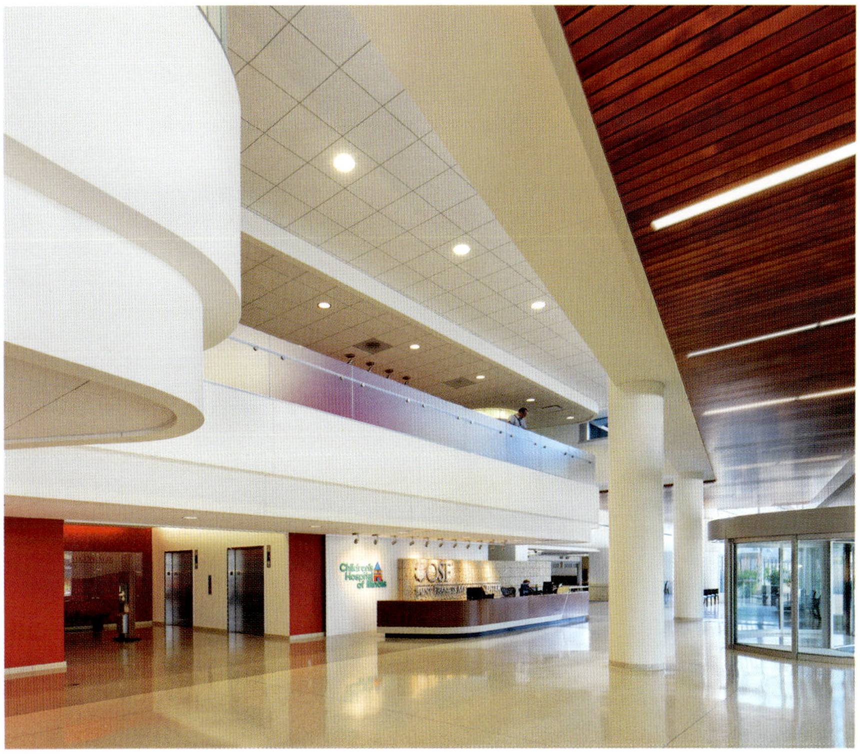

▲ Children's Hospital of Illinois at OSF Saint Francis Medical Center, Peoria, IL
Photo: James Steinkamp

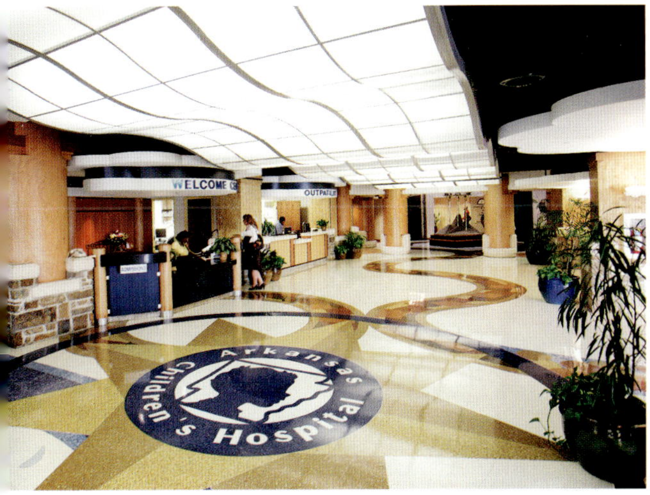

▲ Arkansas Children's Hospital, Little Rock, AR
Photo: Kelley Cooper

▼ Children's Hospital Colorado, Denver, CO
Photo: Eckert & Eckert

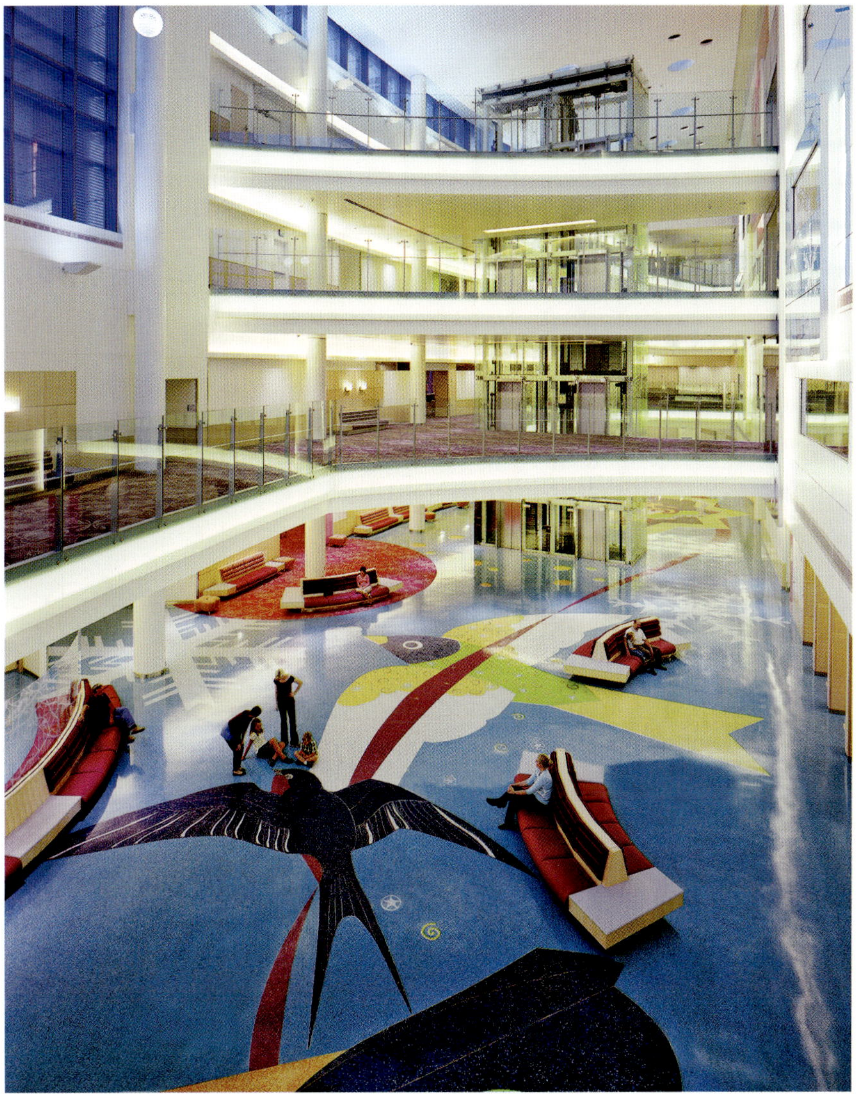

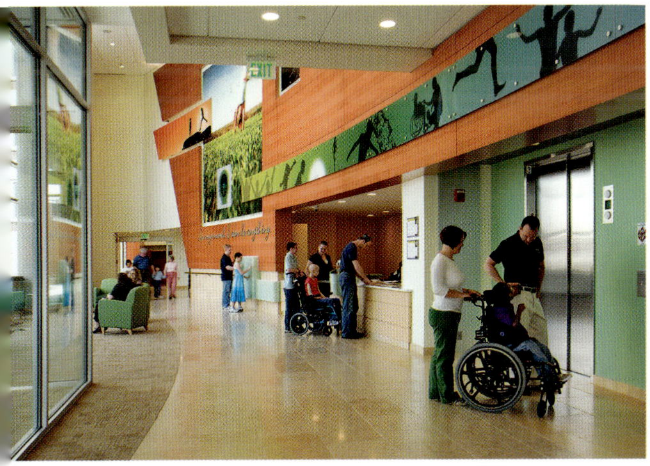

▲ Kennedy Krieger Institute, Kennedy Krieger Children's Hospital, Baltimore, MD
Photo: Jim Roof Creative

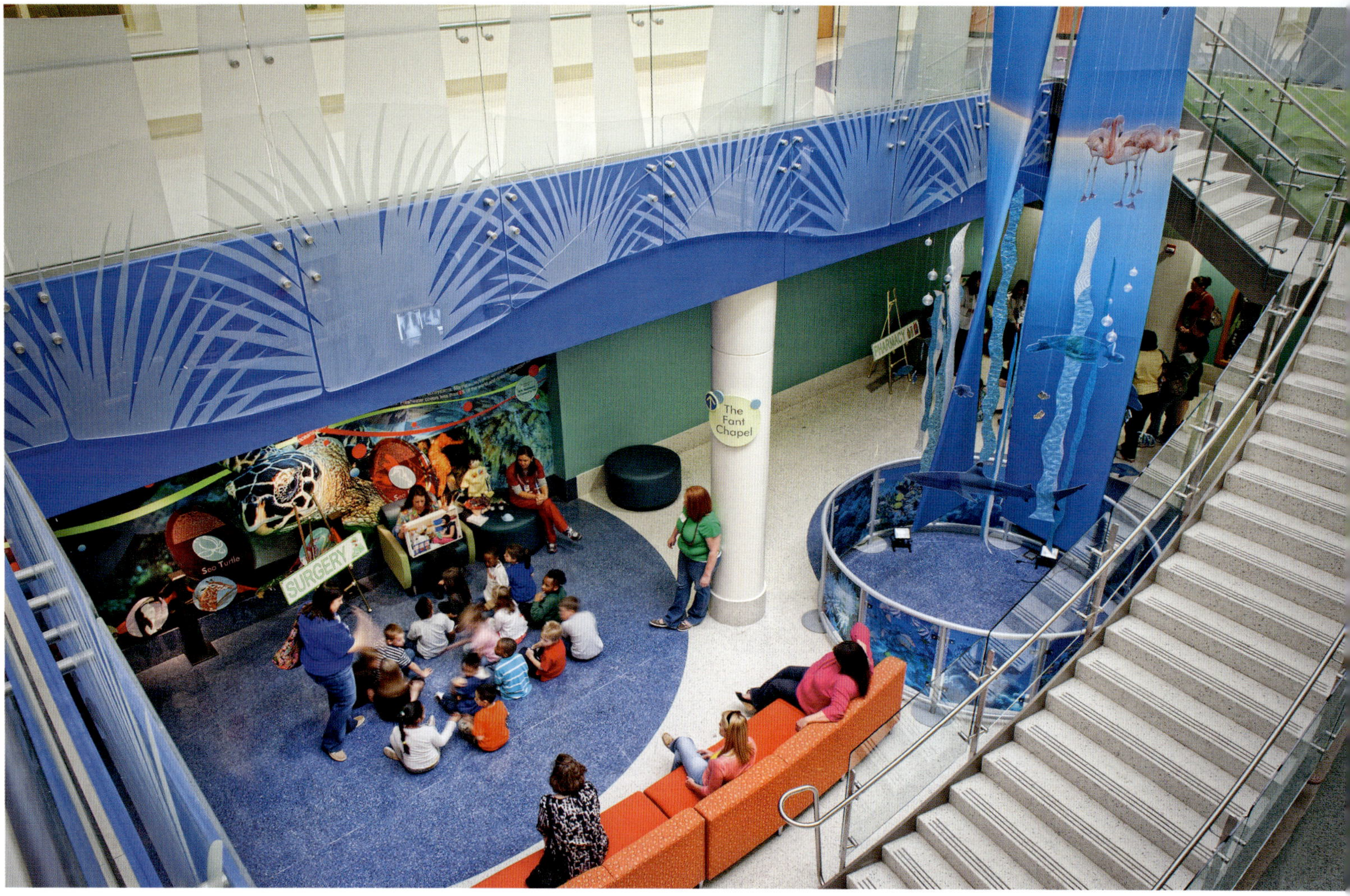

▲ Palmetto Health Children's Hospital, Columbia, SC
▼

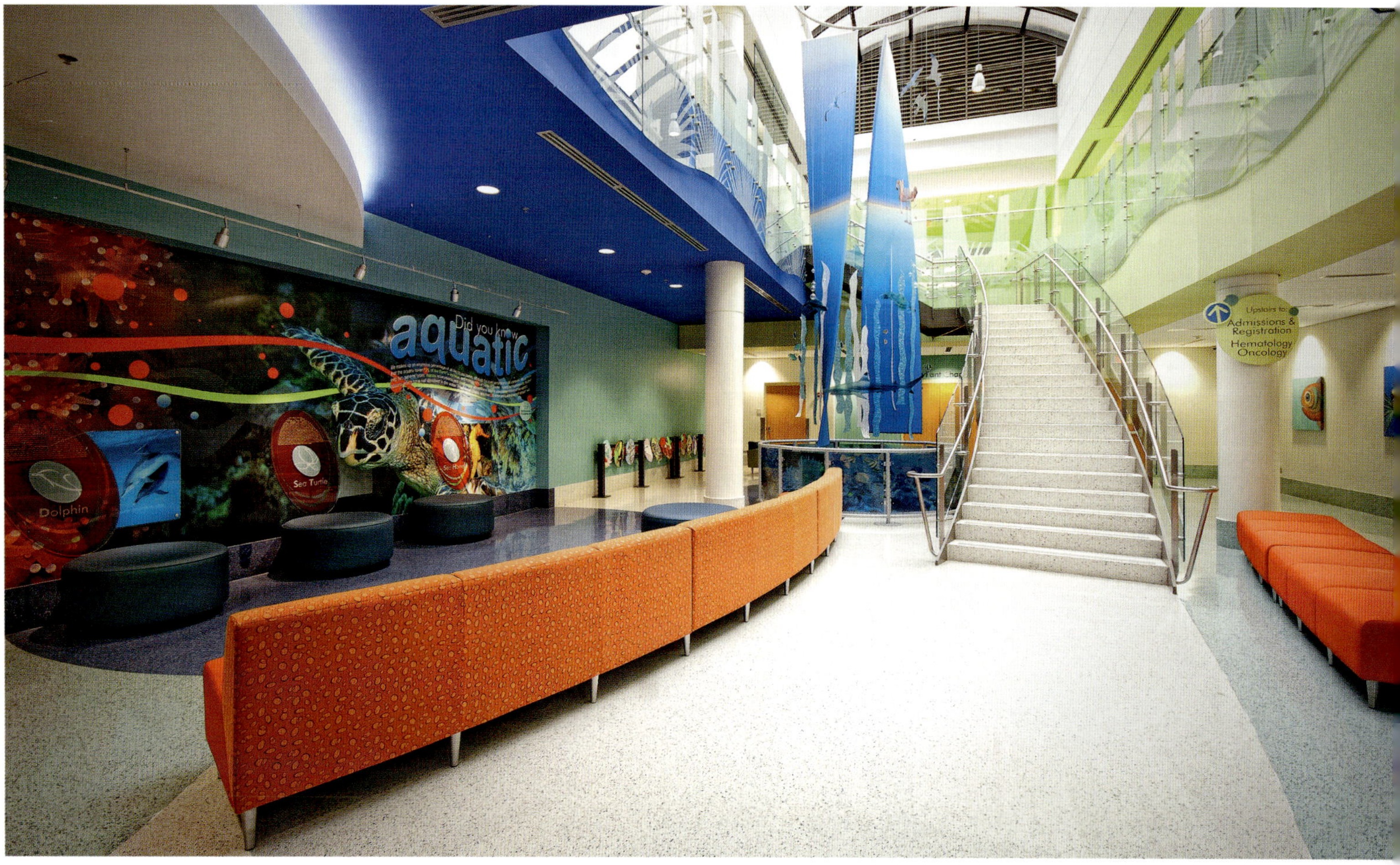

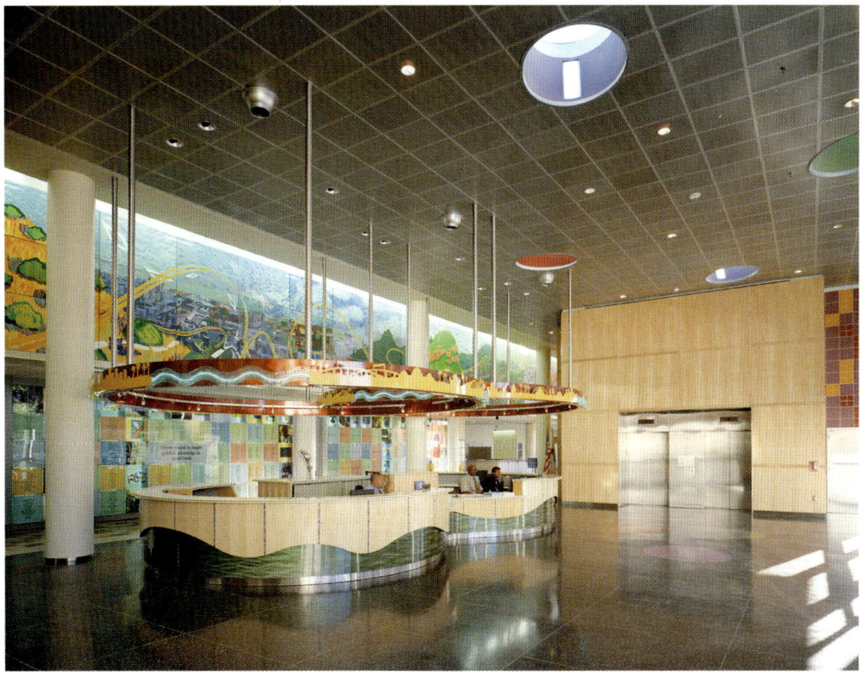

▲ Children's Hospital Los Angeles, CA
Photo: RMA Photography

▼ CHOC Children's Hospital, Orange, CA
Photos: Provided by FKP Architects

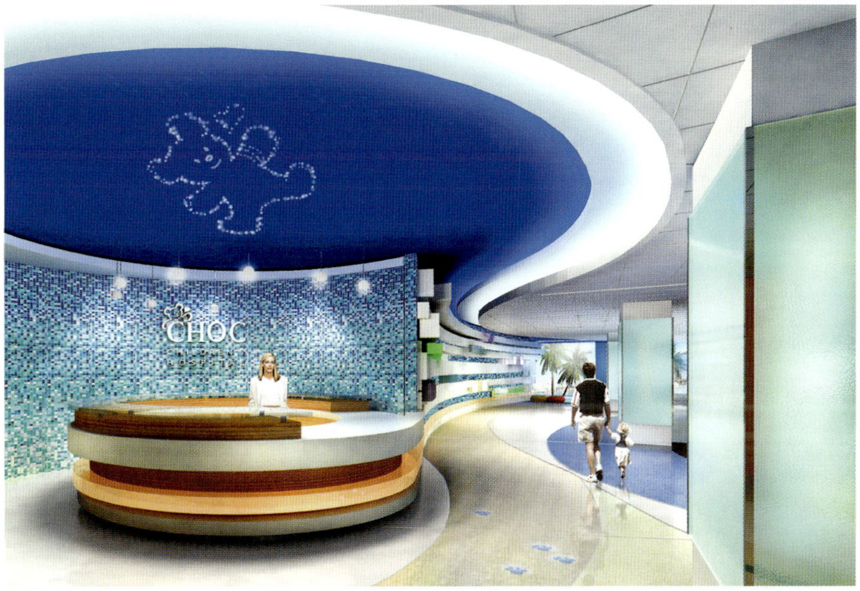

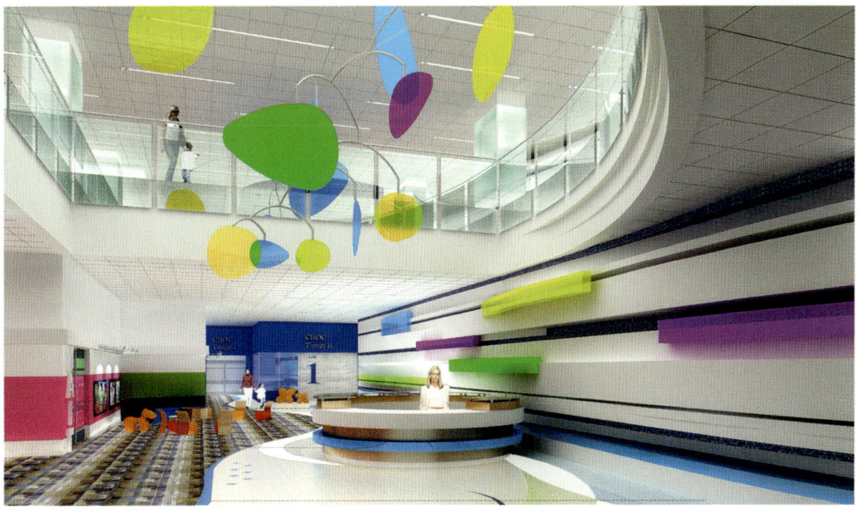

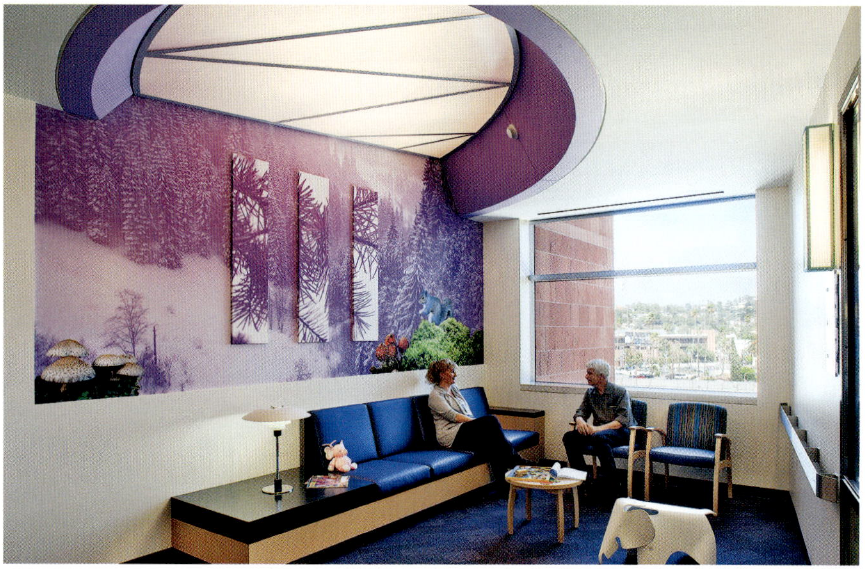

▲ Children's Hospital Los Angeles, CA
Photo: Pete Eckert

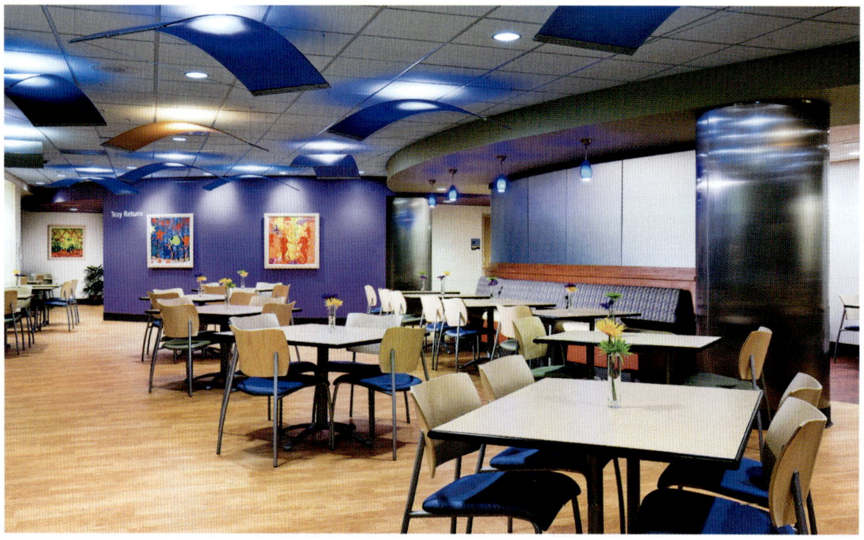

▲ Children's Medical Center, Dallas, TX
Photo: Charles Smith

▼ Holland Bloorview Kids Rehabilitation Hospital, Toronto, Ontario, Canada
Photo: Stantec © Richard Johnson

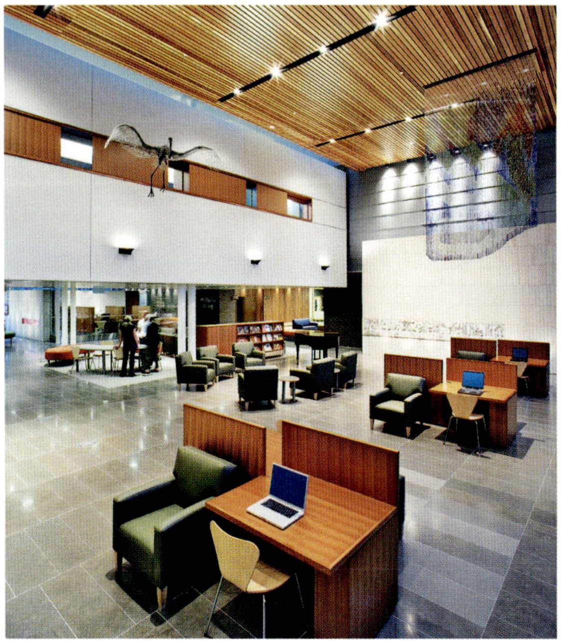

▼ Great Ormond Street Children's Hospital, Octav Botnar Building, London, United Kingdom
Photo: Stantec © Edward Sumner

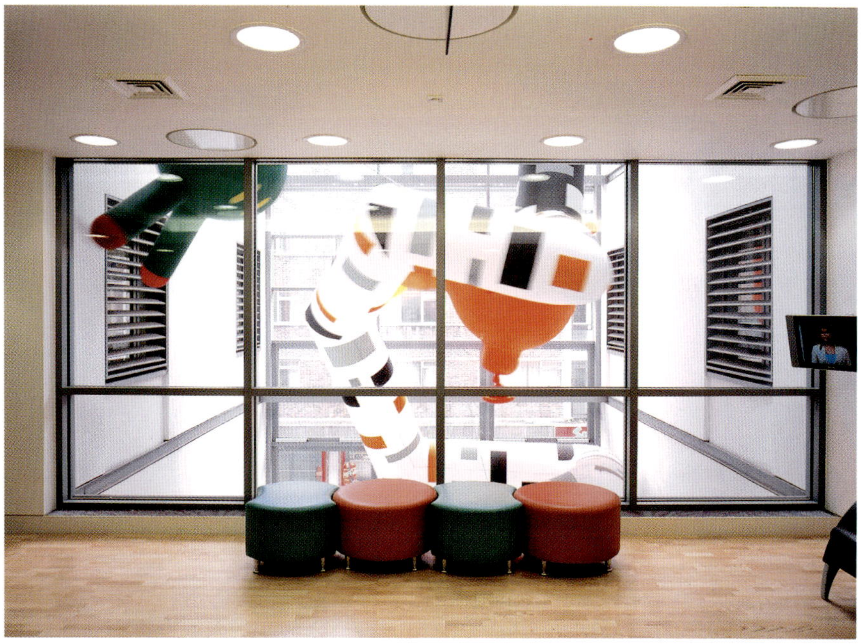

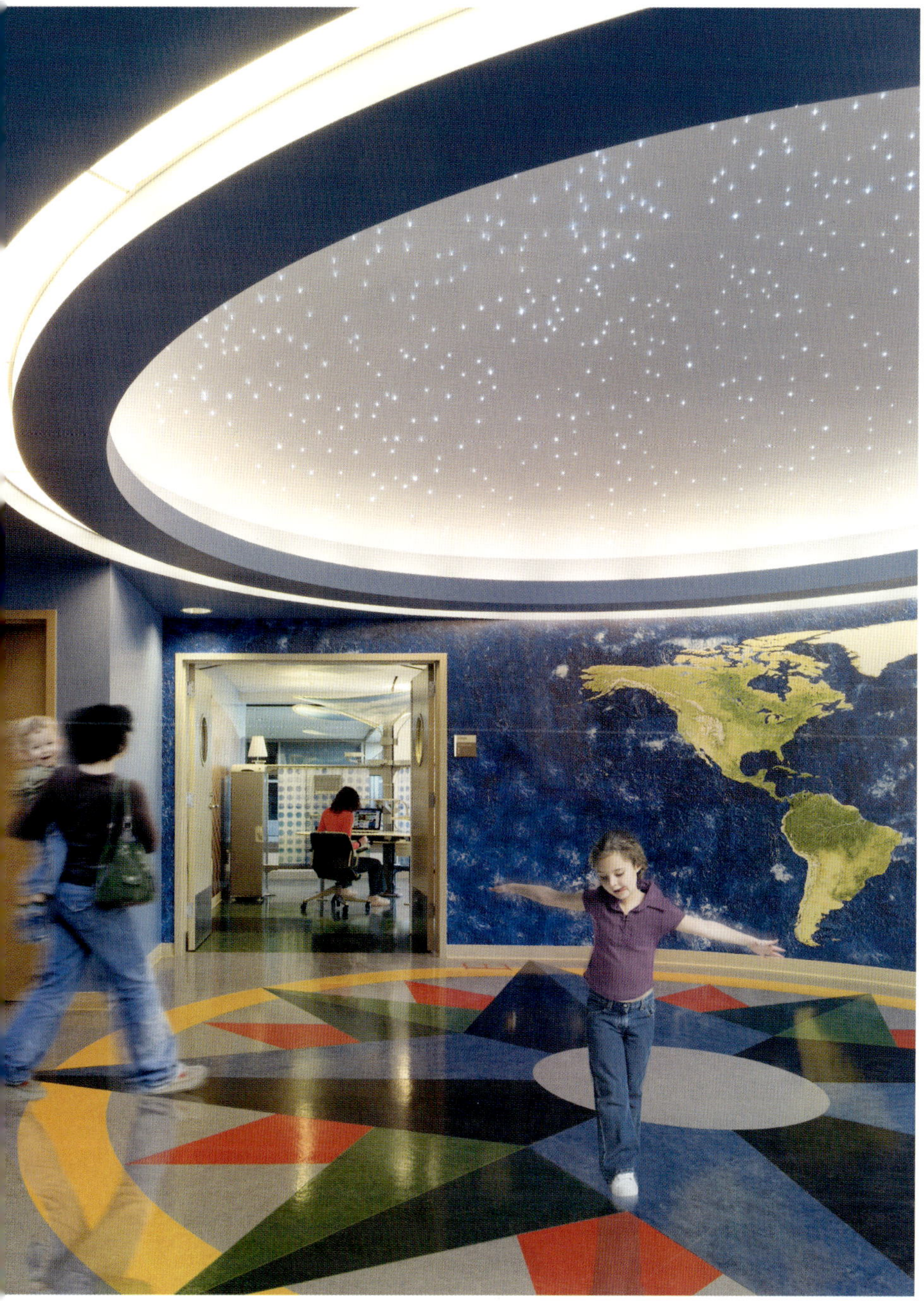

▲ Mattel Children's Hospital UCLA, Los Angeles, CA
Photo: Benny Chan, fotoworks

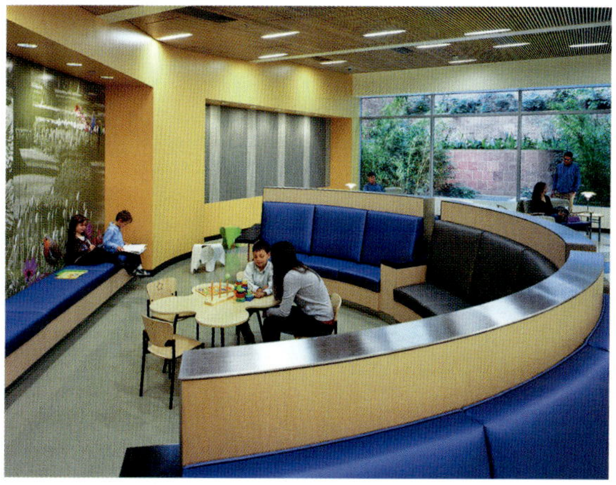

▲ Children's Hospital Los Angeles, CA
Photo: Pete Eckert

▼ Kosair Children's Hospital, Louisville, KY

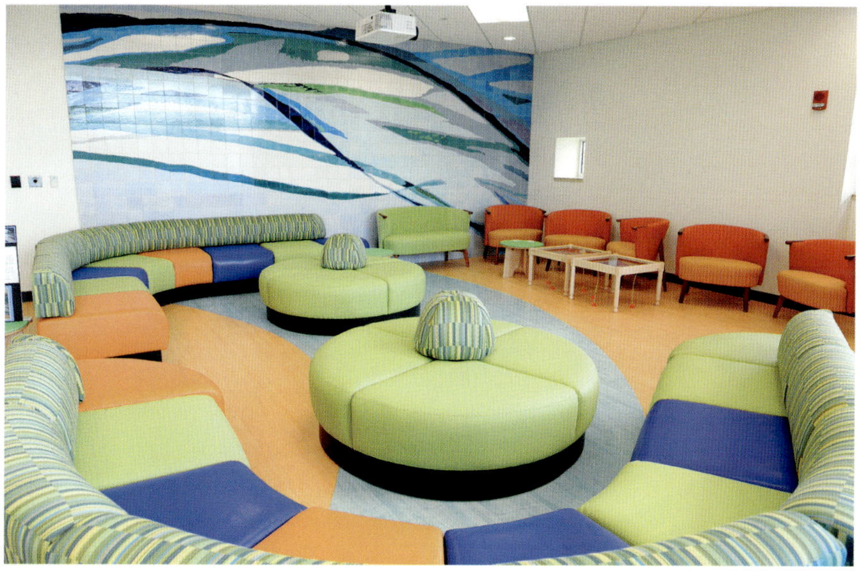

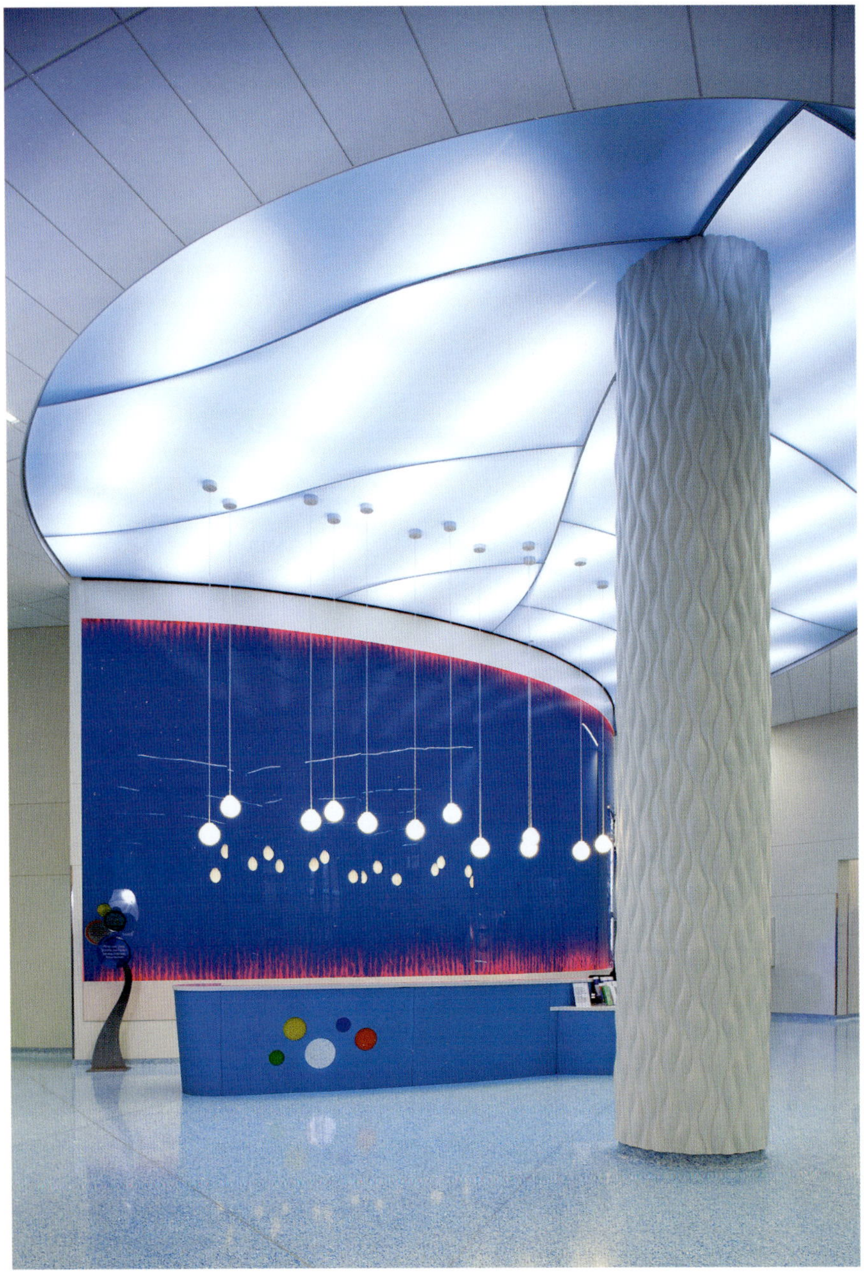

▲ Helen DeVos Children's Hospital, Grand Rapids, MI
Photo: Lucid Architecture, Eric DeWitt

▼ Helen DeVos Children's Hospital, Grand Rapids, MI
Photo: Hedrich Blessing Photography

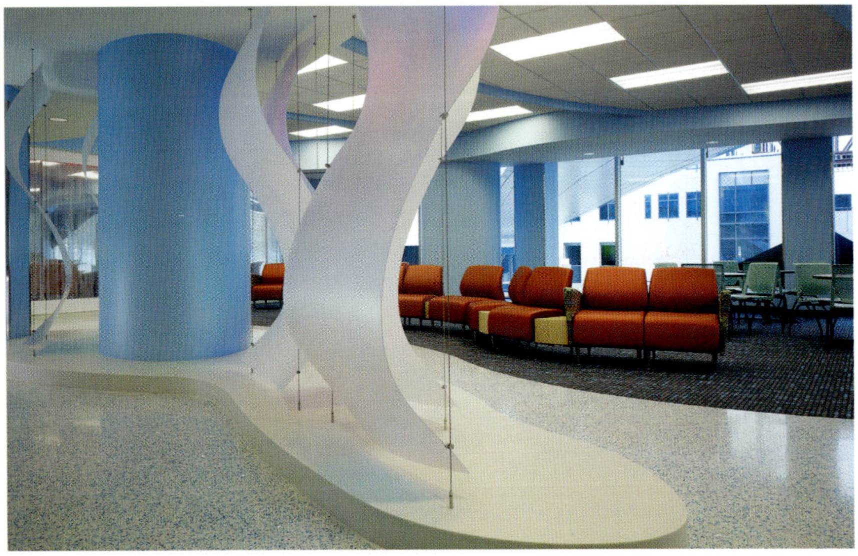

▼ Gillette Children's, Saint Paul, MN
Photos: Terry Mahanna

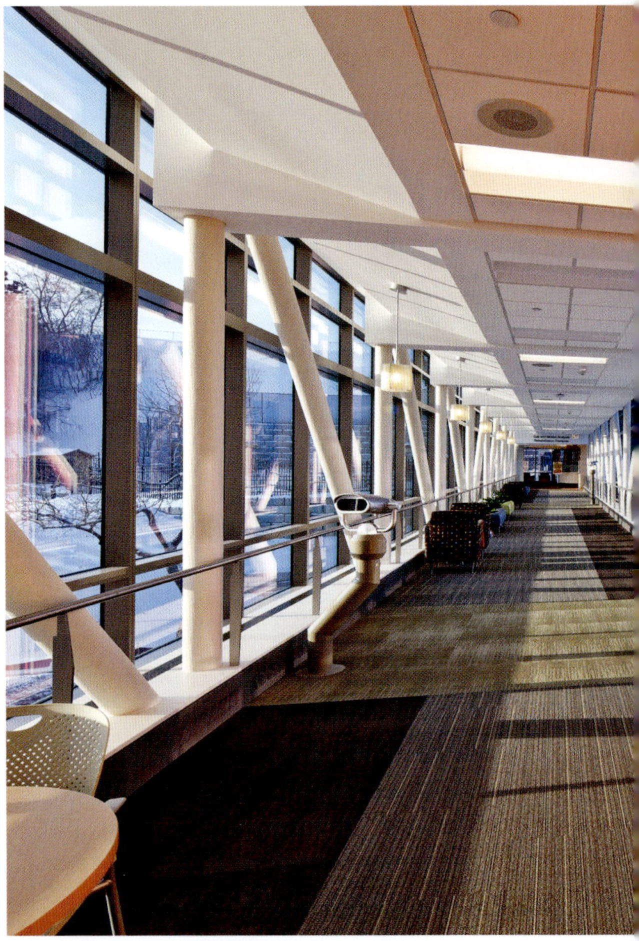

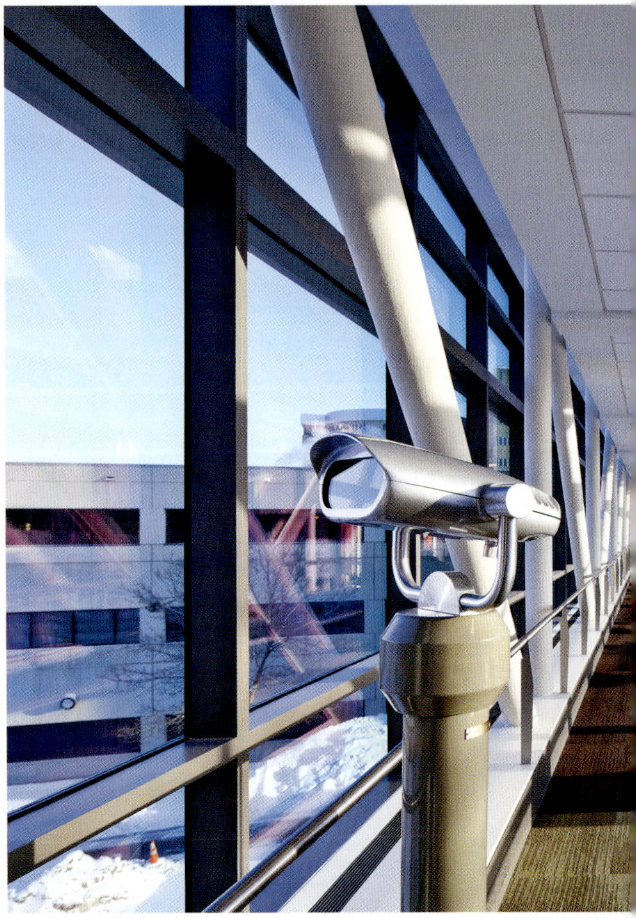

▼ PSE&G Children's Specialized Hospital, New Brunswick, NJ
Photos: Stantec © Tom Crane Photography, Inc.

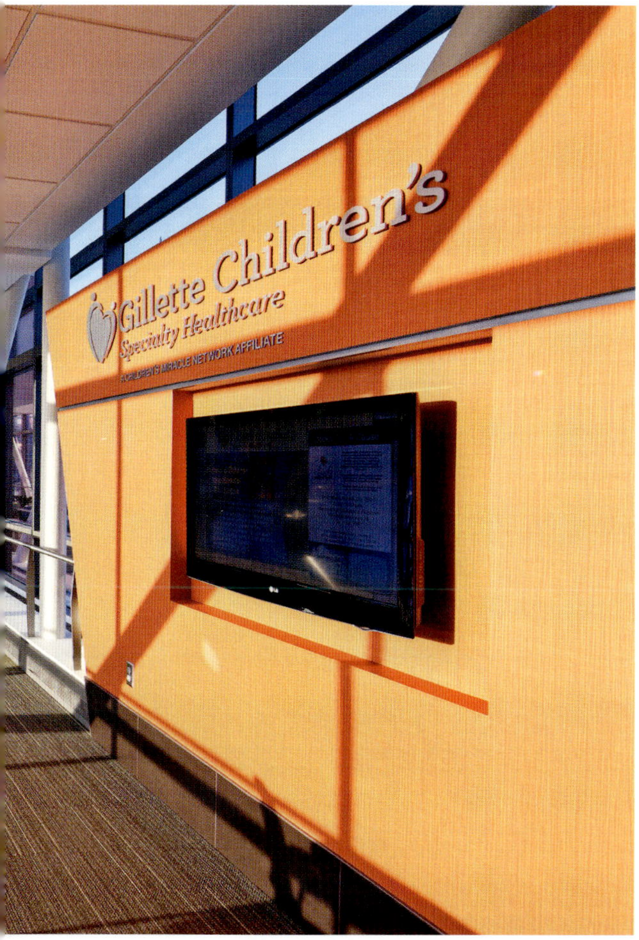

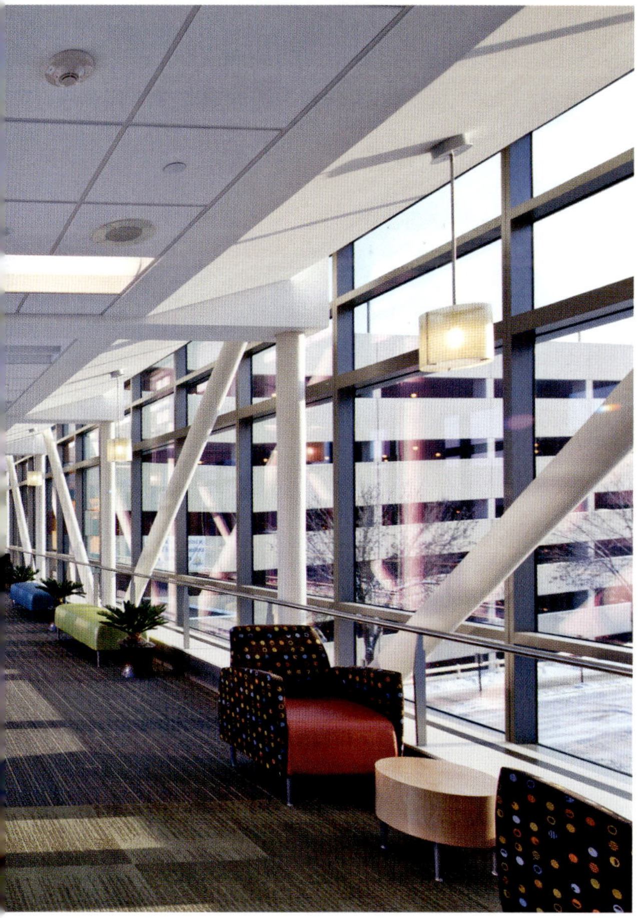

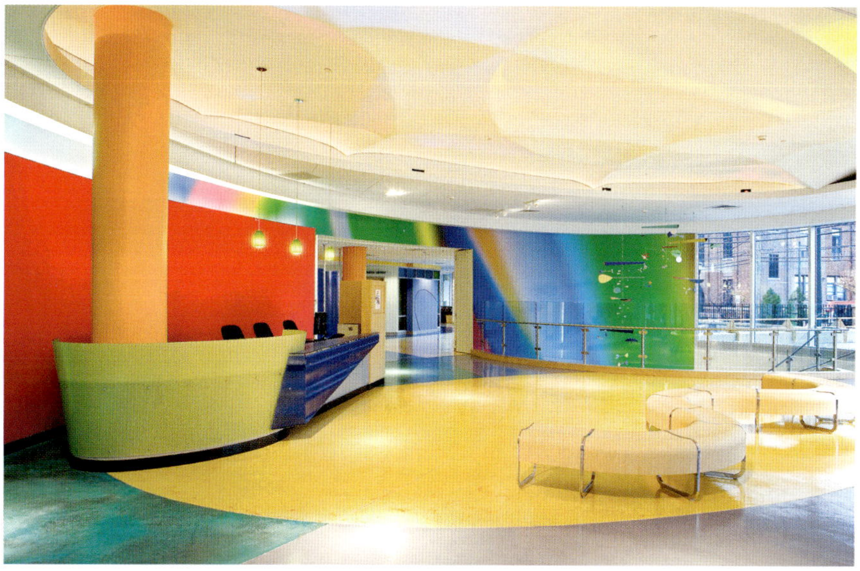

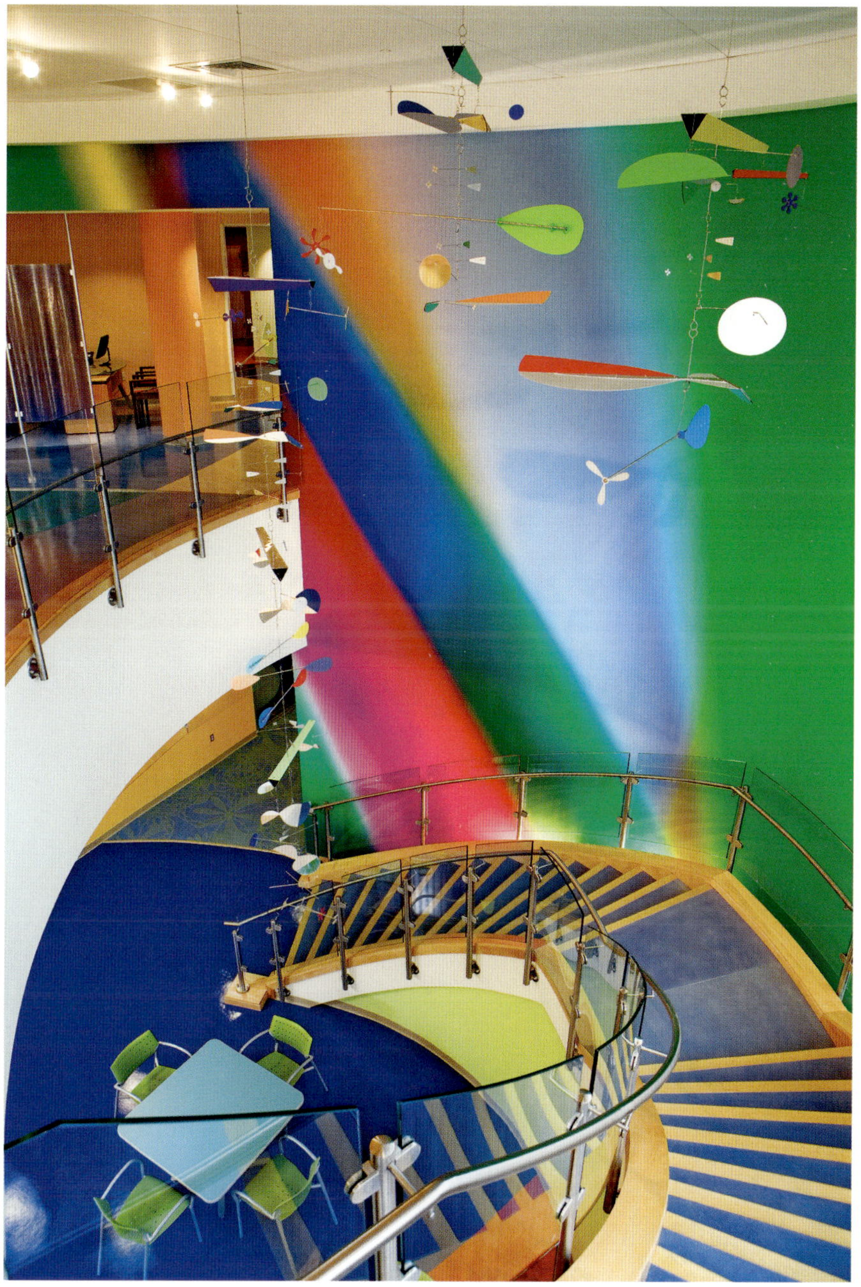

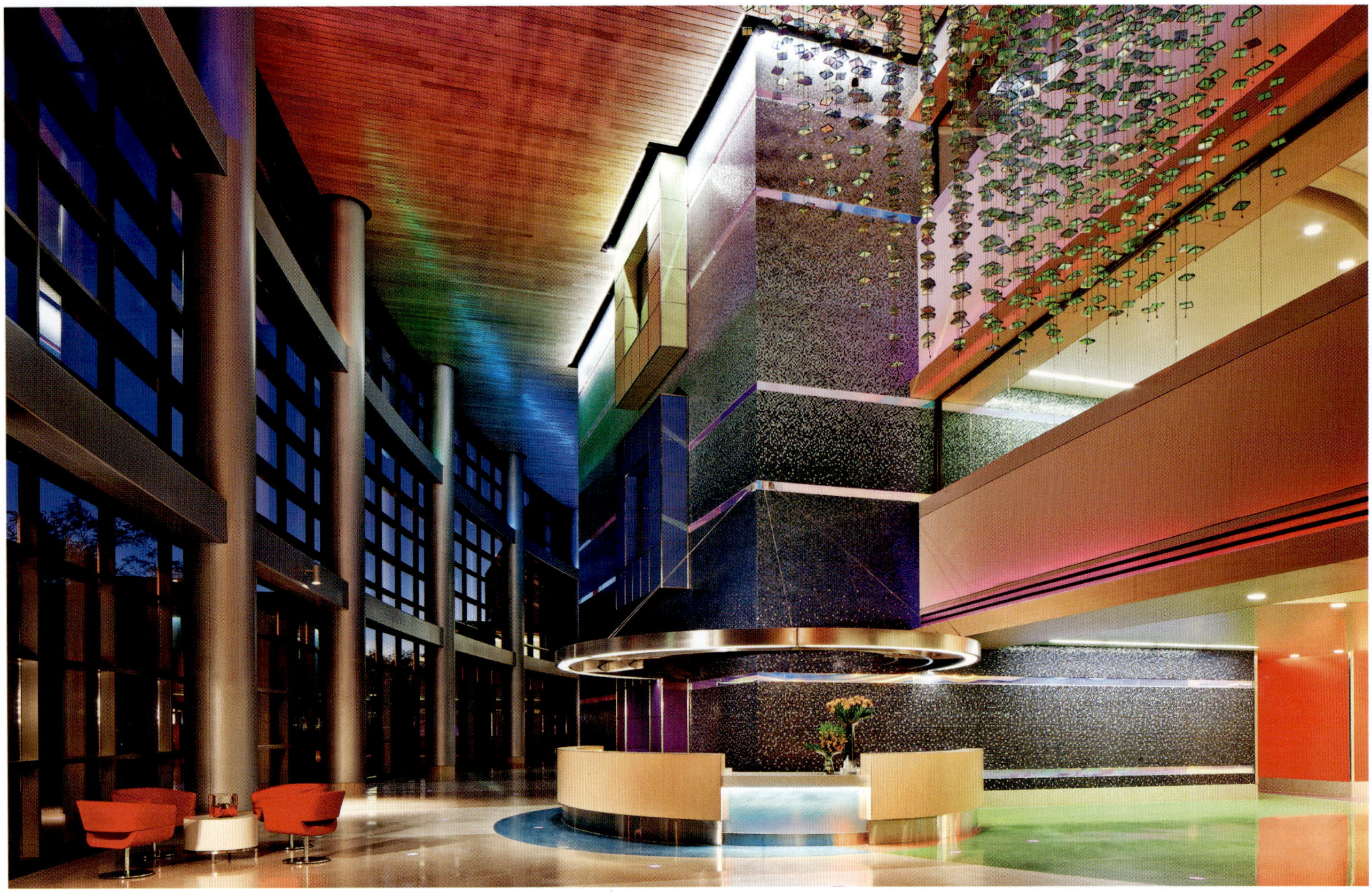

▲ Phoenix Children's Hospital, AZ
Photo: Blake Marvin, HKS

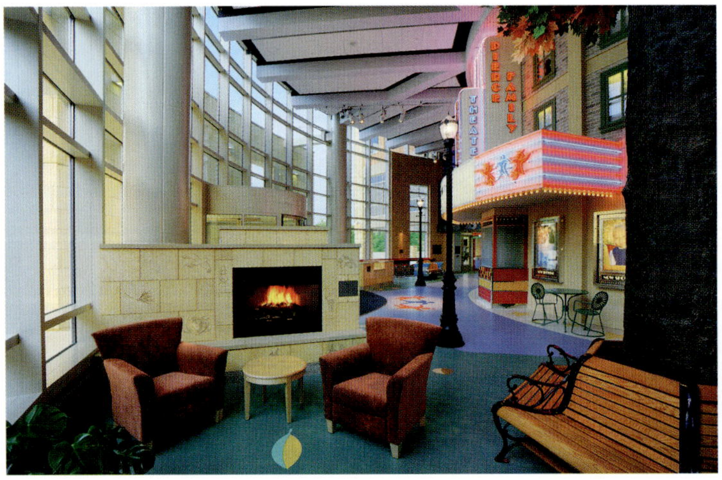

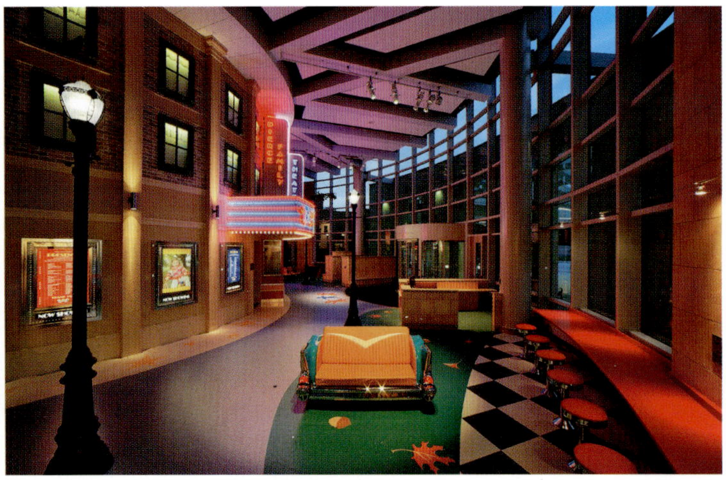

▲ American Family Children's Hospital, Madison, WI
Photos: HDR Architecture, Inc. © 2007 Ballogg Photography Inc., Chicago

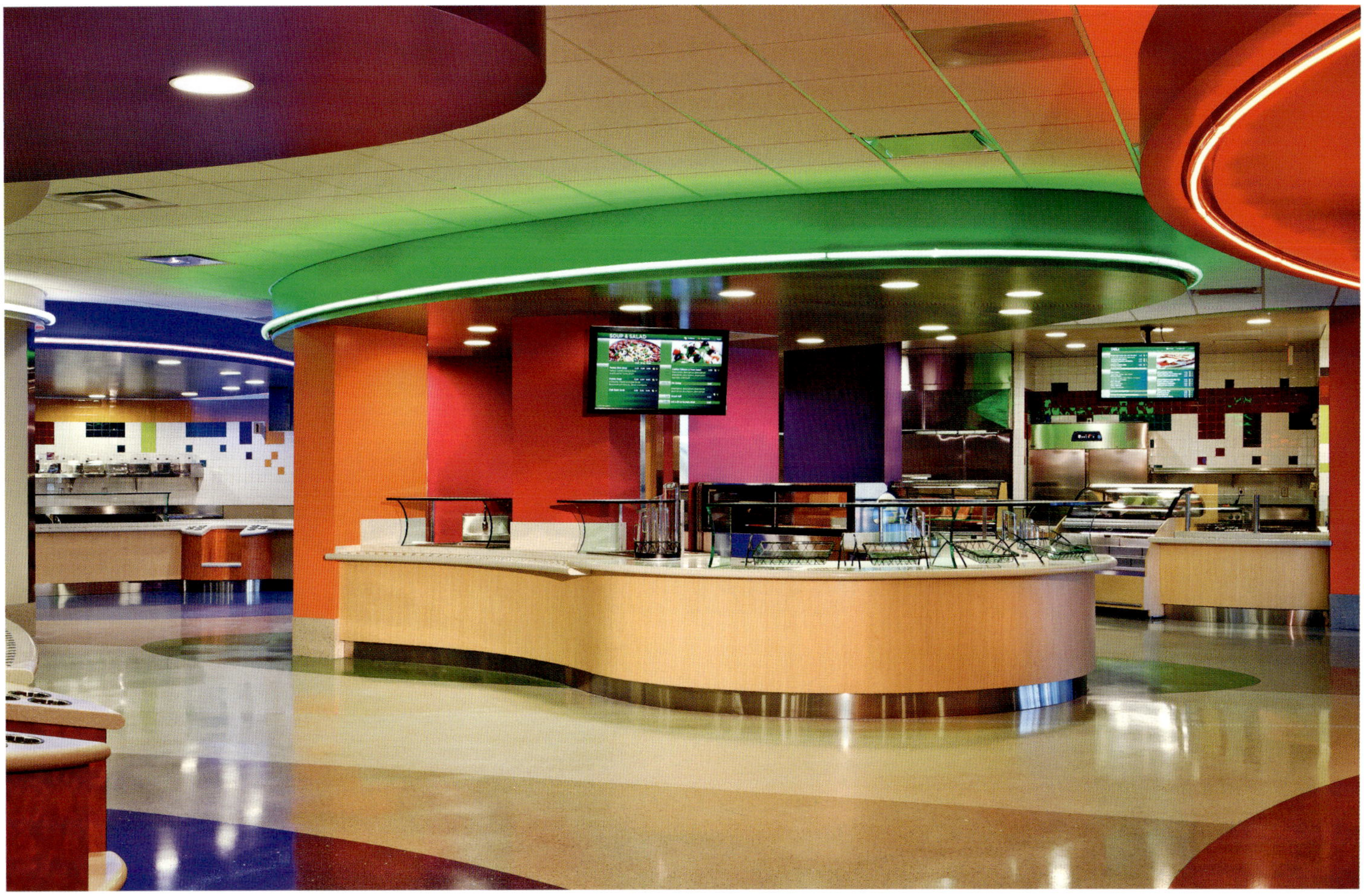

▲ Phoenix Children's Hospital, AZ
Photo: Blake Marvin, HKS

▼ University Medical Center, Tucson, AZ
Photo: Jake Johnson Pictures

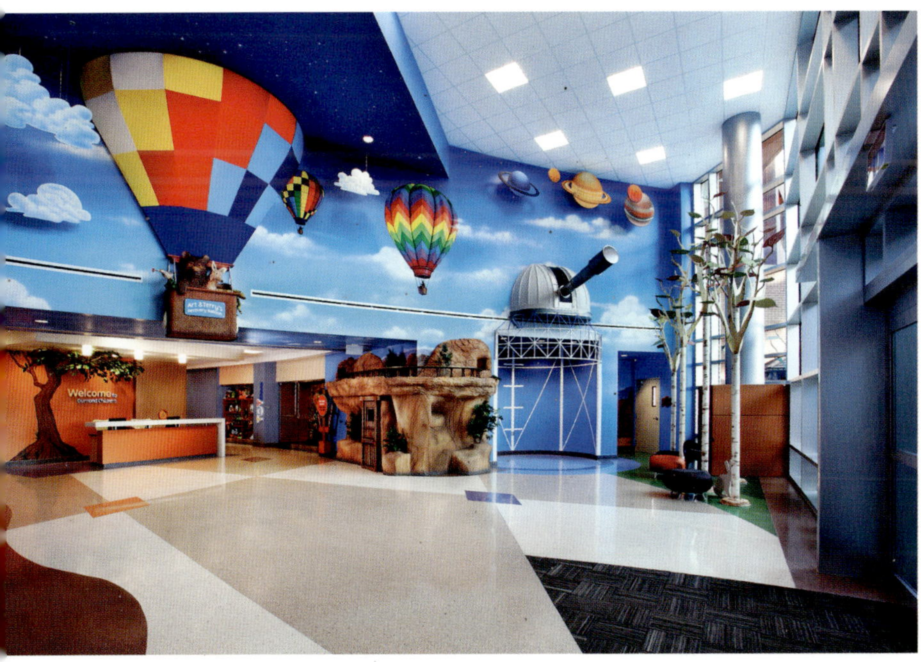

▼ Children's Hospital Omaha, NE
Photo: Matthew Placzek – "Imagine" © 2010 Thomas Grady photography

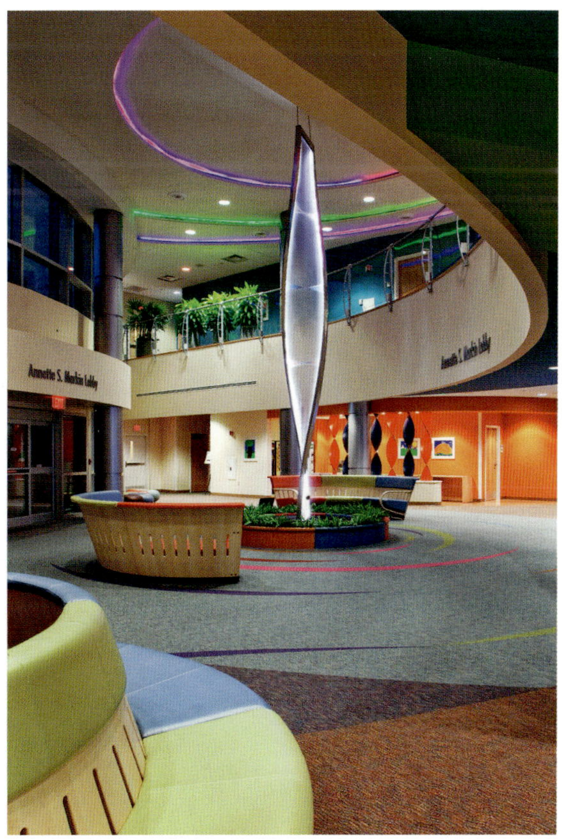

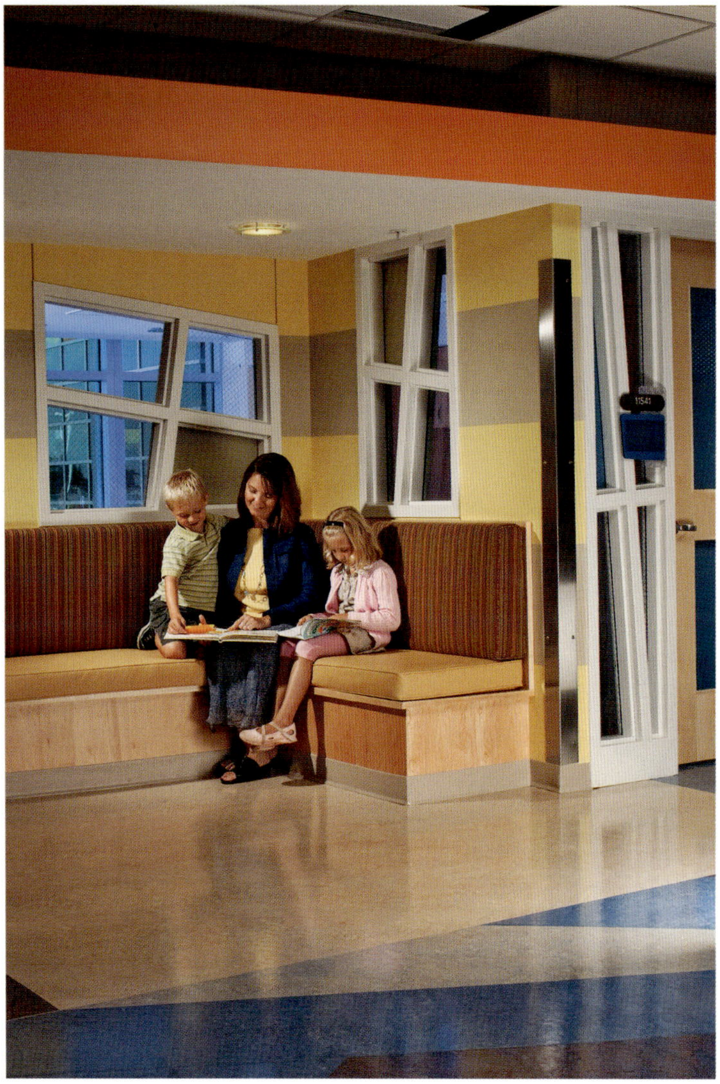

▲ Upstate Golisano Children's Hospital, Syracuse, NY
Photo: Robert Mescavage

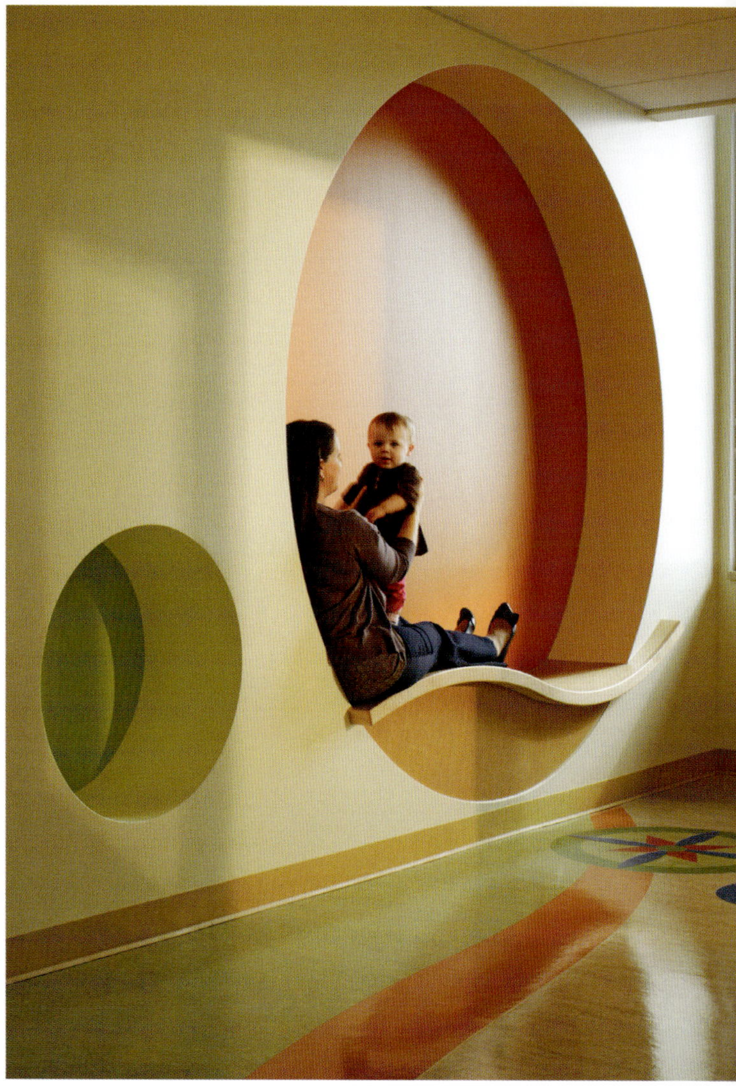

▲ University of Minnesota Amplatz Children's Hospital, Minneapolis, MN
Photo: Hedrich Blessing Photography, Nick Merrick

▼ Children's Medical Center at Legacy, Plano, TX
Photo: Pete Eckert

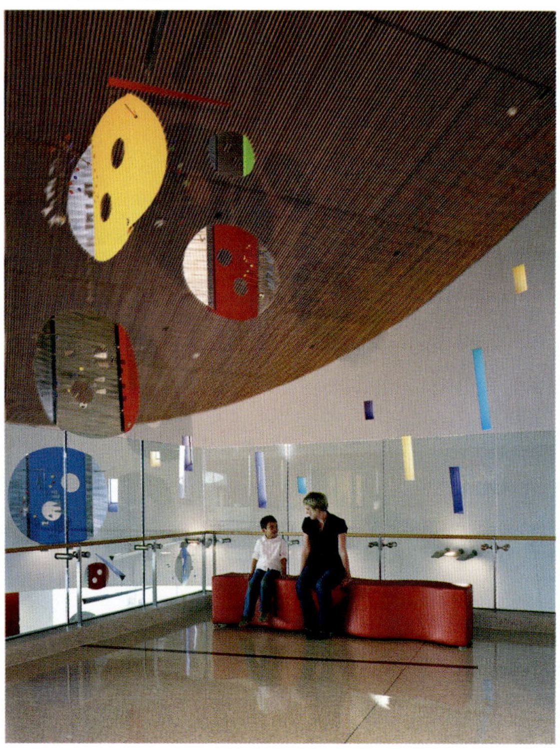

▼ Children's Hospital Colorado, Denver, CO
Photo: Basil Childers

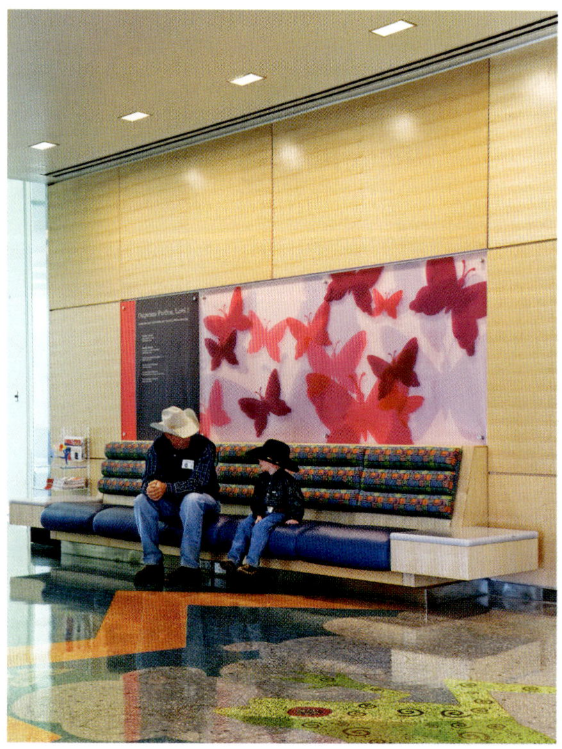

▼ Medical City Children's Hospital, Dallas, TX
Photos: Terry Cockerham

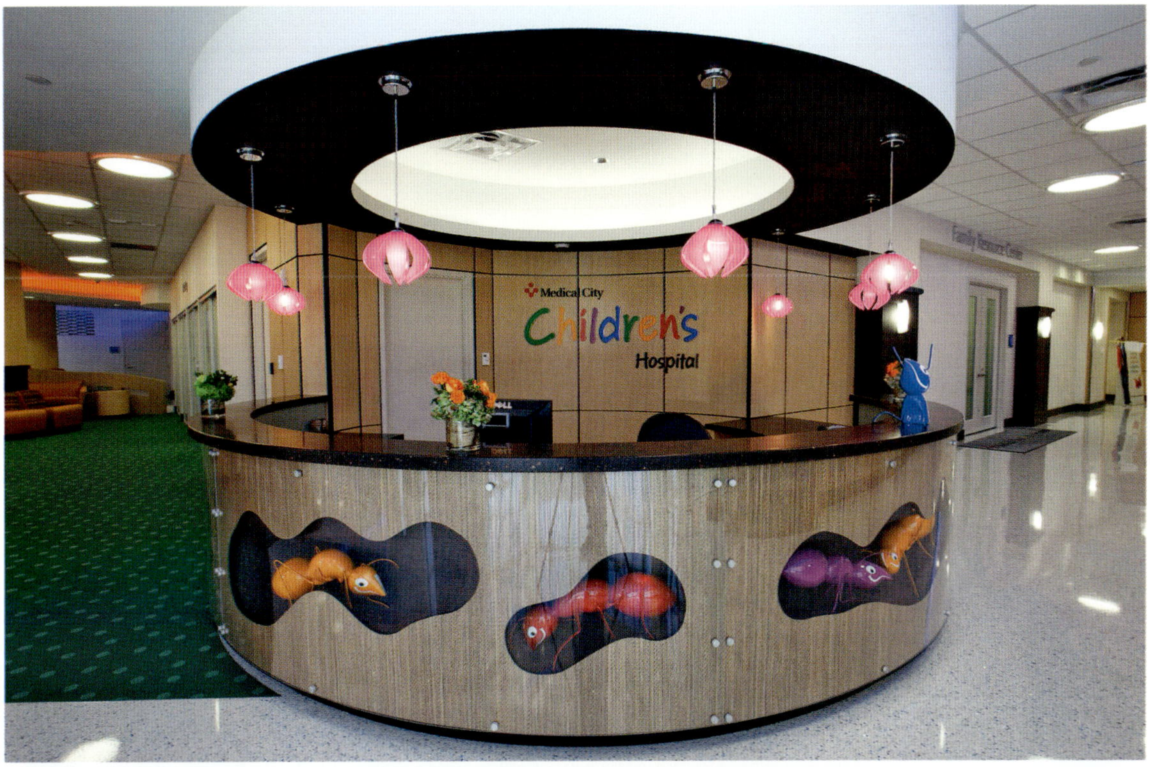

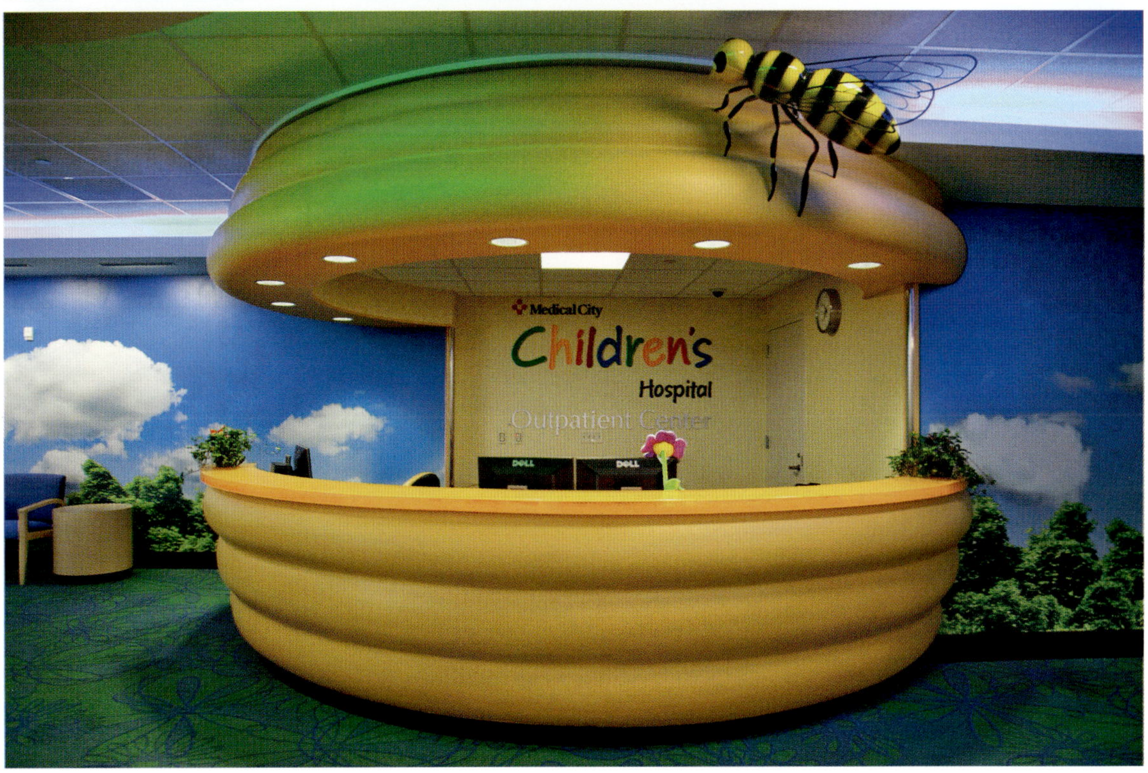

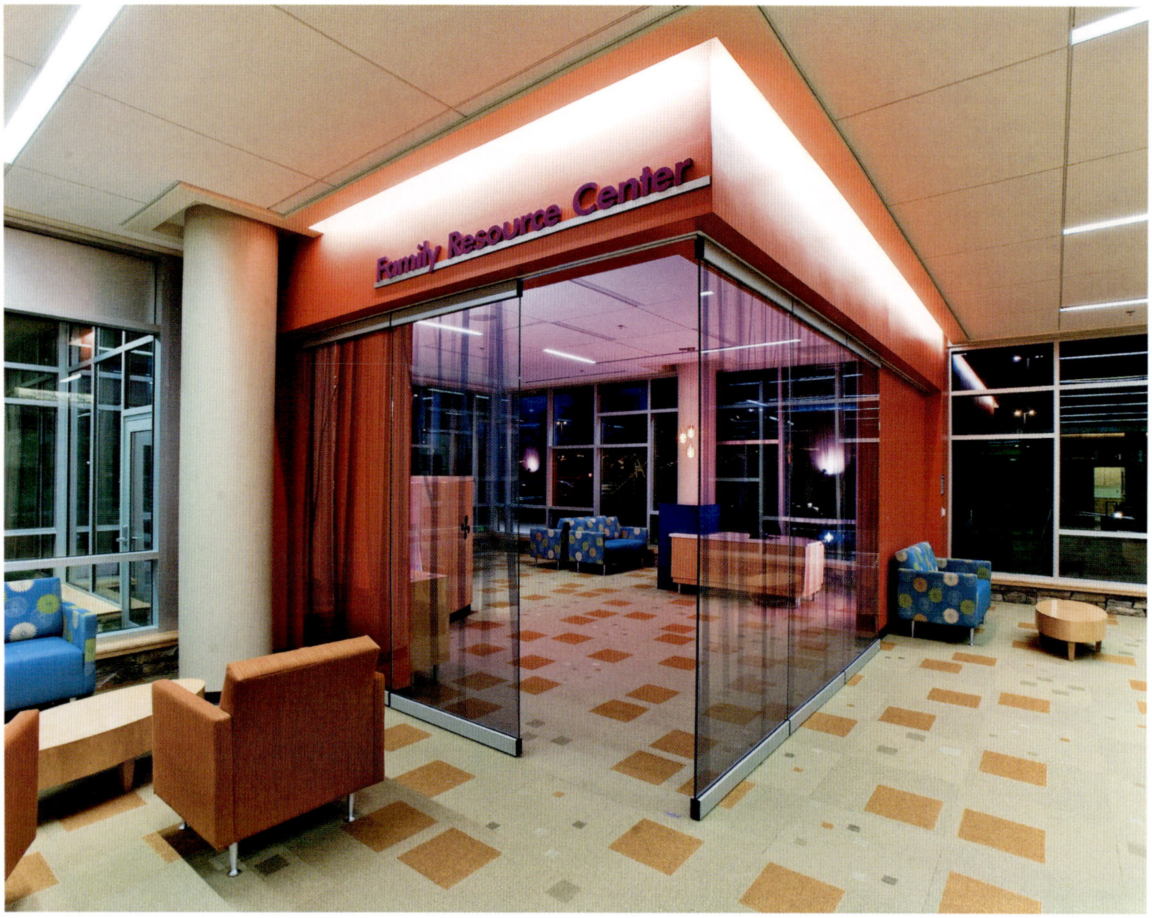

▲ Niswonger Children's Hospital, Johnson City, TN
Photo: Will Griffith

▼ Children's Hospital of Philadelphia, PA
Photo: Children's Hospital of Philadelphia

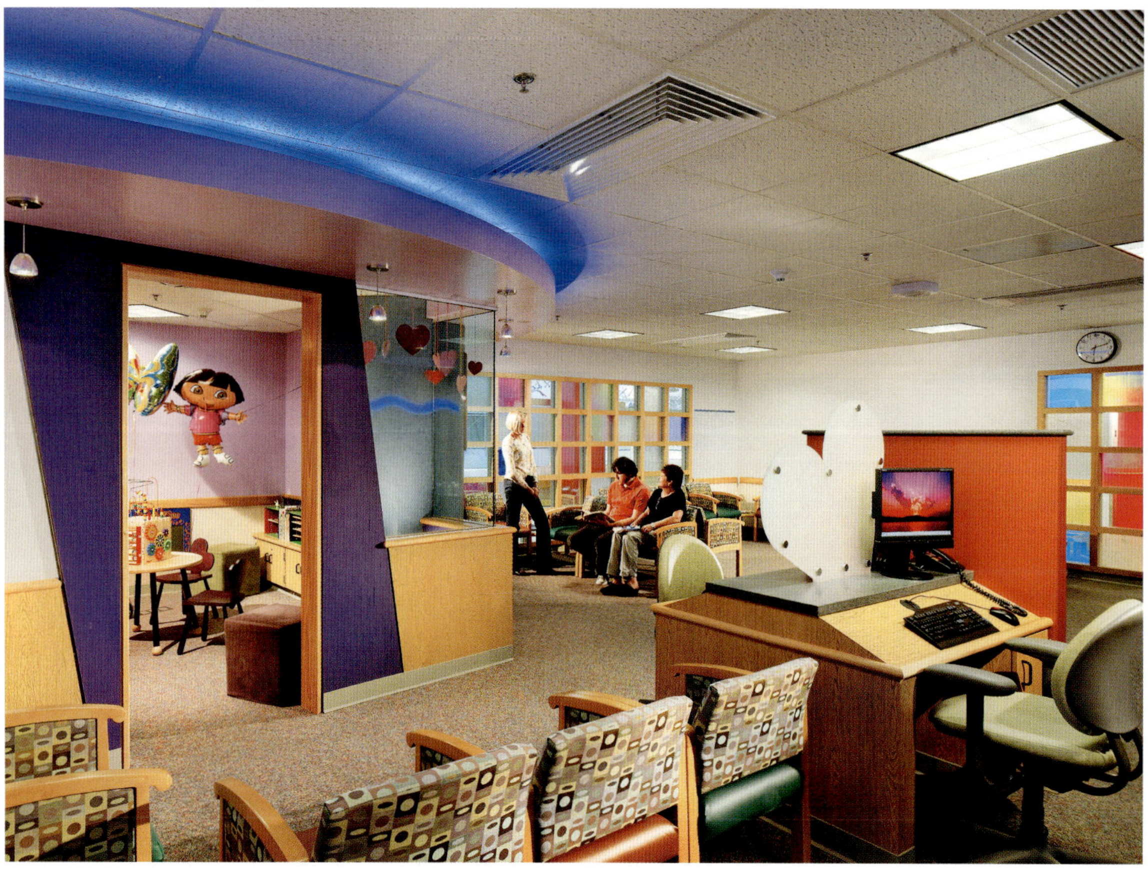

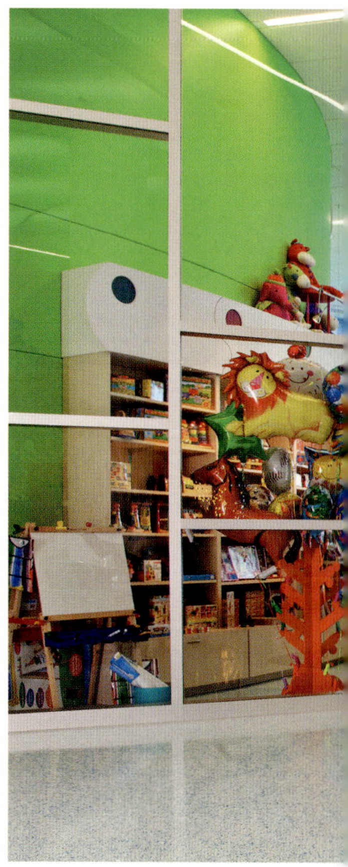

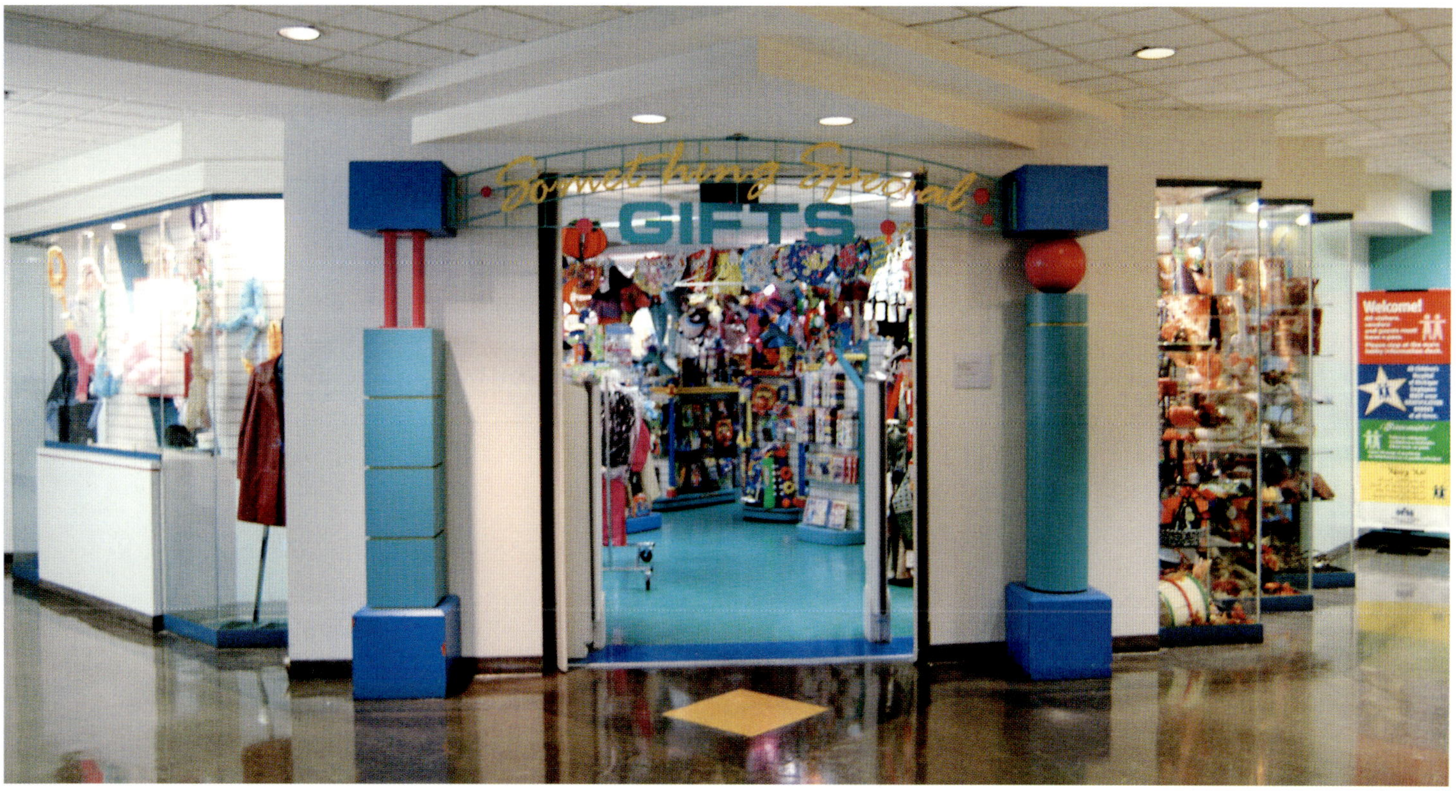

▲ Children's Hospital of Michigan, Detroit, MI

▼ Helen DeVos Children's Hospital, Grand Rapids, MI
Photo: Lucid Architecture, Eric DeWitt

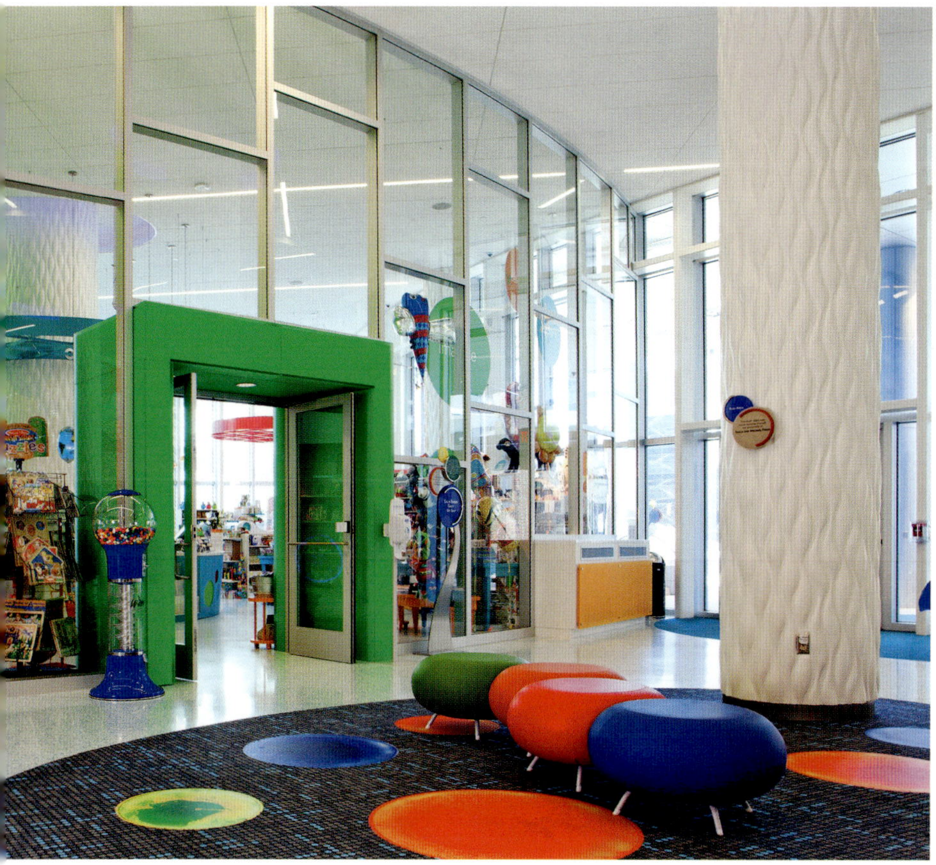

▼ Upstate Golisano Children's Hospital, Syracuse, NY
Photo: William Mueller

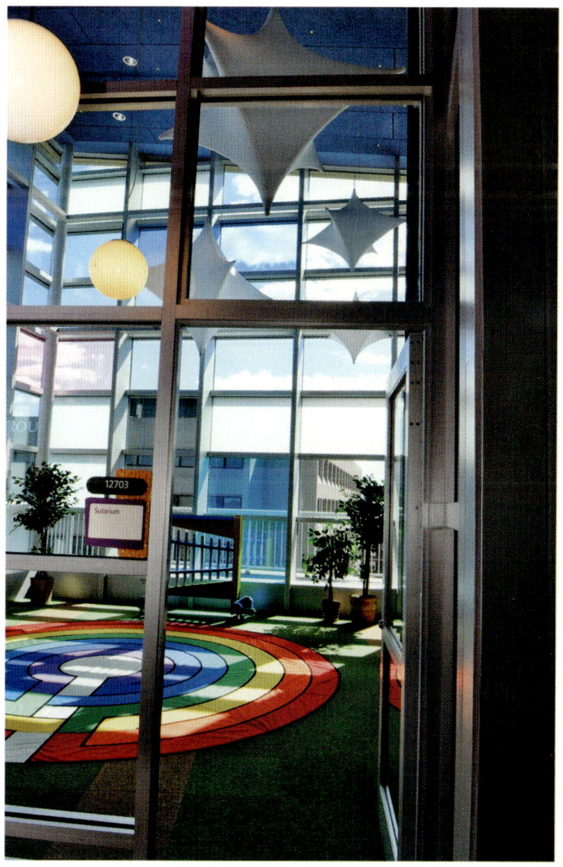

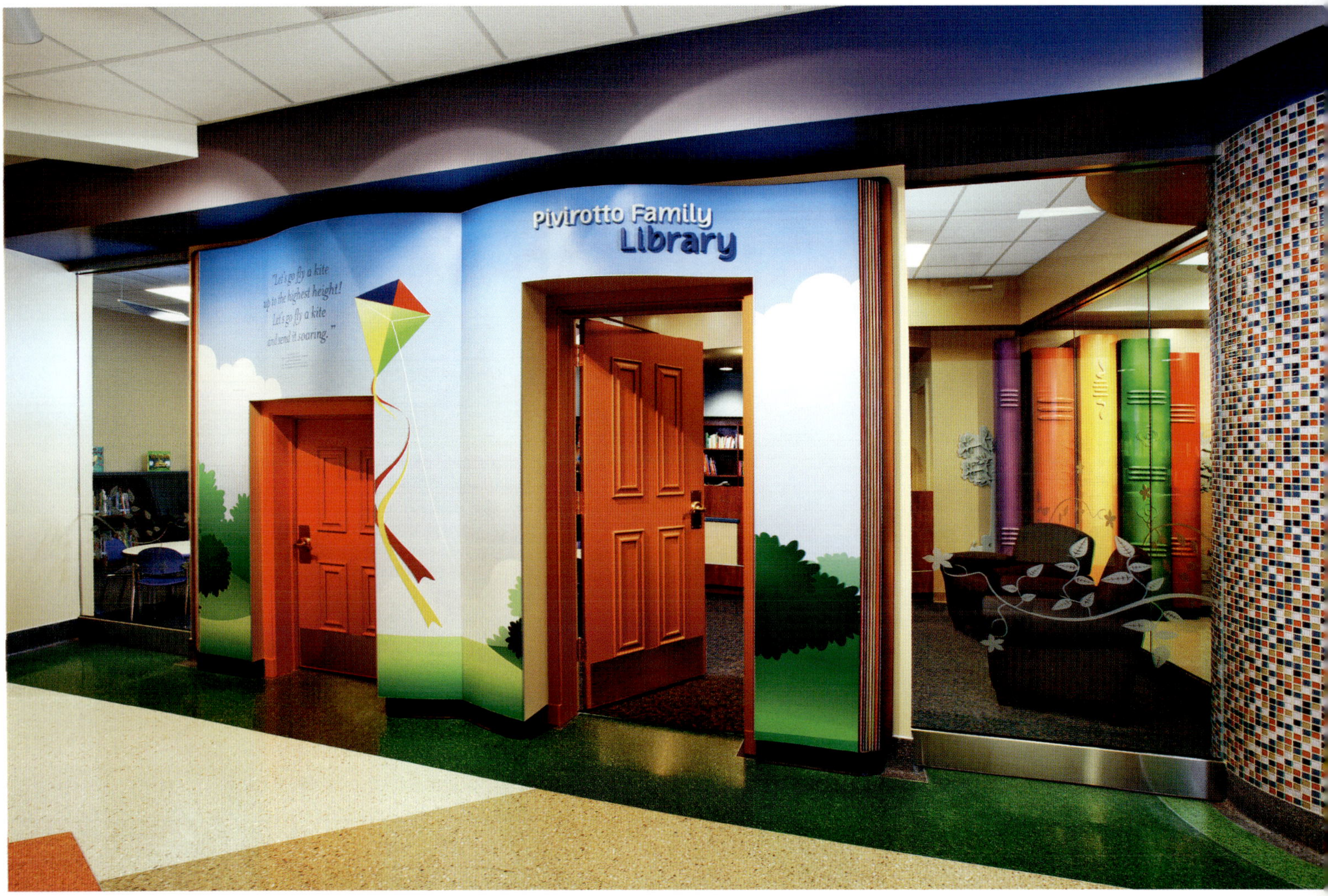

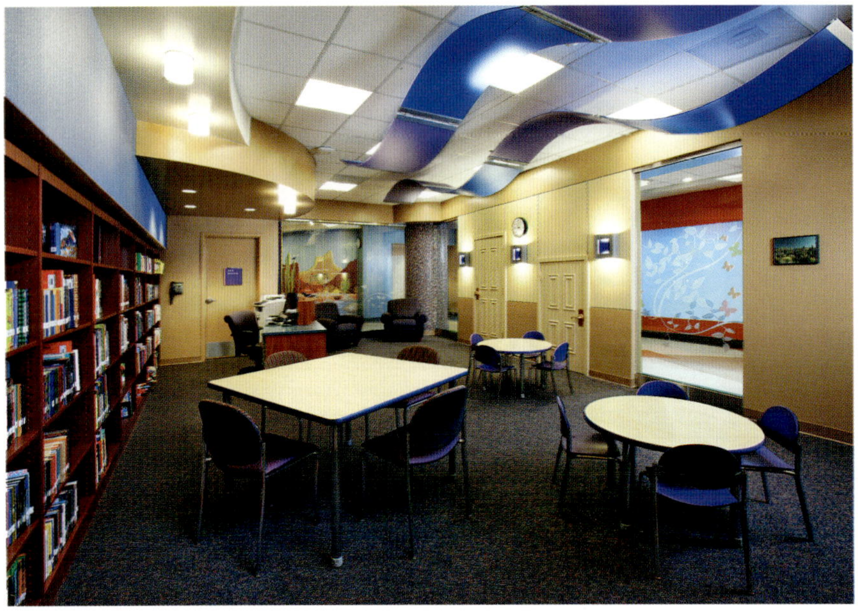

▲ University Medical Center, Tucson, AZ
◀ ***Photos: Jake Johnson Pictures***

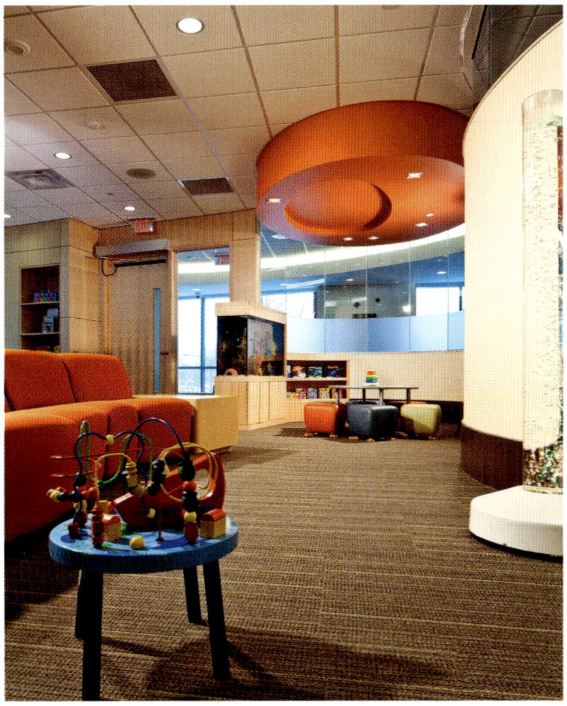

▲ Gillette Children's, Saint Paul, MN
Photo: Terry Mahanna

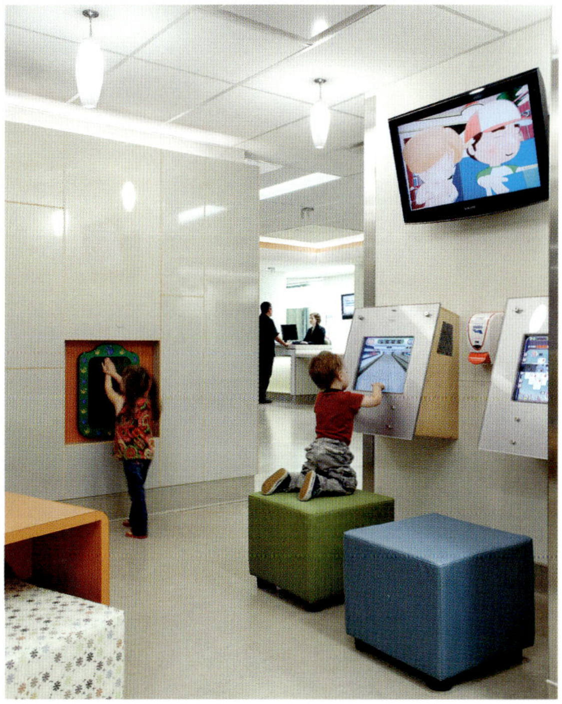

▲ Hospital for Sick Children, Toronto, Ontario, Canada
Photo: Stantec © Richard Johnson

▼ University Medical Center, Tucson, AZ
Photo: Jake Johnson Pictures

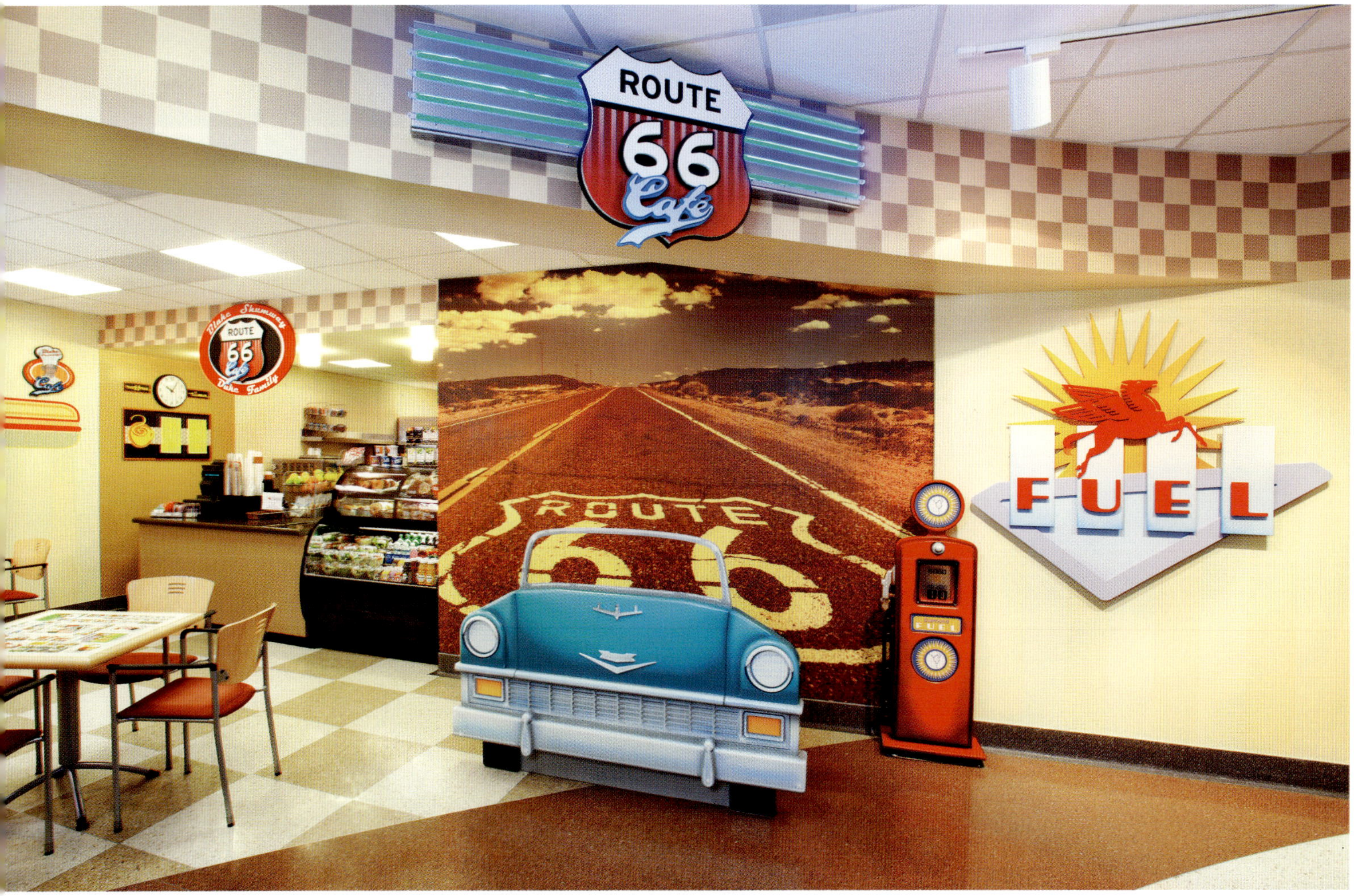

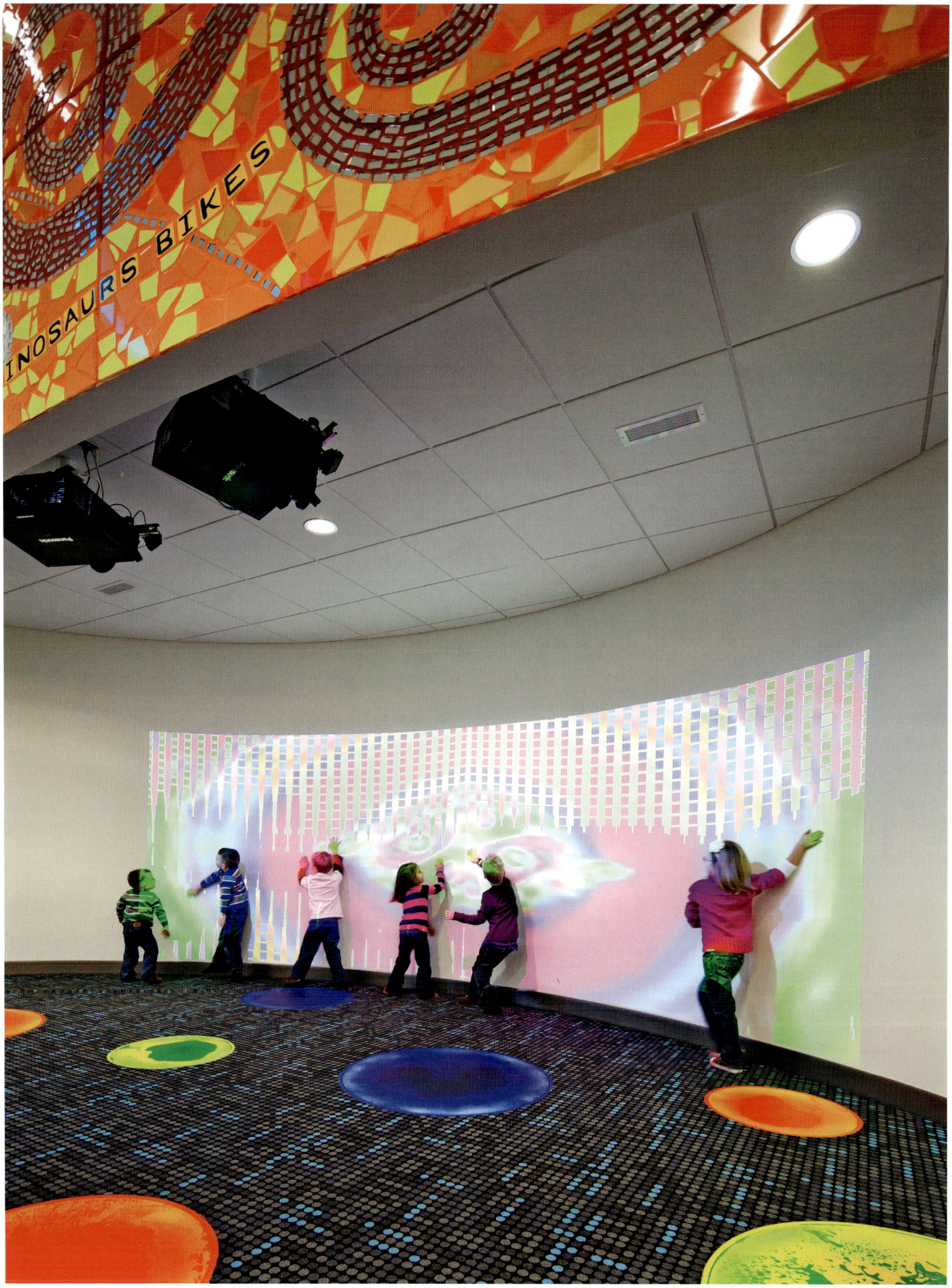

▲ Helen DeVos Children's Hospital, Grand Rapids, MI
Photo: Lucid Architecture, Eric DeWitt

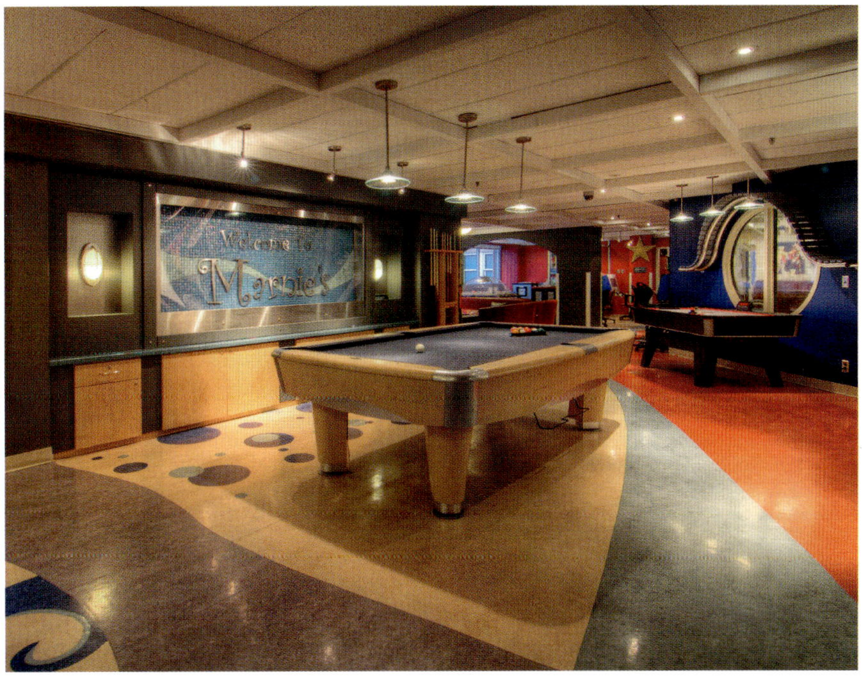

▲ SickKids The Hospital for Sick Children, Toronto, Ontario, Canada
Photo: Diogenes Baena, SickKids

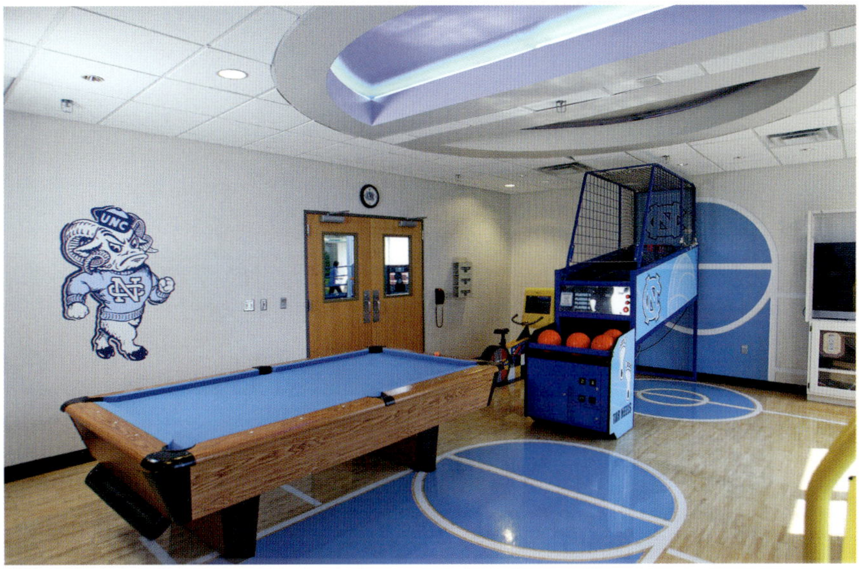

▲ UNC North Carolina Children's Hospital, Chapel Hill, NC
Photo: Brian Strickland

▼ Joseph M. Sanzari Children's Hospital at Hackensack University Medical Center, Hackensack, NJ
Photo: Basil Fargnol

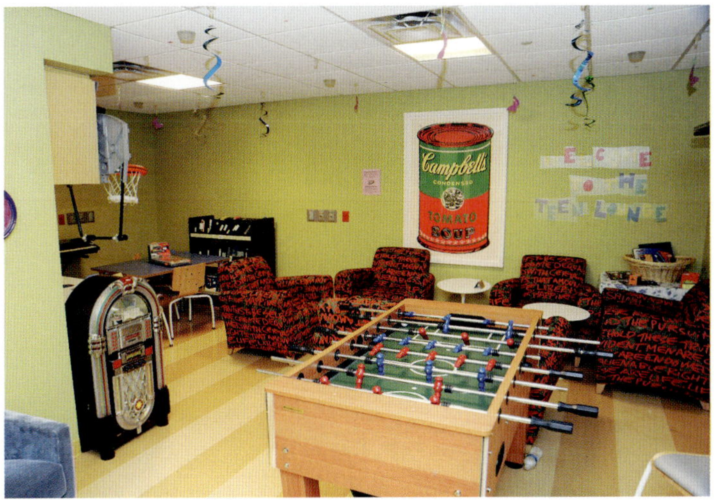

▼ St. Louis Children's Hospital, MO
Photo: Sam Fentress

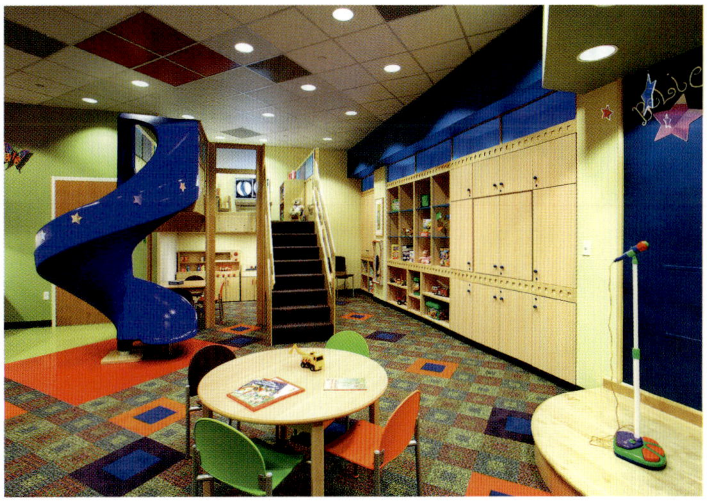

▼ Children's Hospital Colorado, Denver, CO
Photo: Tia Brayman

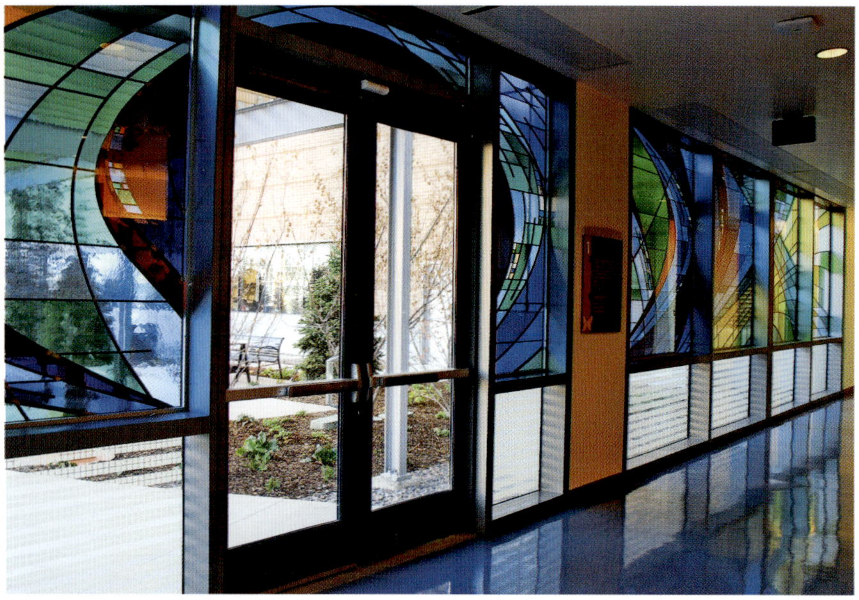

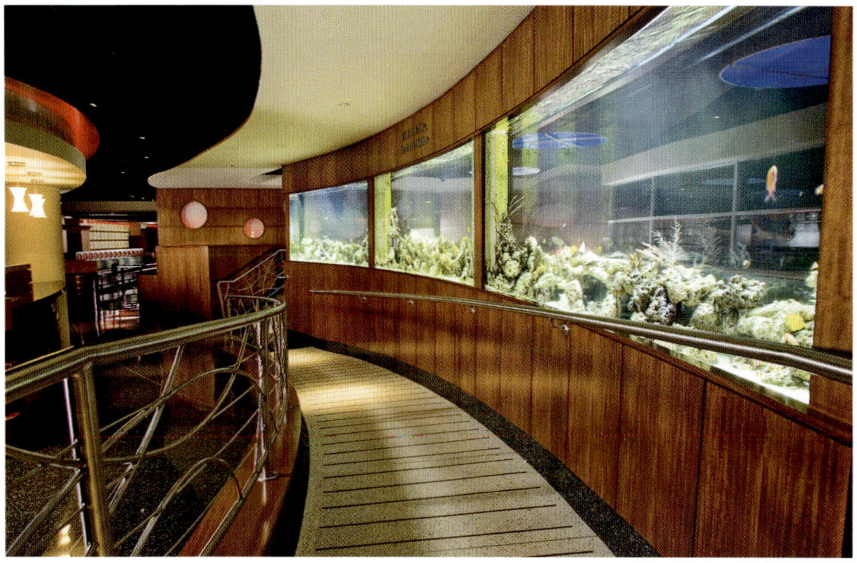

▲ Joseph M. Sanzari Children's Hospital at Hackensack University Medical Center, Hackensack, NJ
Photo: Steve Hockstein, Harvard Studio

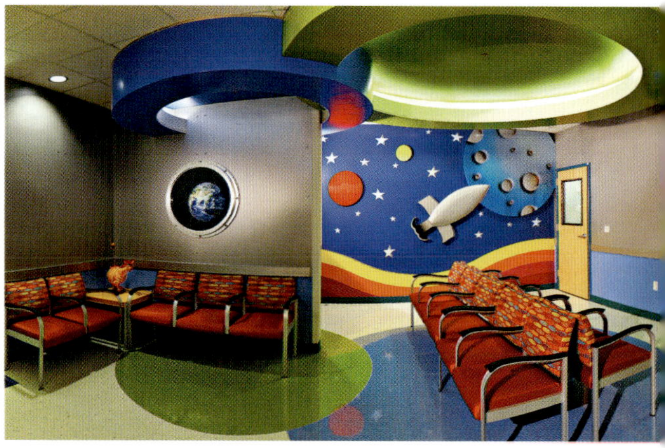

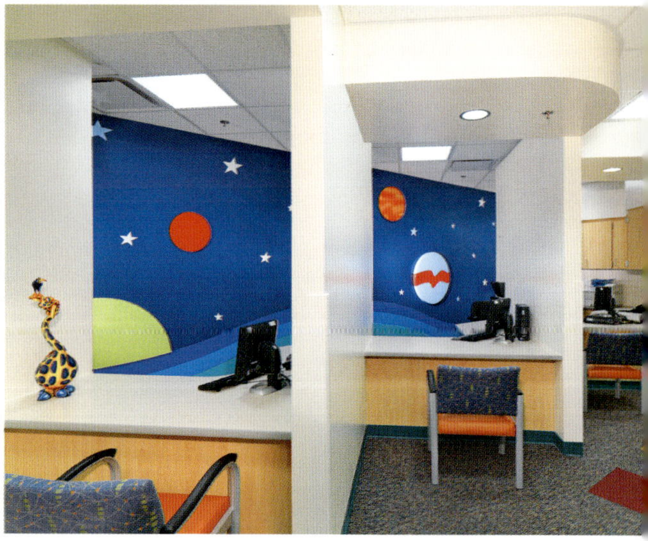

▲ Children's Hospital Central California, Madera, CA
Photos: Mullins Studio

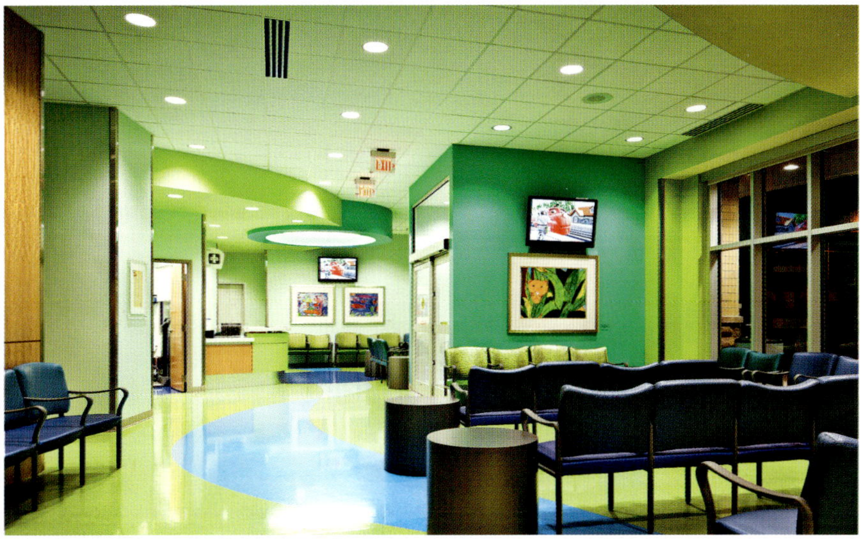

▲ Children's Healthcare of Atlanta, GA
Photo: Blake Marvin

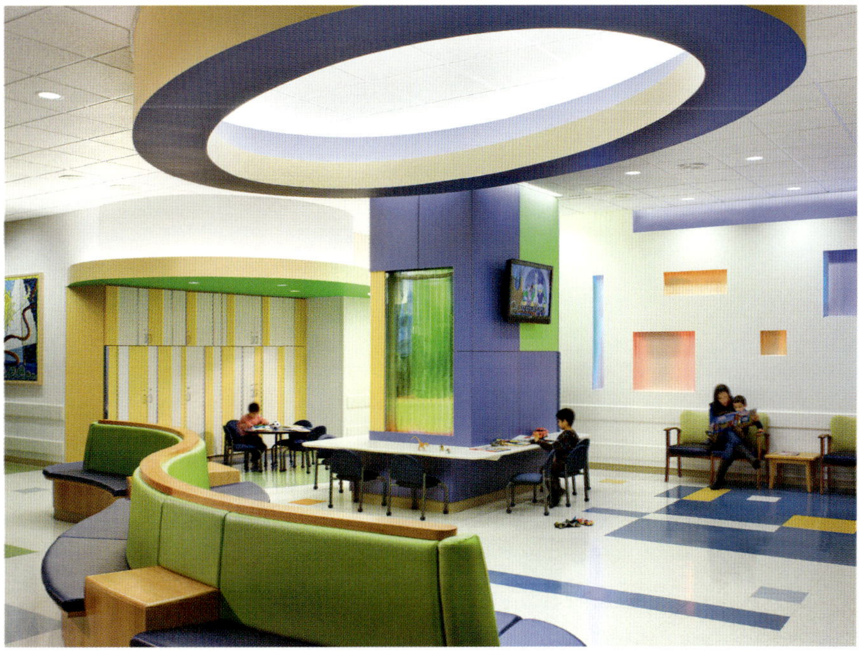

▲ Children's Hospital Boston, MA
Photo: Warren Jagger

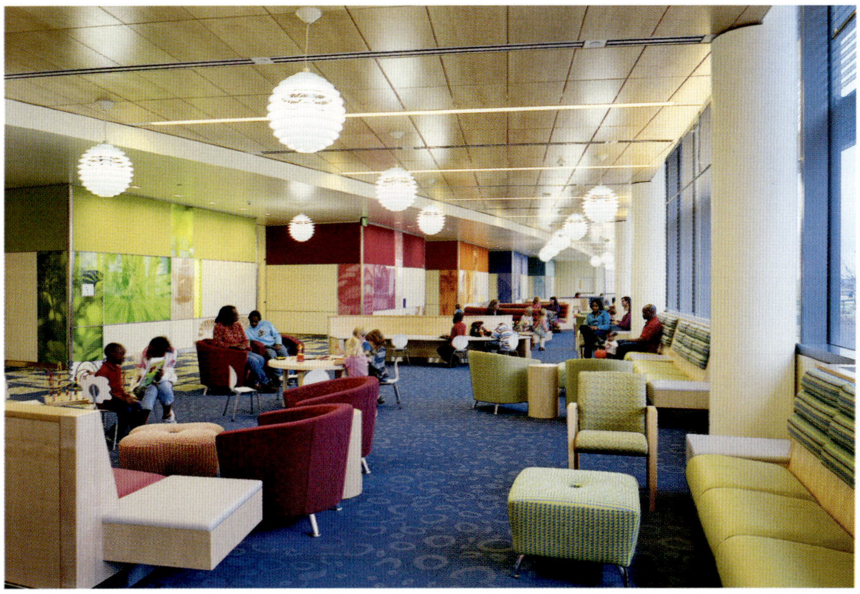

▲ Children's Hospital, Colorado, Denver, CO
Photo: Eckert & Eckert

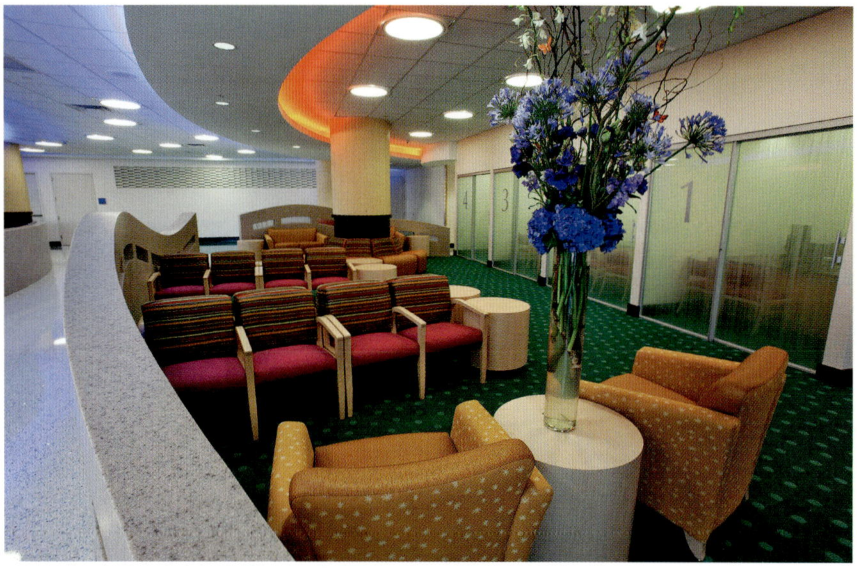

▲ Medical City Children's Hospital, Dallas, TX
Photo: Terry Cockerham

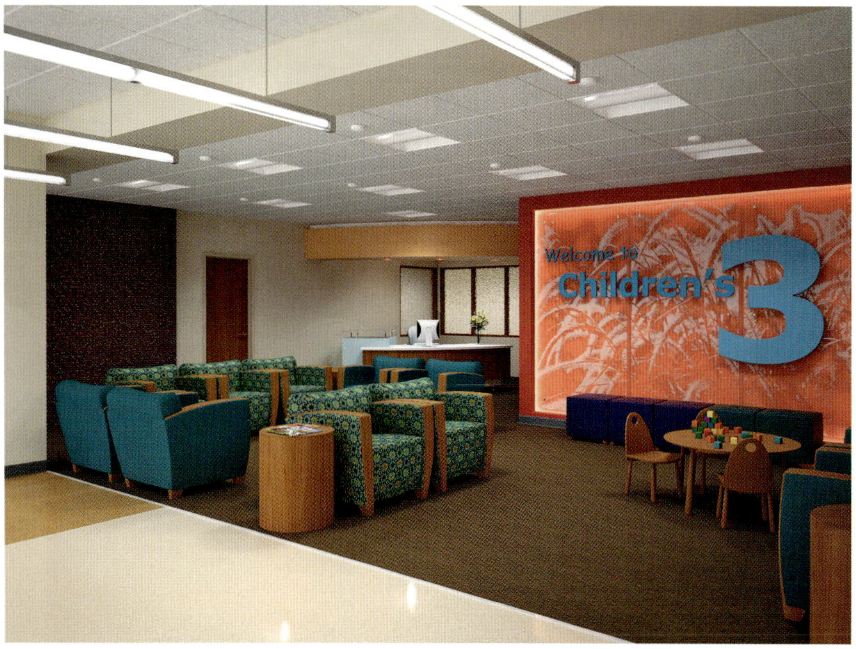

▲ Niswonger Children's Hospital, Johnson City, TN
Photo: Will Griffith

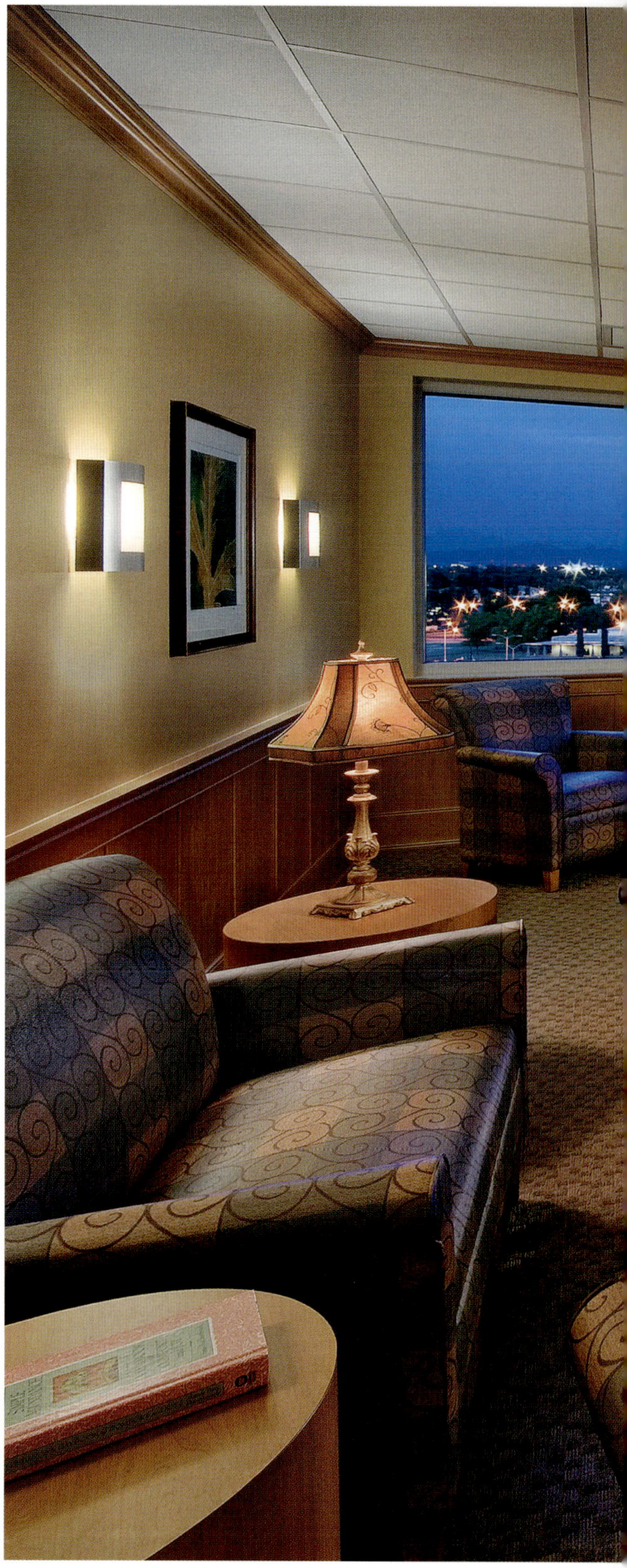

▲ Cardon Children's, Mesa, AZ
Photo: courtesy of HDR Architecture, Inc. © 2010 Mark Boisclair Photography

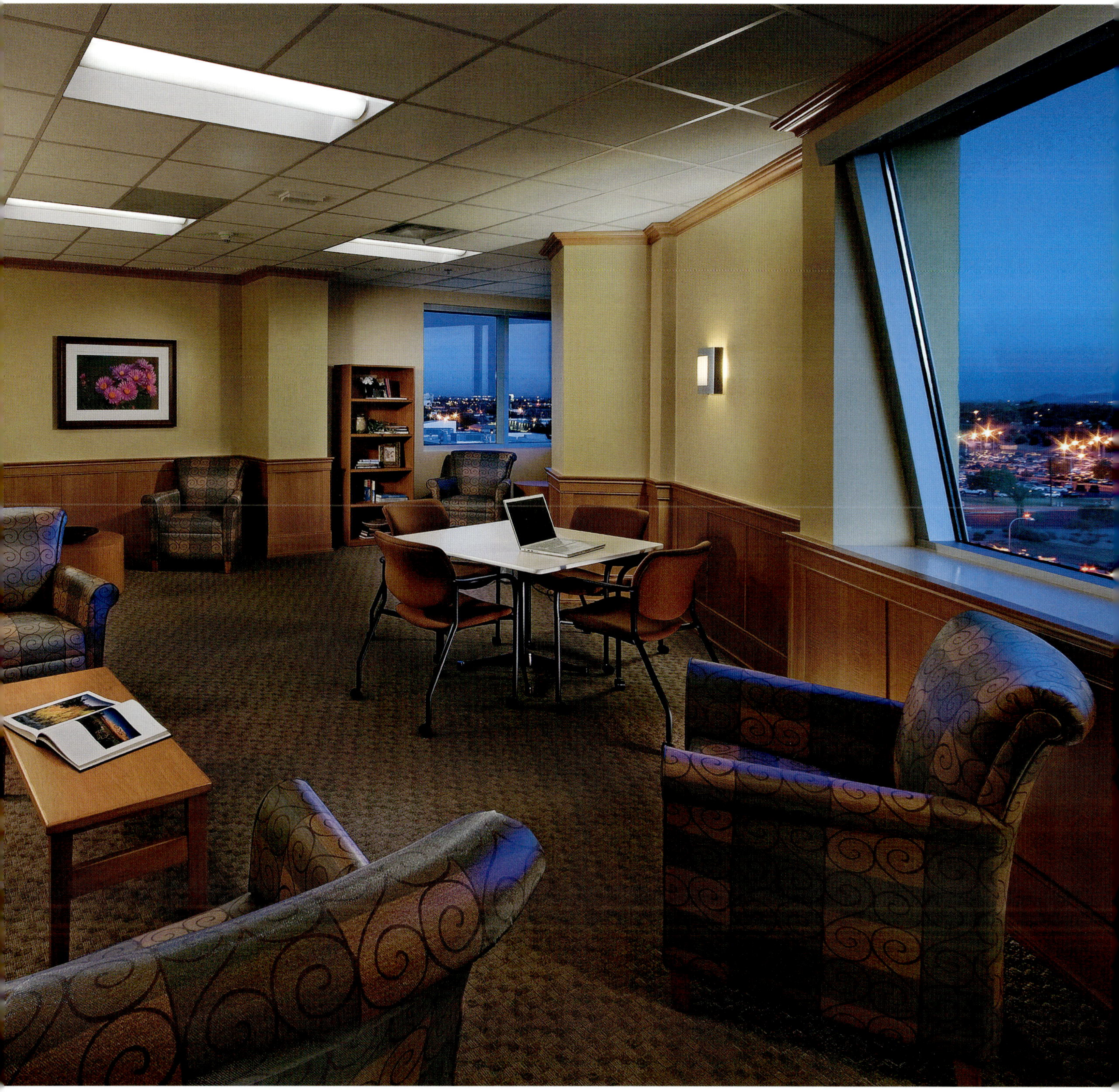

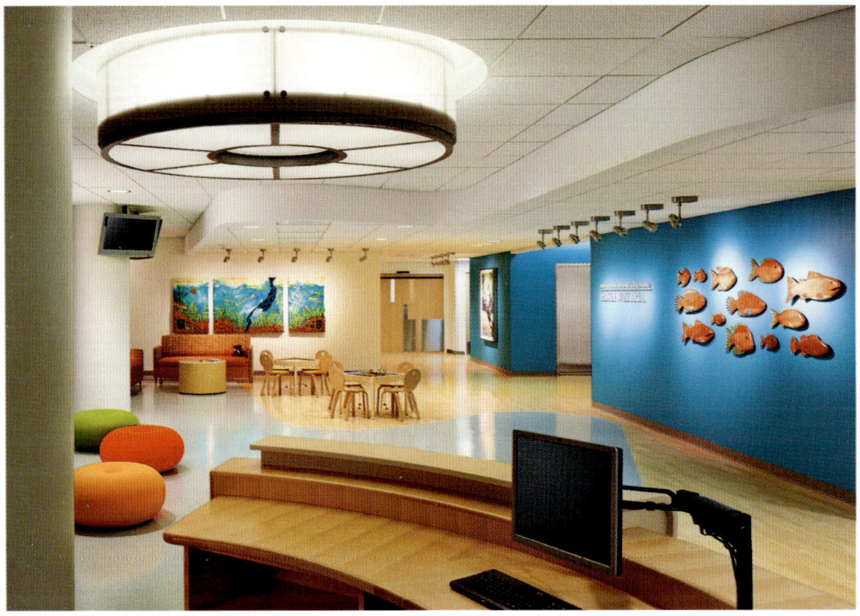

▲ Children's Hospital of Illinois at OSF Saint Francis Medical Center, Peoria, IL
Photo: Christopher Barrett

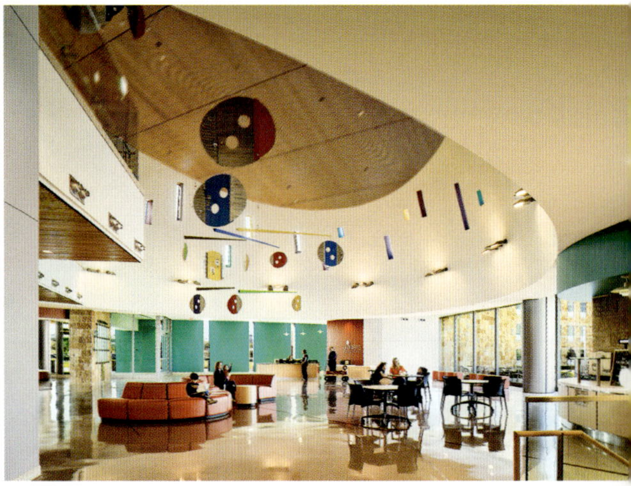

▲ Children's Medical Center at Legacy, Plano, TX
Photo: Robert Canfield

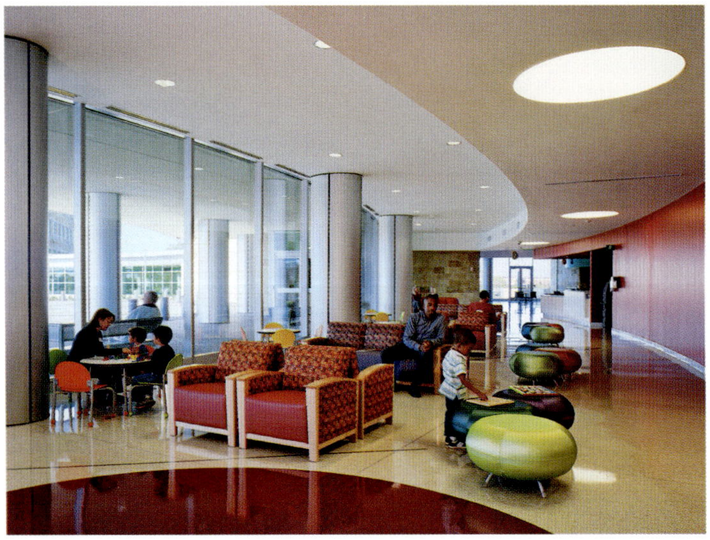

▲ Children's Medical Center at Legacy, Plano, TX
Photo: Eckert & Eckert

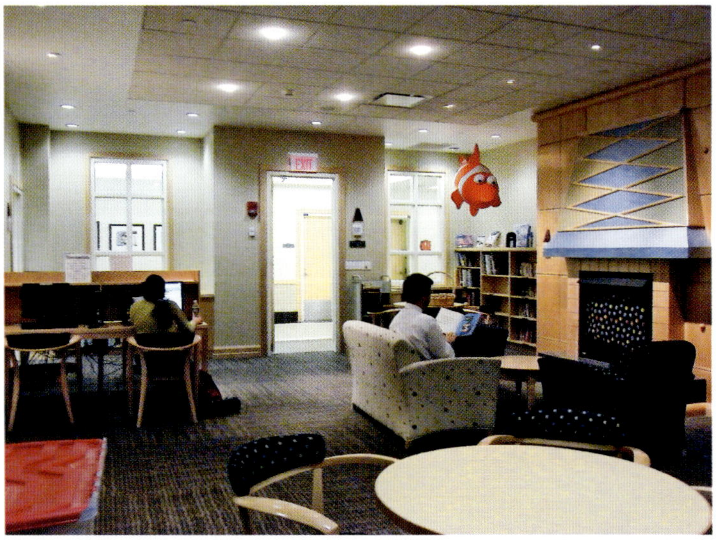

▲ Maria Fareri Children's Hospital, Valhalla, NY
Photo: Westchester Medical Center

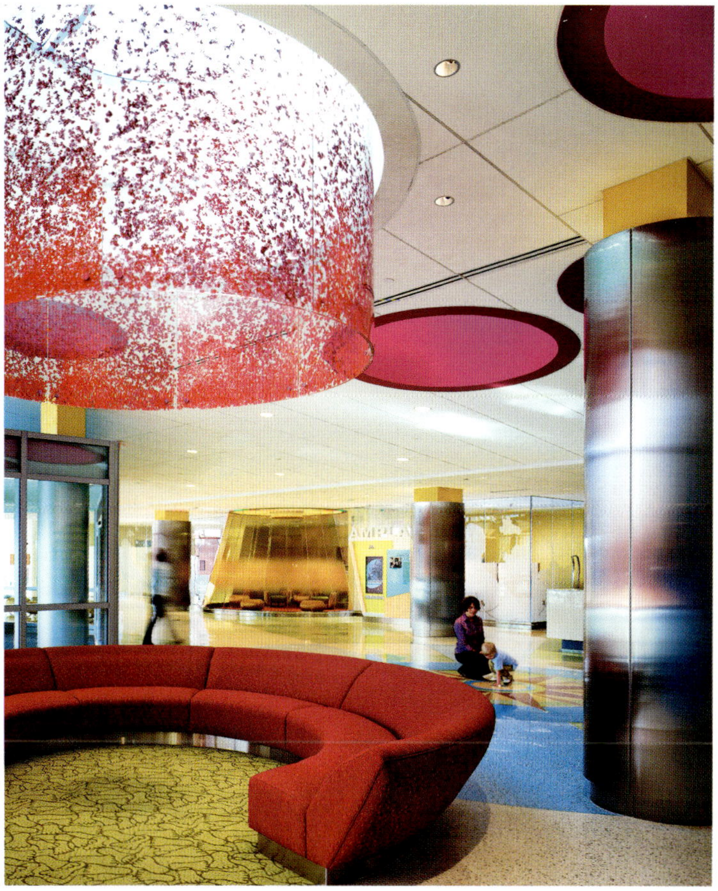

▲ University of Minnesota Amplatz Children's Hospital, Minneapolis, MN
Photo: Hedrich Blessing Photography, Nick Merrick

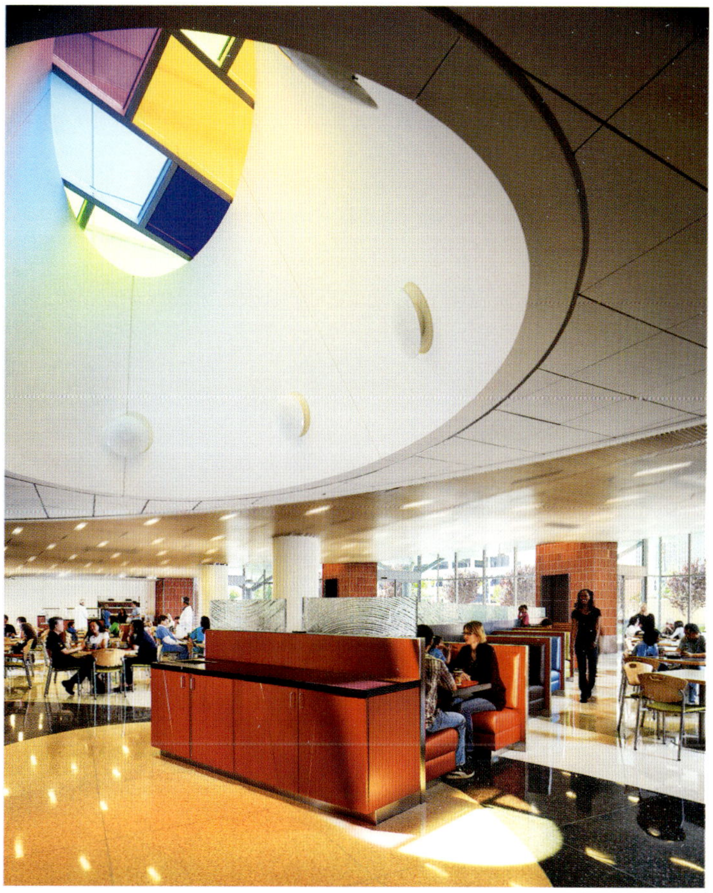

▲ Children's Hospital Los Angeles, CA
Photo: Hedrich Blessing Photography, Nick Merrick

▼ SSM Cardinal Glennon Children's Medical Center, St. Louis, MO
Photo: Christner, Inc.

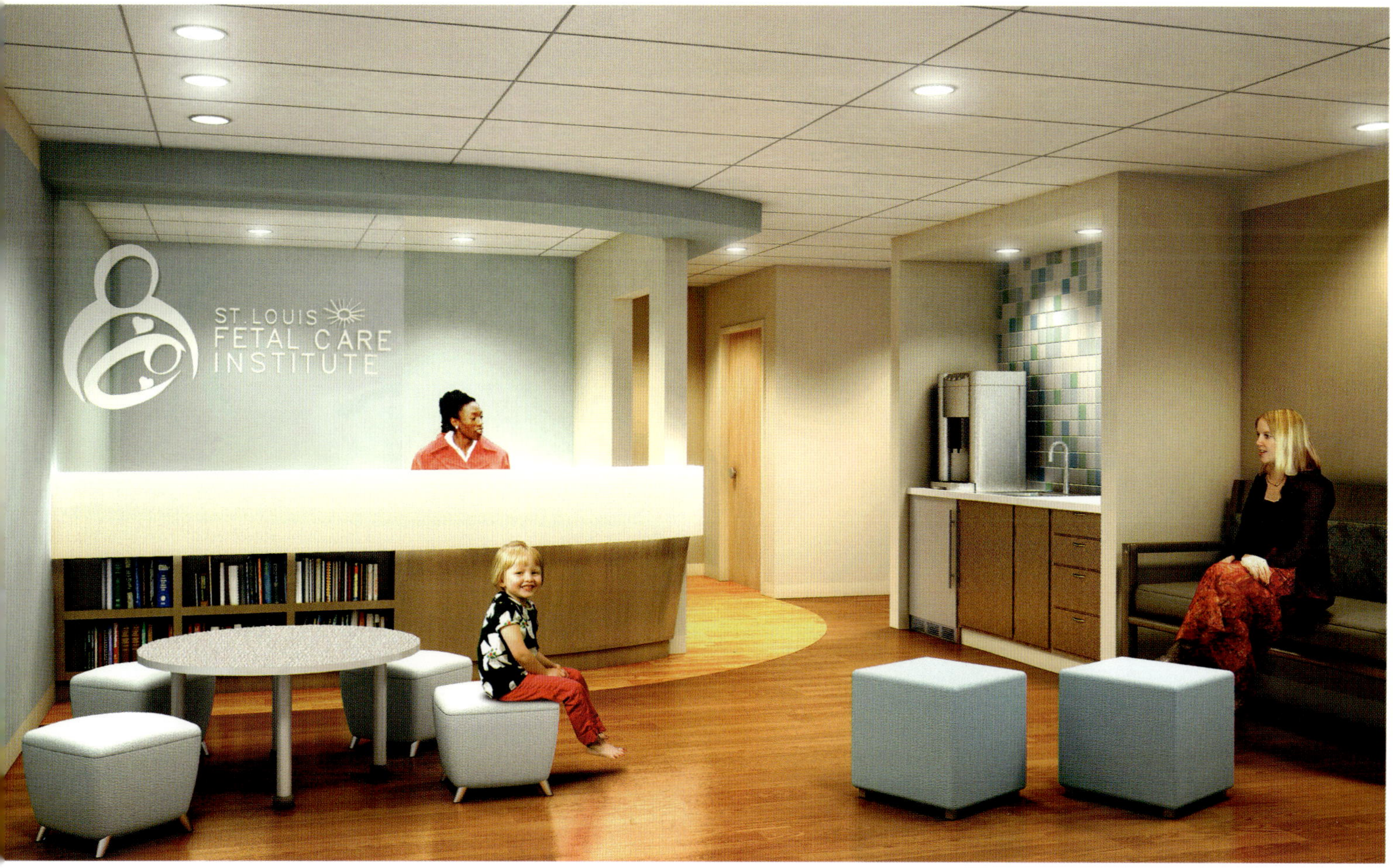

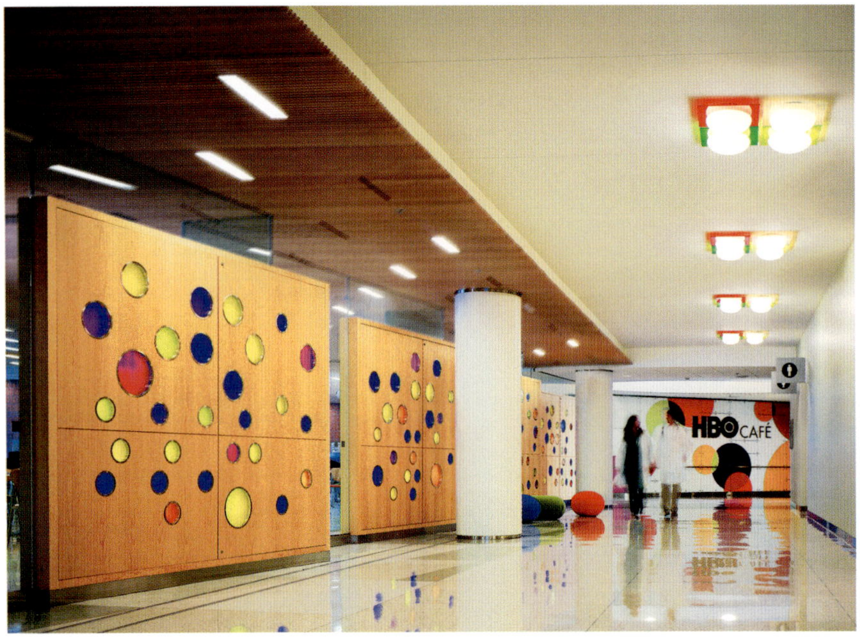

▲ Children's Hospital Los Angeles, CA
Photo: Hedrich Blessing Photography, Nick Merrick

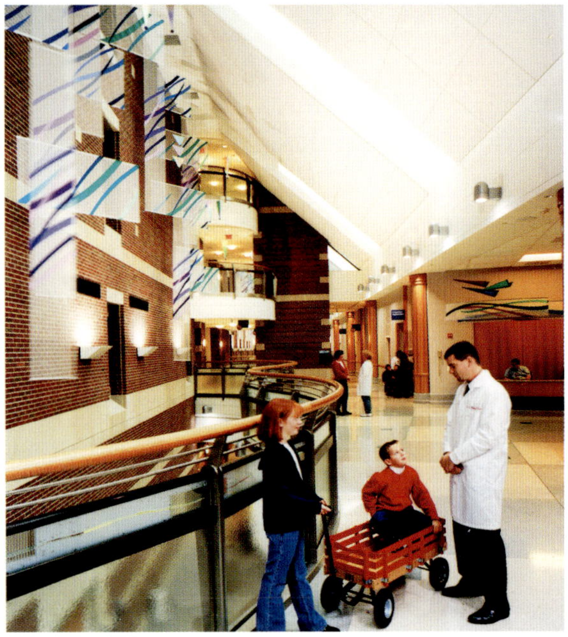

▲ Riley Children's Outpatient Center University of Indiana, Indianapolis, IN
Photo: Michael O'Callahan

▼ Cardon Children's, Mesa, AZ
Photo: courtesy of HDR Architecture, Inc. © 2010 Mark Boisclair Photography Inc.

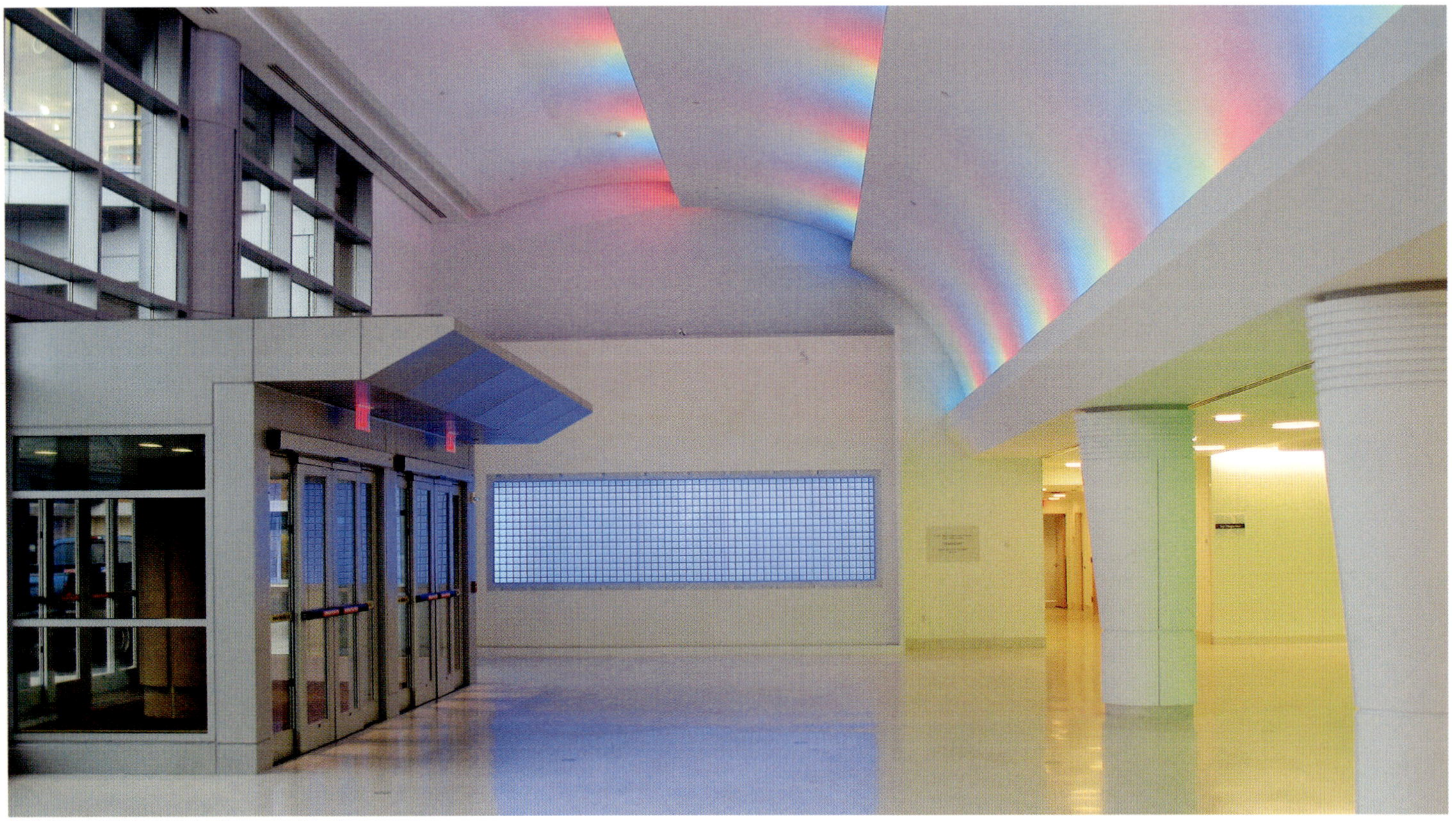

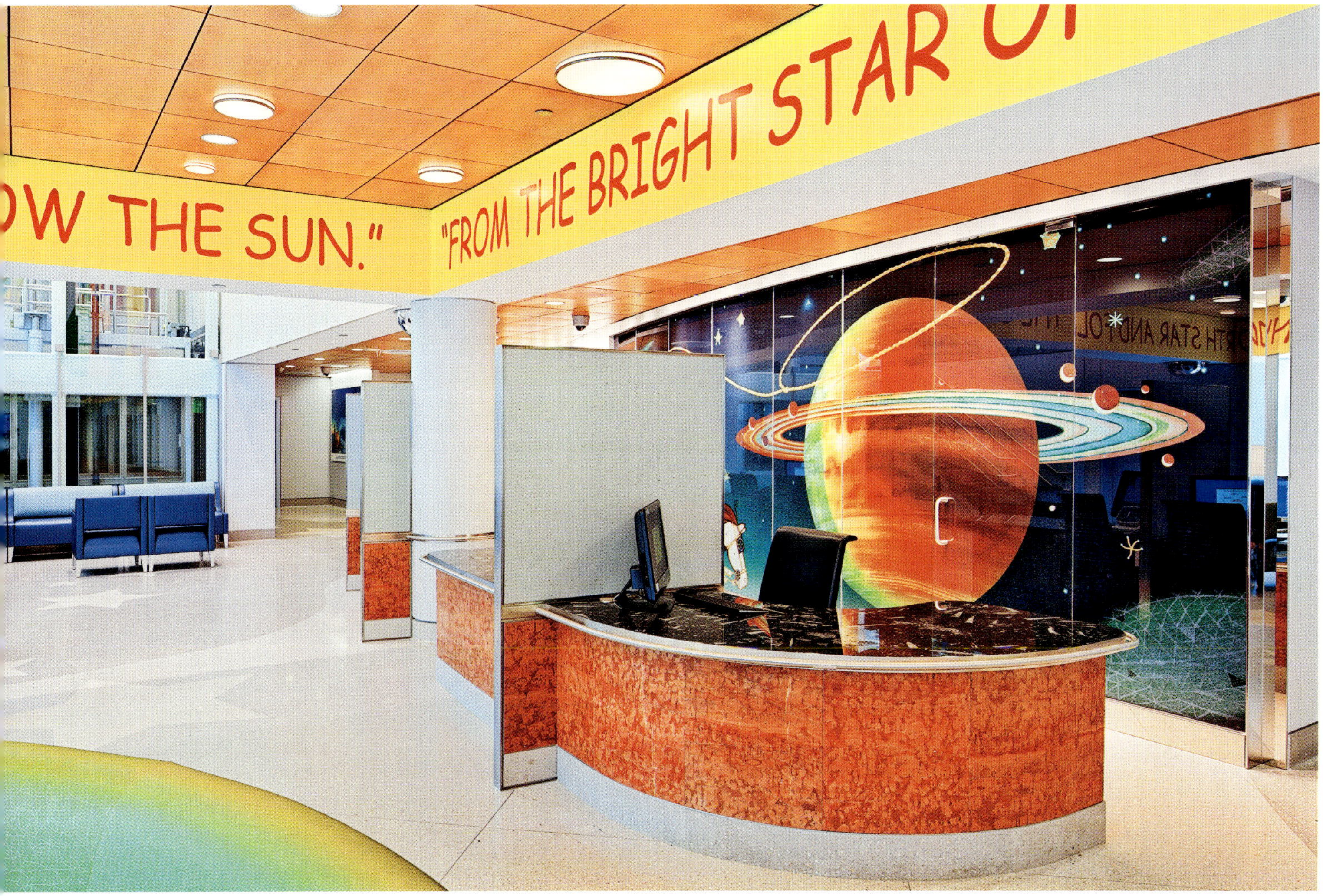

▲ Morgan Stanley Children's Hospital, New York, NY
Photo: Jeffrey Totaro Photographer

▼ Children's Medical Center, Dallas, TX
Photo: Charles Smith

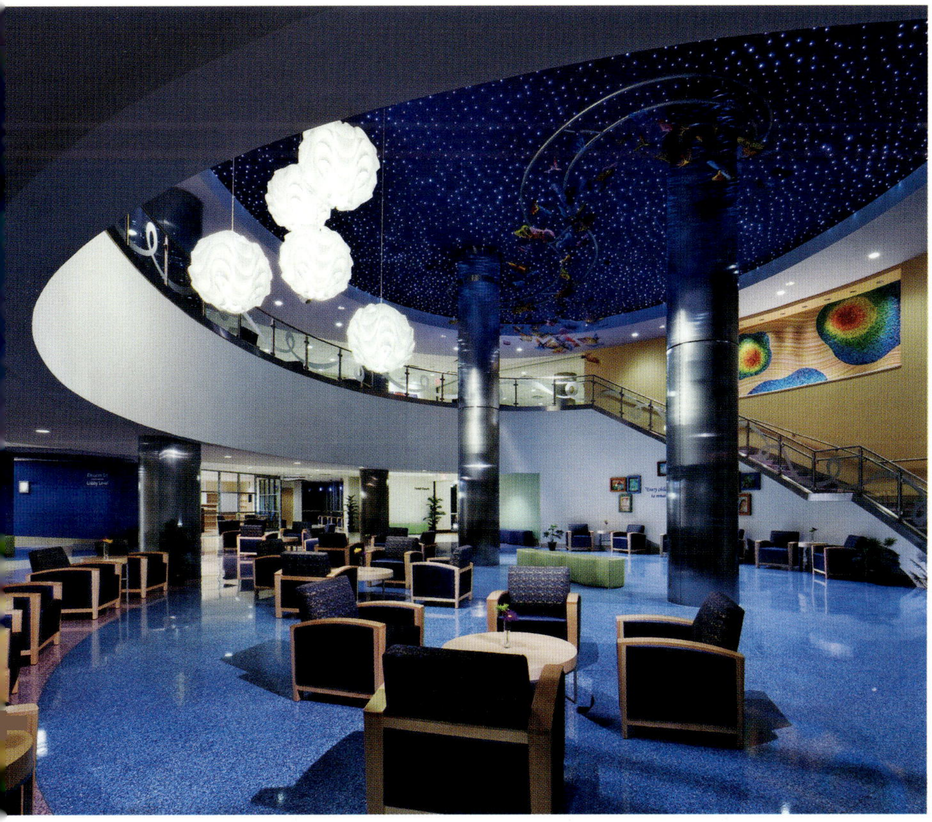

▼ Phoenix Children's Hospital, AZ
Photo: Blake Marvin, HKS

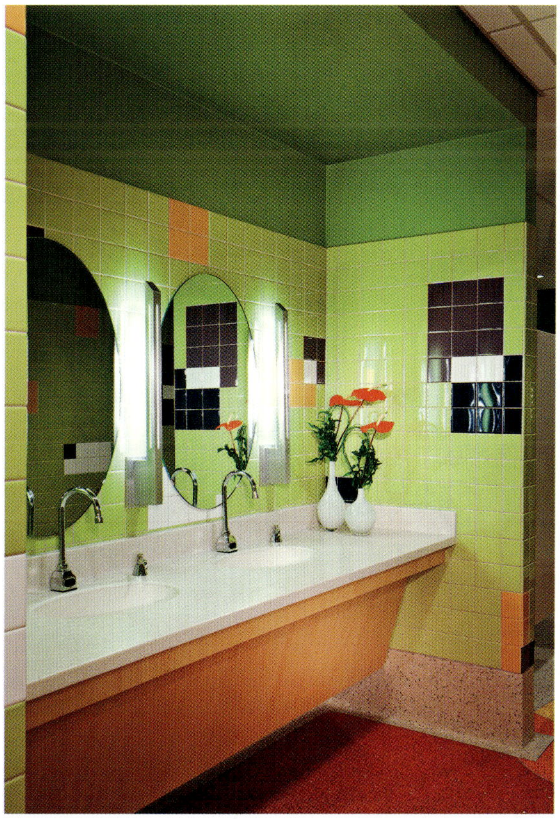

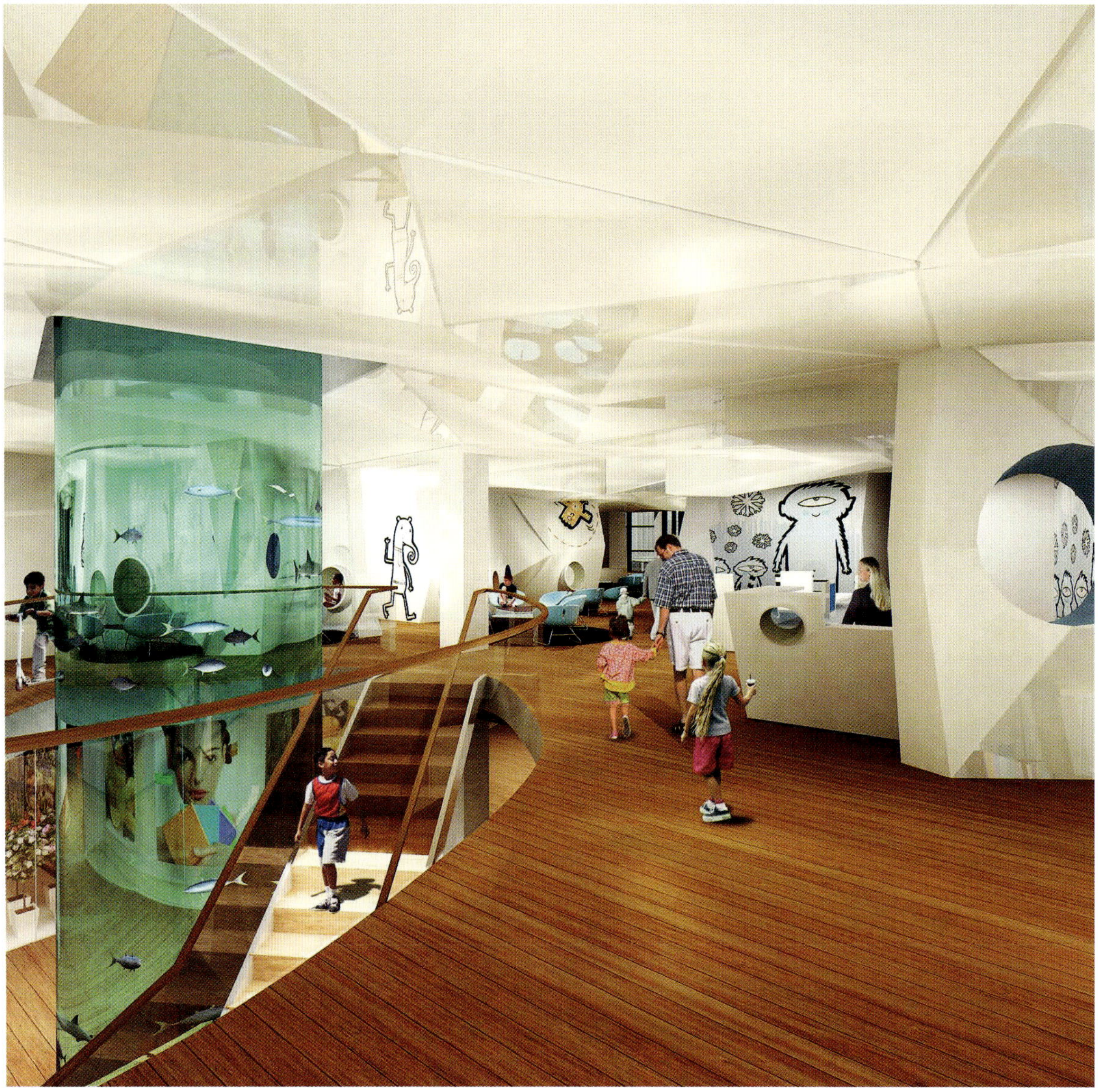

▲ University of Melbourne Hospital, Melbourne, Victoria, Australia
Photo: Stantec ©

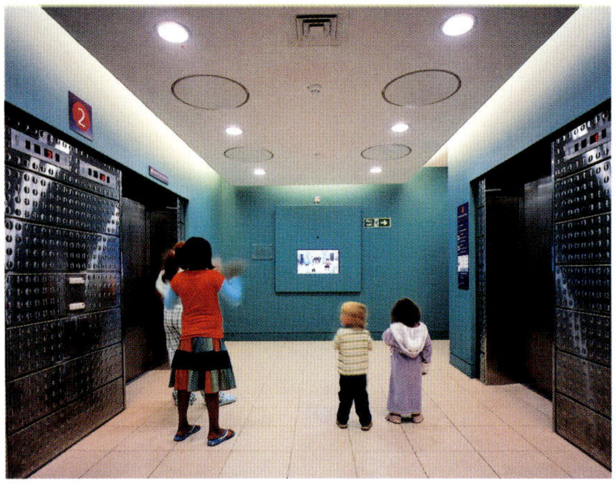

▲ Great Ormond Street Children's Hospital, Octav Botnar Building, London, United Kingdom
Photo: Stantec © Edward Sumner

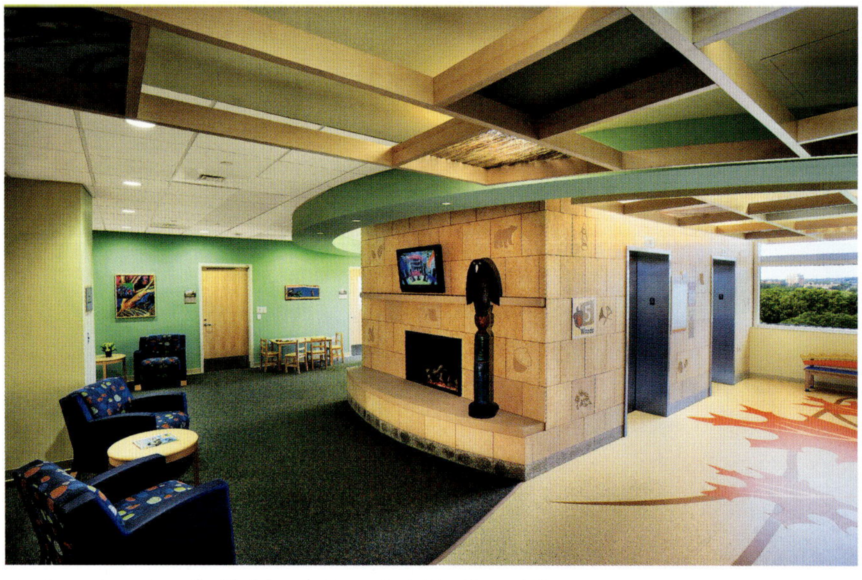

▲ American Family Children's Hospital, Madison, WI
Photo: HDR Architecture, Inc. © 2007 Ballogg Photography Inc., Chicago

▼ Children's Healthcare of Atlanta, GA
Photo: Blake Marvin

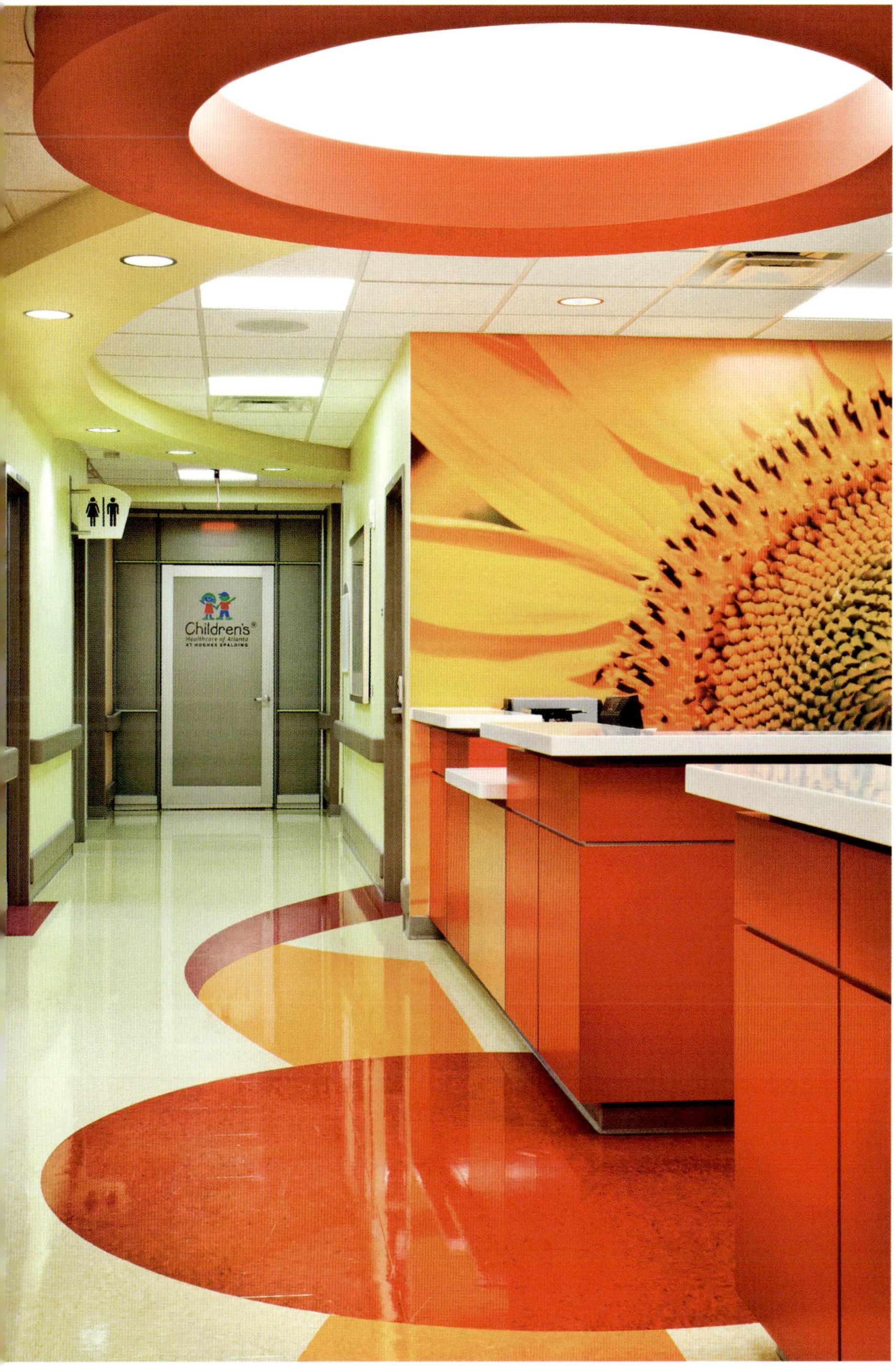

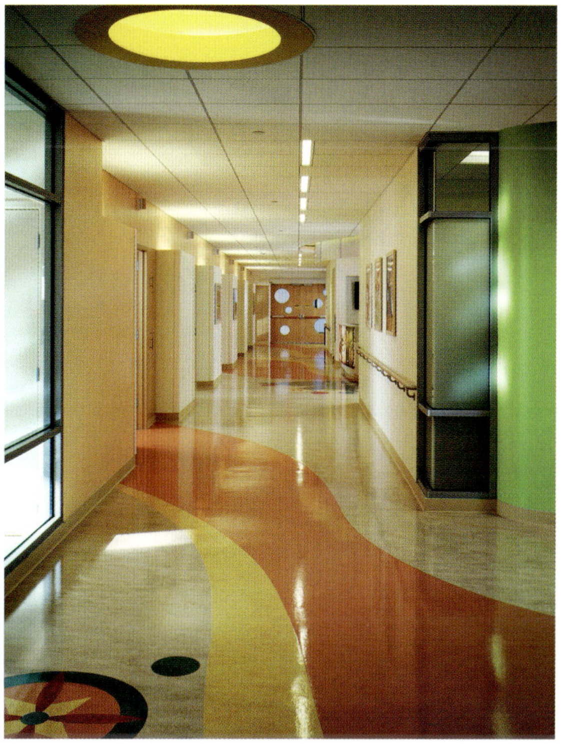

▲ University of Minnesota Amplatz Children's Hospital, Minneapolis, MN
Photo: Hedrich Blessing Photography, Nick Merrick

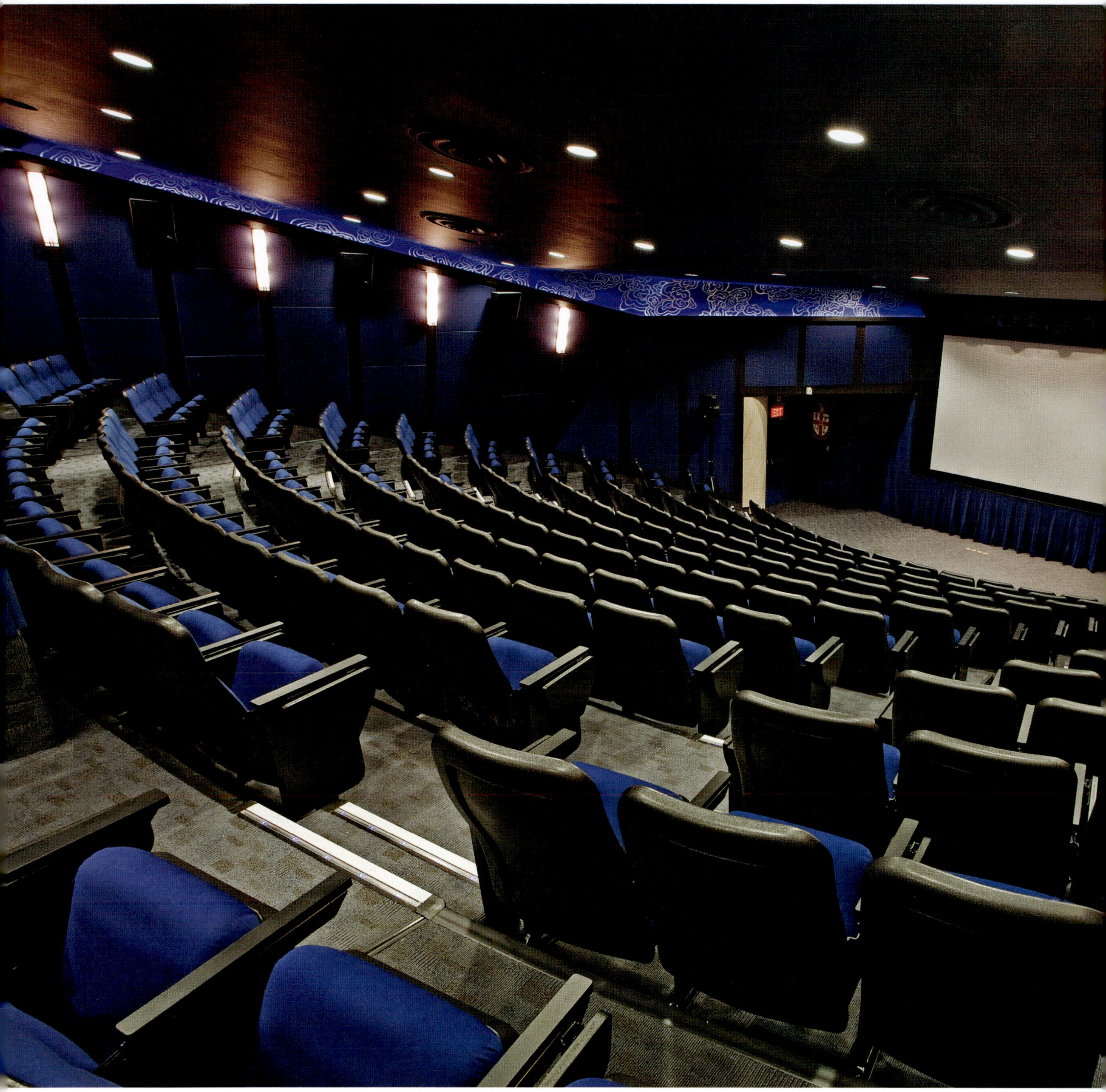

▲ SickKids The Hospital for Sick Children, Toronto, Ontario, Canada
Photo: Diogenes Baena, SickKids

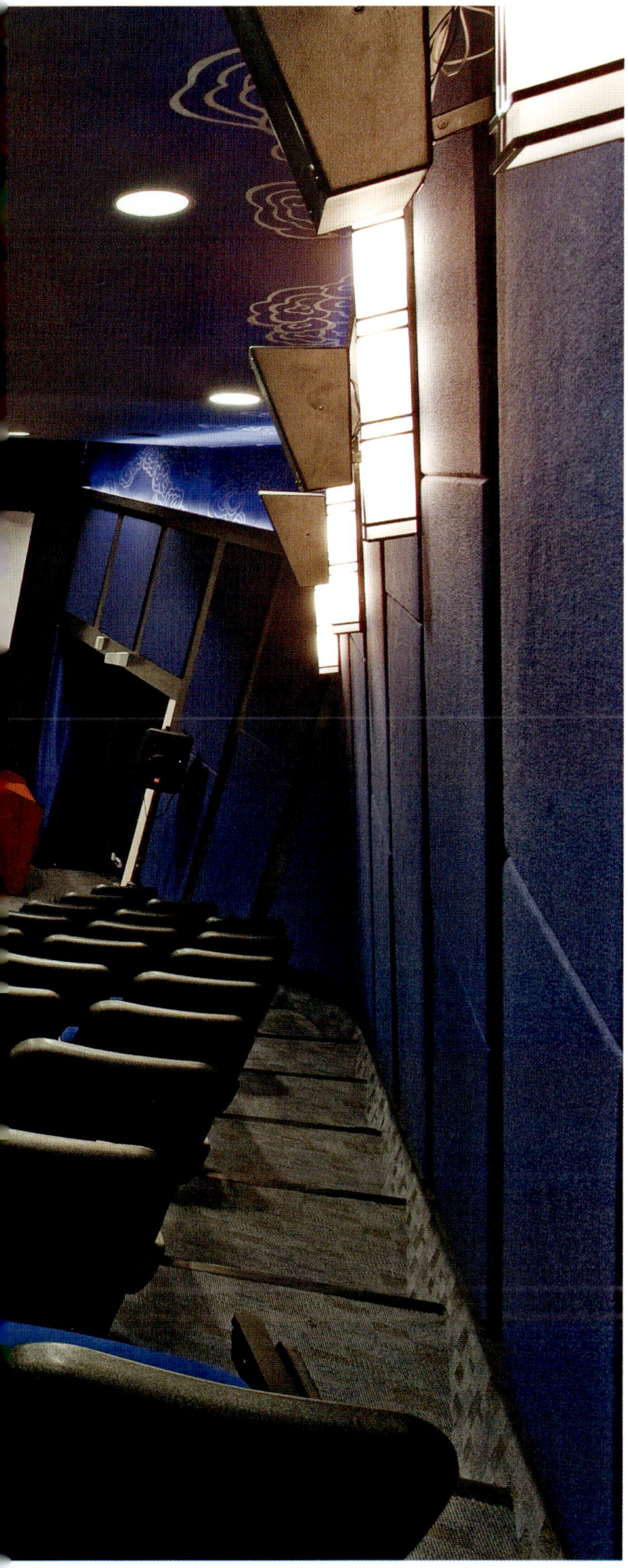

▼ Memorial Sloan-Kettering Cancer Center, New York, NY
Photo: Stantec © Paul Warchol

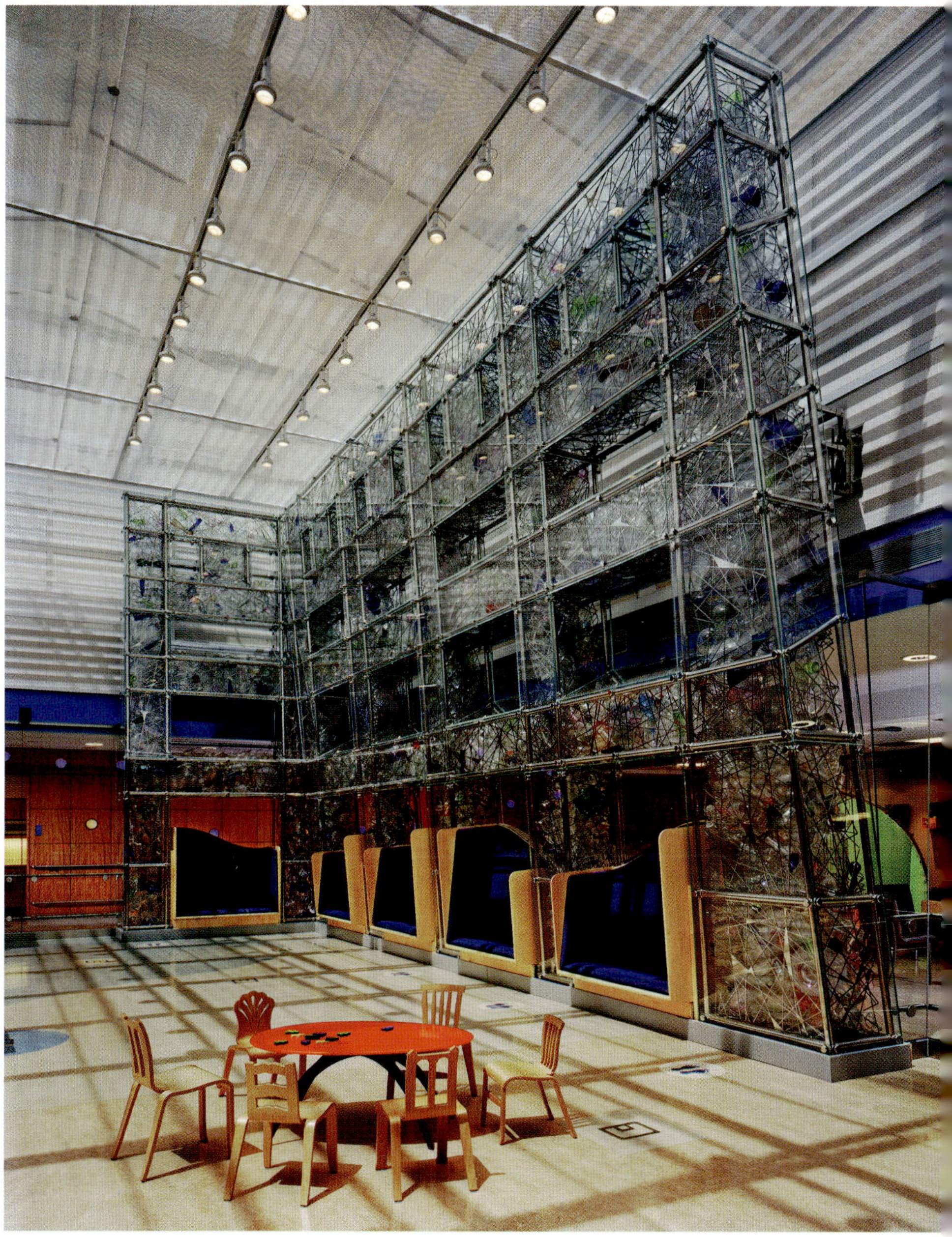

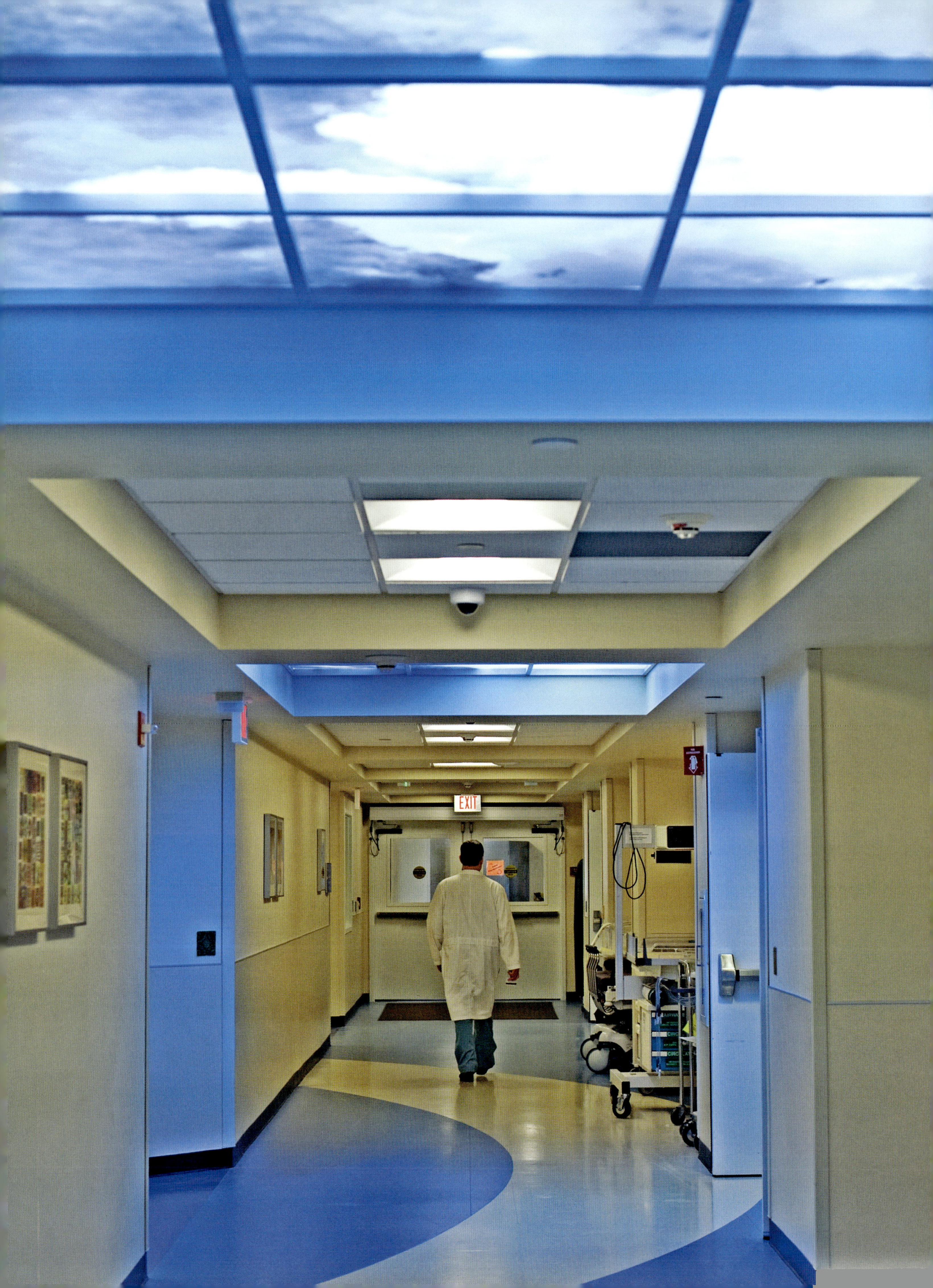
EXIT

Patient Care Spaces

Maya Angelou, famed American poet, echoed the feelings of many healthcare consumers when she said, "I've learned that people will forget what you said, people will forget what you did, but people will never forget how you made them feel."

As the quality of healthcare has improved, exemplary care has become the new normal. This in turn has led patients and families to demand more from healthcare providers. In response, many providers are expanding their focus to include the optimal patient experience.

The patient experience includes everything from the interactions a patient has with a hospital, to the ways a patient's emotional, spiritual, and medical needs are met. In pediatric design, the key to creating a positive patient experience is following a patient/family-centered care model and ensuring that all patient areas are healing environments. As these concepts are continually enhanced by Lean, LEED, and evidence-based strategies, the patient experience will evolve and become the genesis for the design of future pediatric spaces.

The future will challenge us to create spaces that enhance the patient experience—where form not only follows function, but feelings as well, and where laughter or a smile might just become a key measure of success.

Jim Hohenstein, AIA
HDR

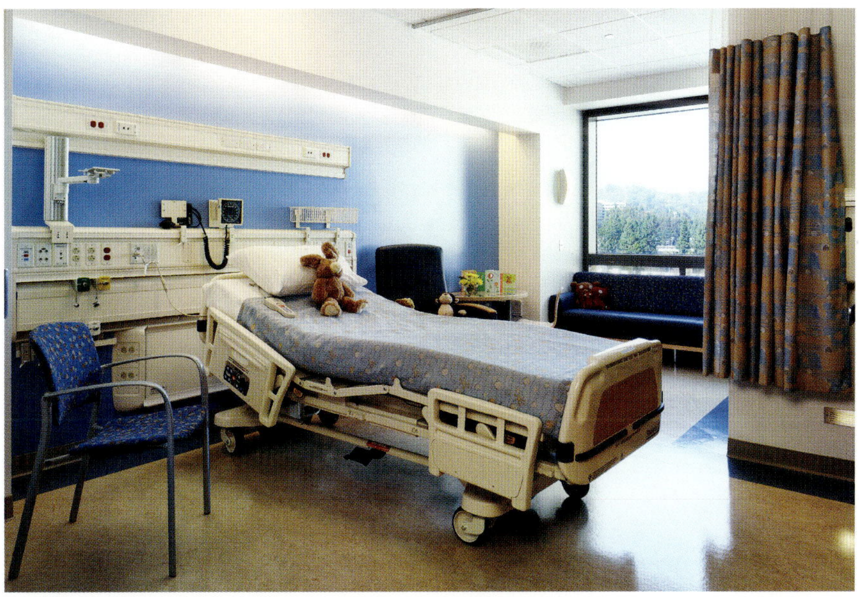

▲ Mattel Children's Hospital UCLA, Los Angeles, CA
Photo: Benny Chan, fotoworks

◀ Dayton Children's, OH
Photo: Ken Shory

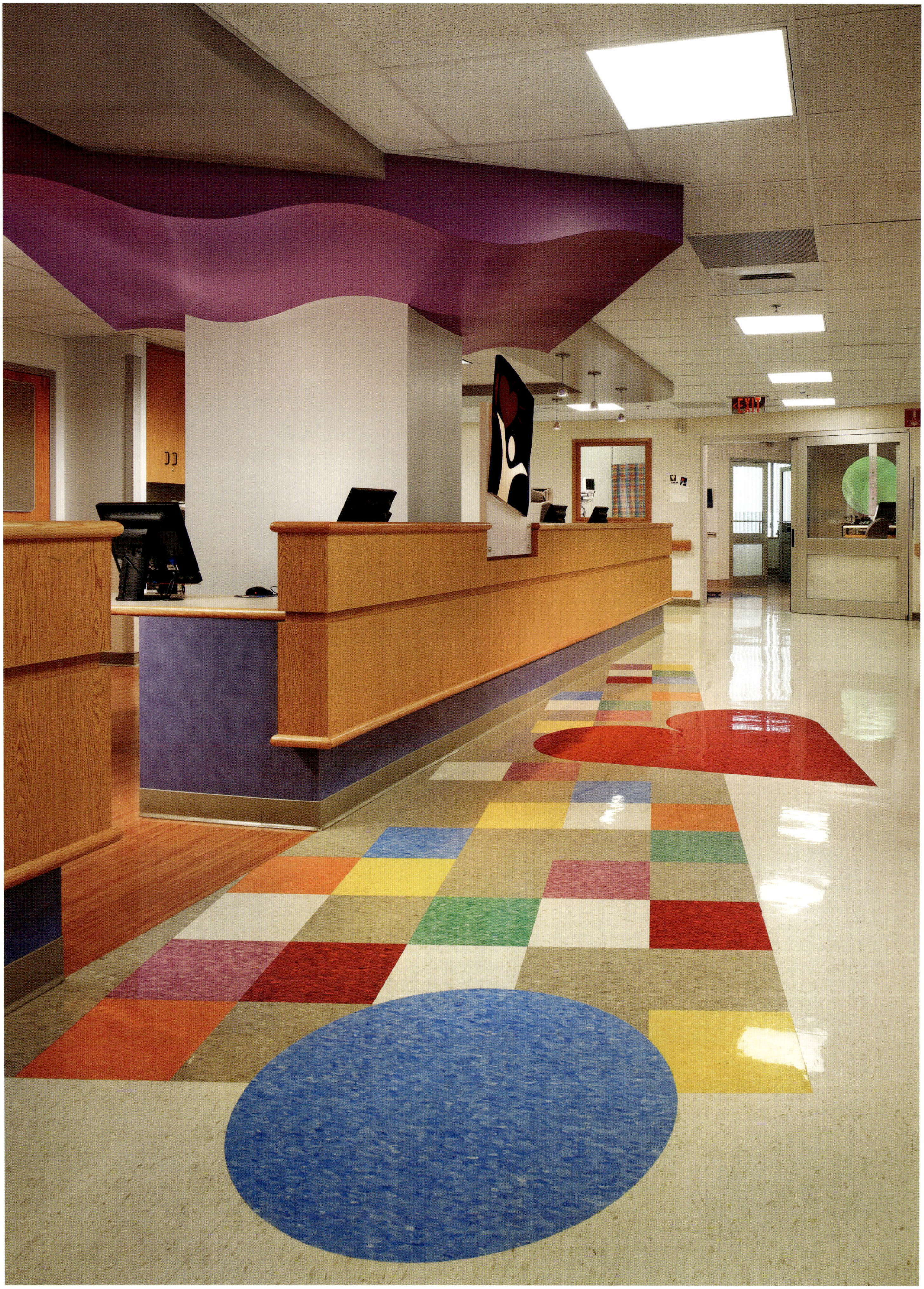
EXIT

◀ Children's Hospital of Philadelphia, PA
Photo: The Children's Hospital of Philadelphia

▼ Phoenix Children's Hospital, AZ
Photo: Blake Marvin, HKS

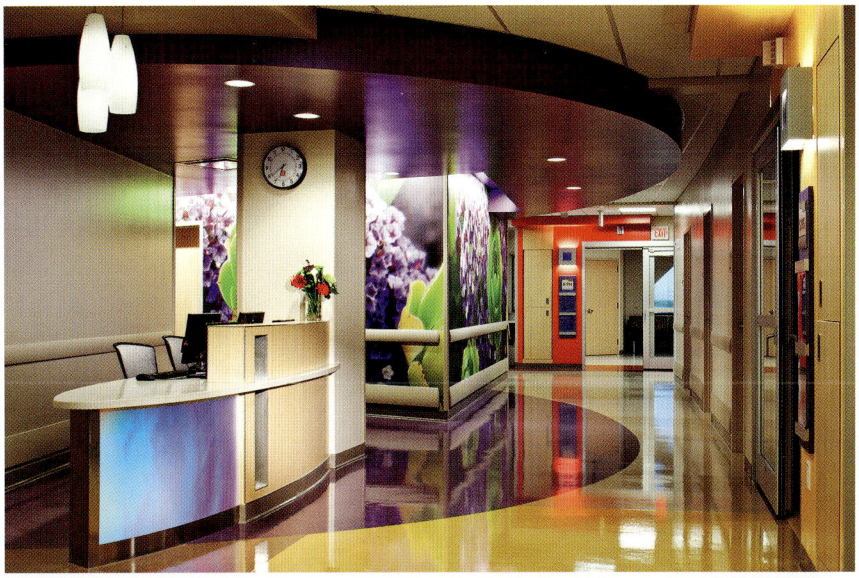

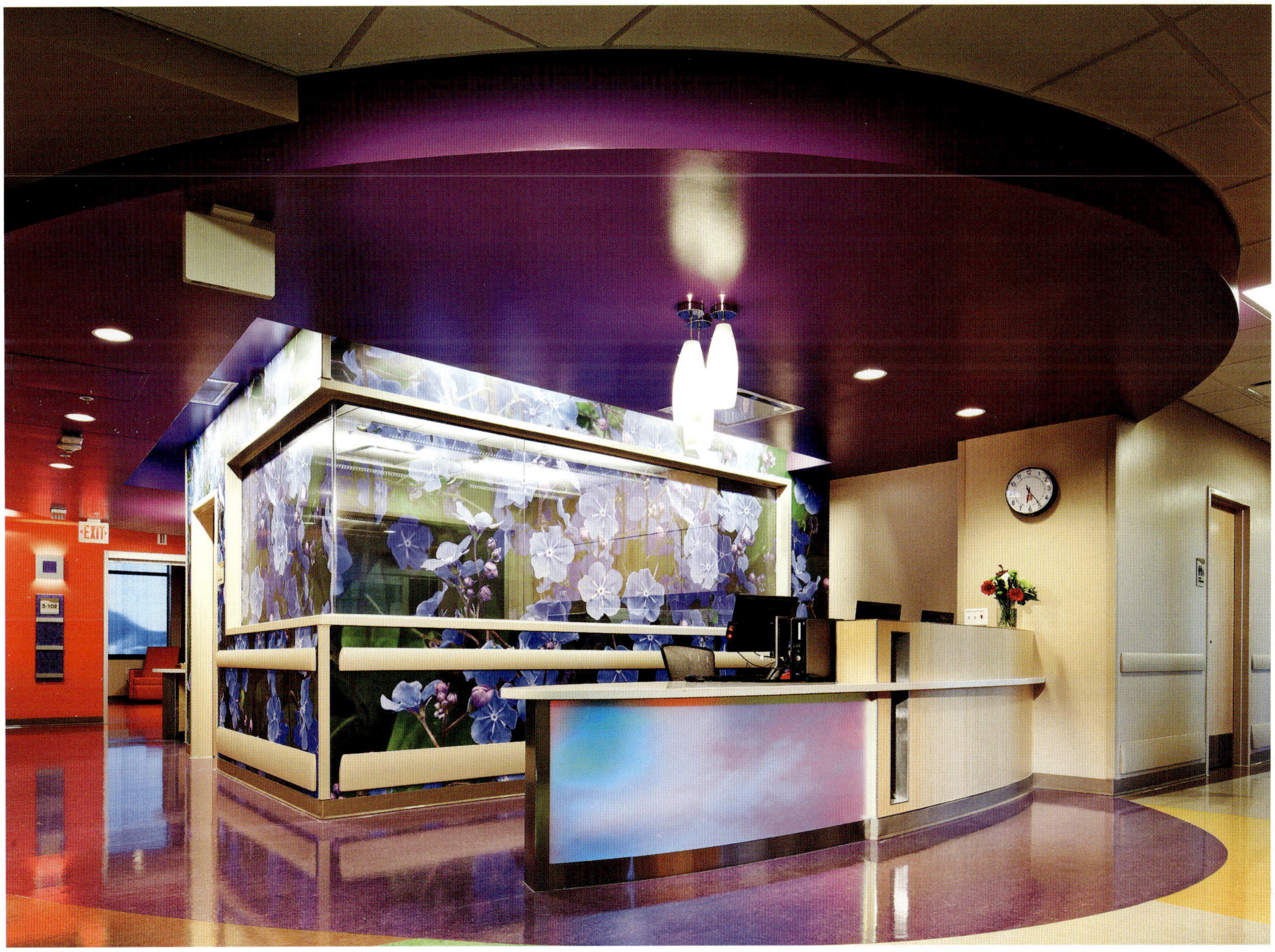

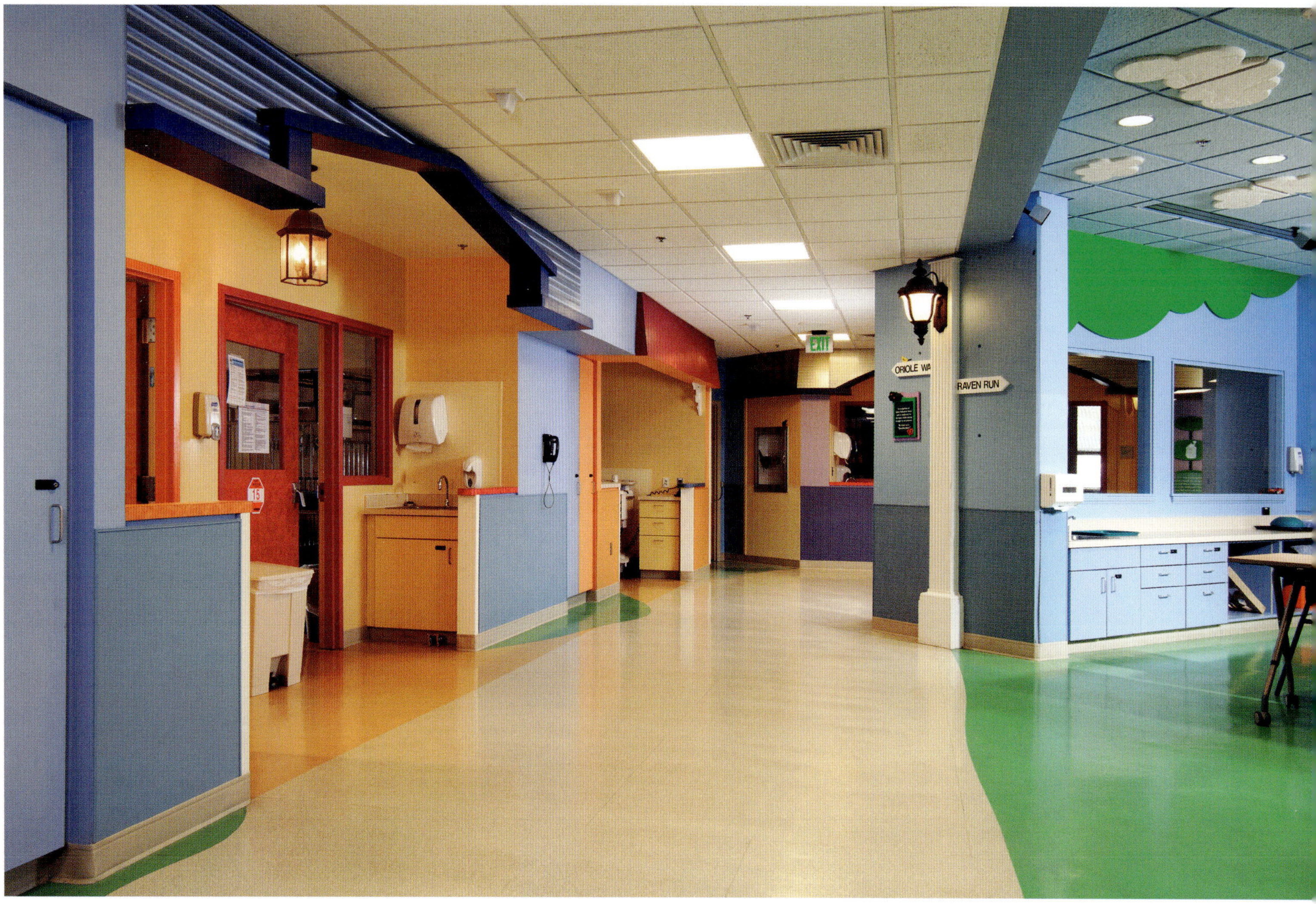

▲ Mt. Washington Pediatric Hospital, Baltimore, MD
Photo: Jeffrey Totaro Photographer

▼ Arkansas Children's Hospital, Little Rock, AR
Photo: Kelley Cooper

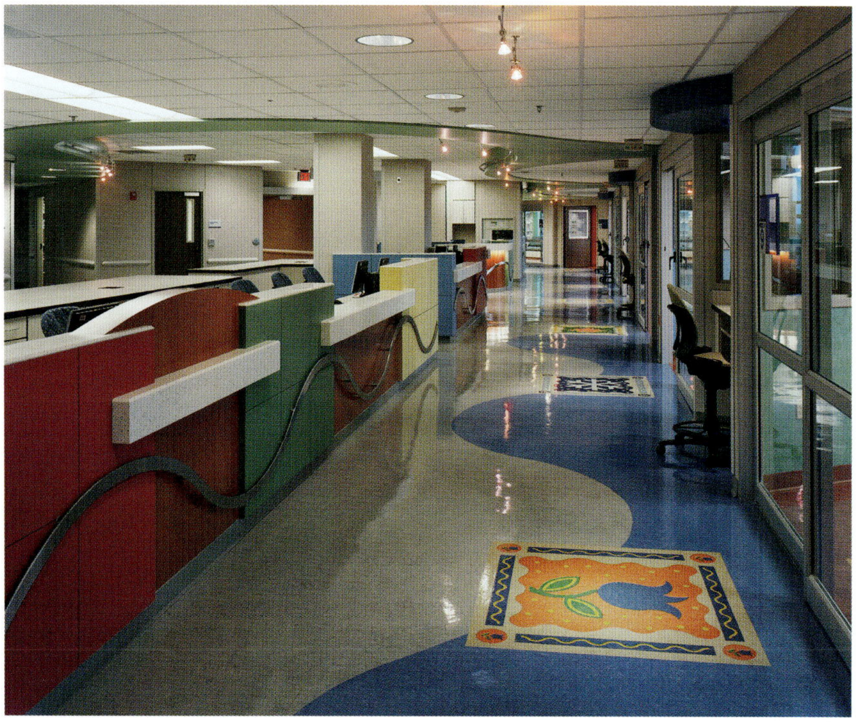

▼ Helen DeVos Children's Hospital, Grand Rapids, MI
Photo: Lucid Architecture, Eric DeWitt

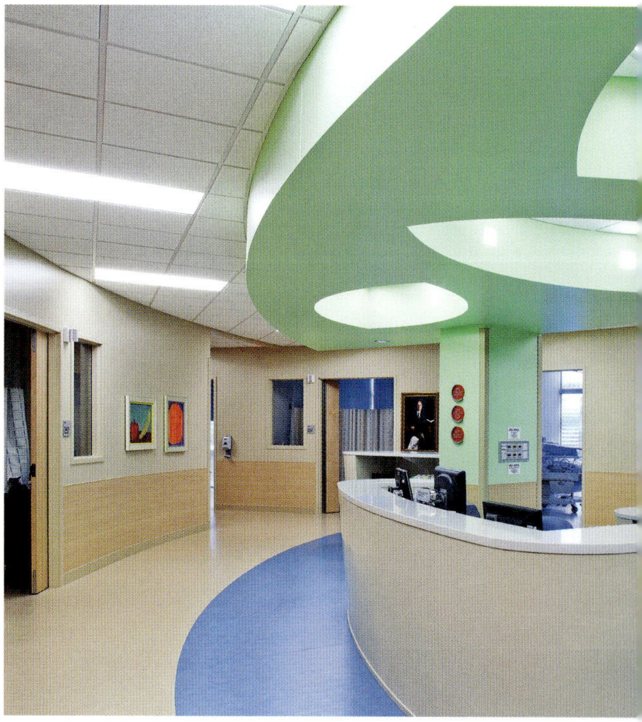

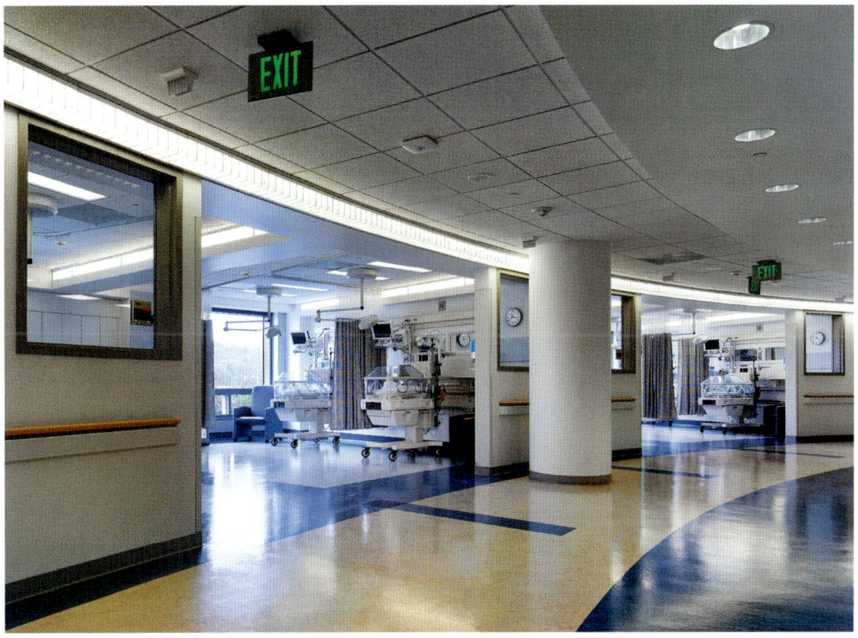

▲ Mattel Children's Hospital UCLA, Los Angeles, CA
Photo: Benny Chan, fotoworks

▼ Morgan Stanley Children's Hospital, New York, NY
Photo: Jeffrey Totaro Photographer

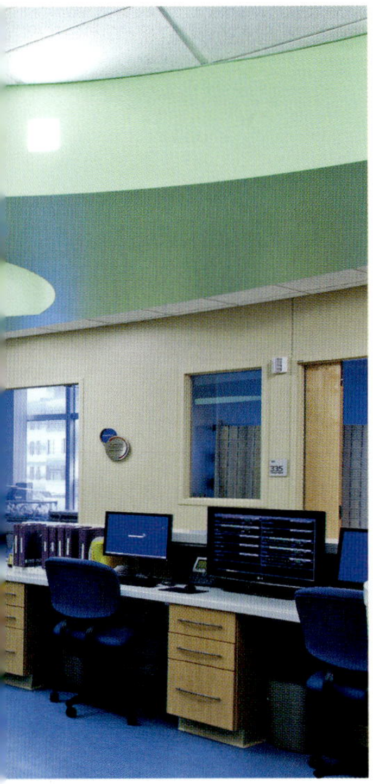

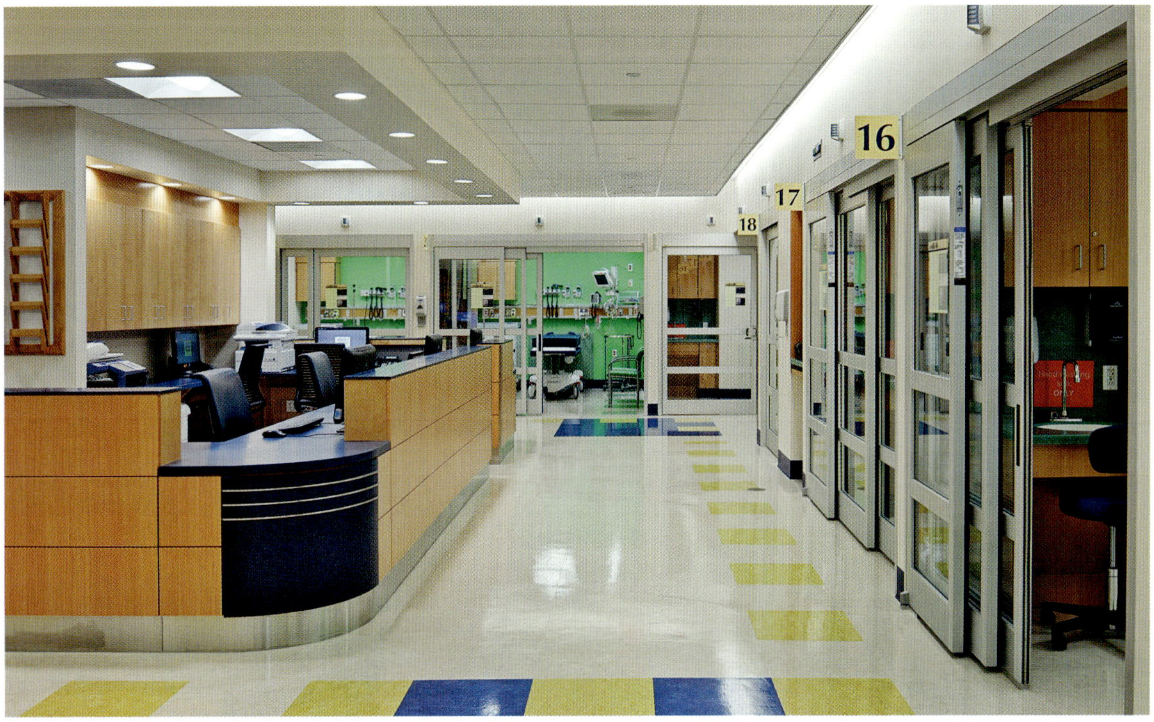

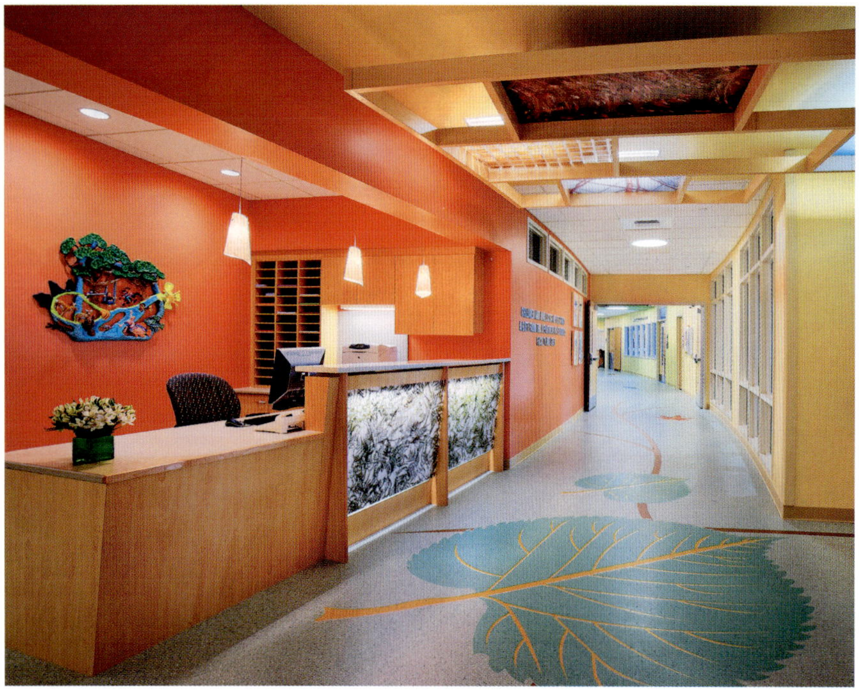

▲ American Family Children's Hospital, Kellogg, WI
Photo: HDR Architecture, Inc. © 2007 Ballogg Photography Inc., Chicago

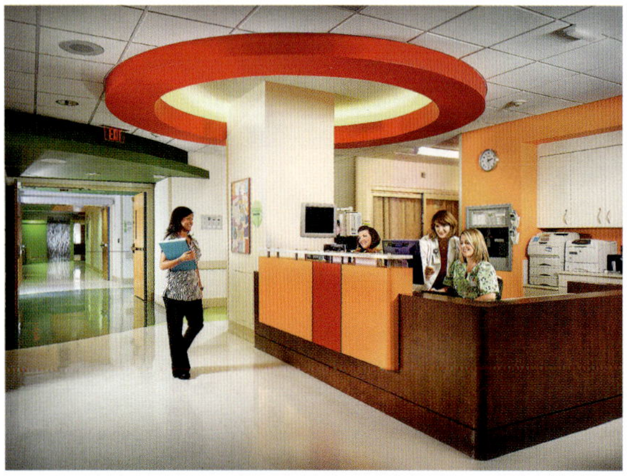

▲ Palmetto Health Children's Hospital, Columbia, SC

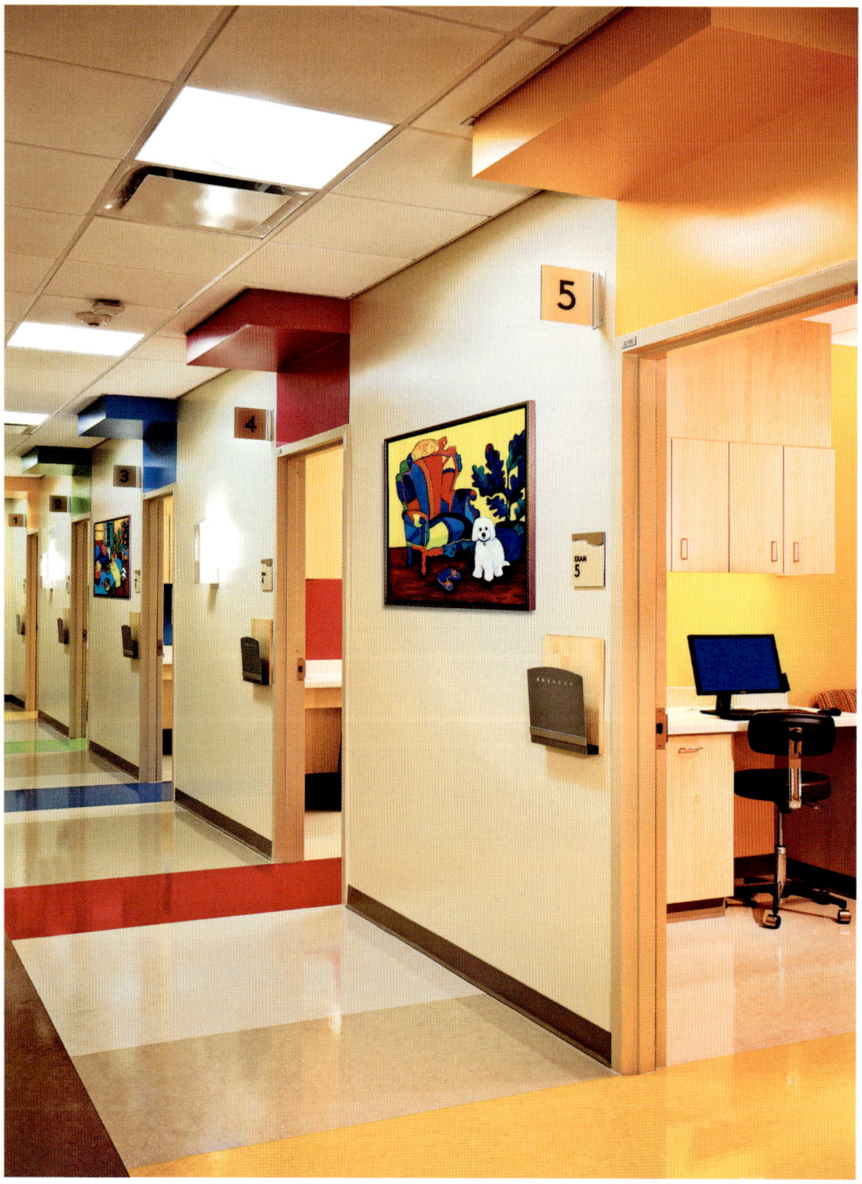

Phoenix Children's Hospital, AZ ▶
Photo: Blake Marvin, HKS

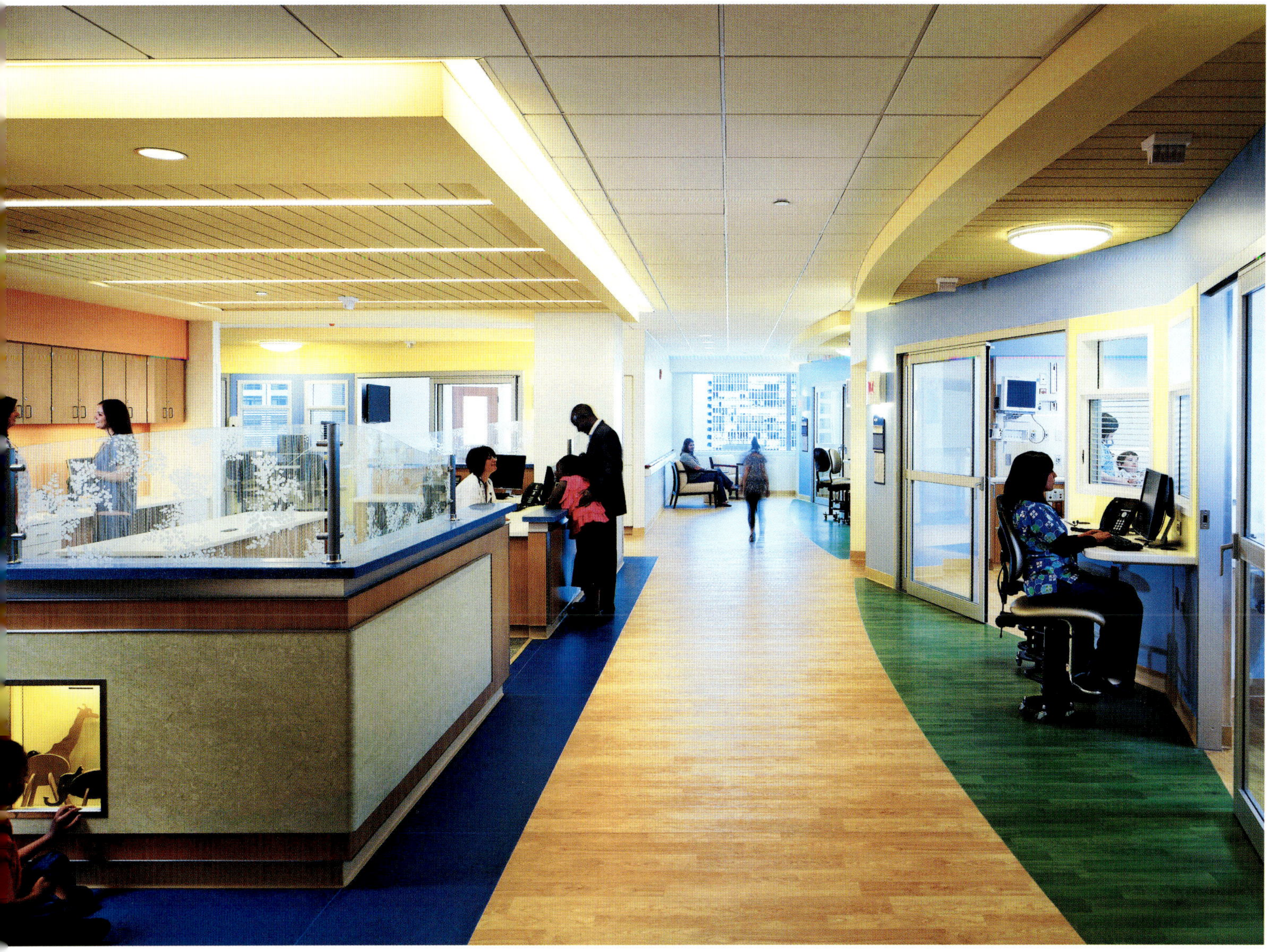

▲ Ann & Robert H. Lurie Children's Hospital of Chicago, IL
Photo: Hedrich Blessing Photography, Nick Merrick

▼ Dayton Children's, OH
Photo: Ken Shory

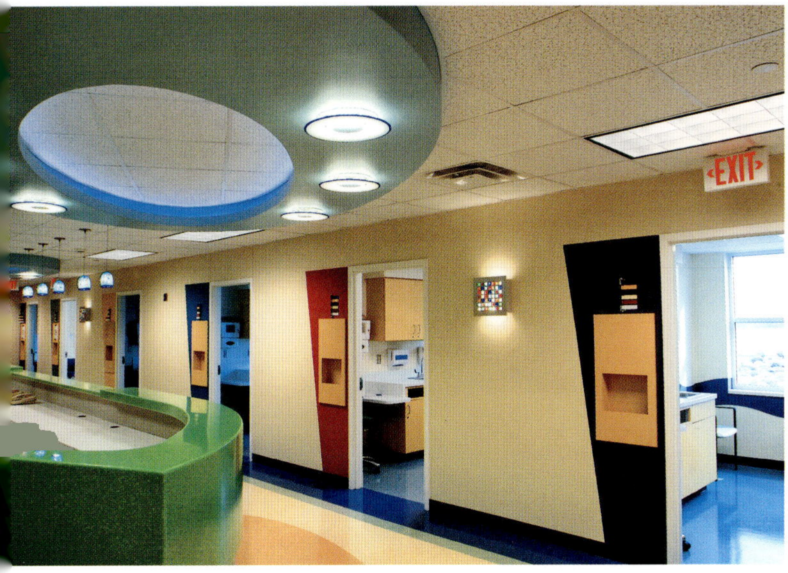

▼ Children's Hospital of Philadelphia, PA
Photo: Barry Halkin

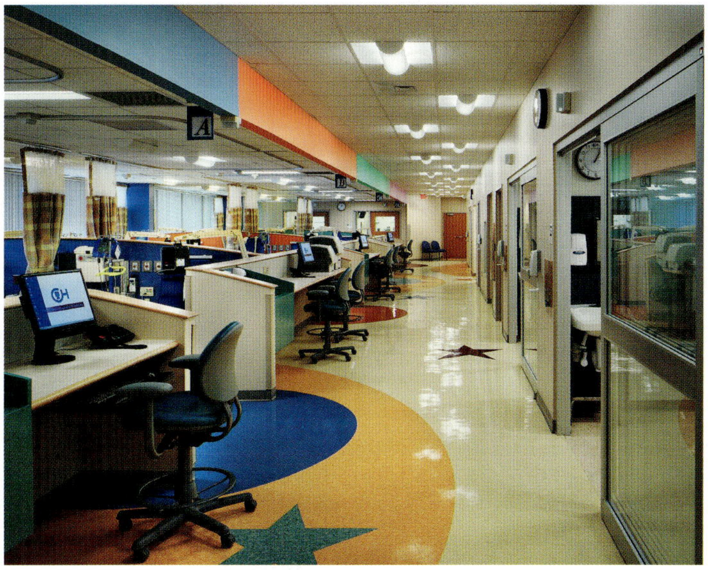

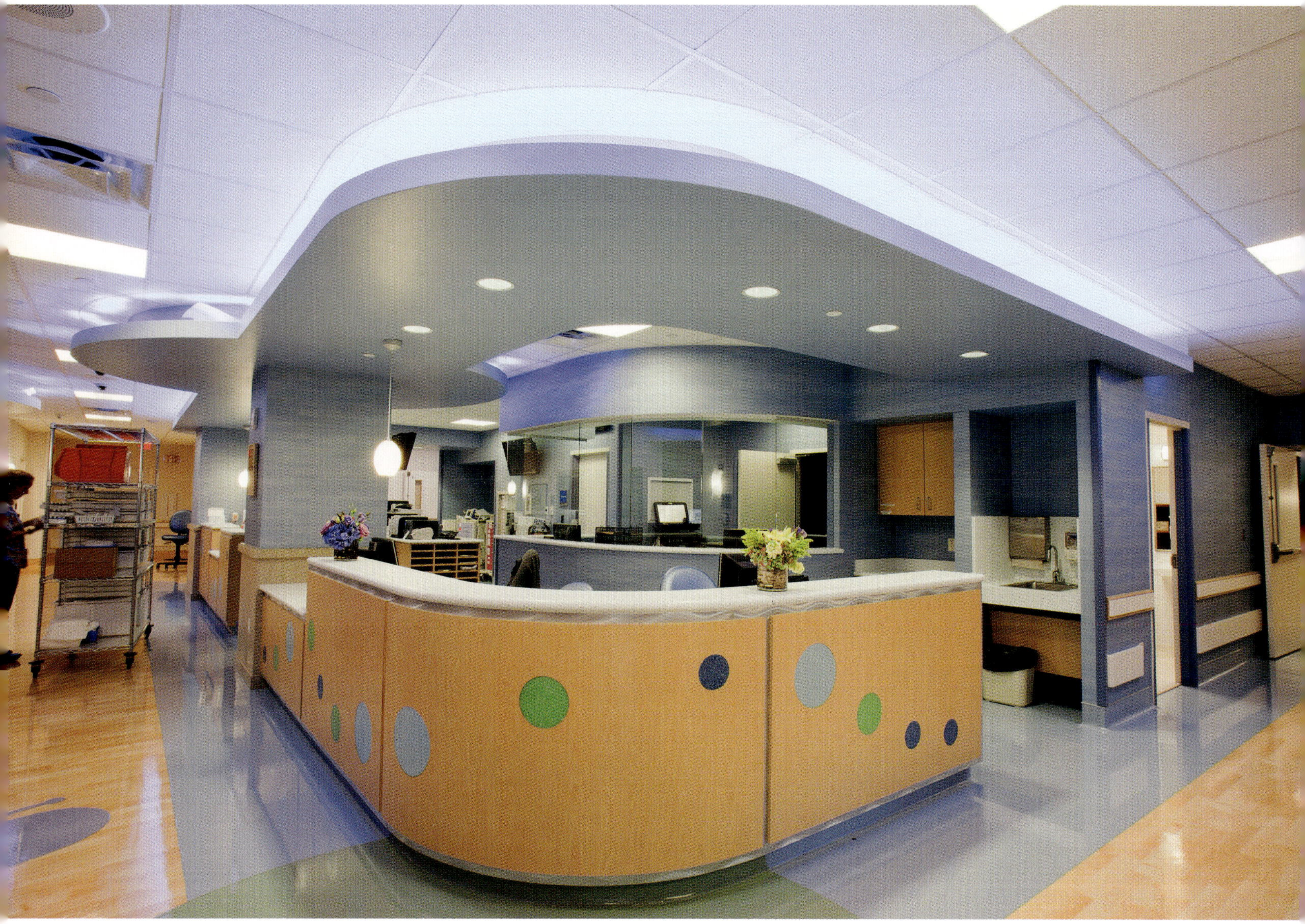

▲ Medical City Children's Hospital, Dallas, TX
Photo: Terry Cockerham

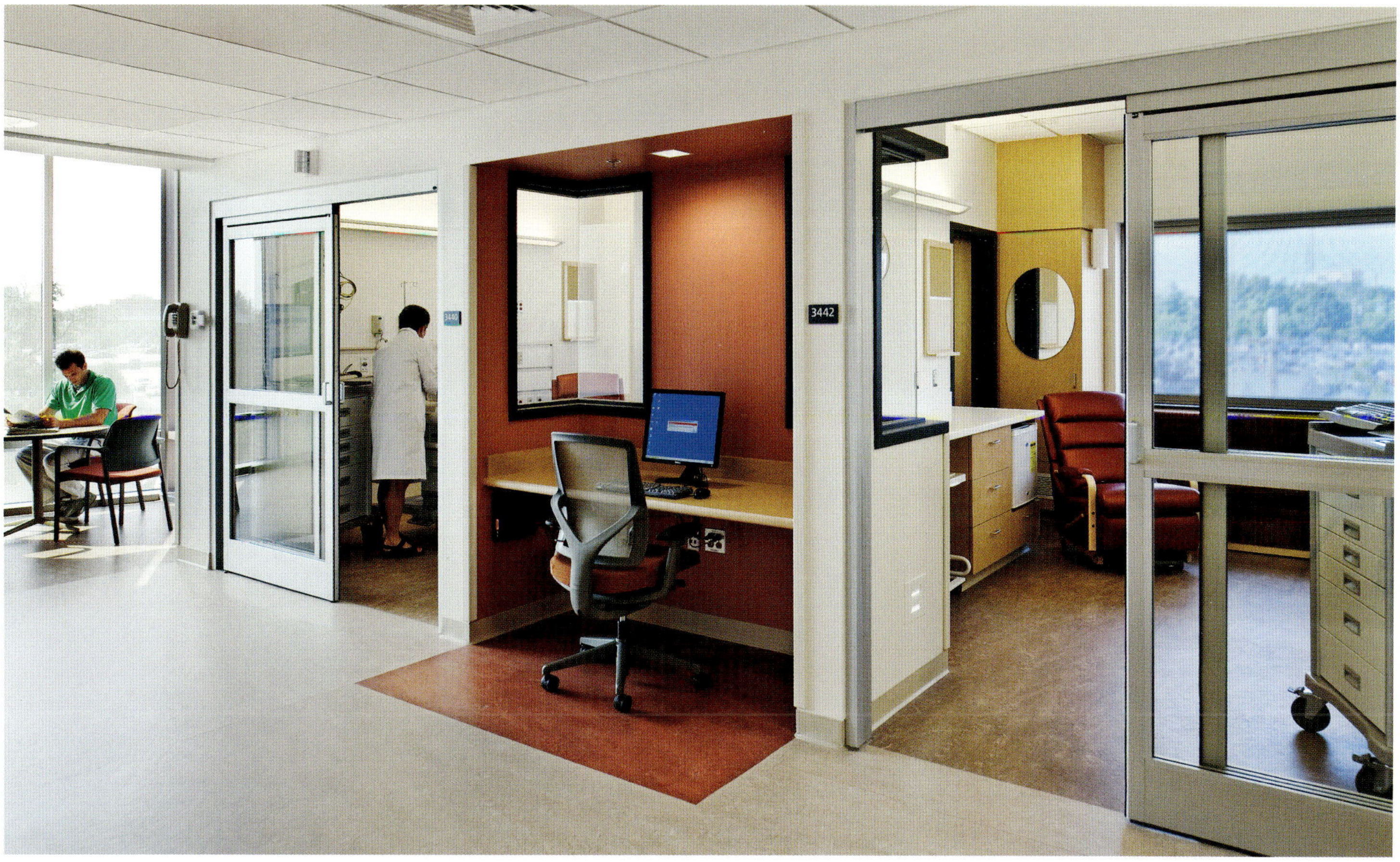

▲ Women & Infant's Hospital Clinical Services Building, Providence, RI
Photo: Stantec © Anton Grassl/Esto Photographics

▼ American Family Children's Hospital, Kellogg, WI
Photo: HDR Architecture, Inc. © 2007 Ballogg Photography Inc., Chicago

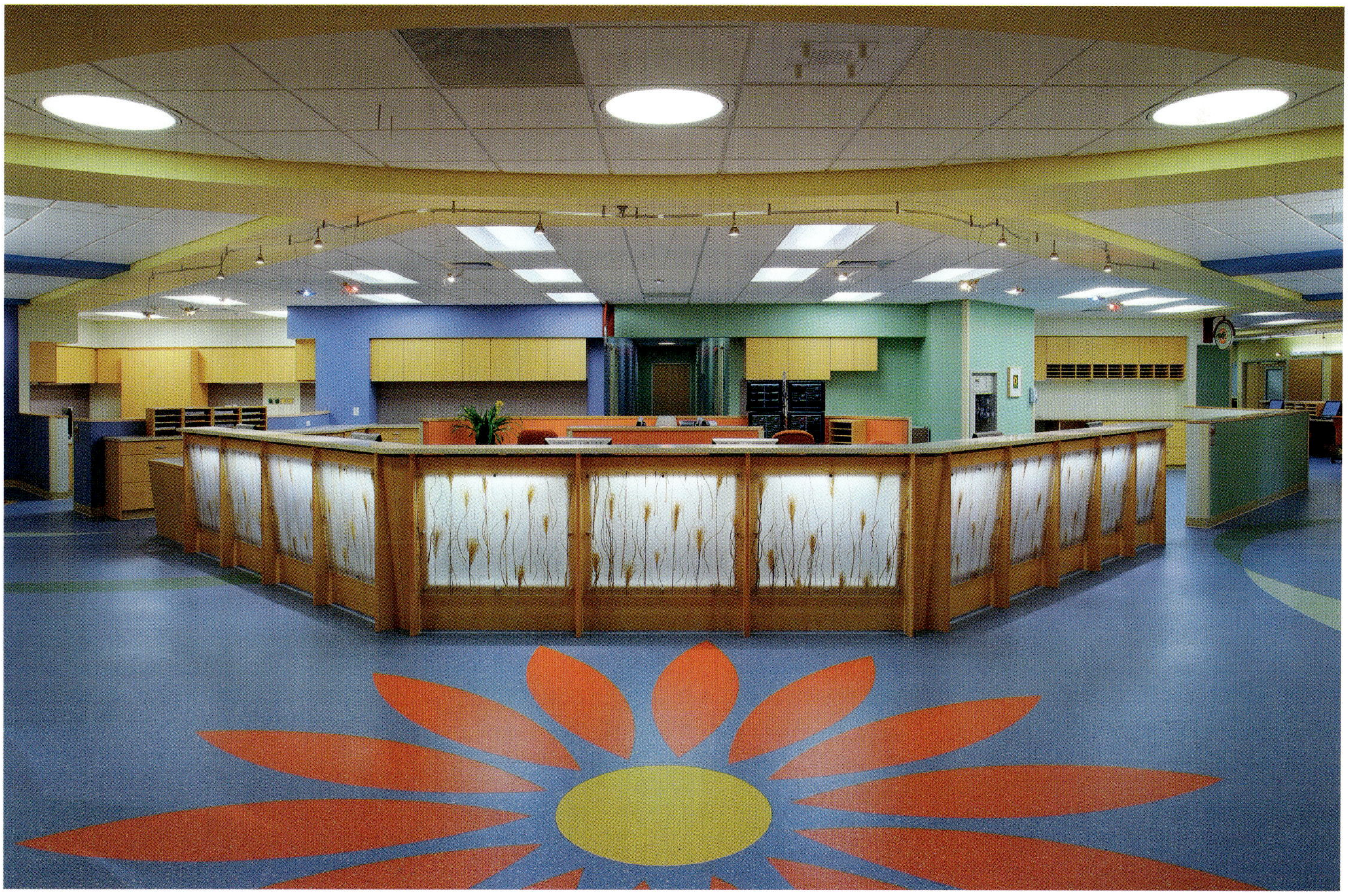

American Family Children's Hospital, Kellogg, WI ▶
Photo: HDR Architecture, Inc. © 2007 Ballogg Photography Inc., Chicago

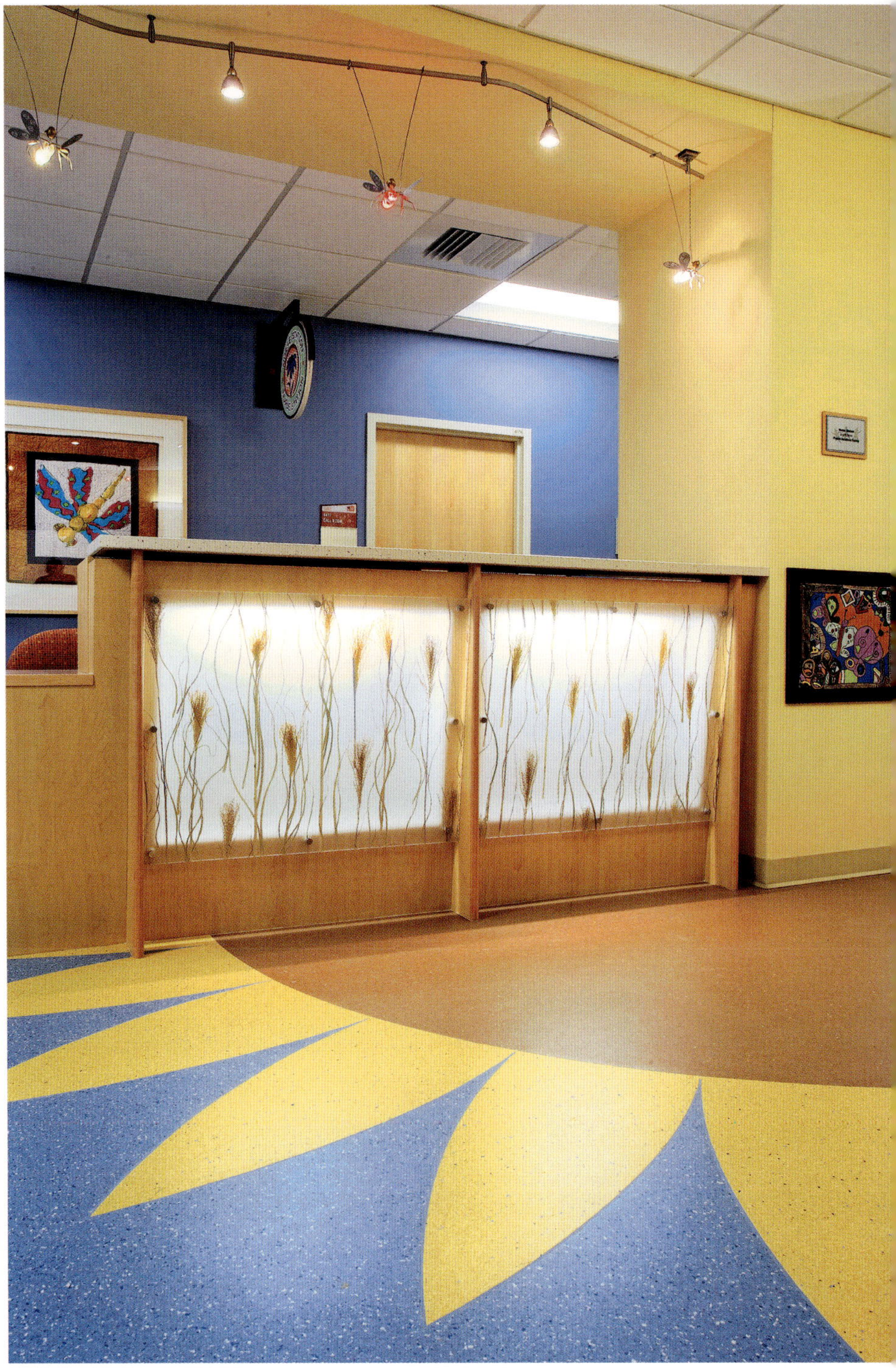

▼ Rady Children's Hospital, San Diego, CA
Photo: Stantec © RMA Photography

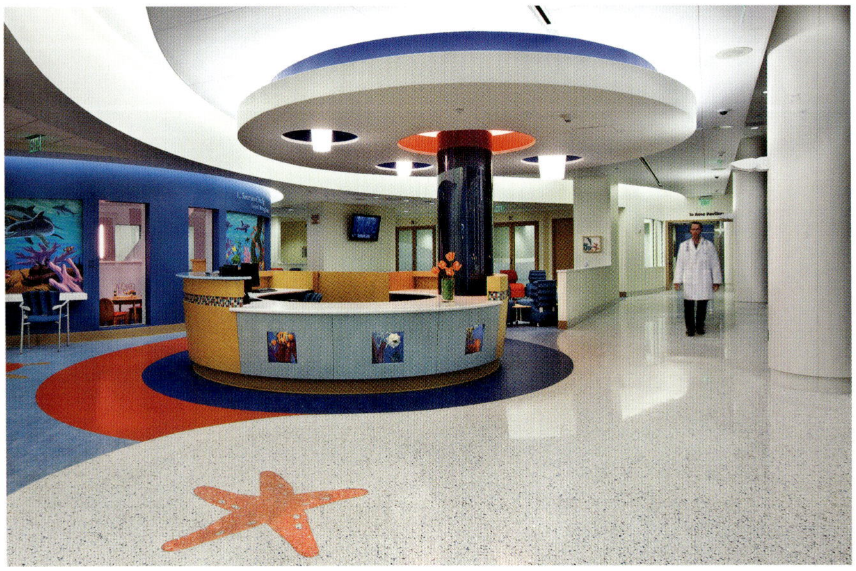

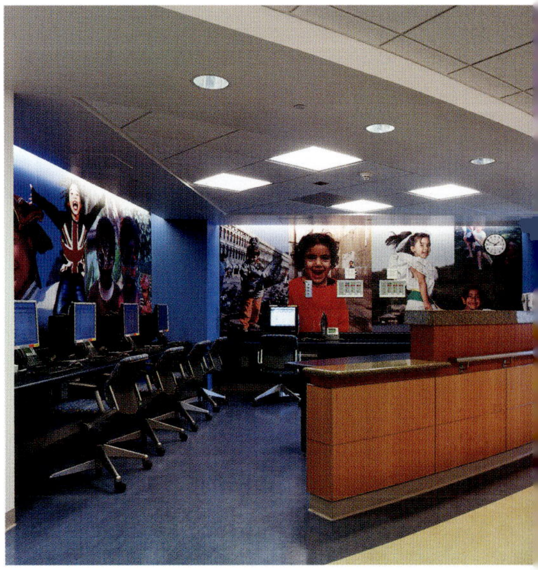

▼ Mattel Children's Hospital UCLA, Los Angeles, CA
Photo: Benny Chan, fotoworks

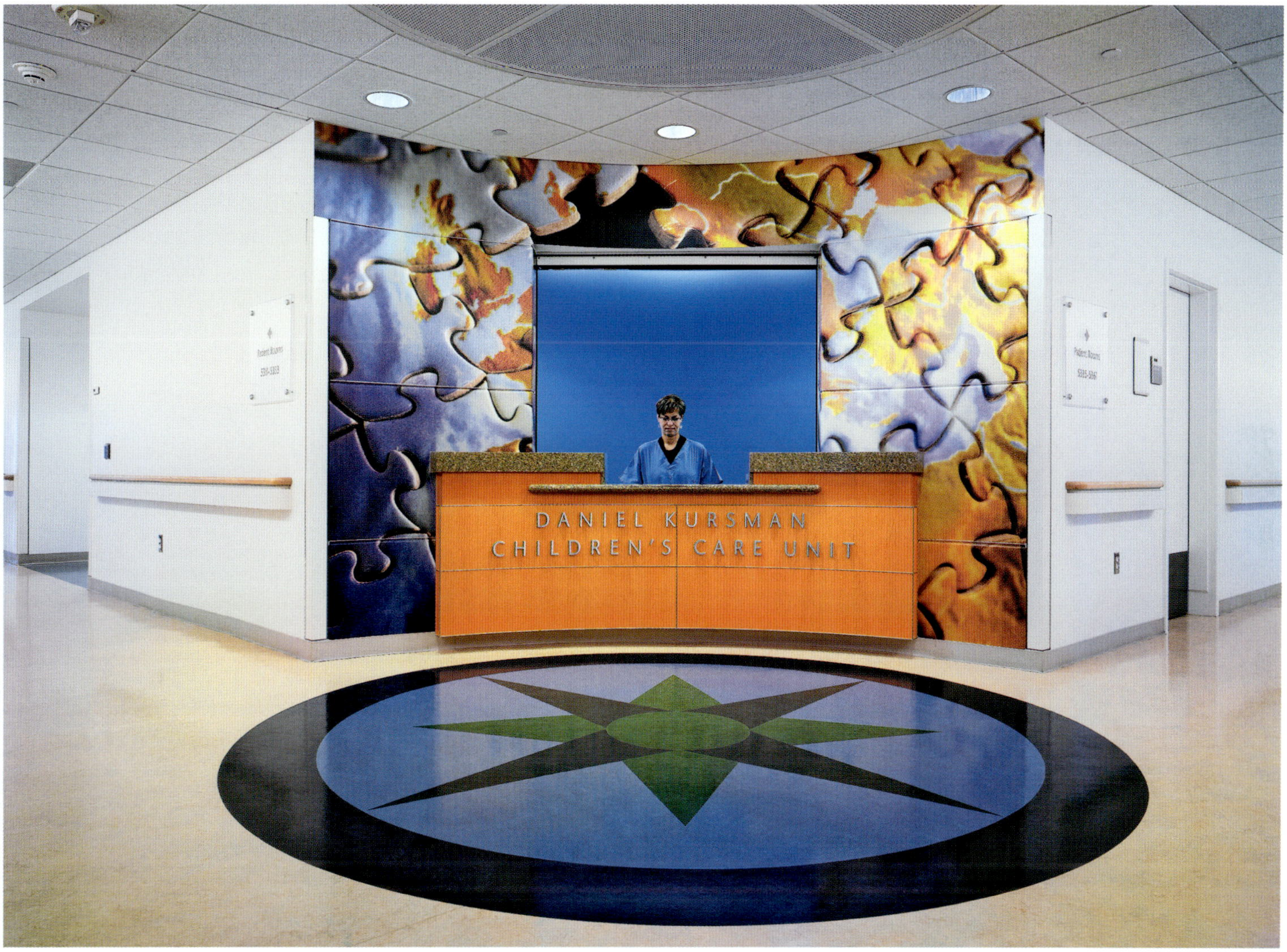

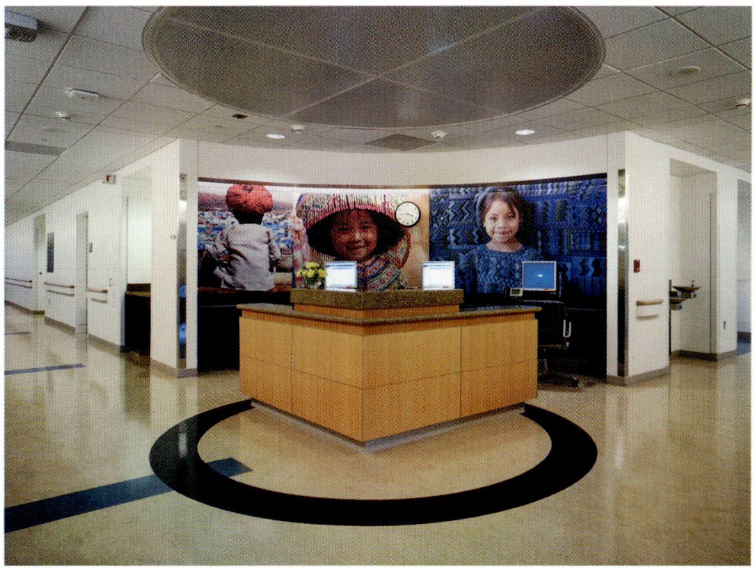

◀ Mattel Children's Hospital UCLA, Los Angeles, CA
Photo: Benny Chan, fotoworks

Following pages: Gaston Memorial Hospital, Gastonia, NC
Photo: Tim Griffith Photography

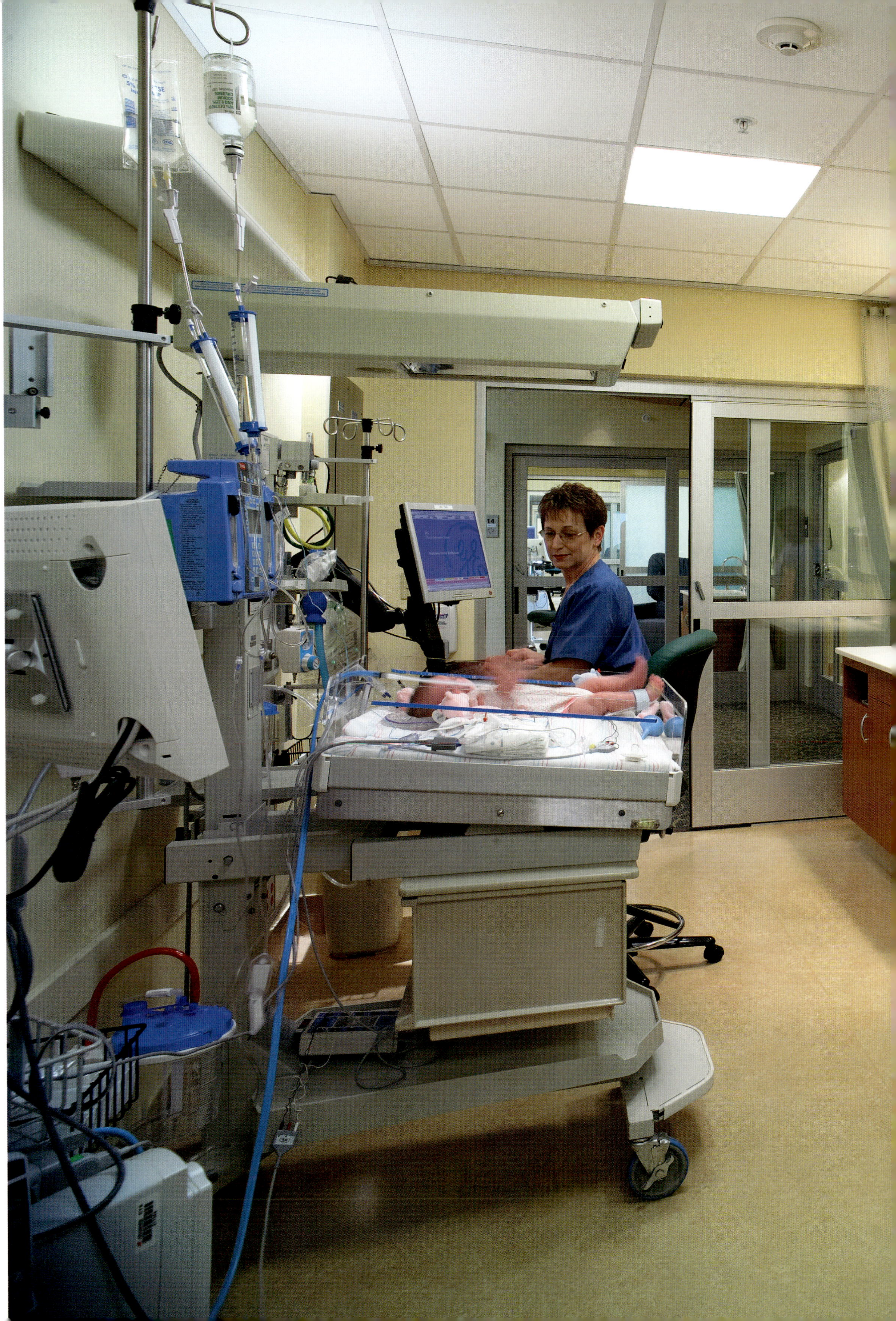

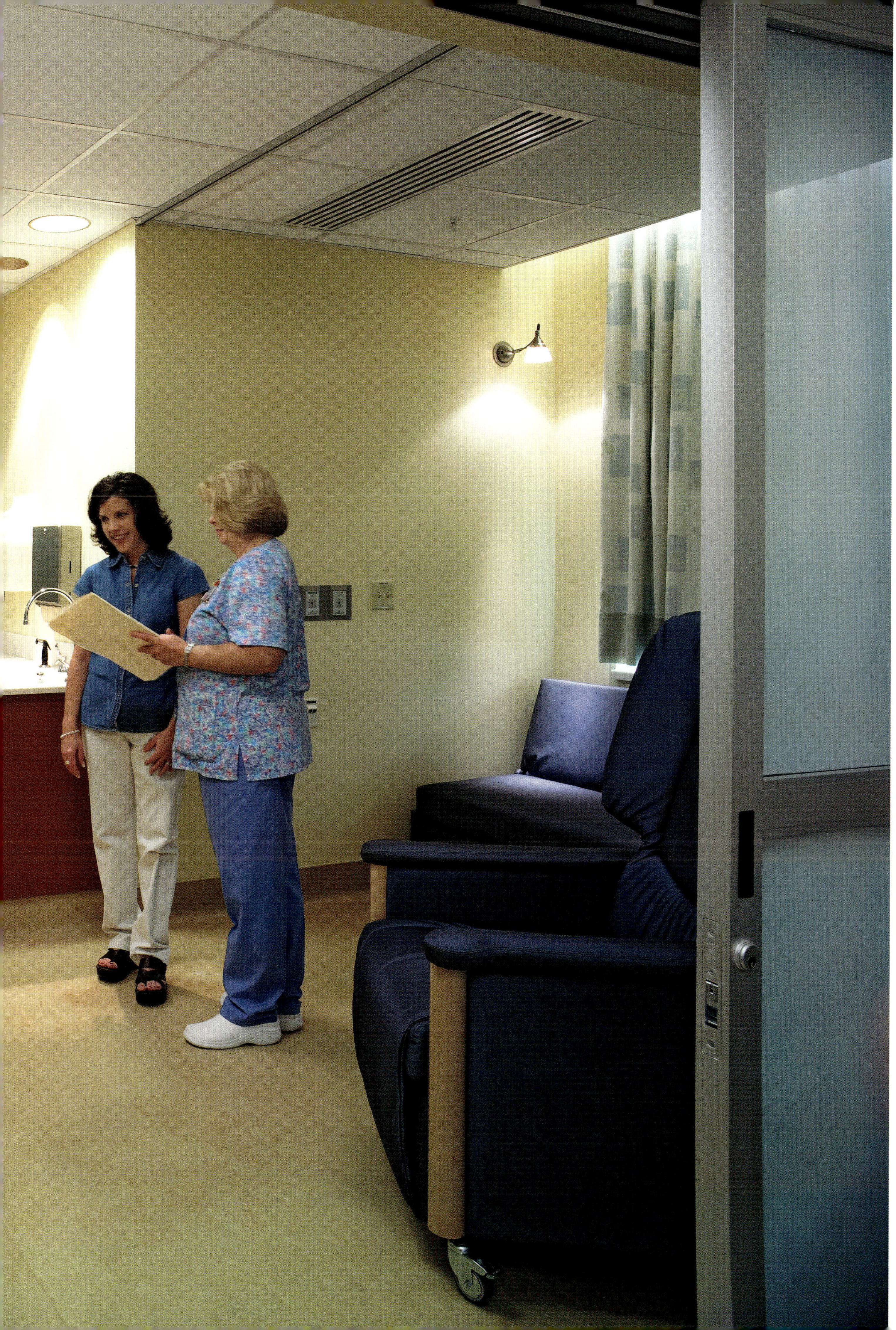

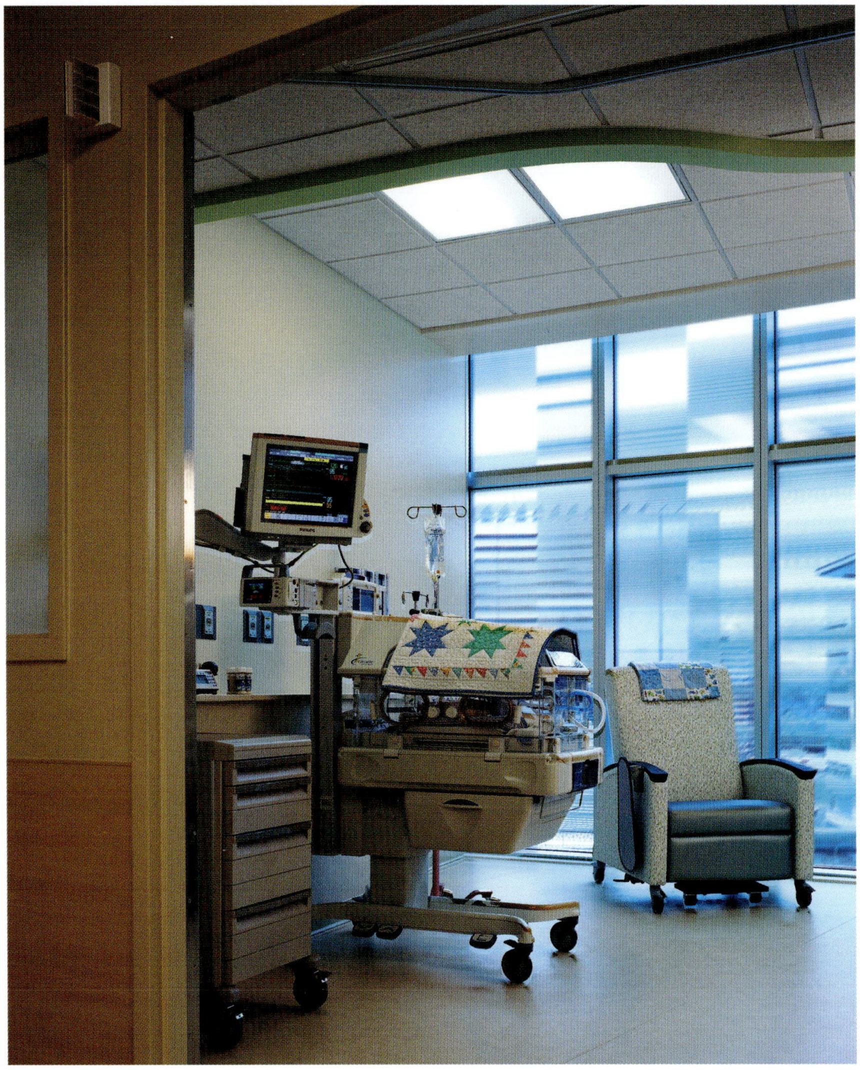

▲ Helen DeVos Children's Hospital, Grand Rapids, MI
Photo: Hedrich Blessing

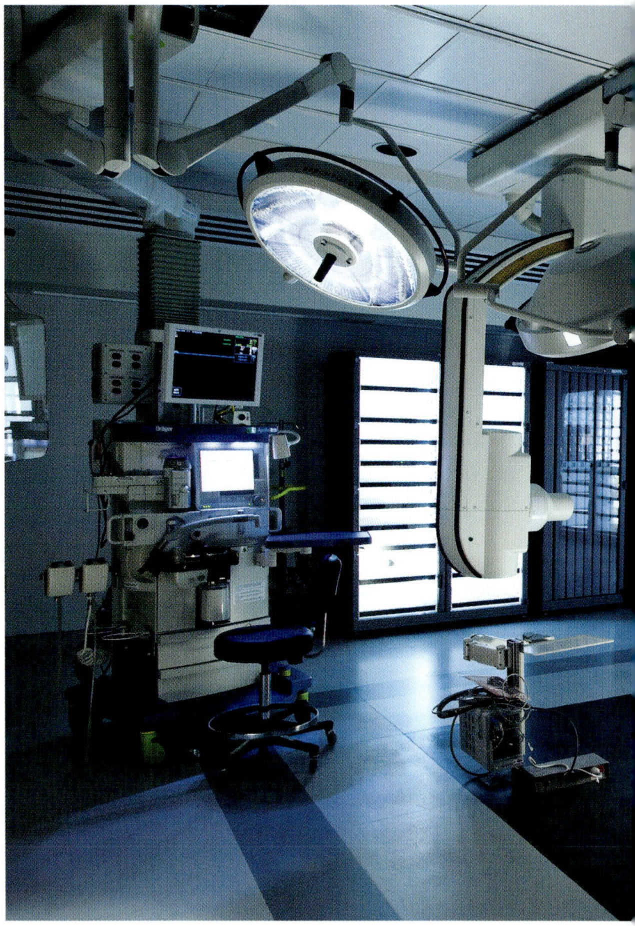

▲ Children's Hospital of Philadelphia, PA
Photo: Paul Crane

▼ Medical City Children's Hospital, Dallas, TX
Photo: Terry Cockerham

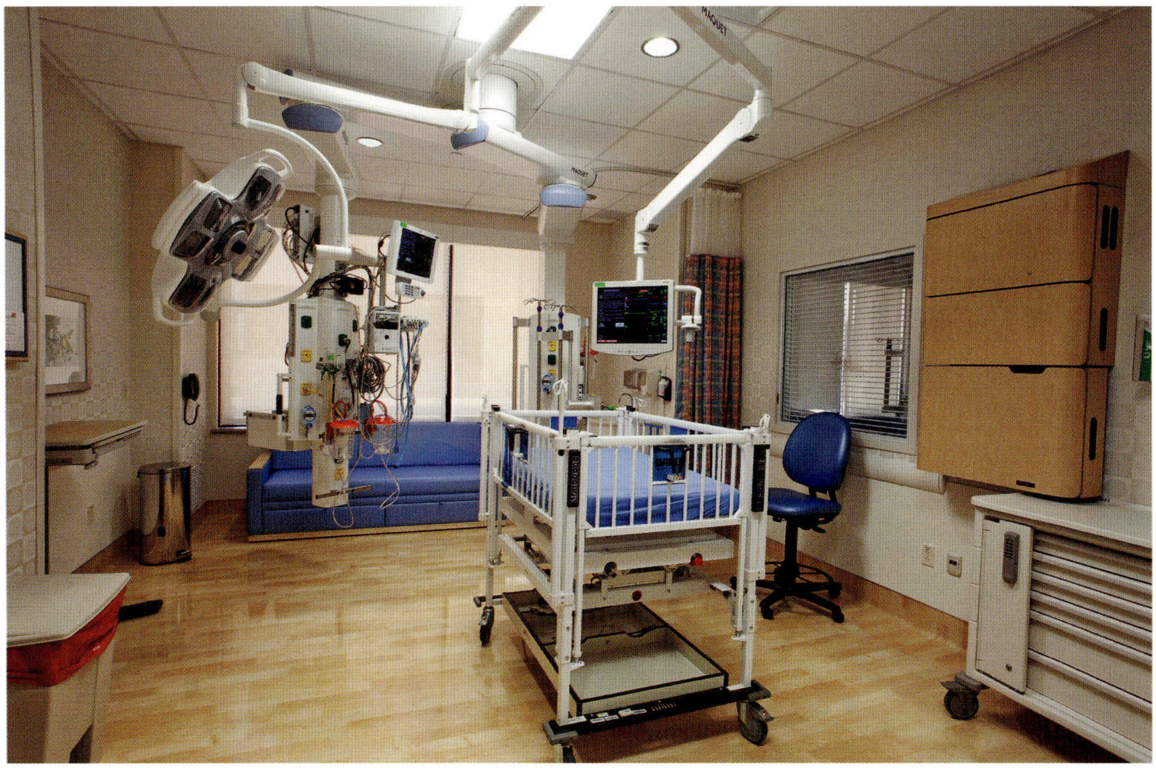

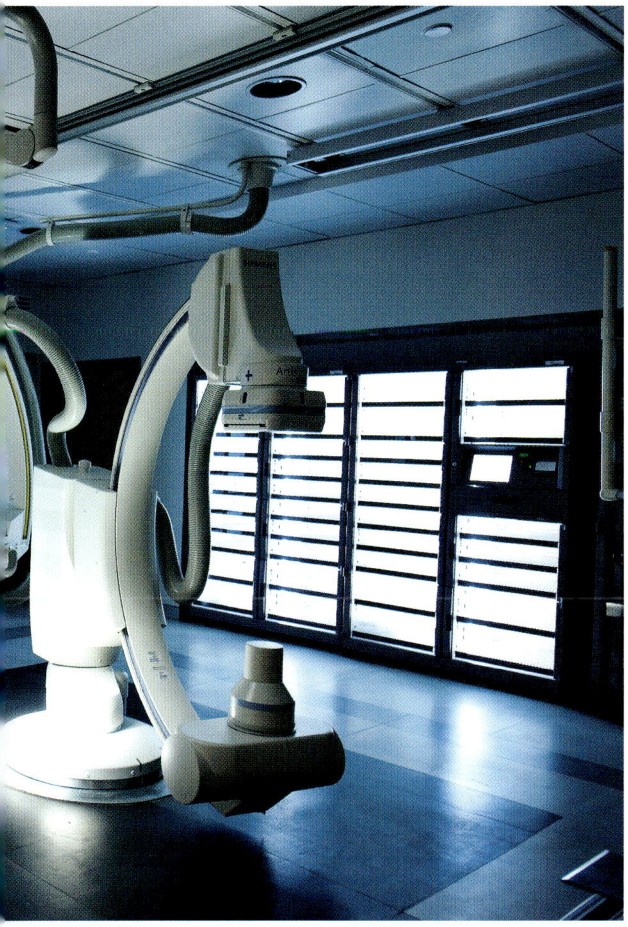

▼ Rady Children's Hospital, San Diego, CA
Photo: Stantec © RMA Photography

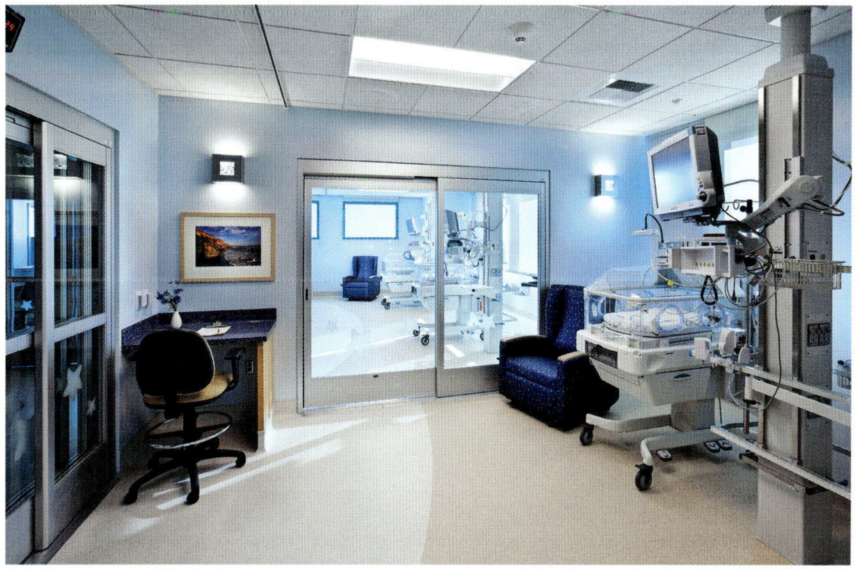

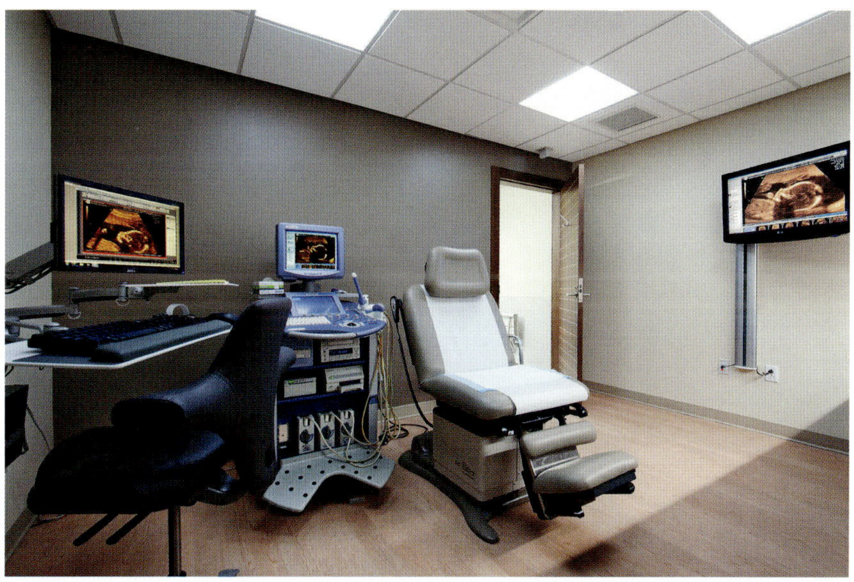

▲ Morgan Stanley Children's Hospital, New York, NY
Photo: Jeffrey Totaro Photographer

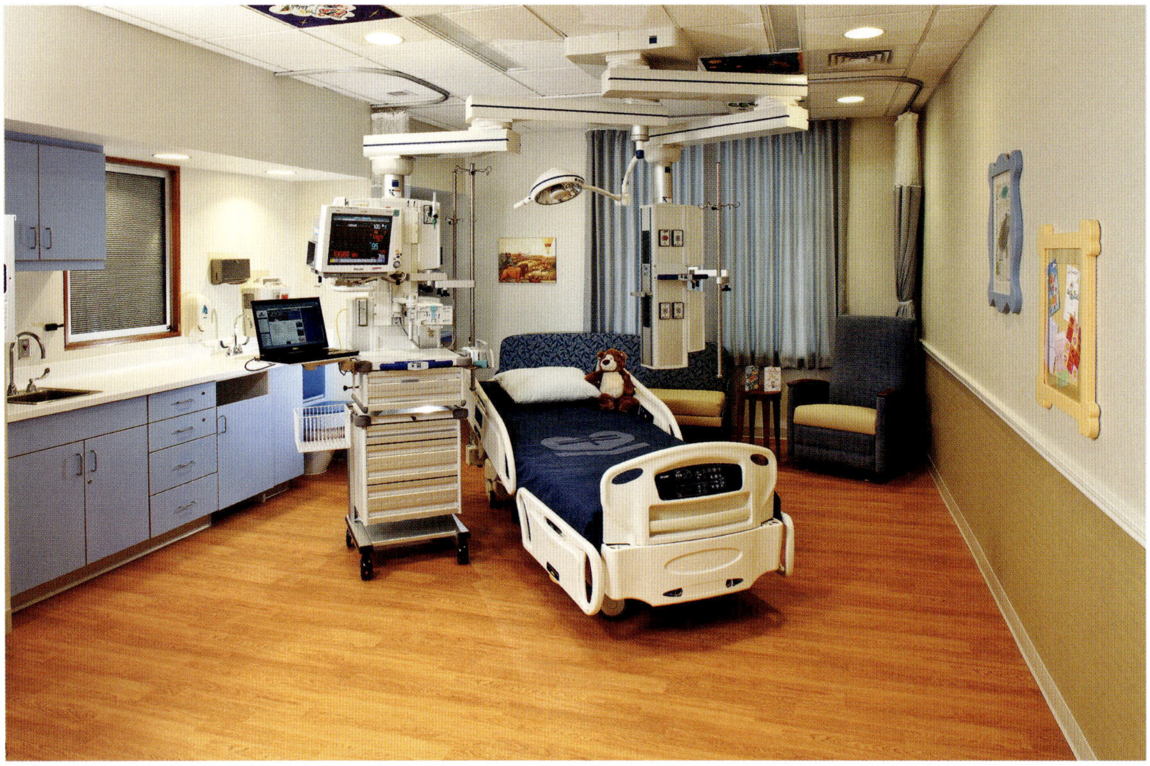

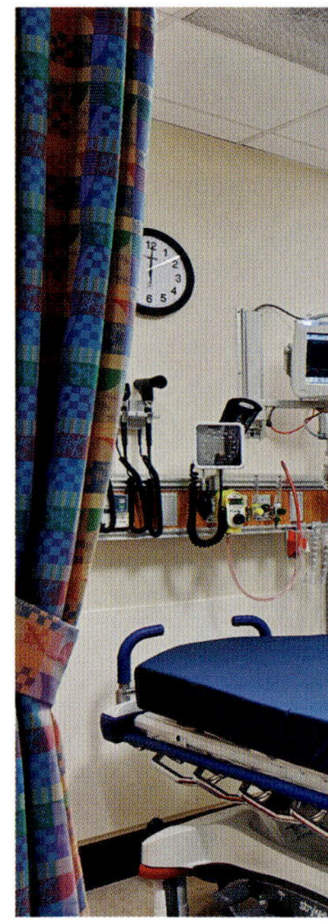

▲ Sanford Children's Hospital, Sioux Falls, SD

▼ Kosair Children's Hospital, Louisville, KY

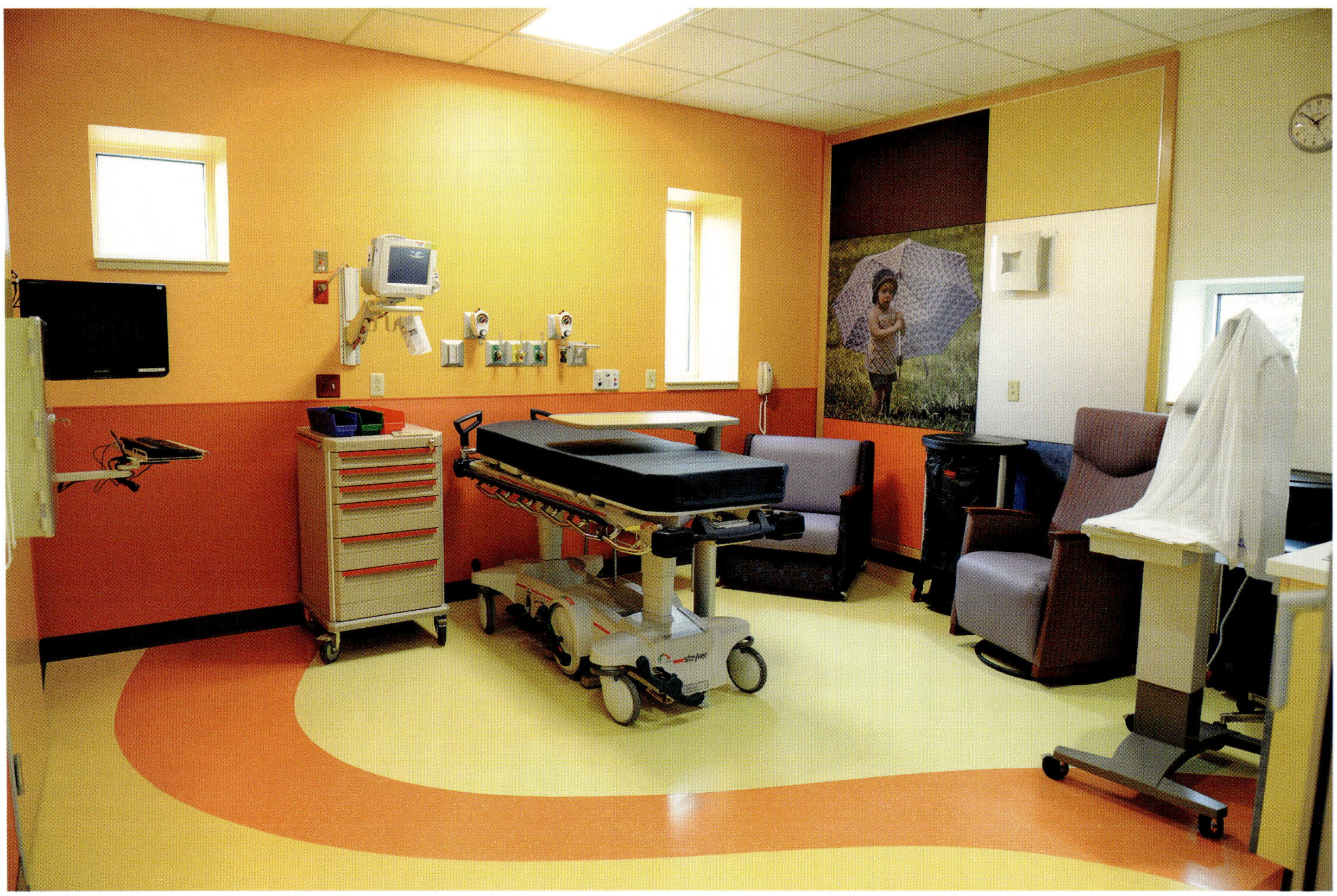

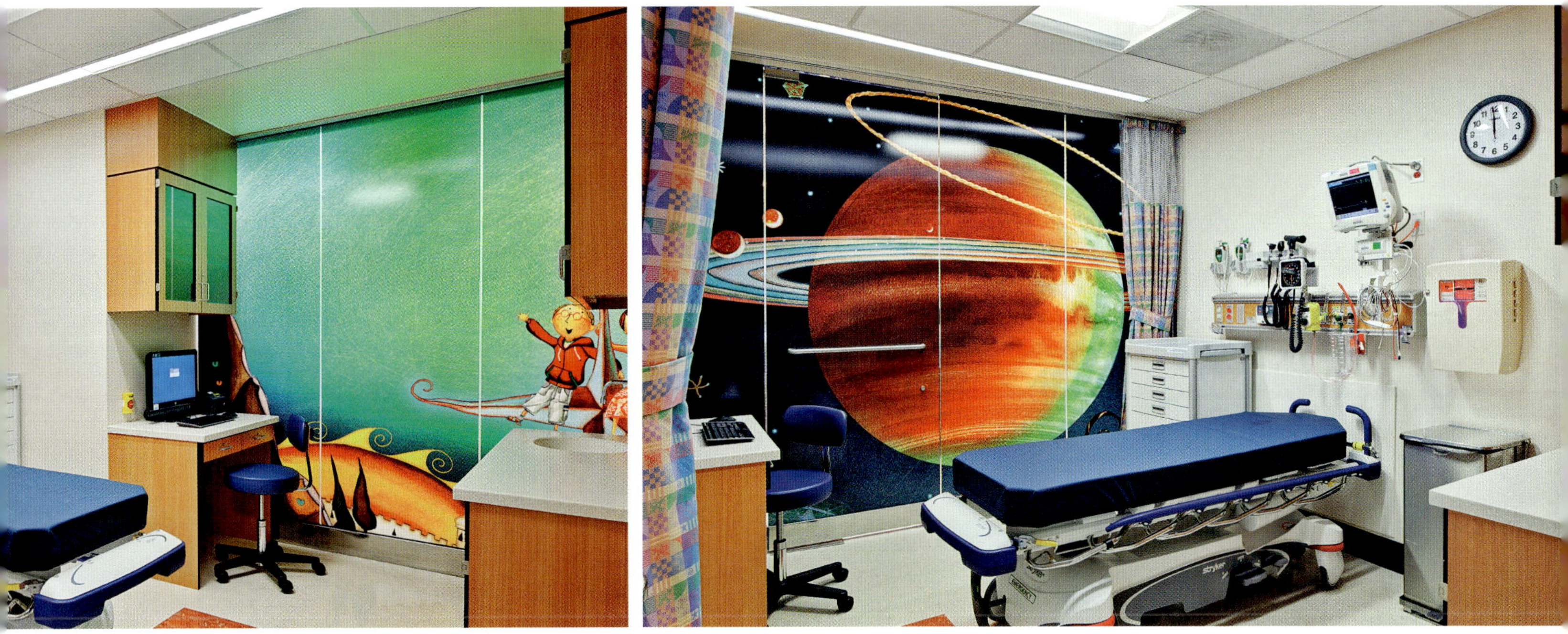

▲ Morgan Stanley Children's Hospital, New York, NY
Photos: Jeffrey Totaro Photographer

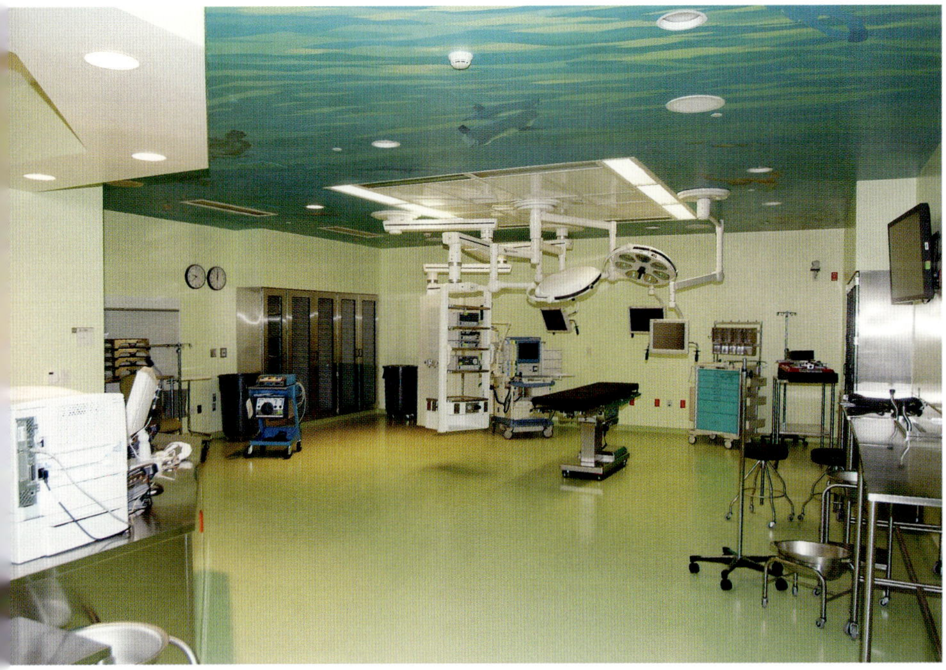

▲ Joseph M. Sanzari Children's Hospital at Hackensack University Medical Center, Hackensack, NJ
Photo: Basil Fargnoli

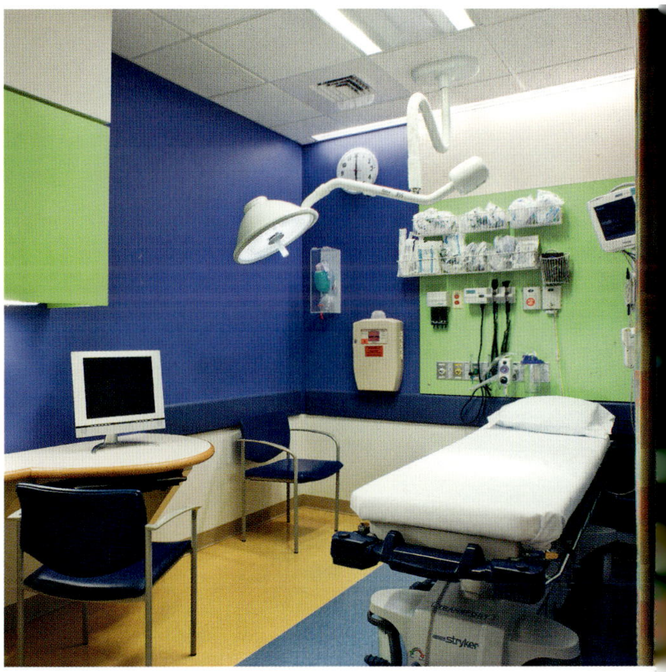

▲ Children's Hospital Boston, MA
Photo: Warren Jagger

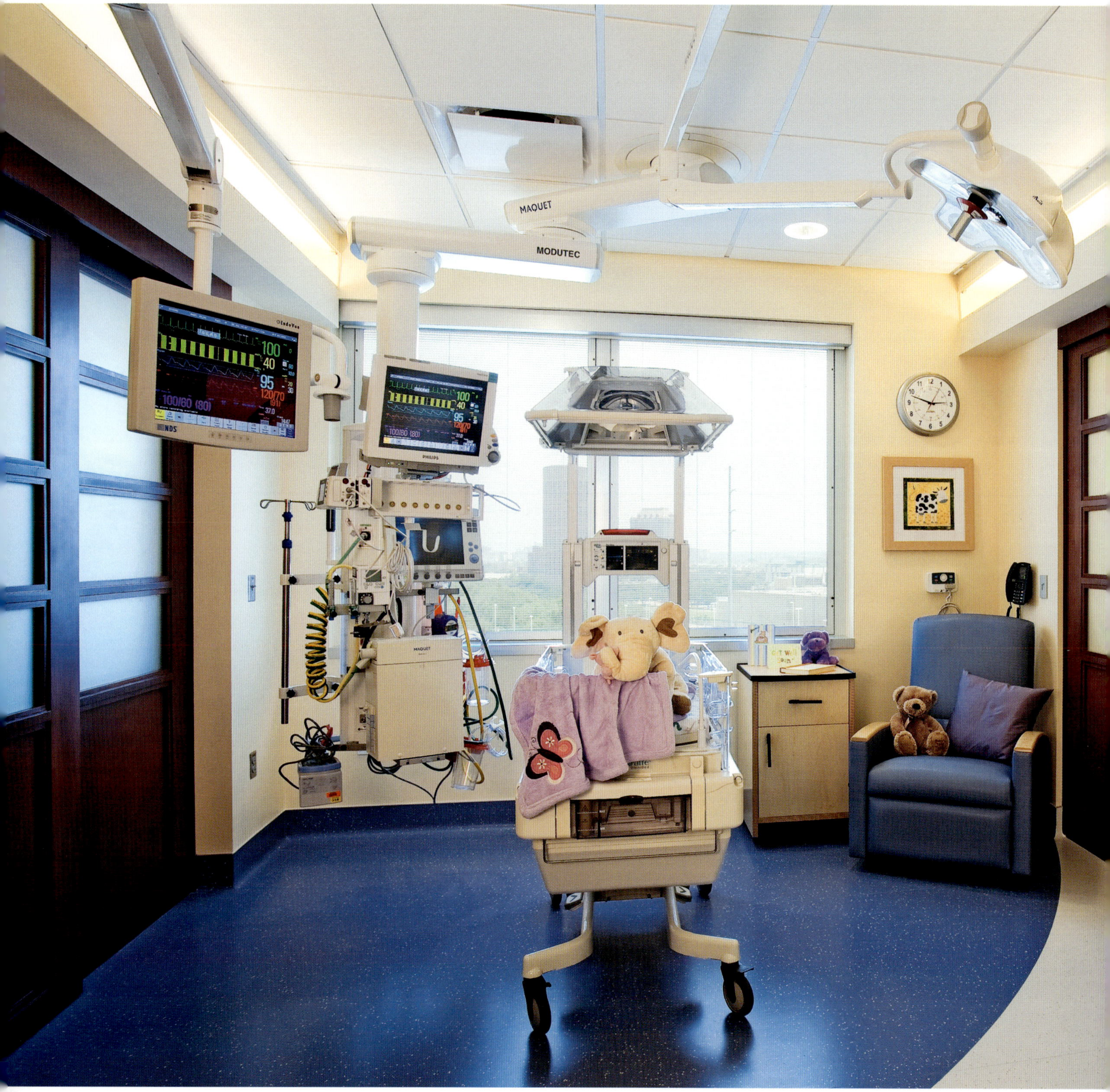

▲ Children's Medical Center, Dallas, TX
Photo: Charles Smith

Women & Infants Hospital Clinical Services Building, Providence, RI ▶
Photo: Stantec © Anton Grassl/Esto Photographics

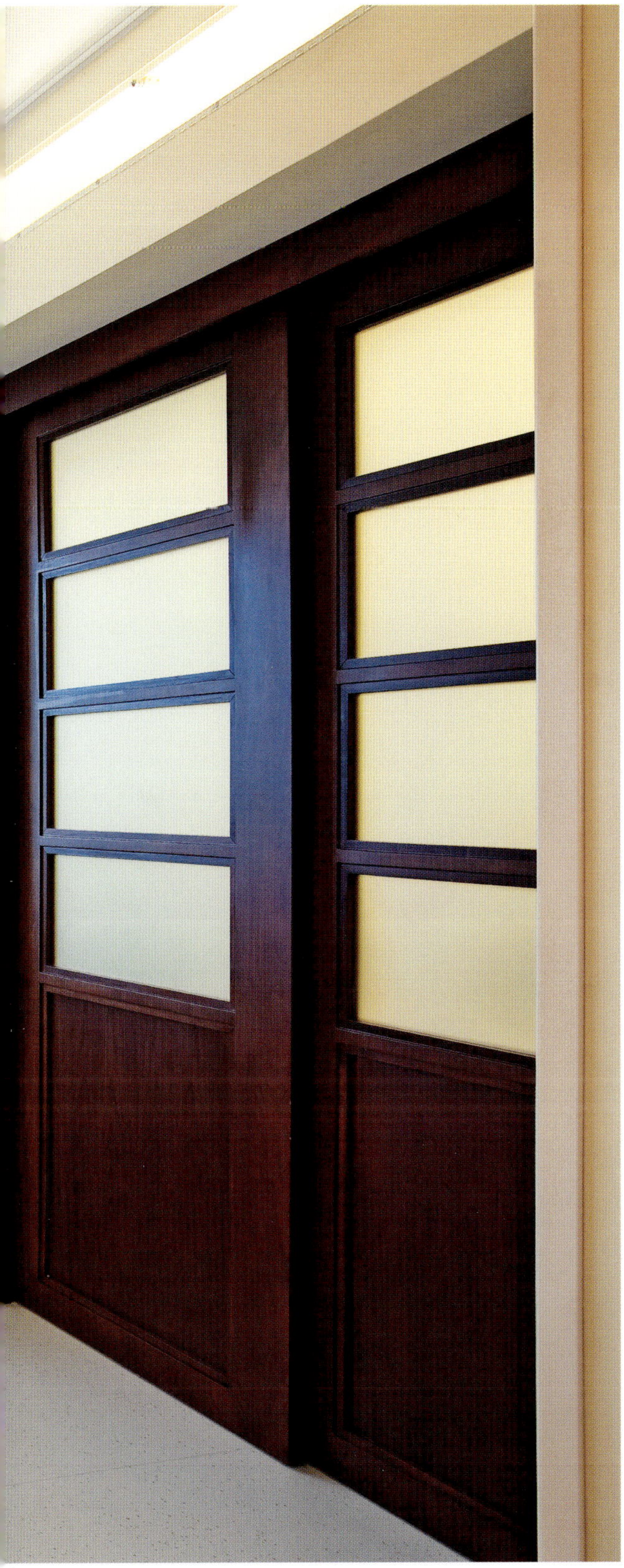

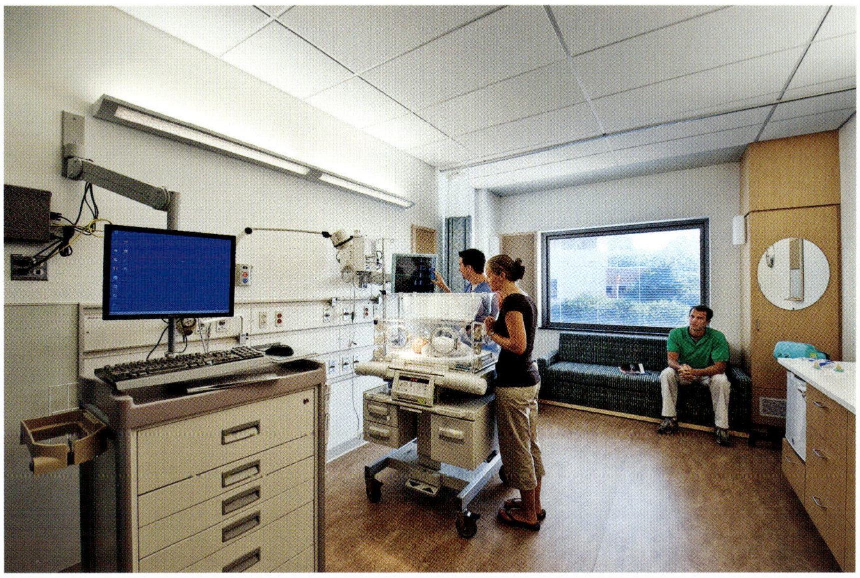

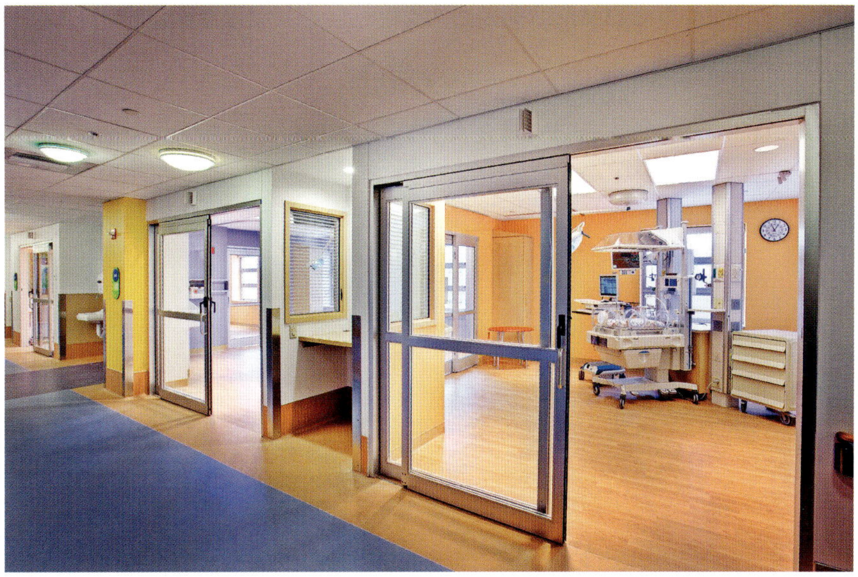

▲ Children's Hospital, Pittsburgh, PA
Photo: Alexander Denmarsh

▼ Medical City Children's Hospital, Dallas, TX
Photo: Terry Cockerham

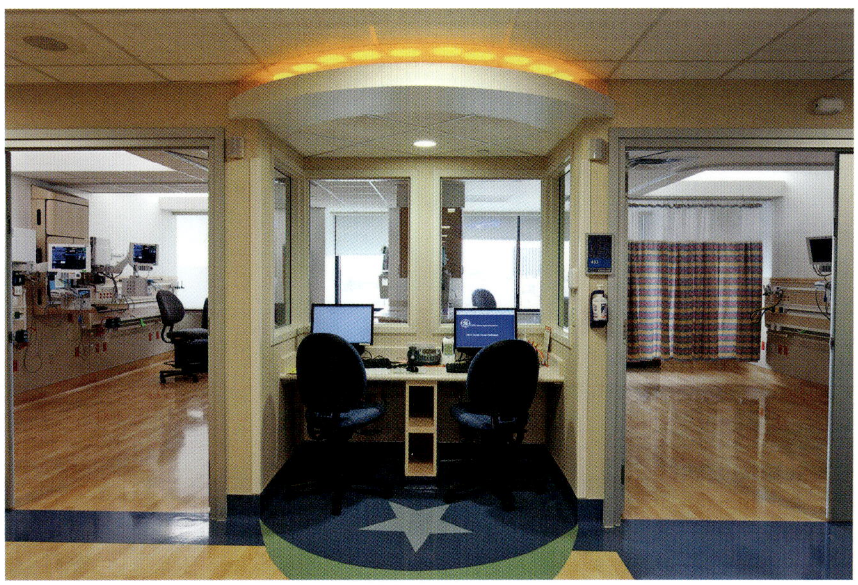

Following pages: Helen DeVos Children's Hospital, Grand Rapids, MI
Photo: Lucid Architecture, Eric DeWitt

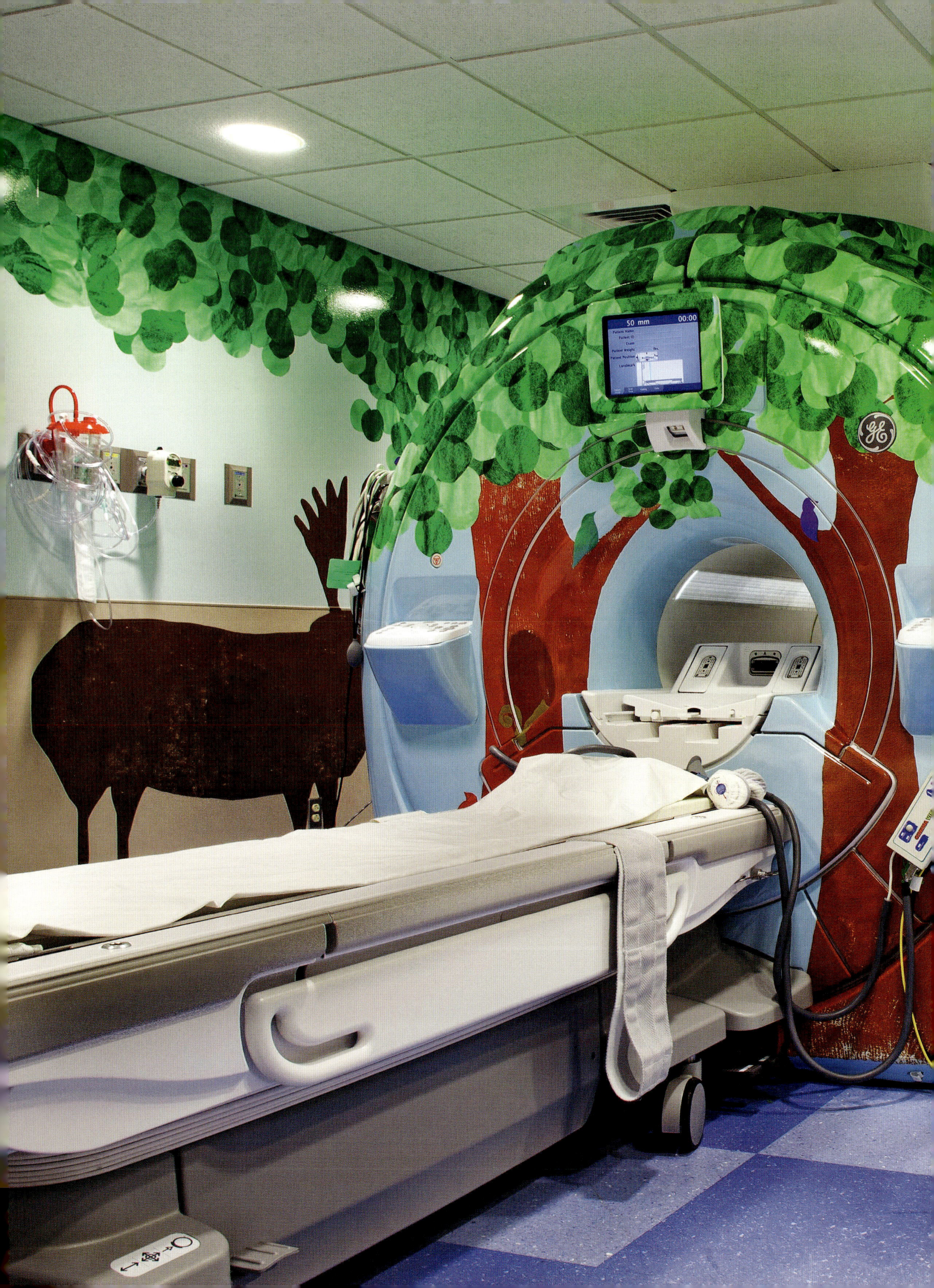
50 mm
00:00

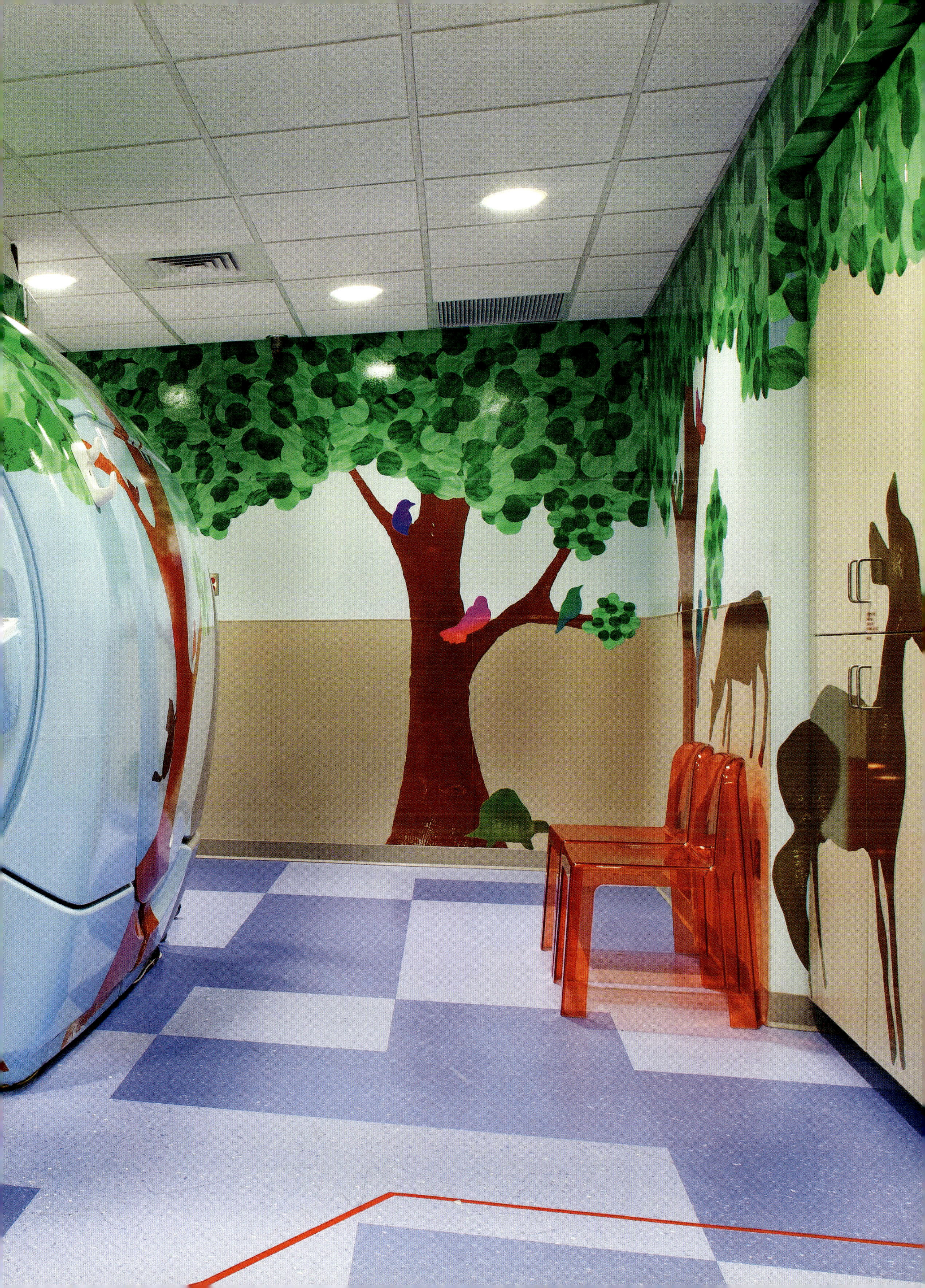

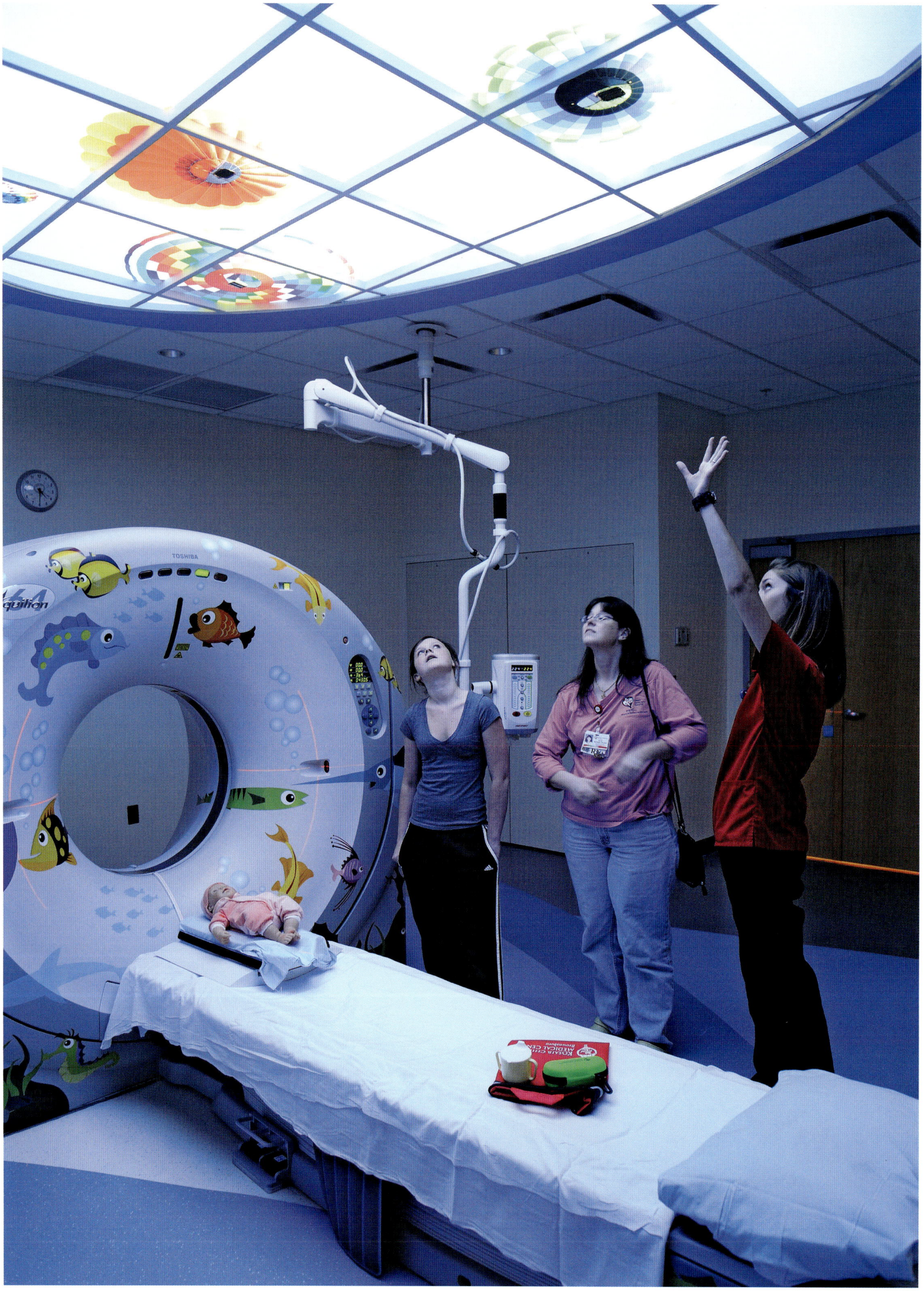
TOSHIBA

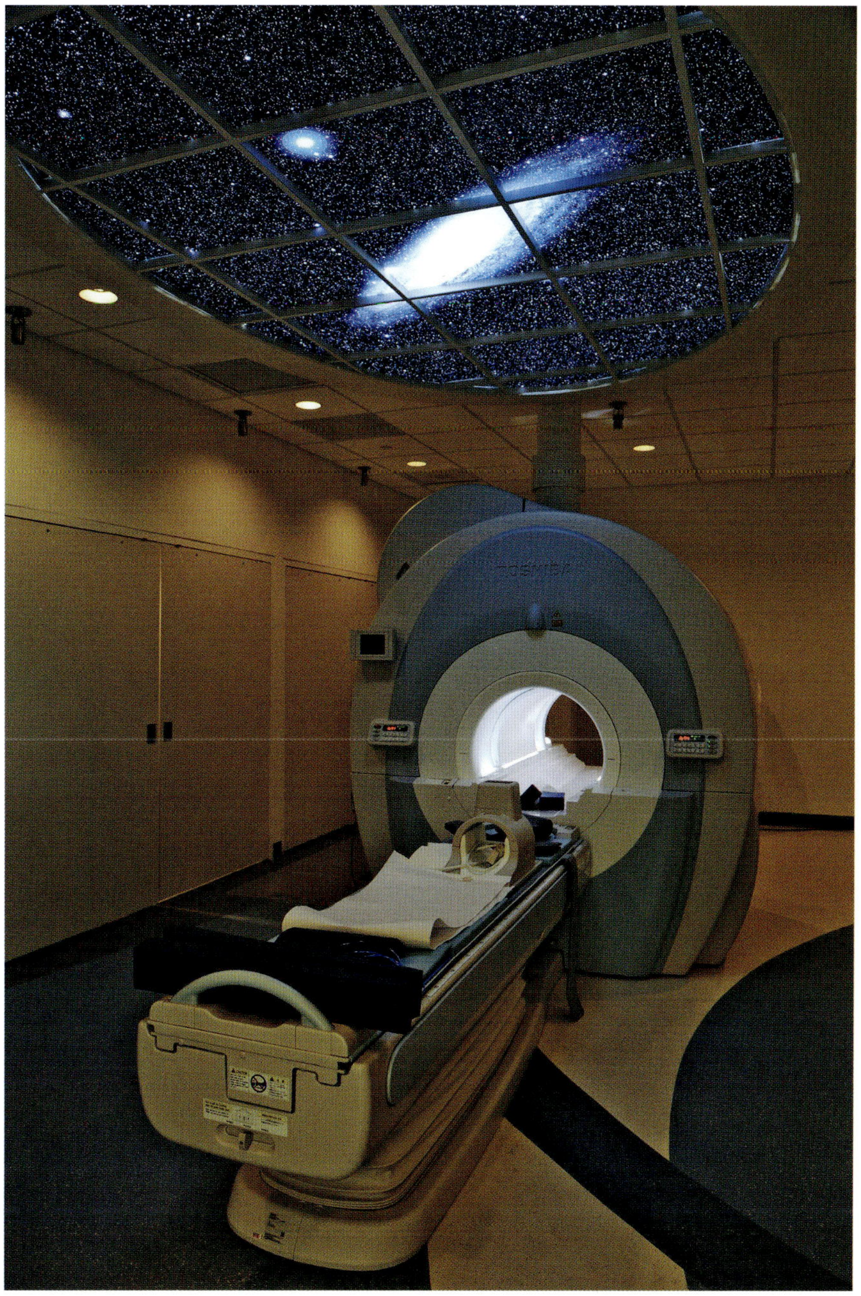

▲ Kosair Children's Hospital, Louisville, KY
◀

▼ Children's Medical Center at Legacy, Plano, TX
Photo: Robert Canfield

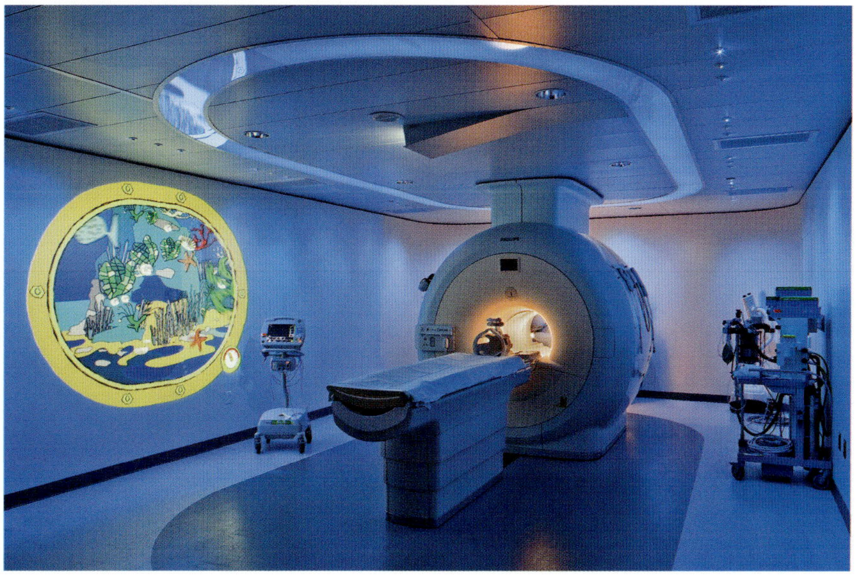

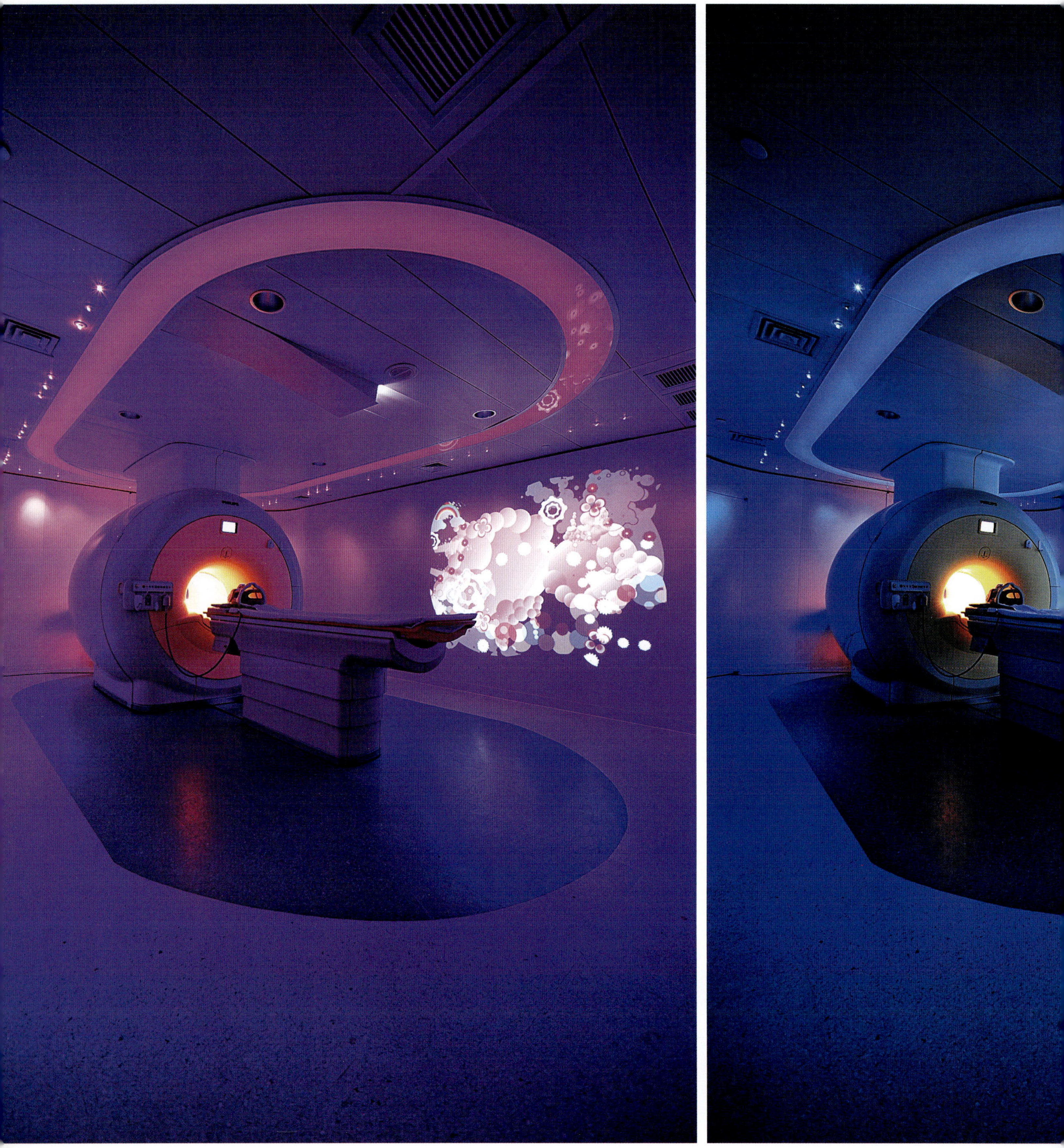

▲ Texas Children's Health Center, Sugar Land, Houston, TX
Photo: Aker Imaging

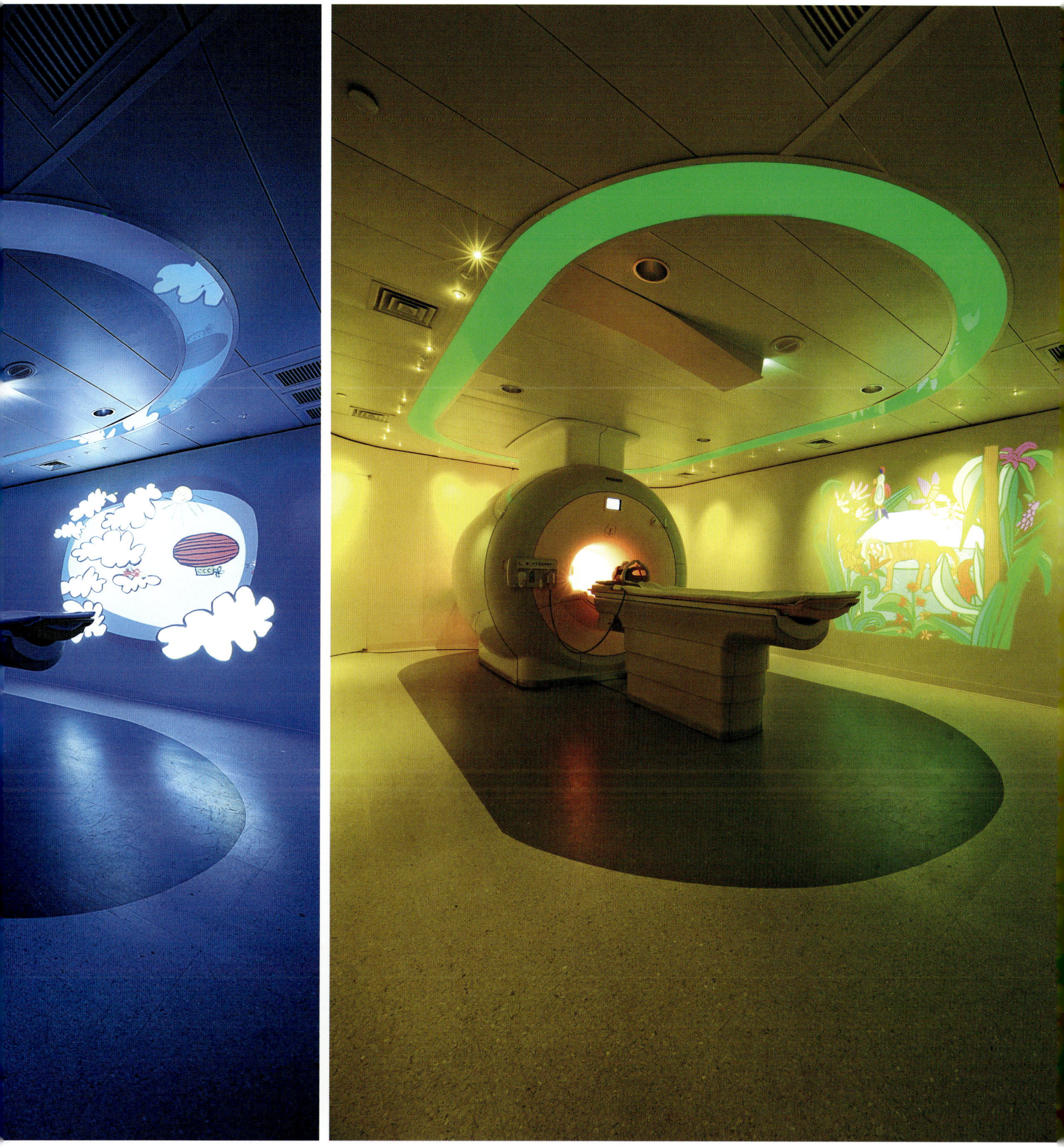

▲ Texas Children's Health Center, Sugar Land, Houston, TX
Photo: Aker Imaging

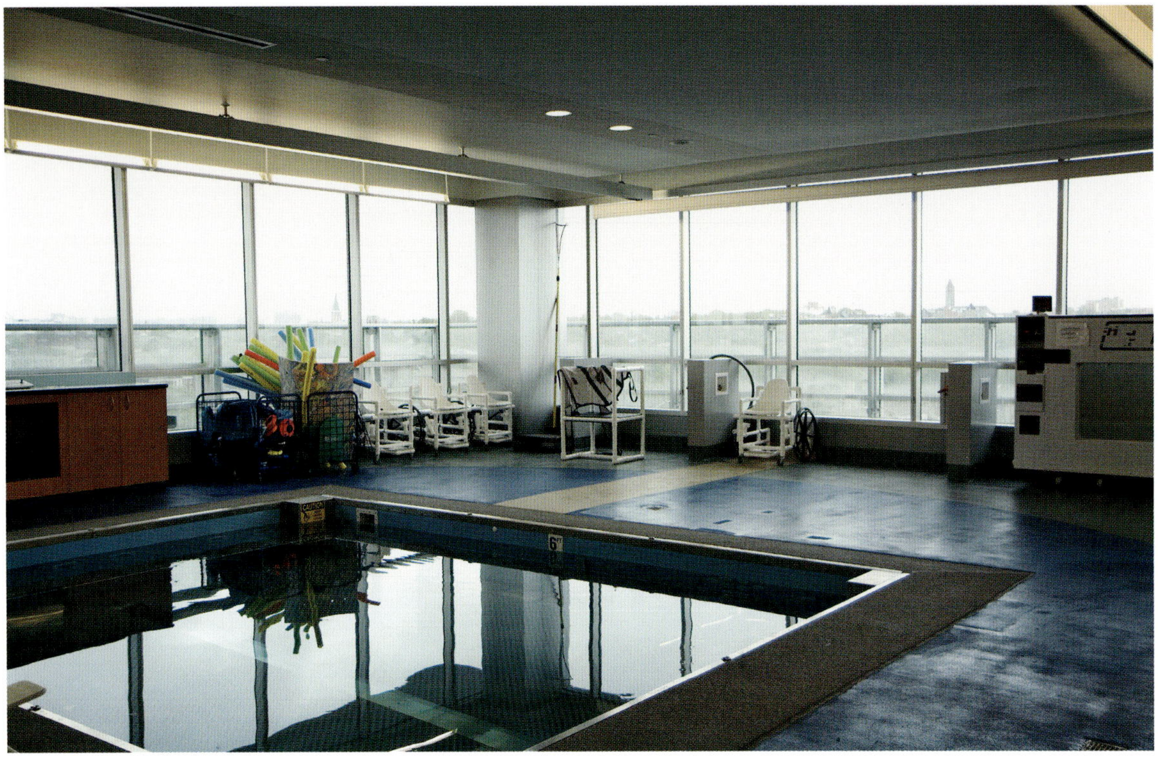

▲ Kennedy Krieger Institute Kennedy Krieger Children's Hospital, Baltimore, MD
▼ ***Photo: Jim Roof Creative (below)***

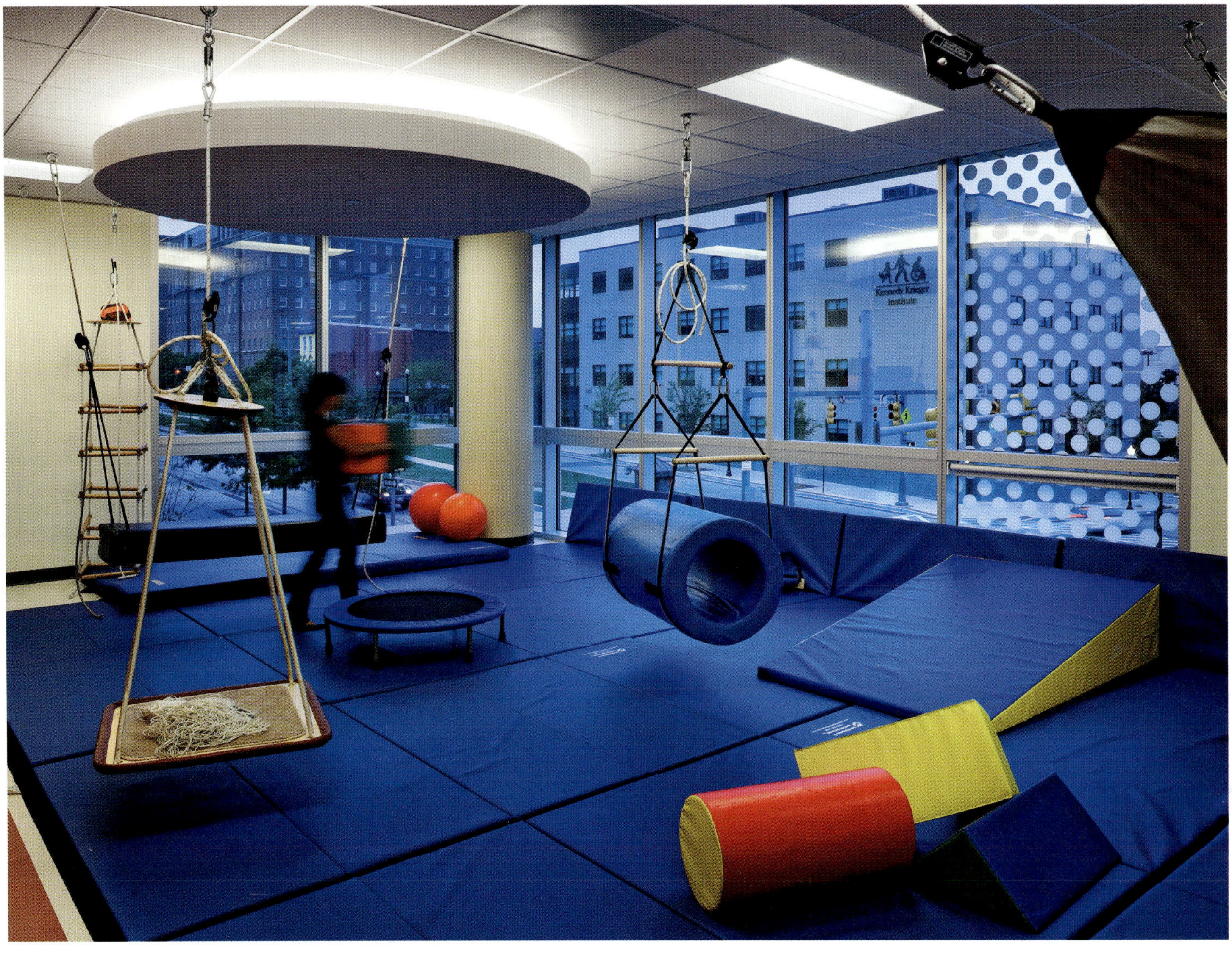

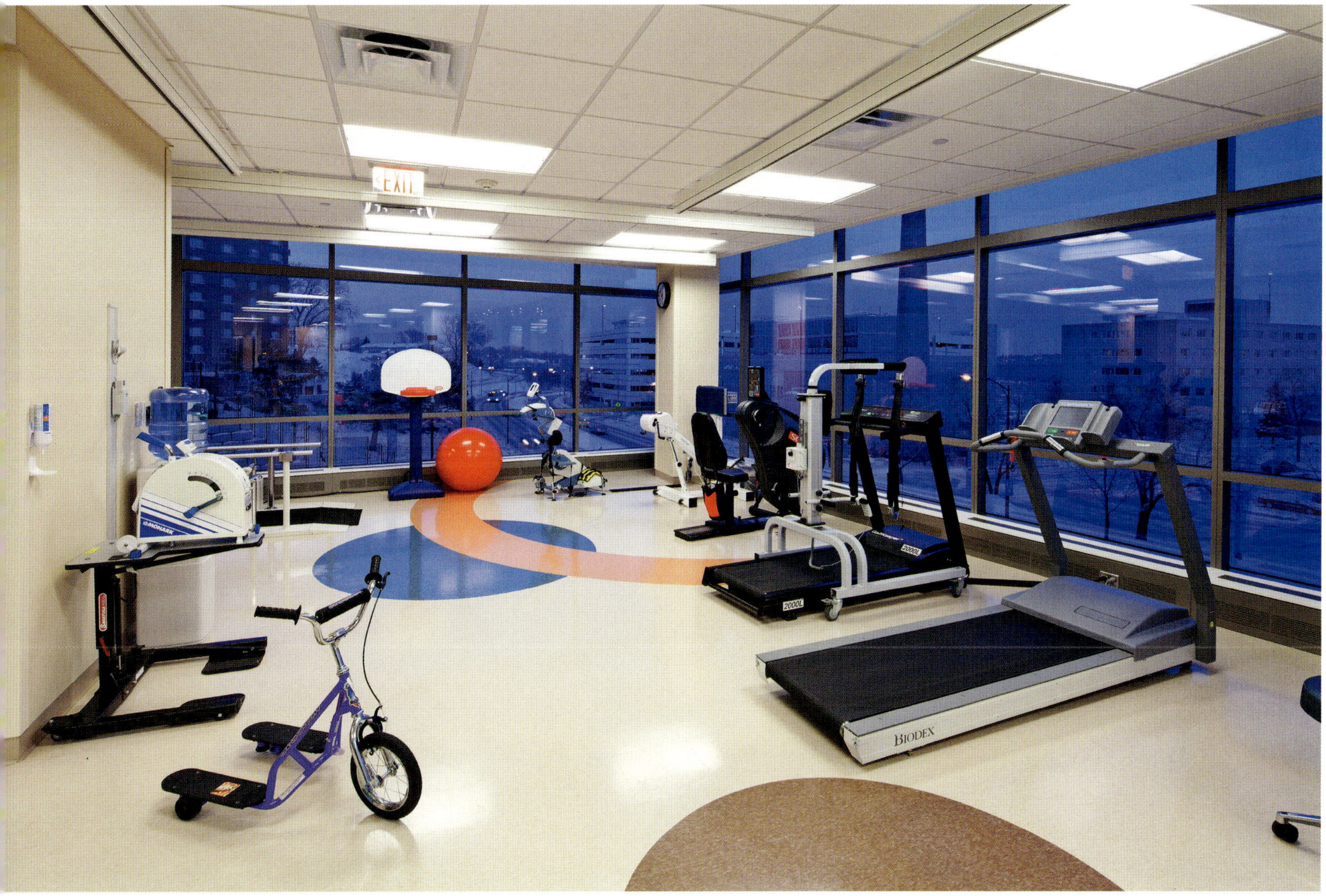

▲ Gillette Children's, Saint Paul, MN
Photo: Terry Mahanna

▼ Nemours/Alfred I. duPont Hospital for Children, Wilmington, DE
Photo: Karl Richeson

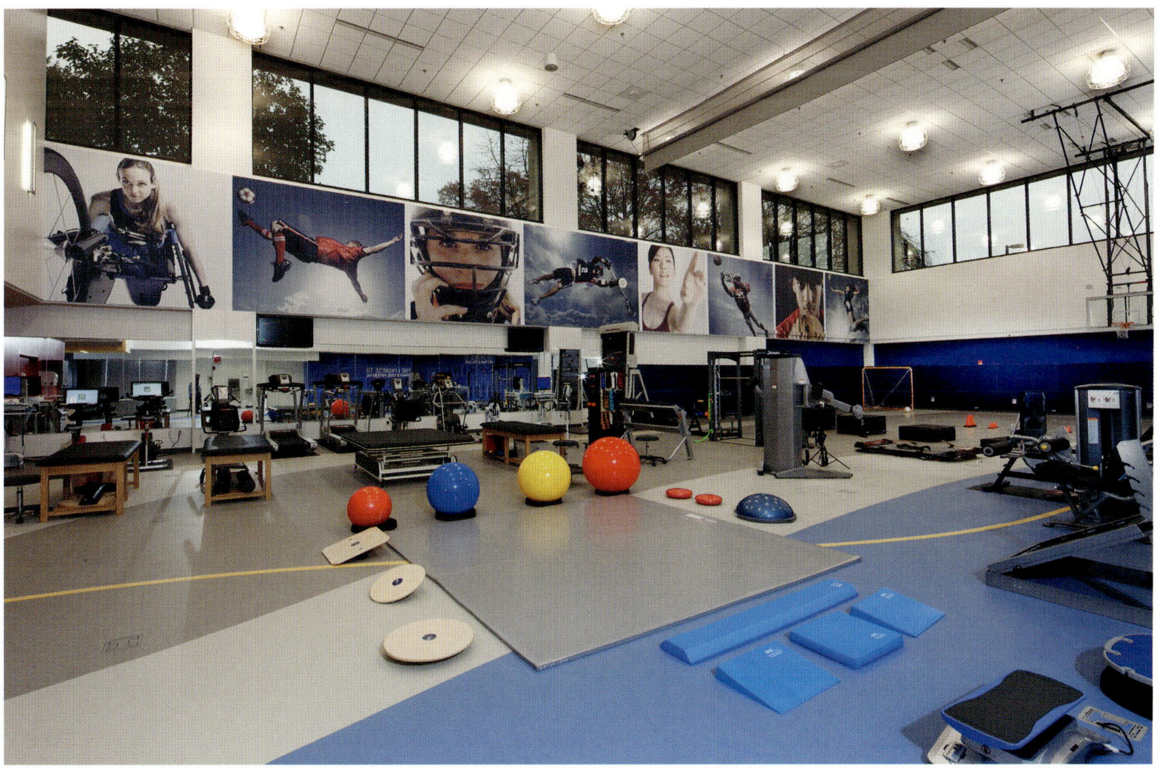

▼ Children's Hospital Colorado, Denver, CO
Photos: Eckert & Eckert

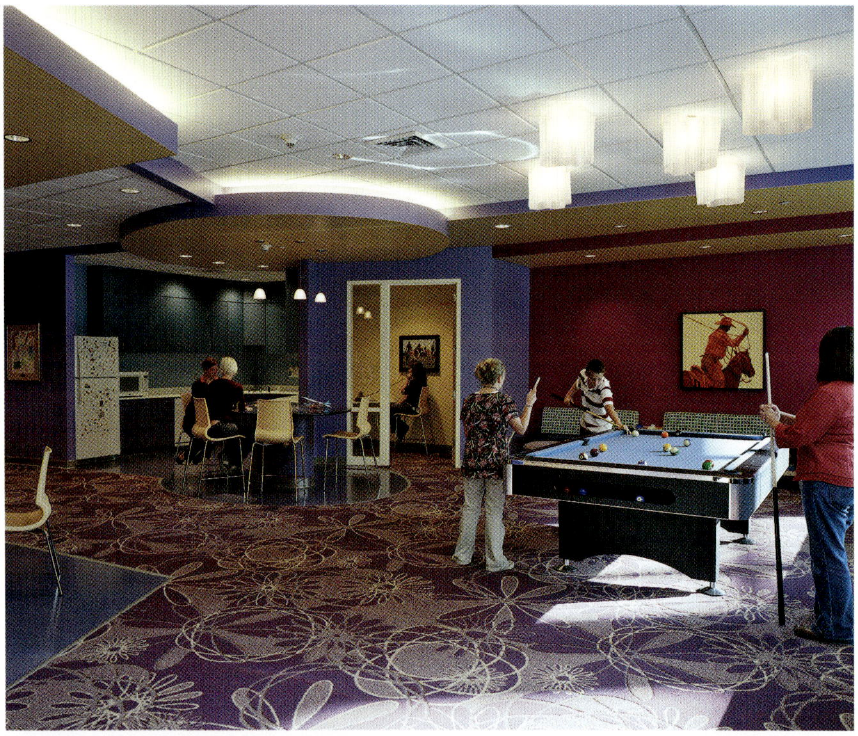

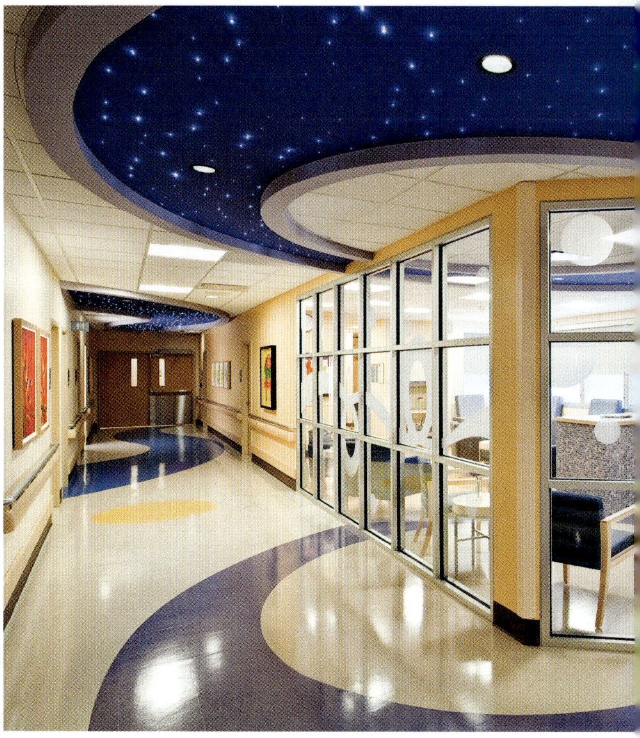

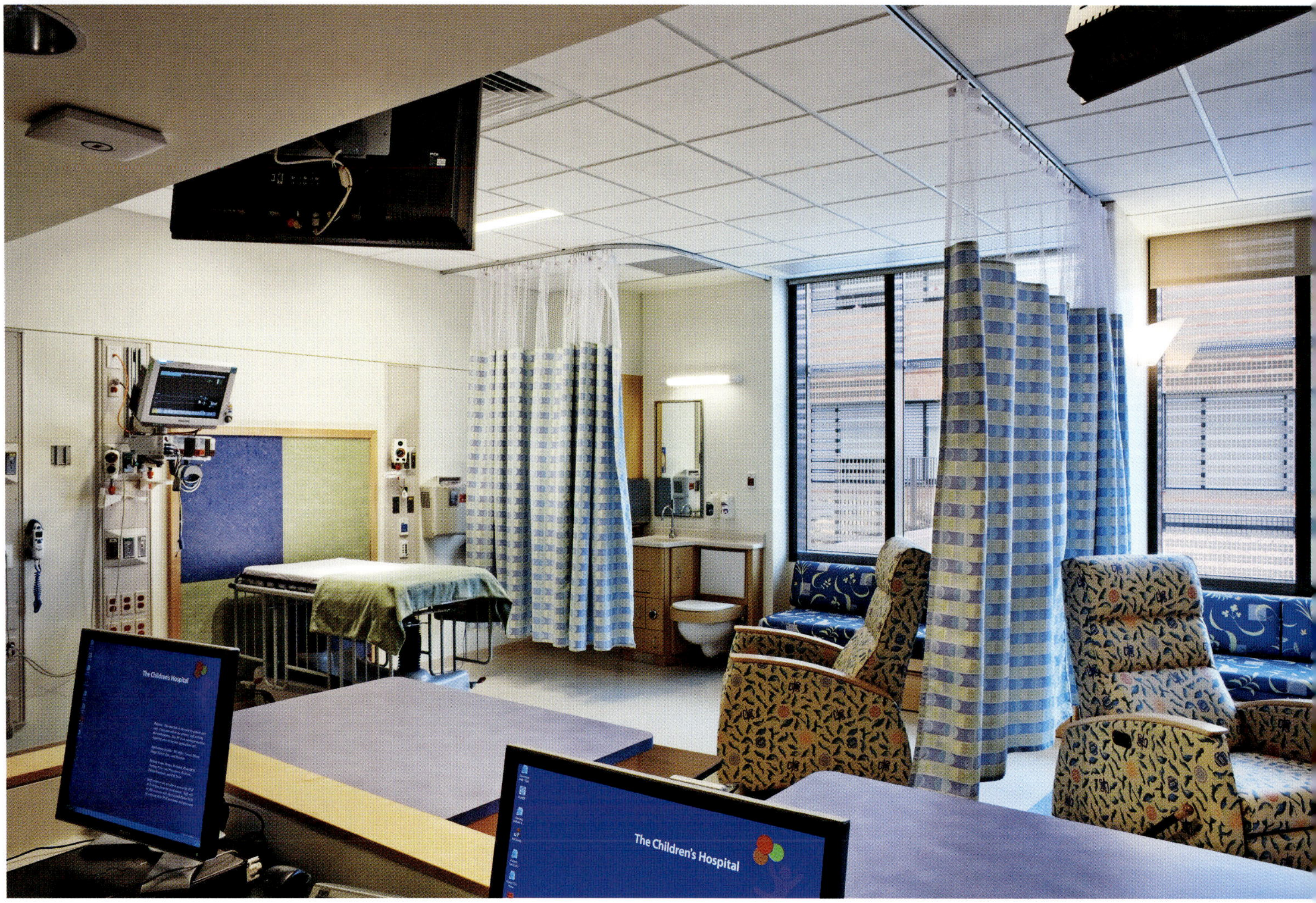

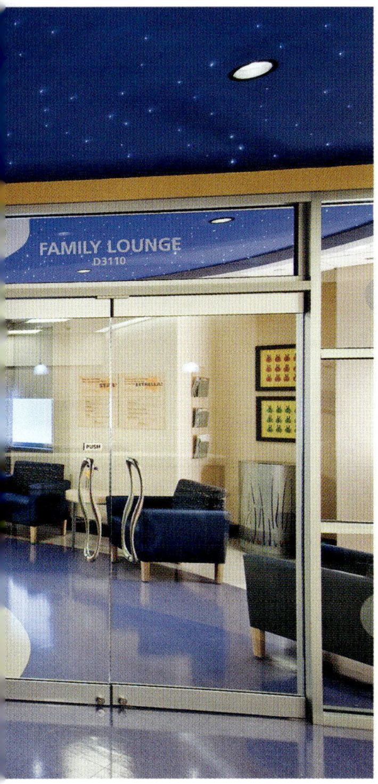

◀ Children's Medical Center, Dallas, TX
▼ ***Photos: Charles Smith***

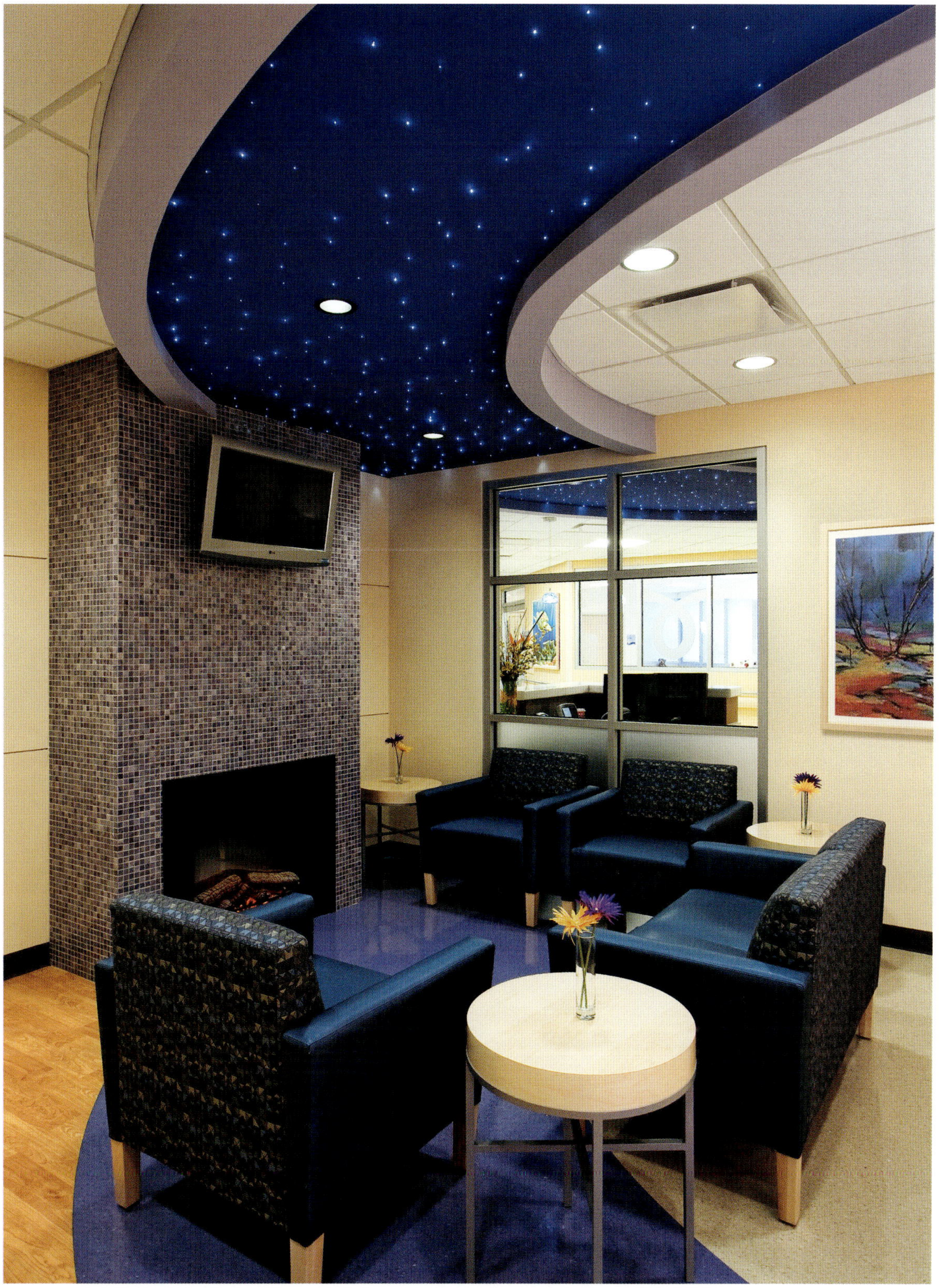

Following pages: Children's Healthcare of Atlanta, GA
Photo: Blake Marvin

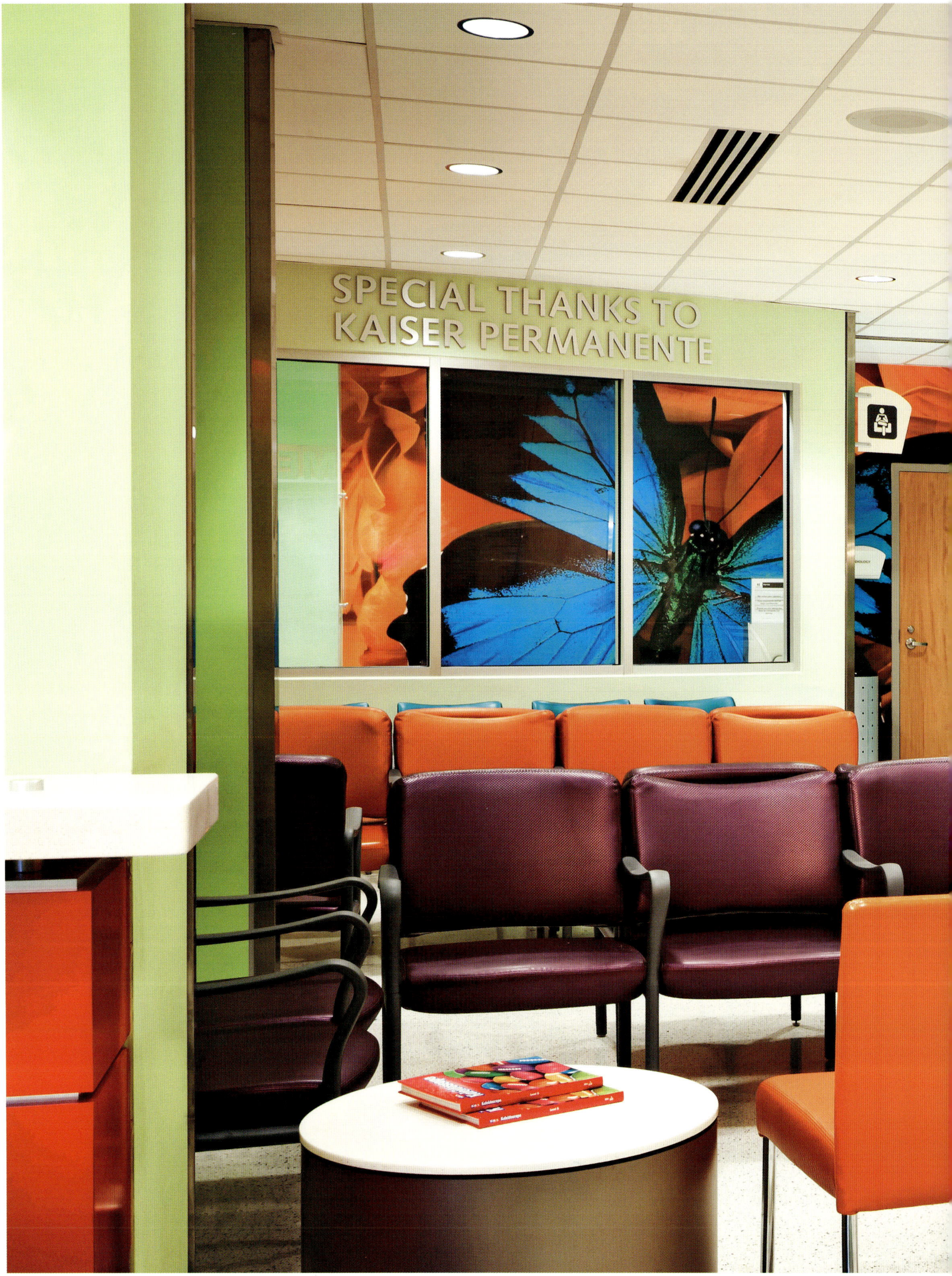
SPECIAL THANKS TO
KAISER PERMANENTE

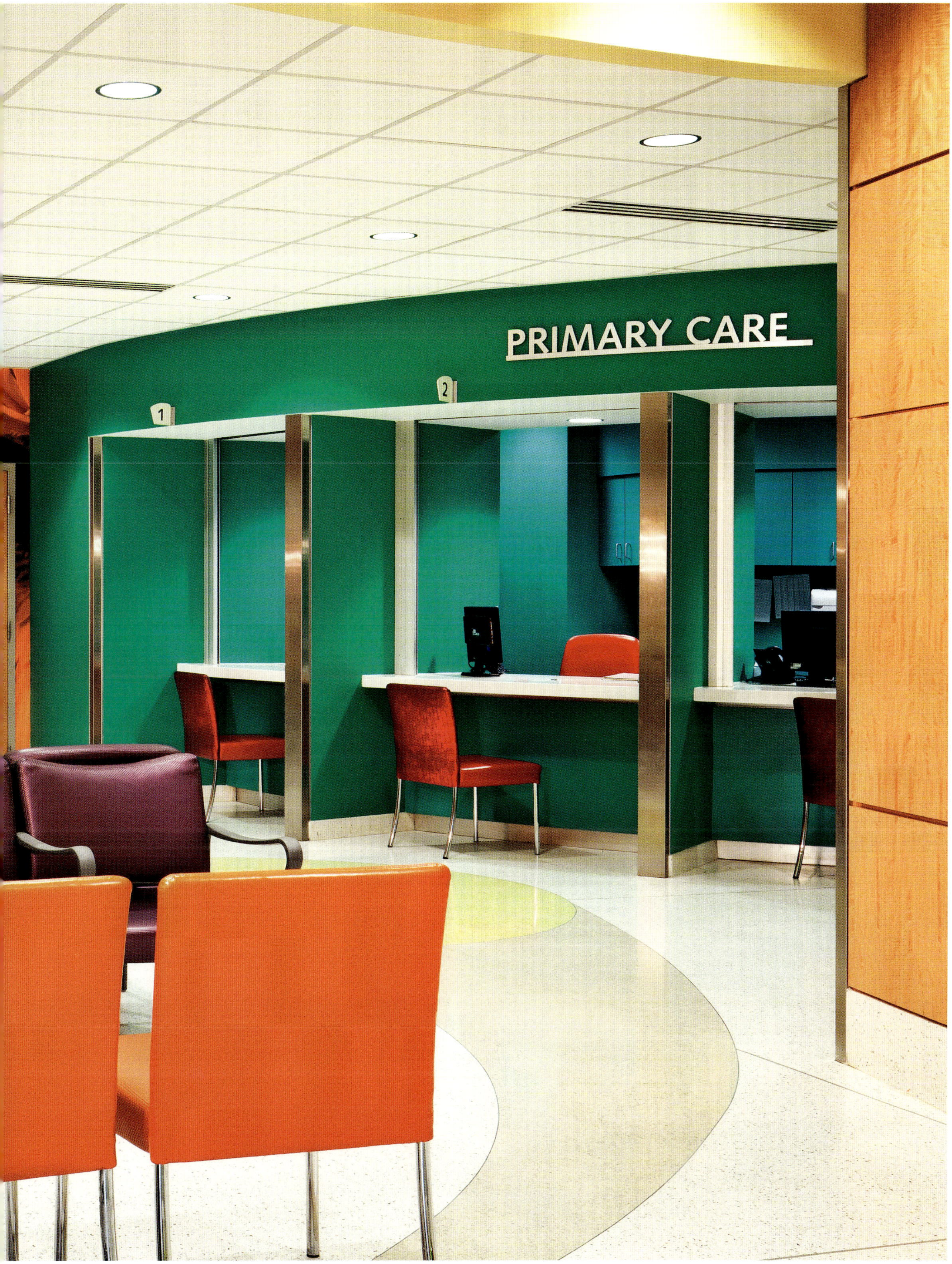
PRIMARY CARE
1
2

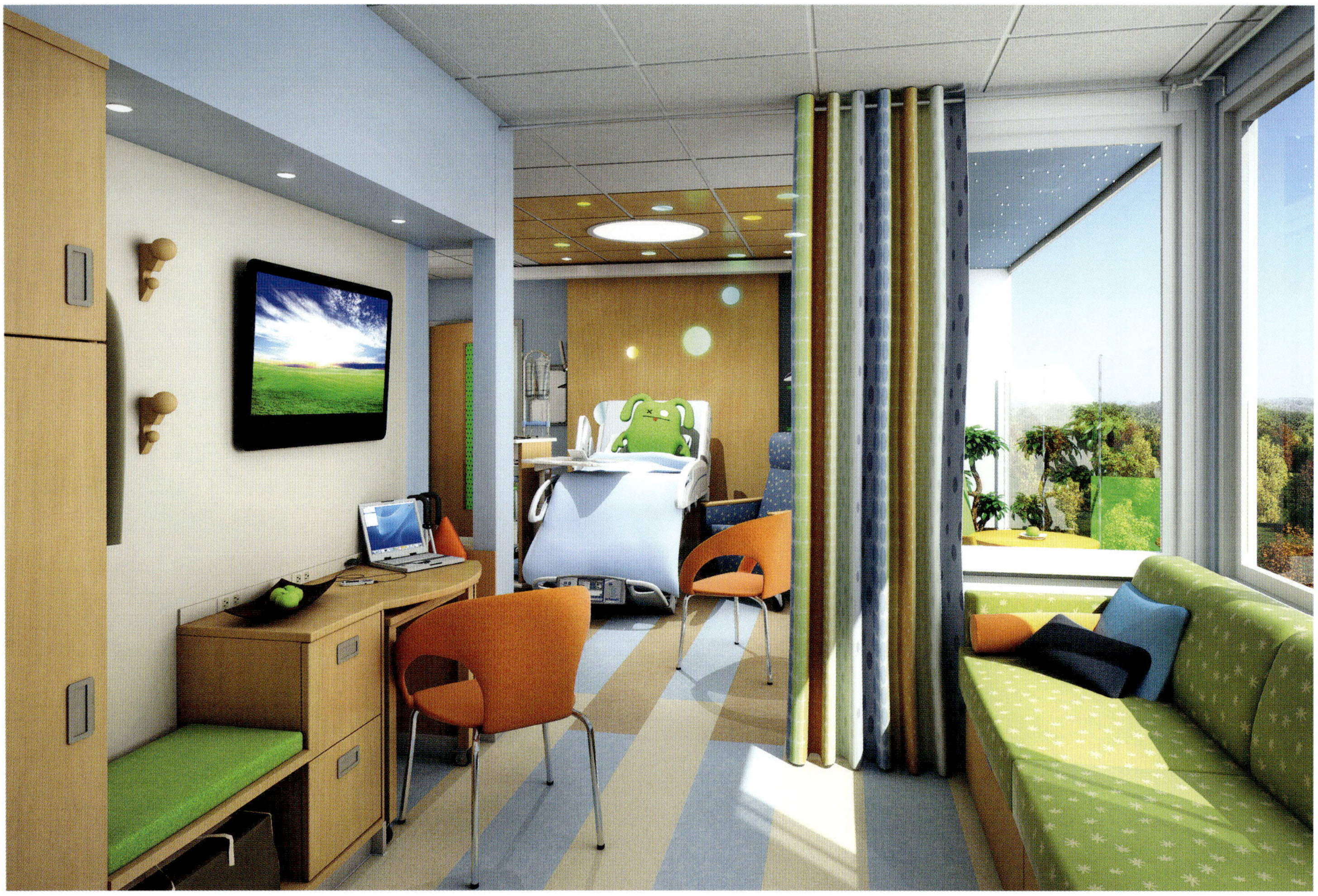

▲ Green Patient Lab

▼ ***Photos: Stantec ©***

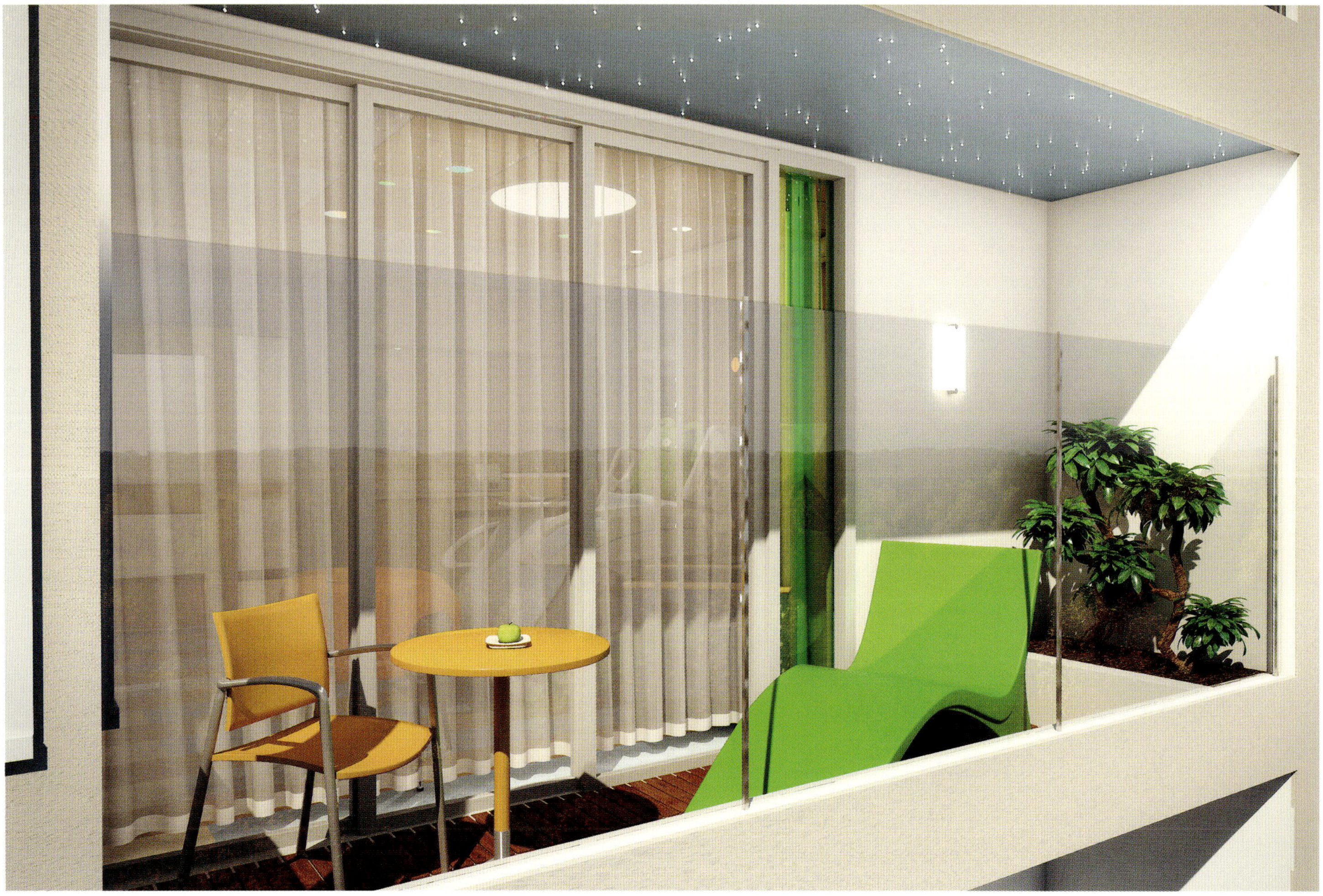

▼ Children's Medical Center at Legacy, Plano, TX
Photo: Robert Canfield

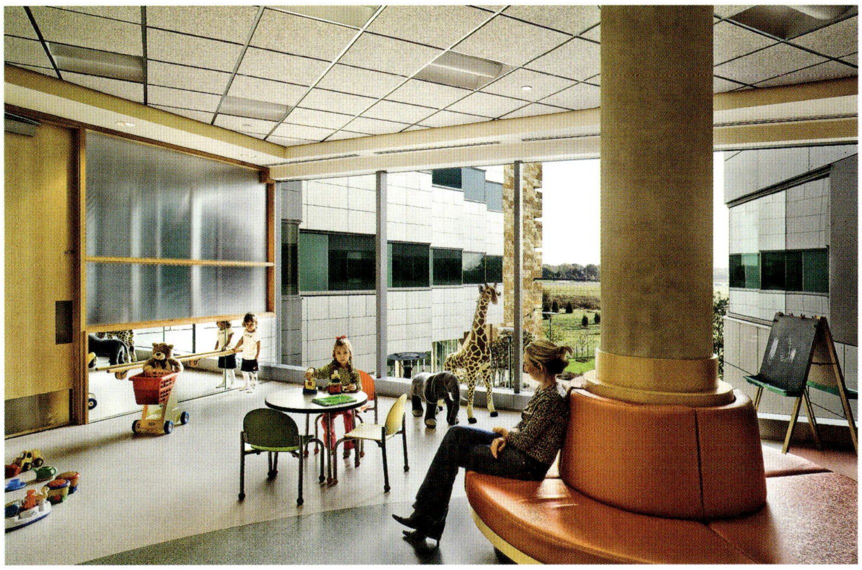

▼ Phoenix Children's Hospital, AZ
Photo: Blake Marvin, HKS

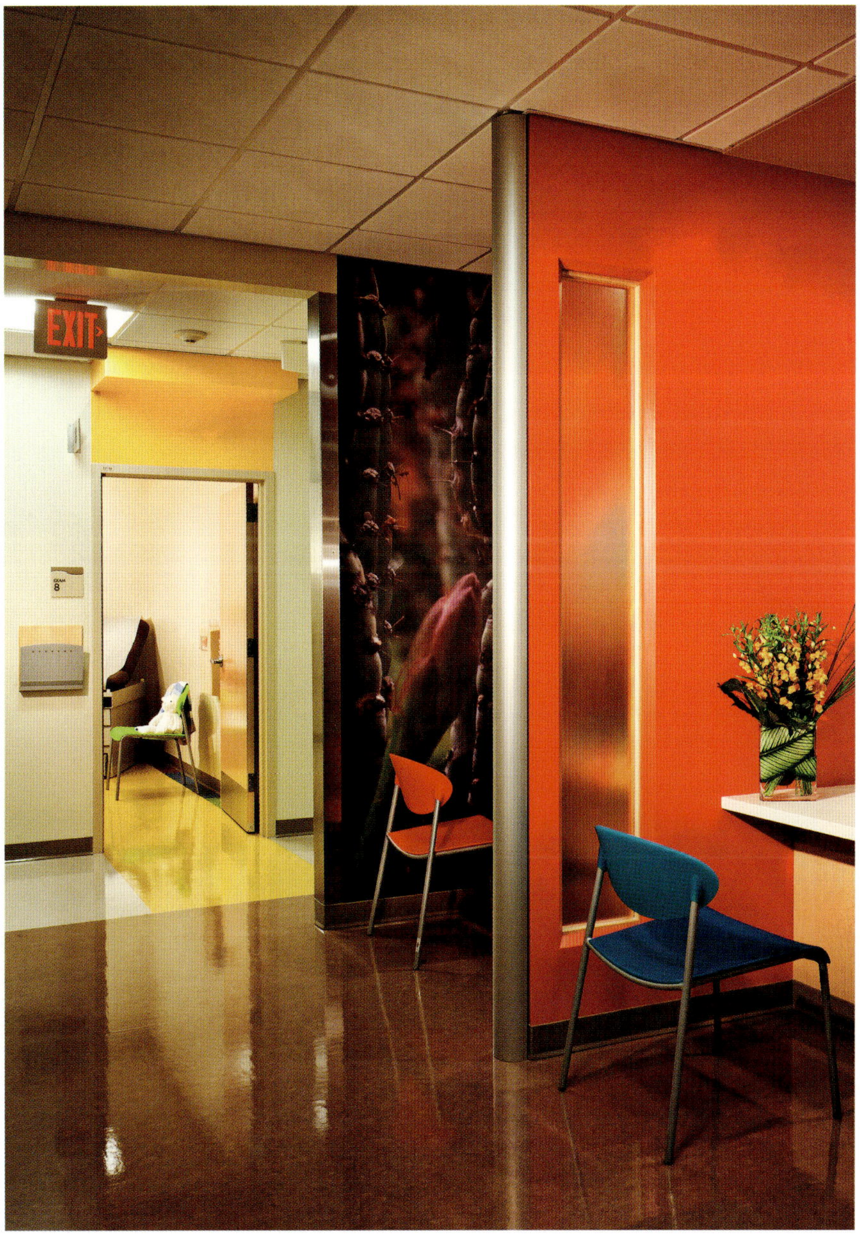

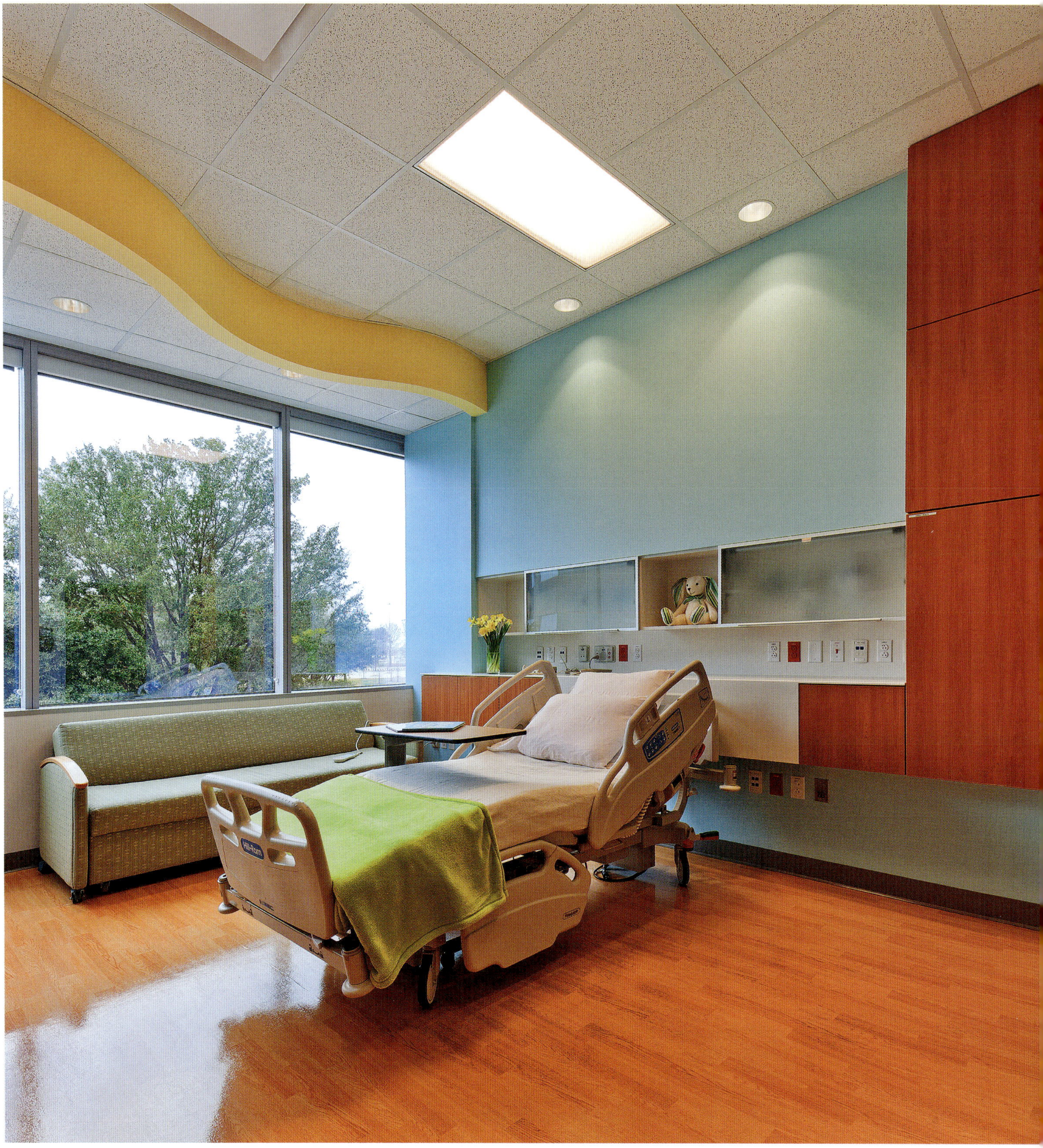

▲ Texas Children's Hospital West Campus, Houston, TX
Photo: Geoff Dyon, G. Dyon Photography

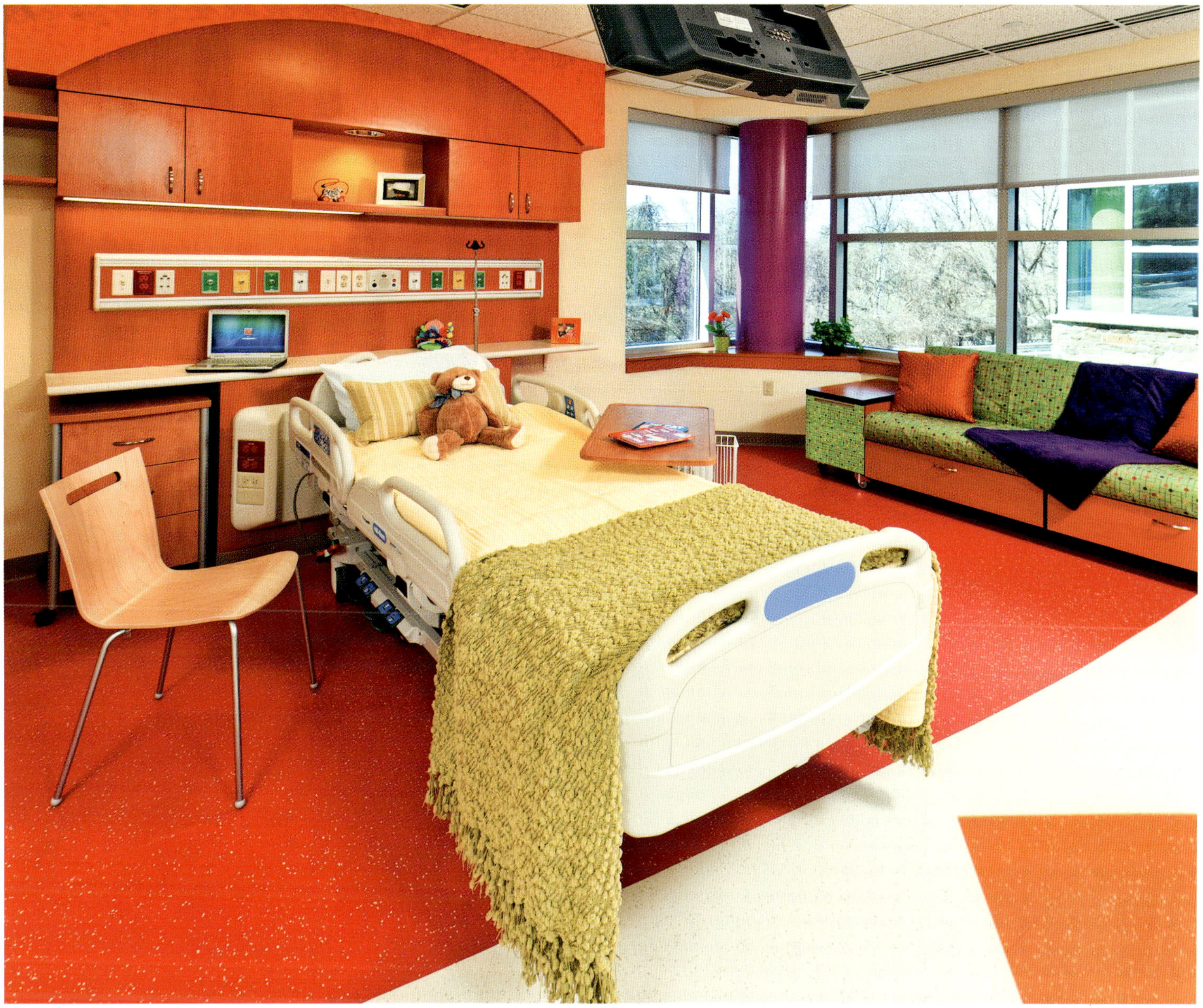

▲ Blythedale Children's Hospital, Valhalla, NY
Photo: Copyright 2010 © Jeff Smith Photography

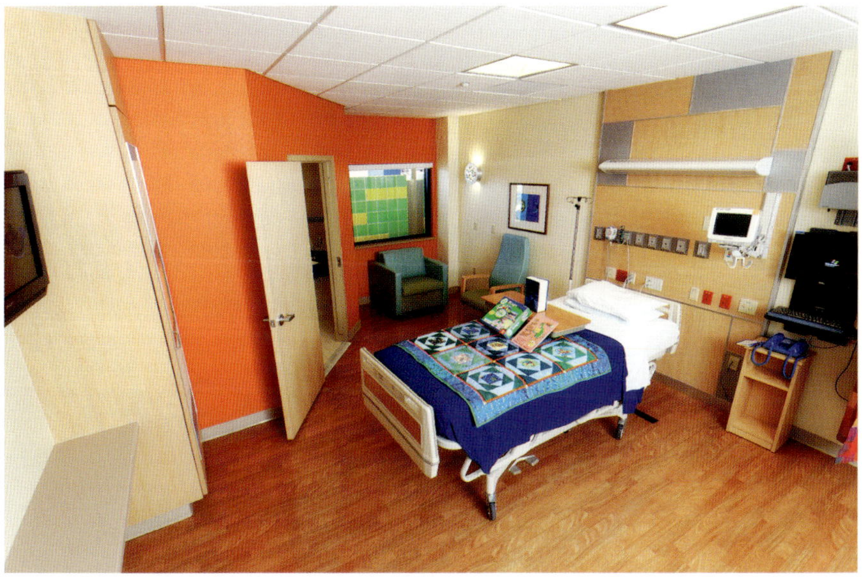

▲ Tucson Medical Center, AZ
Photo: Eric Suhm

▼ Helen DeVos Children's Hospital, Grand Rapids, MI
Photo: Hedrich Blessing

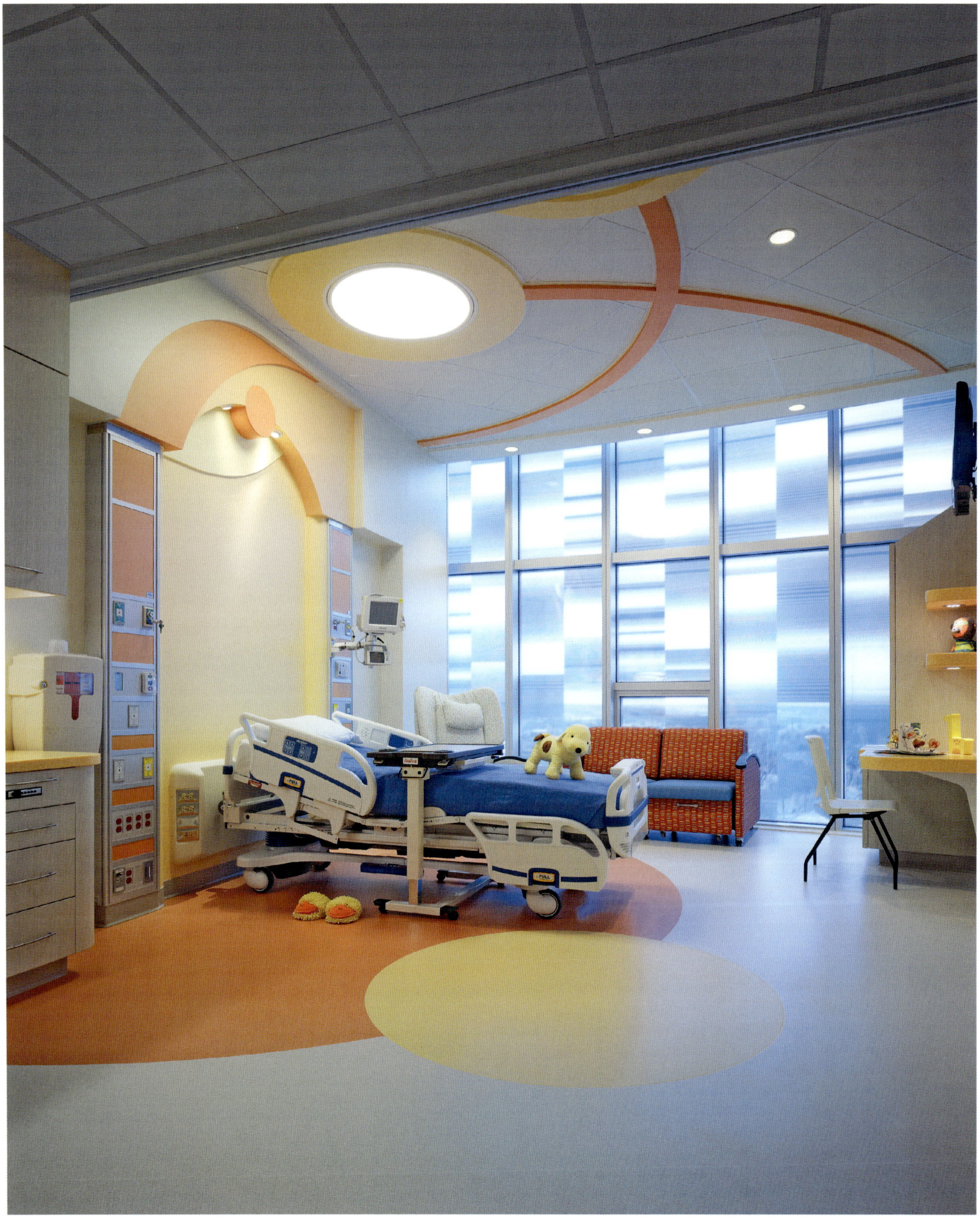

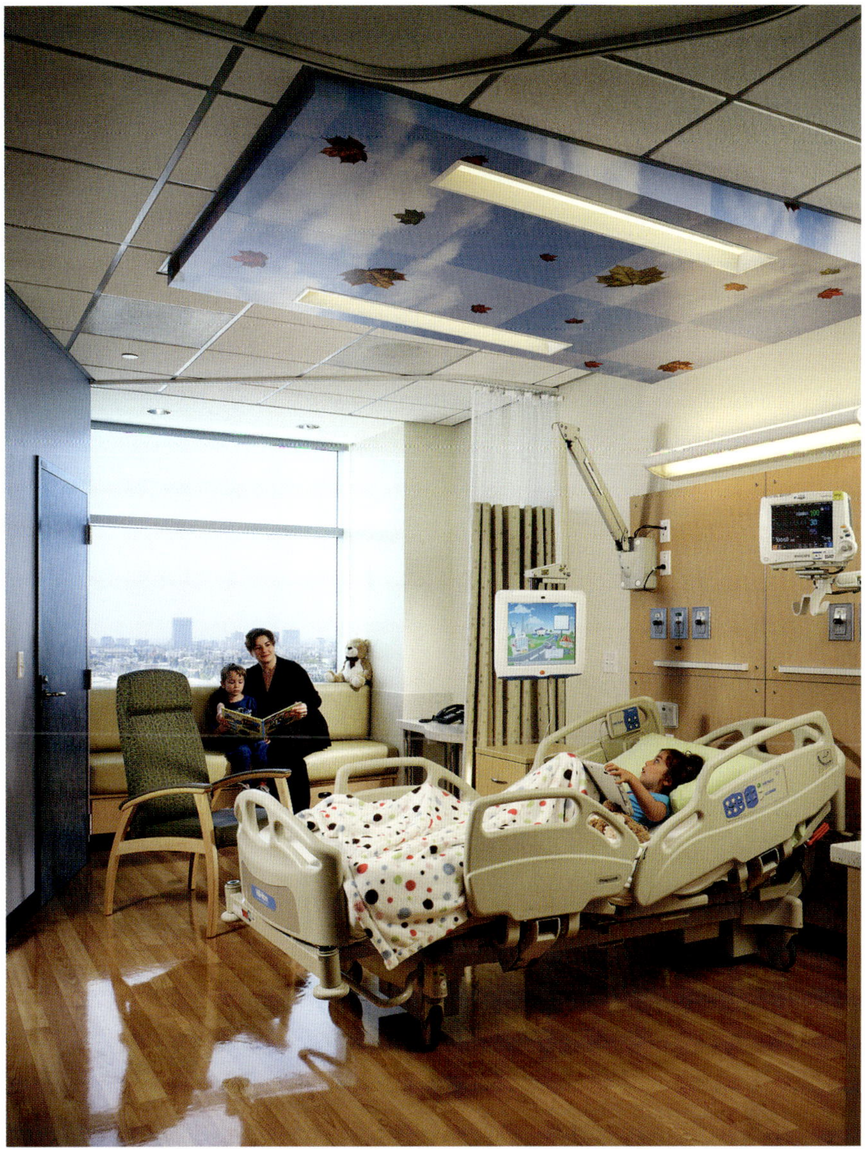

▲ Children's Hospital Los Angeles, CA
Photo: Hedrich Blessing Photography, Nick Merrick

▼ Palmetto Health Children's Hospital, Columbia, SC

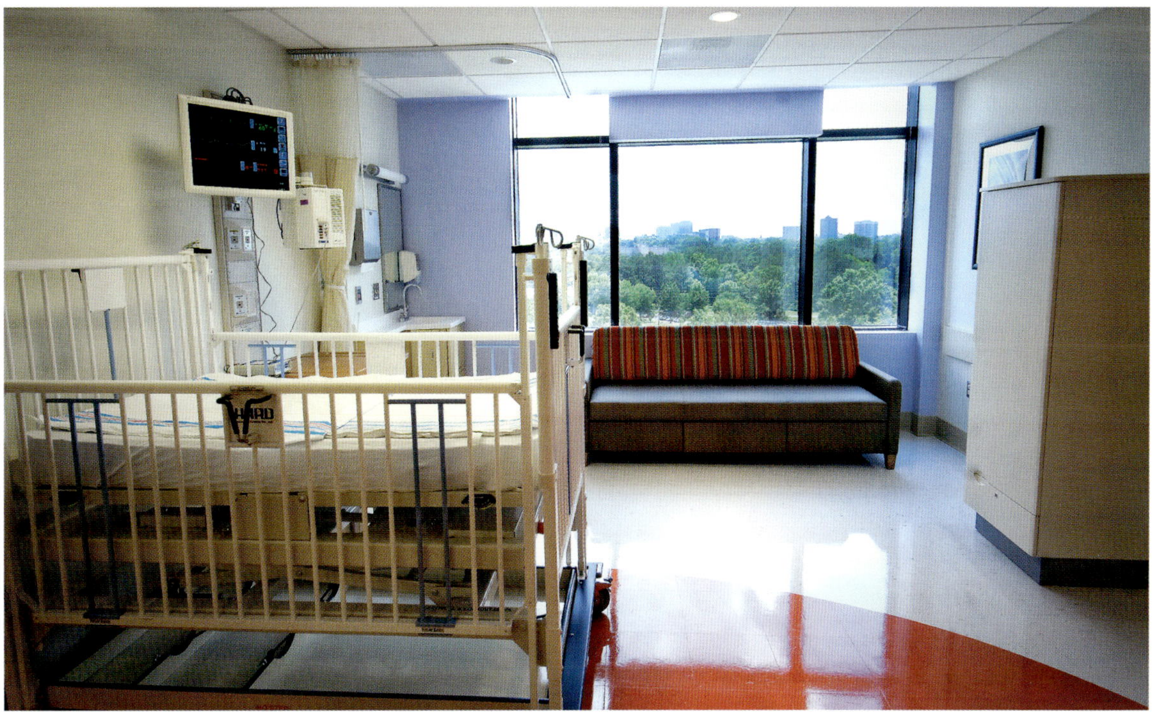

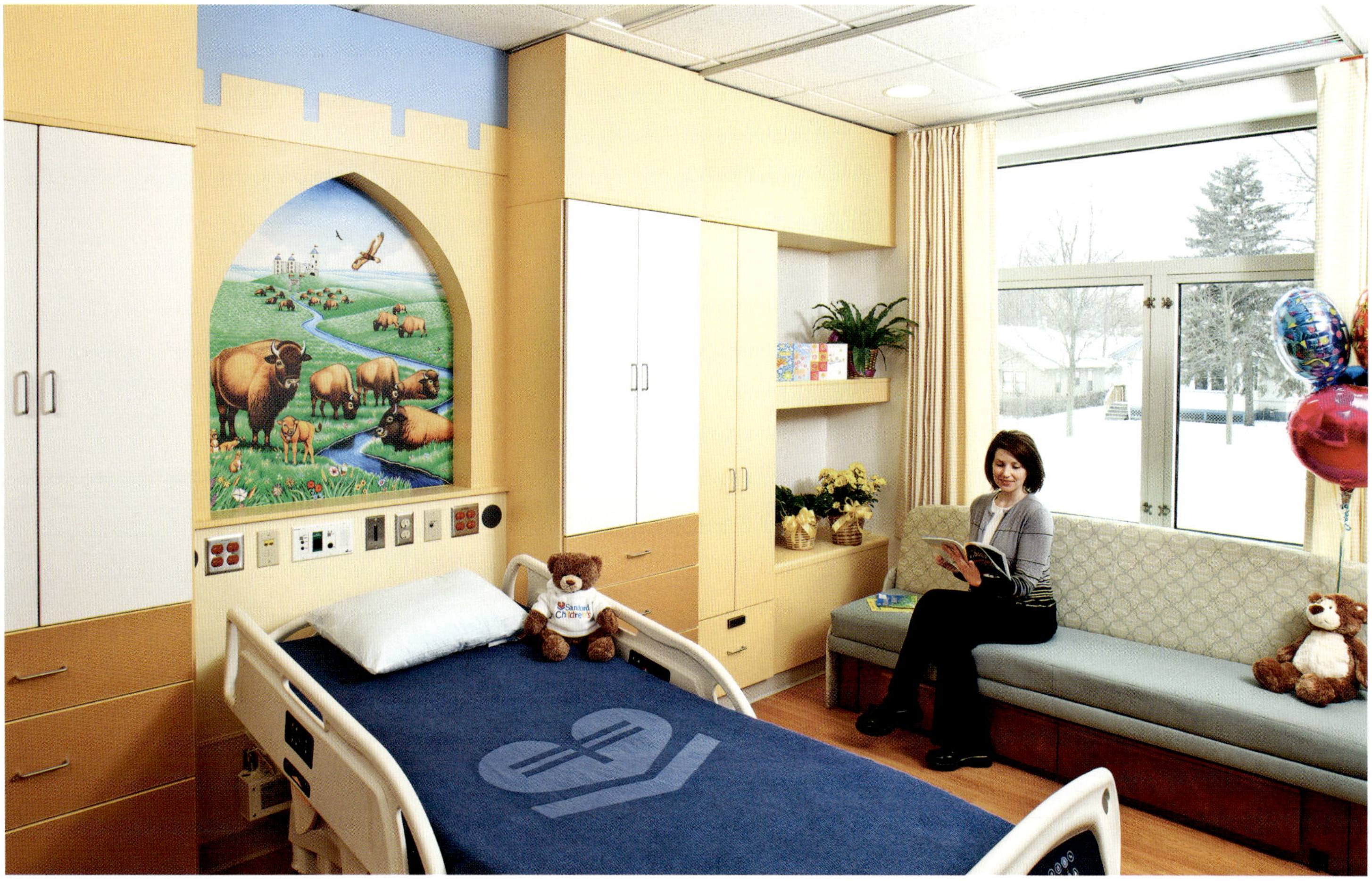

▲ Sanford Children's Hospital, Sioux Falls, SD

▼ Dayton Children's, OH
Photo: Ken Shory

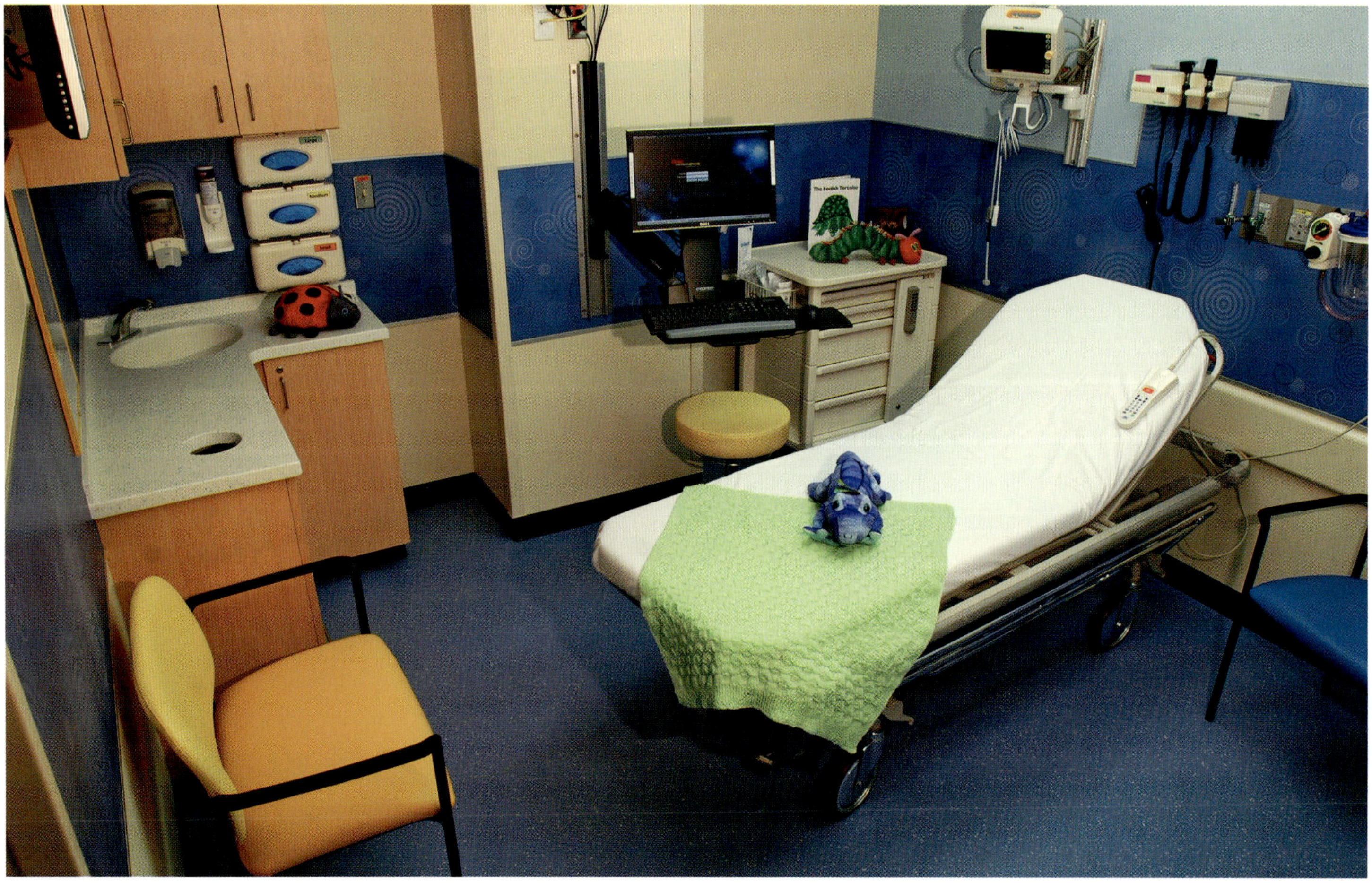

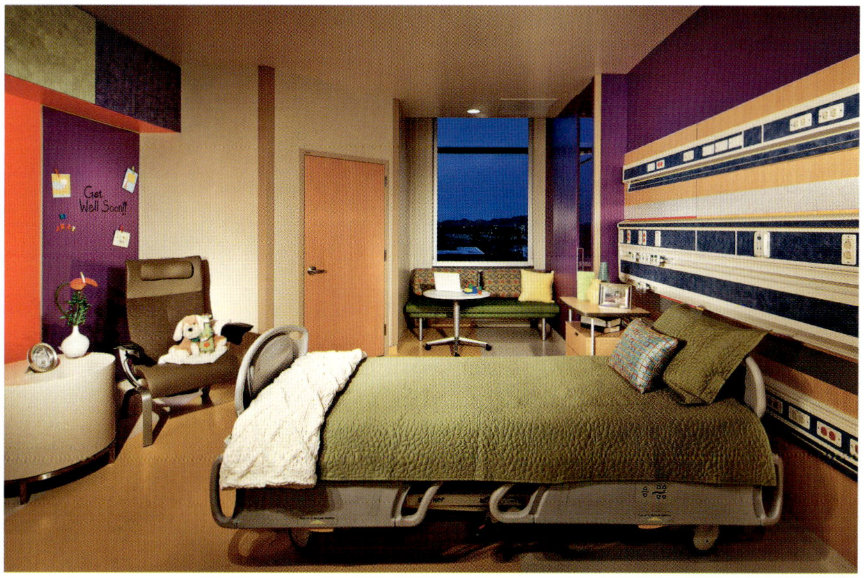

▲ Phoenix Children's Hospital, AZ
Photo: Blake Marvin, HKS

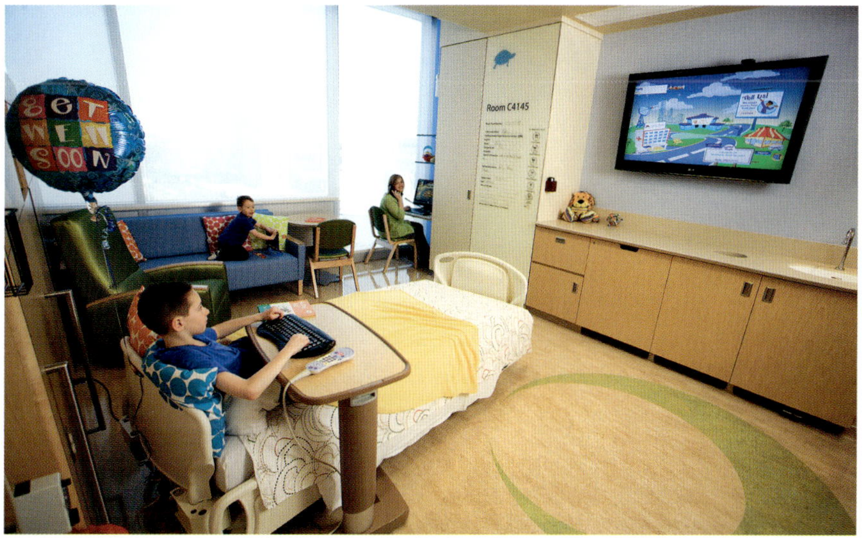

▲ University of Minnesota Amplatz Children's Hospital, Minneapolis, MN
Photo: Hedrich Blessing Photography, Nick Merrick

▼ Ann & Robert H. Lurie Children's Hospital of Chicago, IL
Photo: Hedrich Blessing Photography, Nick Merrick

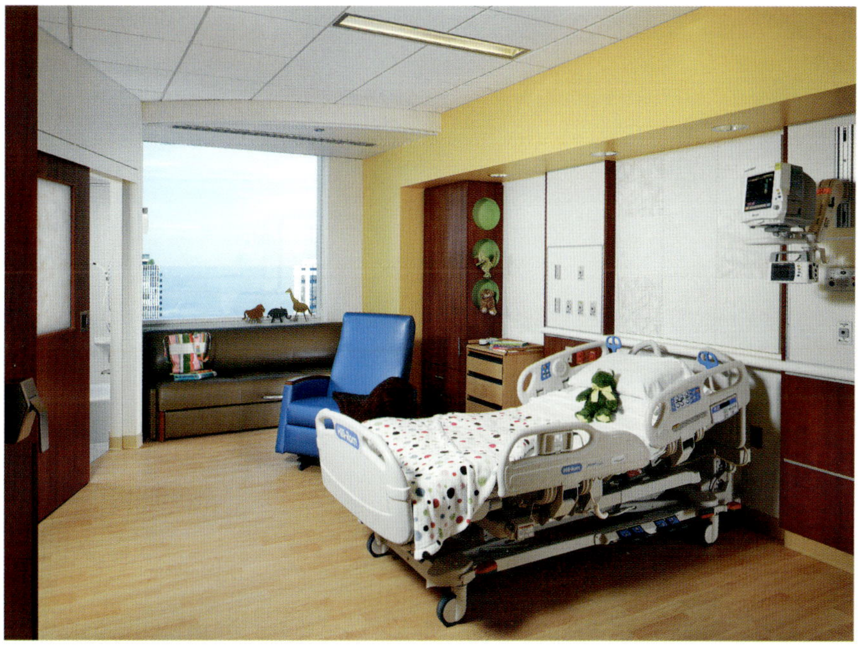

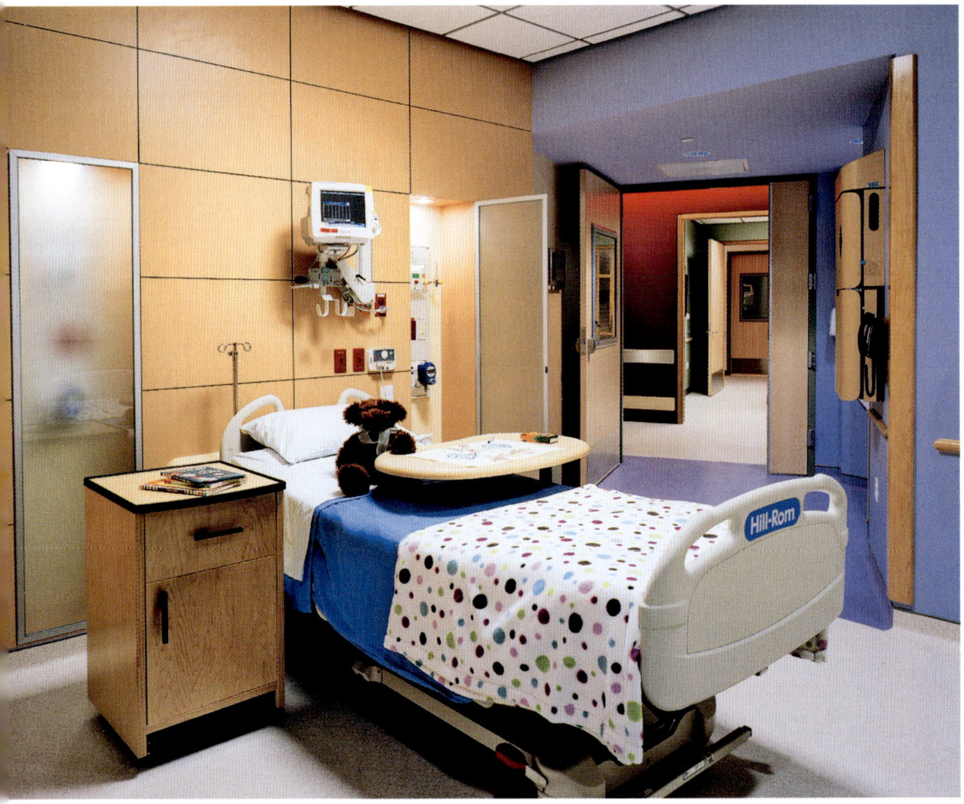

▲ Children's Medical Center at Legacy, Plano, TX
Photo: Eckert & Eckert

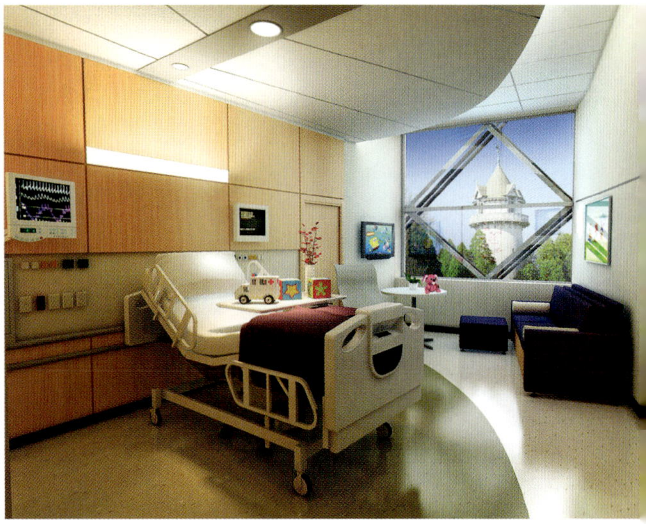

▲ Nemours/Alfred I. duPont Hospital for Children, Wilmington, DE
Photo: FKP Architects

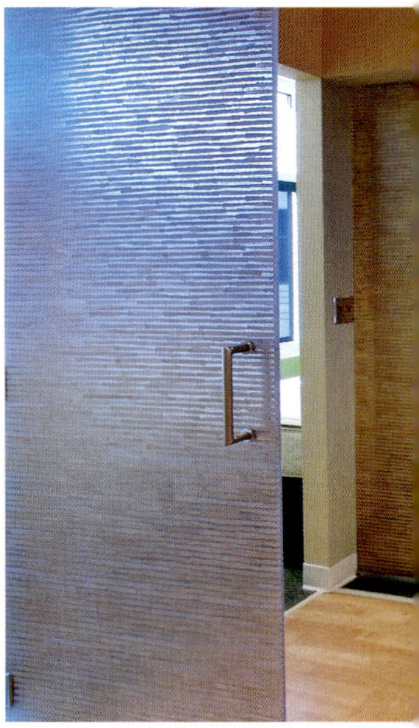

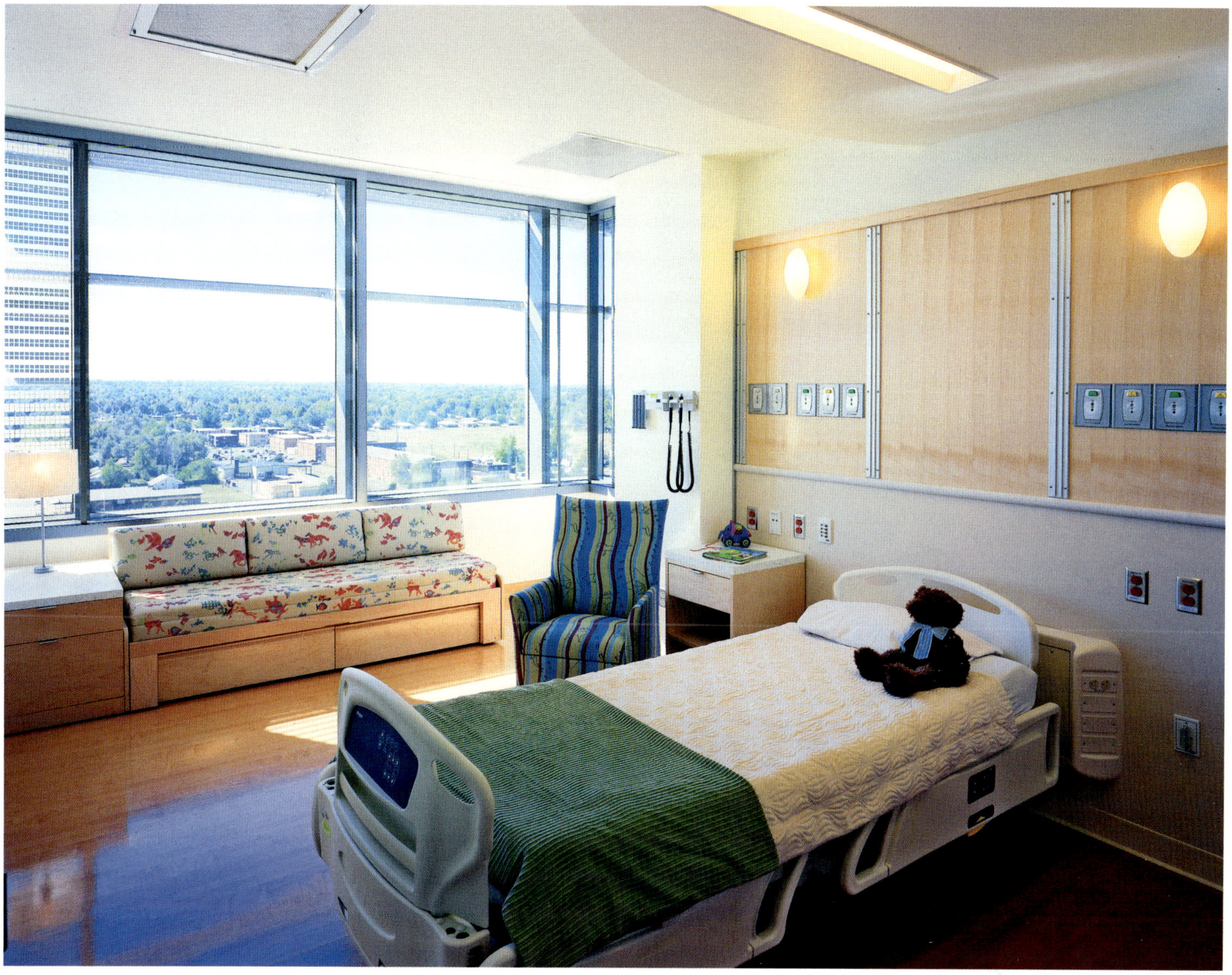

▲ Children's Hospital Colorado, Denver, CO
Photo: Eckert & Eckert

▼ CHOC Children's Hospital, Orange, CA
Photos: Joy Gonzales and Kevin Makowski

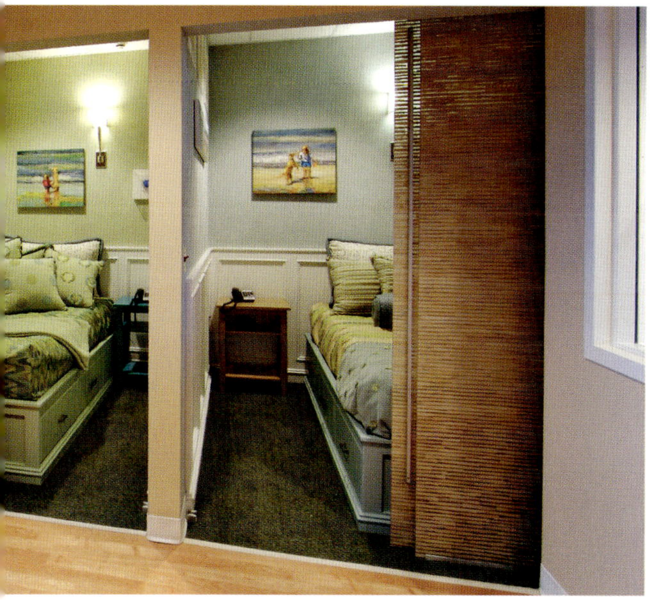

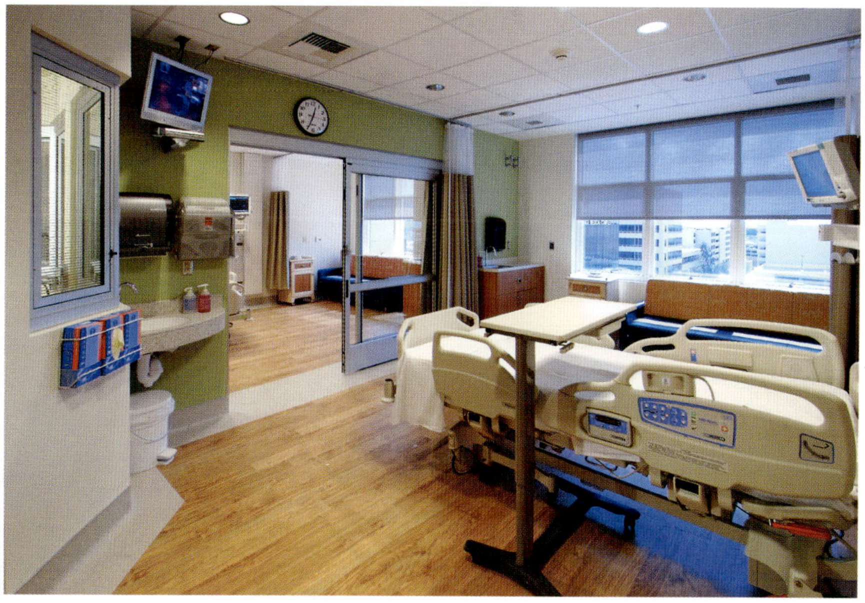

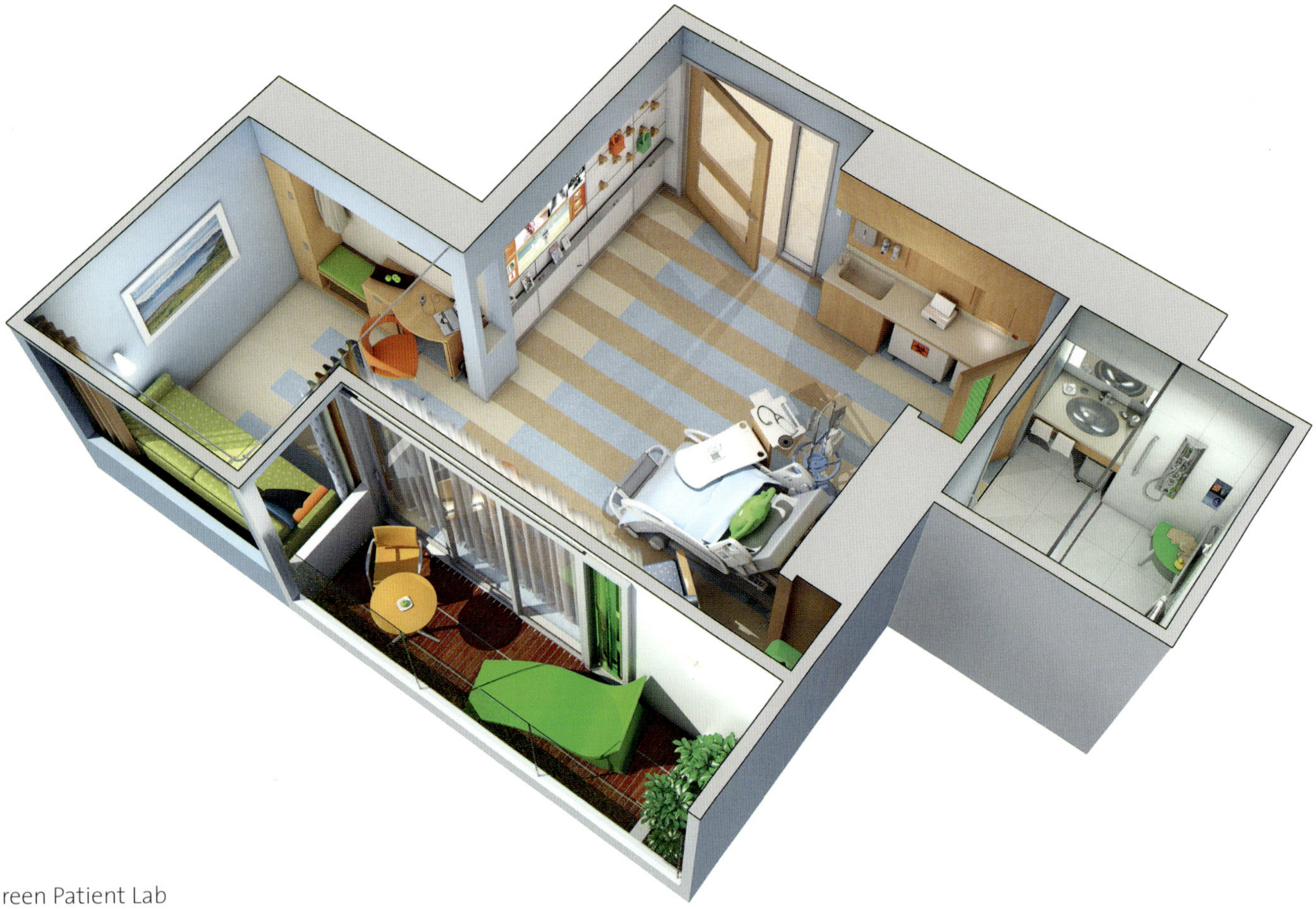

▲ Green Patient Lab
▼ *Photos: Stantec ©*

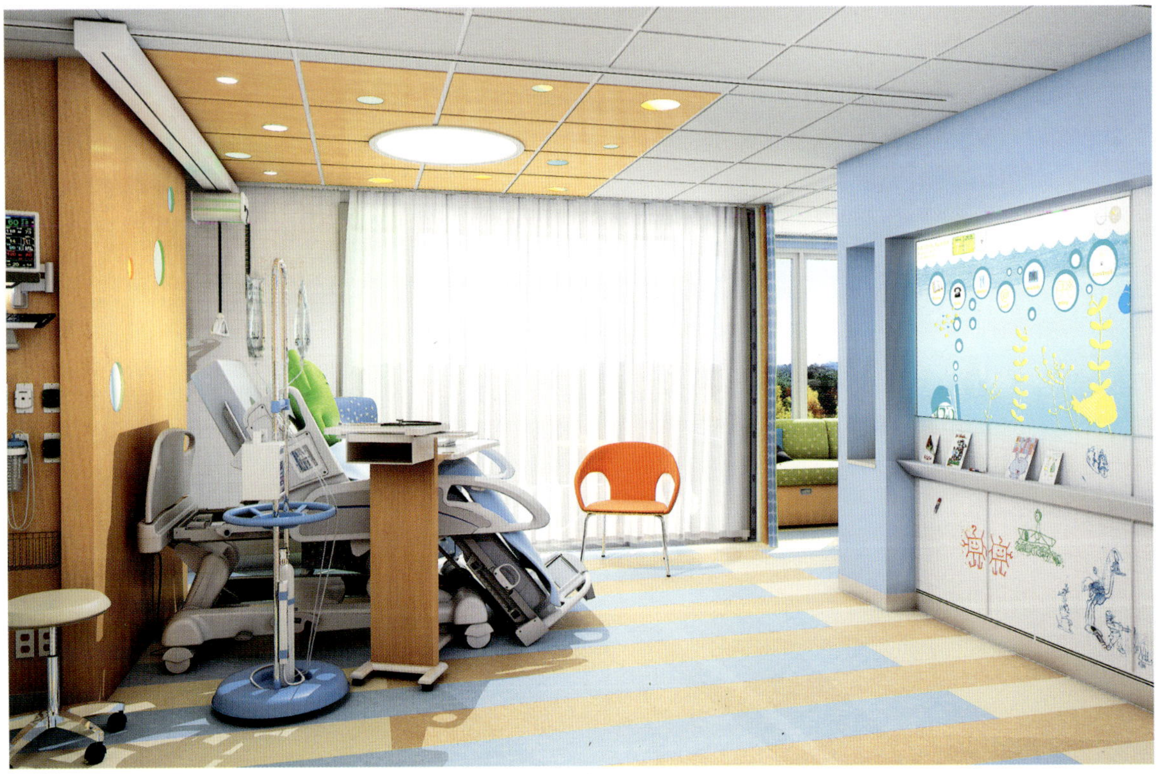

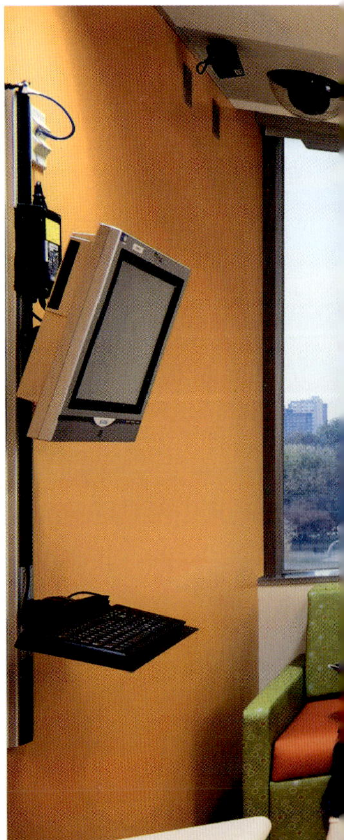

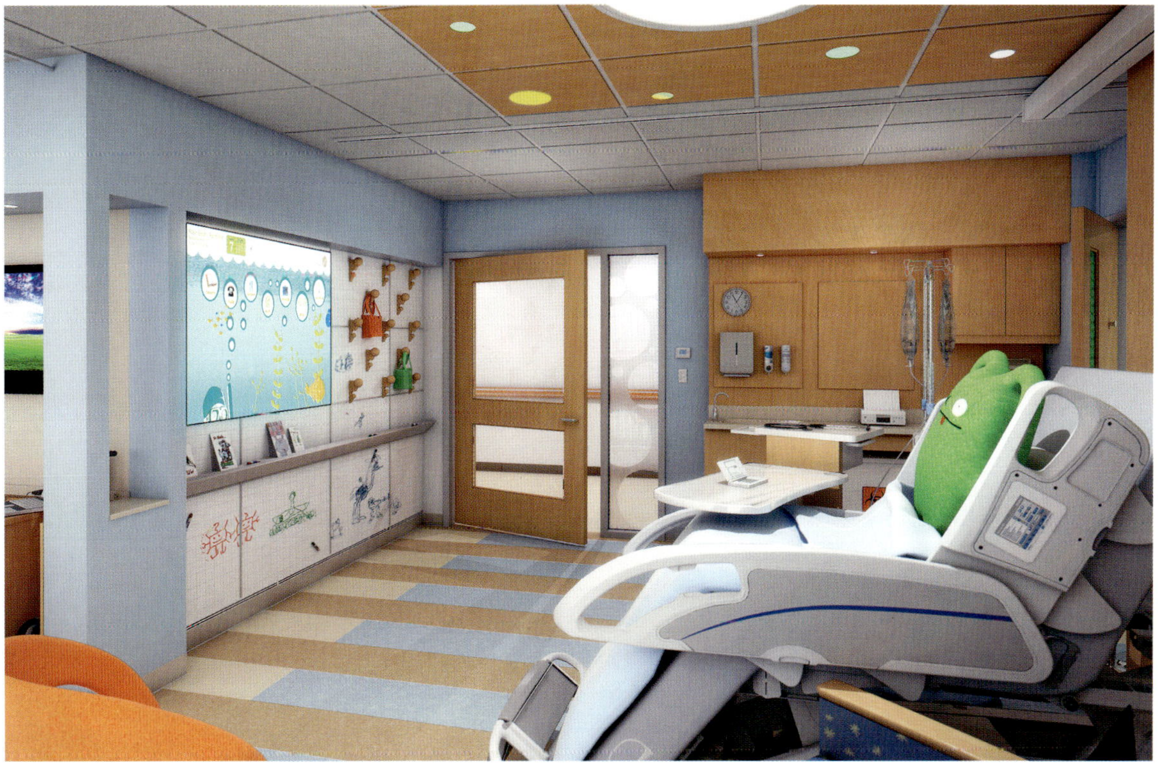

▲ Green Patient Lab
Photo: Stantec ©

▼ Le Bonheur Children's Hospital, Memphis, TN
Photo: Aker Imaging

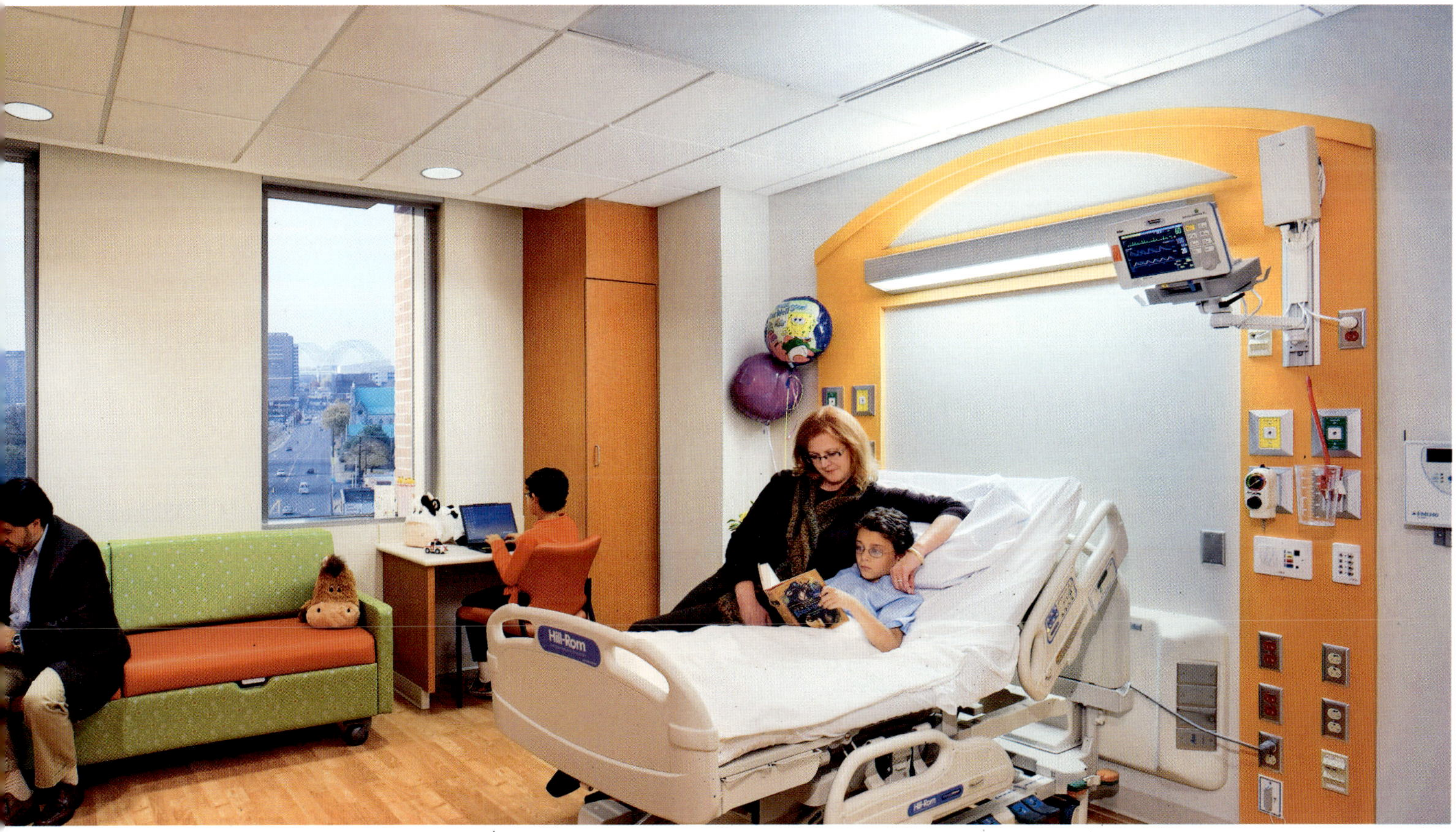

▼ Rady Children's Hospital, San Diego, CA
Photo: Stantec © Brian Kitts

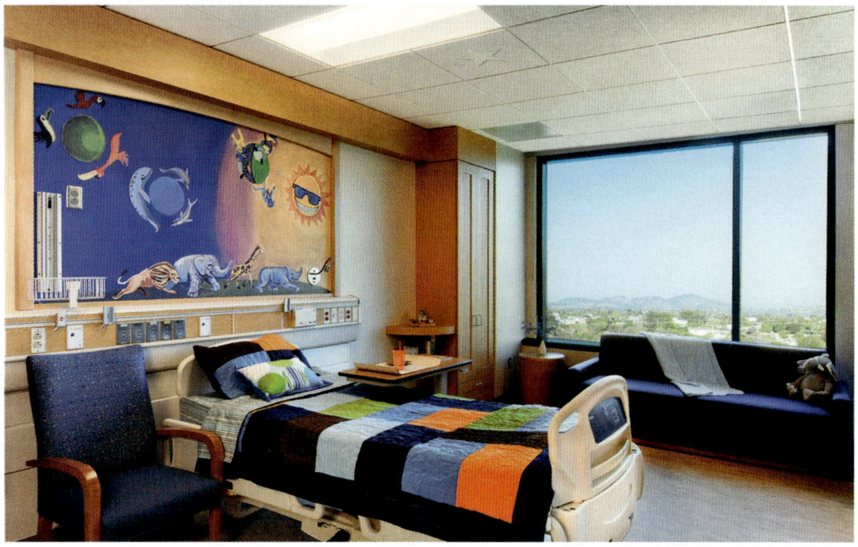

▼ Riverton Hospital Primary Children's Medical Center, Riverton, UT
Photo: Stantec © David Wakely Photography

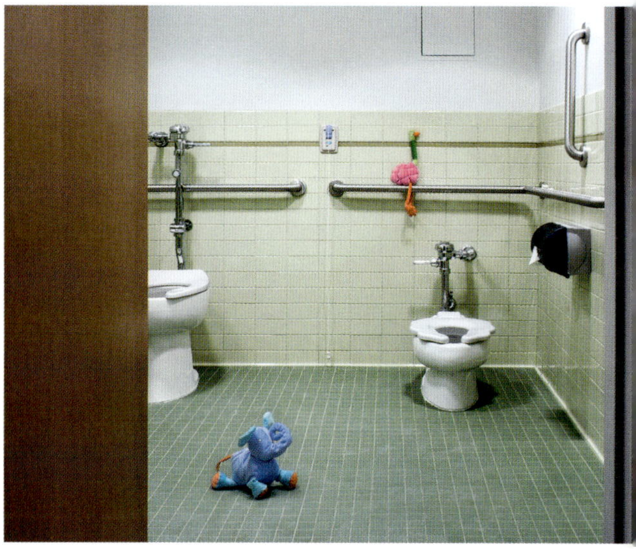

▼ University of Melbourne Hospital, Melbourne, Victoria, Australia
Photo: Stantec ©

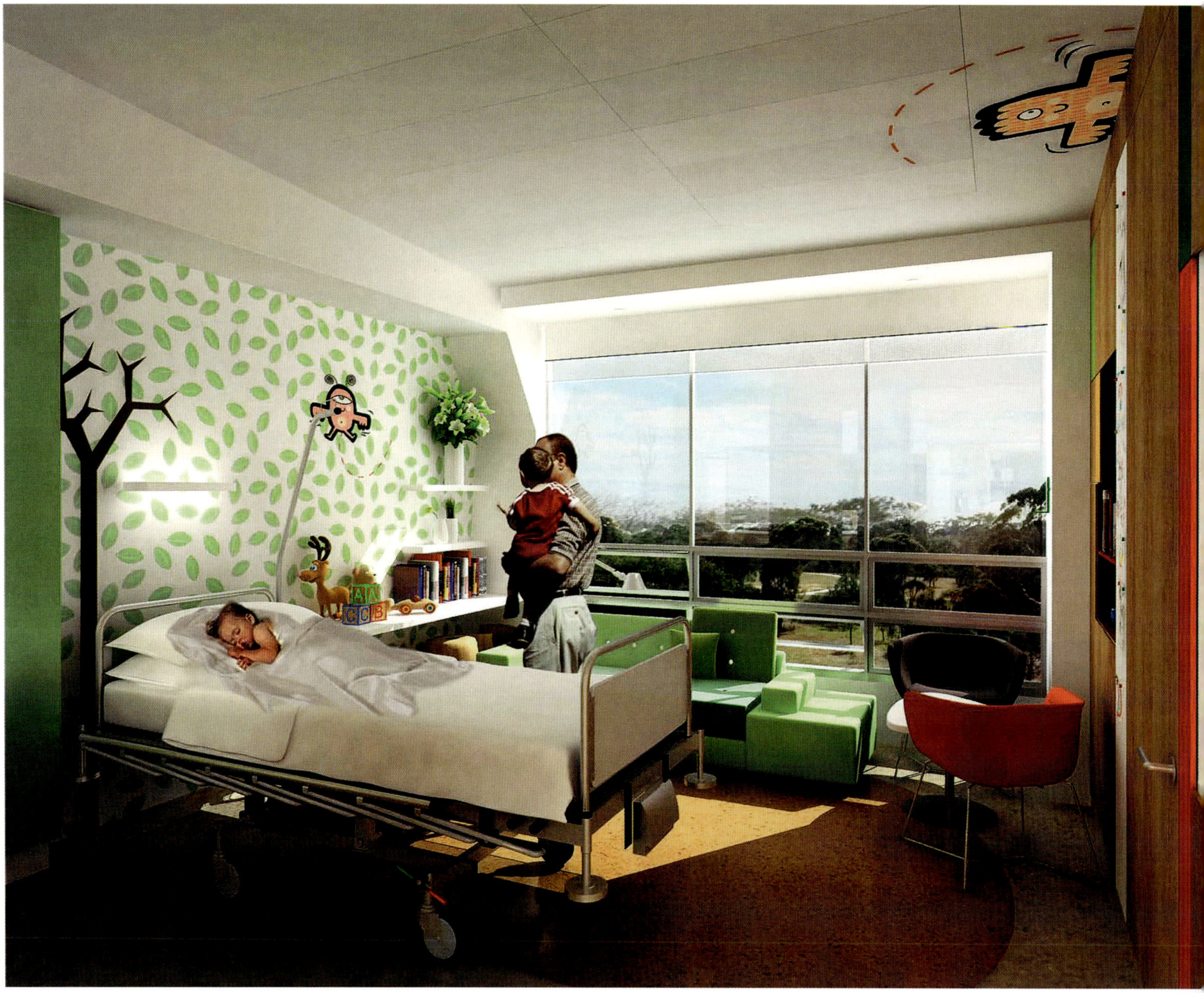

▼ American Family Children's Hospital, Kellogg, WI
Photo: HDR Architecture, Inc. © 2007 Ballogg Photography Inc., Chicago

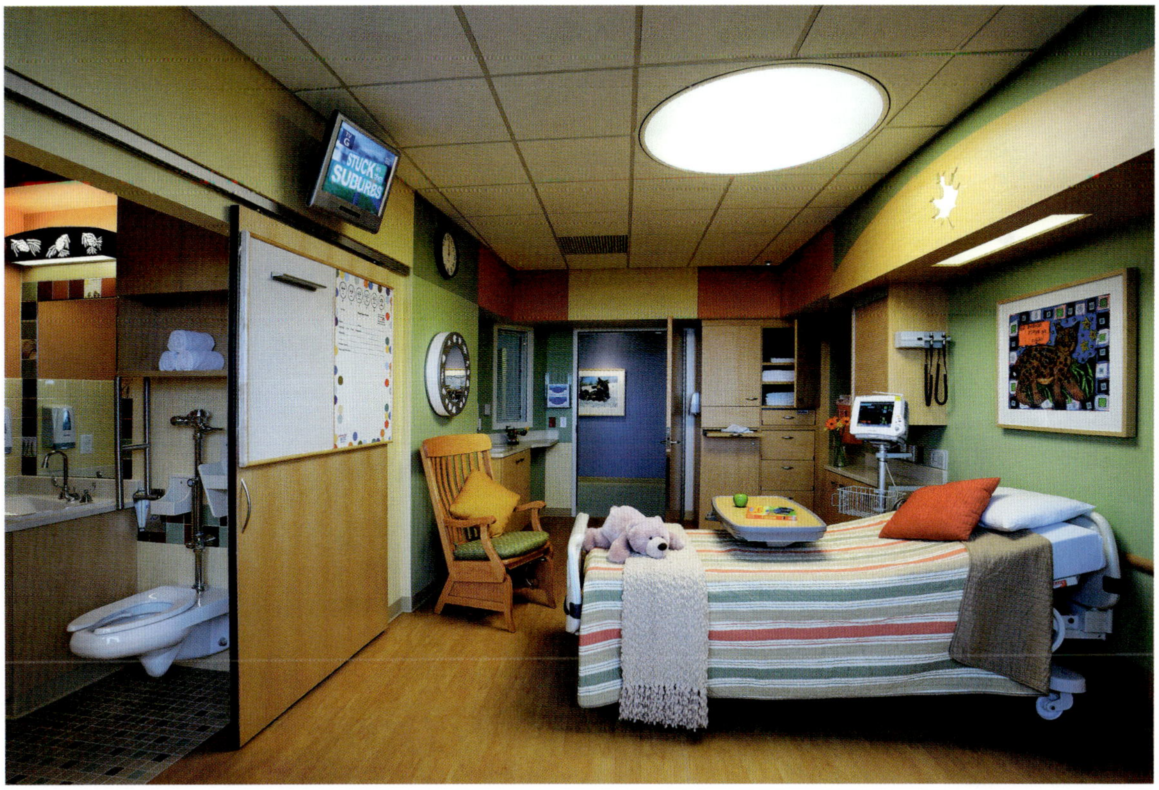

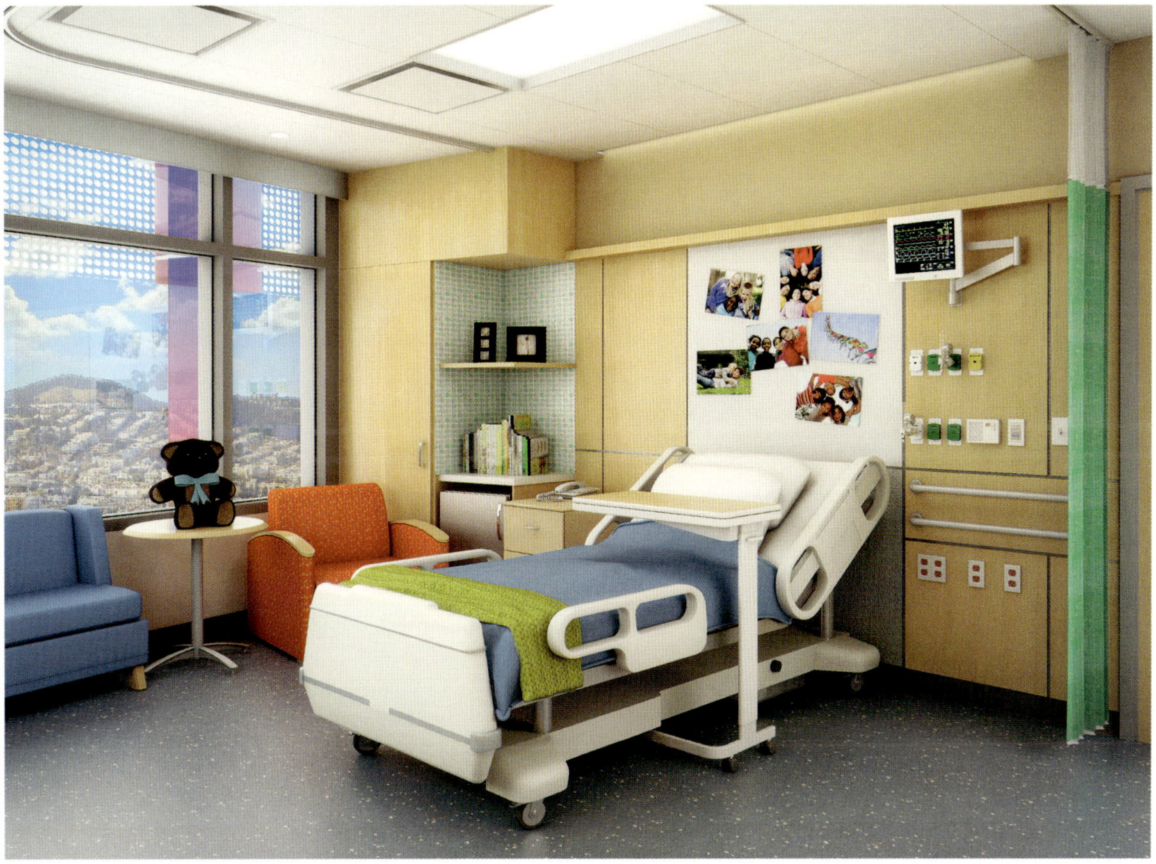

▲ UCSF Benioff Children's Hospital, San Francisco, CA
Photo: Stantec ©

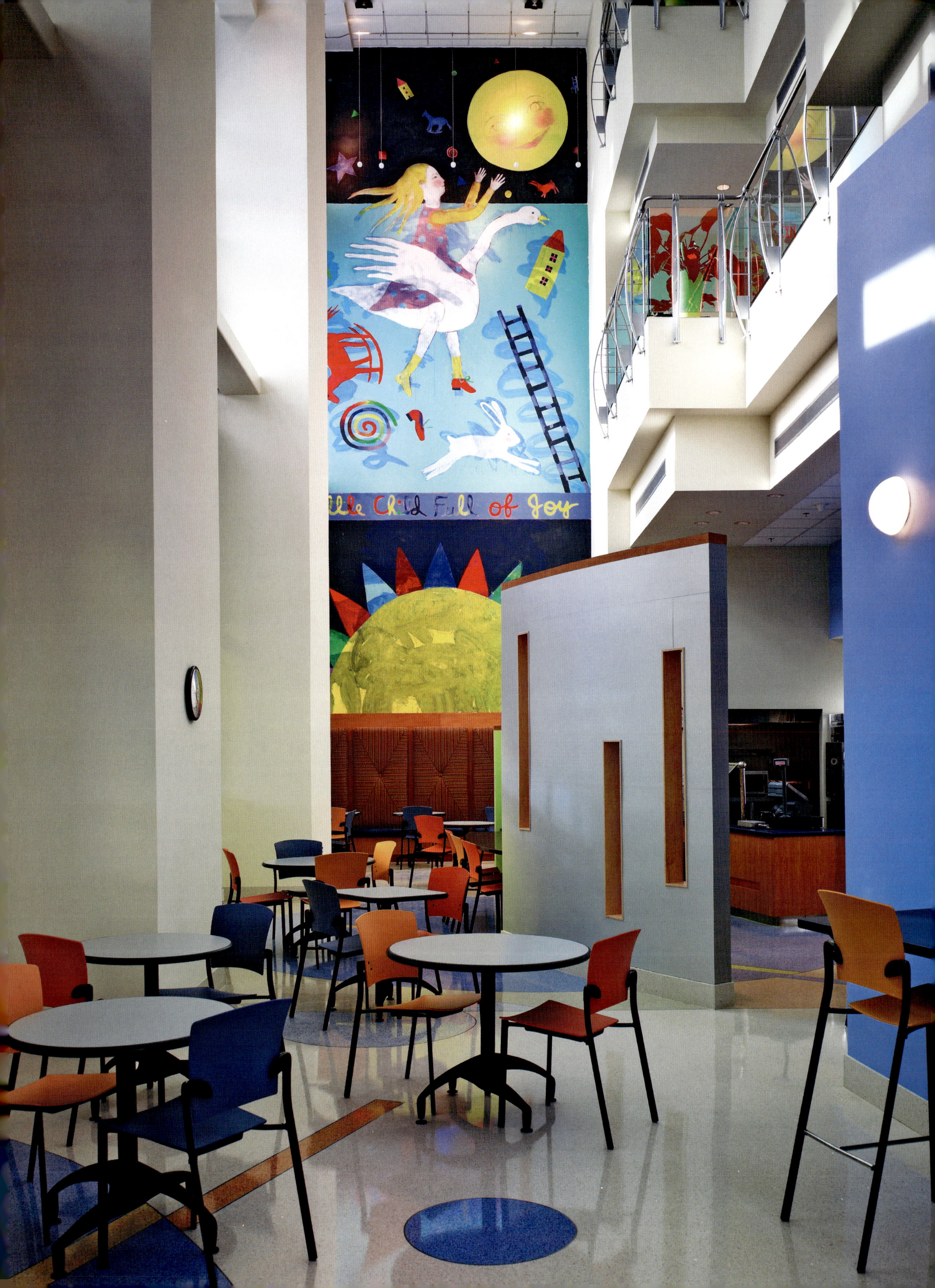
Child Full of Joy

Art and Community Involvement

Bringing art and community into children's hospitals is all about the perpetual transfer of positive energy. Art is instinctively personal, with boundless possibilities for interpretation. Every emotion it arouses is individual and unique; it lifts spirits, evokes thought, and spurs emotion. Done right, it is used to create positive energy. Artwork, in all its forms, crafts both a distraction and an escape from everyday stressors—an essential element in fulfilling a true healing environment.

These aspirations have moved the display of artwork in children's hospitals through the years, from simple framed prints adorning the walls and the display of children's personal artwork, to robust curated programs incorporating a range of media generating interactive spaces.

Experience with art is unique for all ages and genders. Whether the art is expressed in sculpture, painting or photography, variety is key to a successful art program. Adjusting the size, color and placement of artwork within the hospital provides an intriguing blend of encounters as it complements the architecture and empowers the patient experience. Keeping the art displays fresh with new work will continue to uplift the spirit as they provide returning visitors or long-term patients with new interactions.

Kristin Ledet, IIDA
FKP Architects

◀ Levine Children's Hospital, Charlotte, NC
Photo: Brad Feinknopf

▼ Helen DeVos Children's Hospital, Grand Rapids, MI
Photo: Lucid Architecture, Eric DeWitt

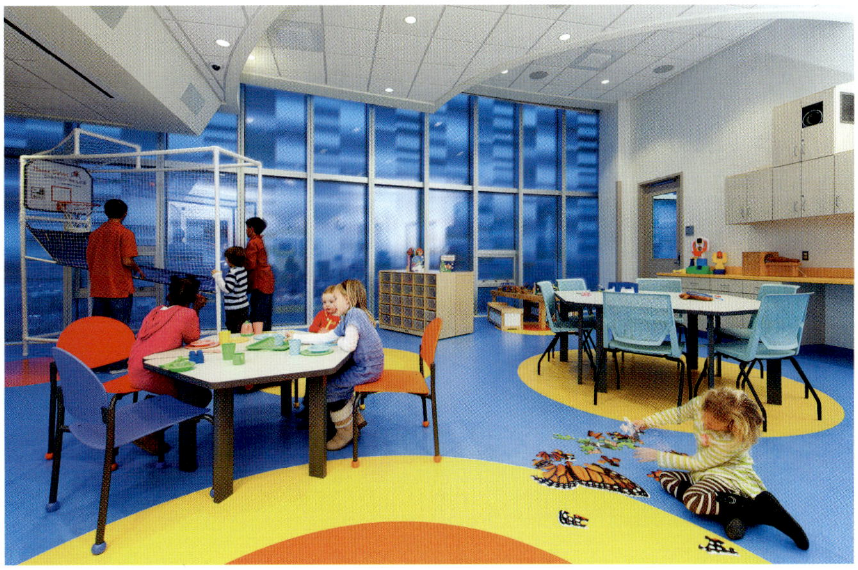

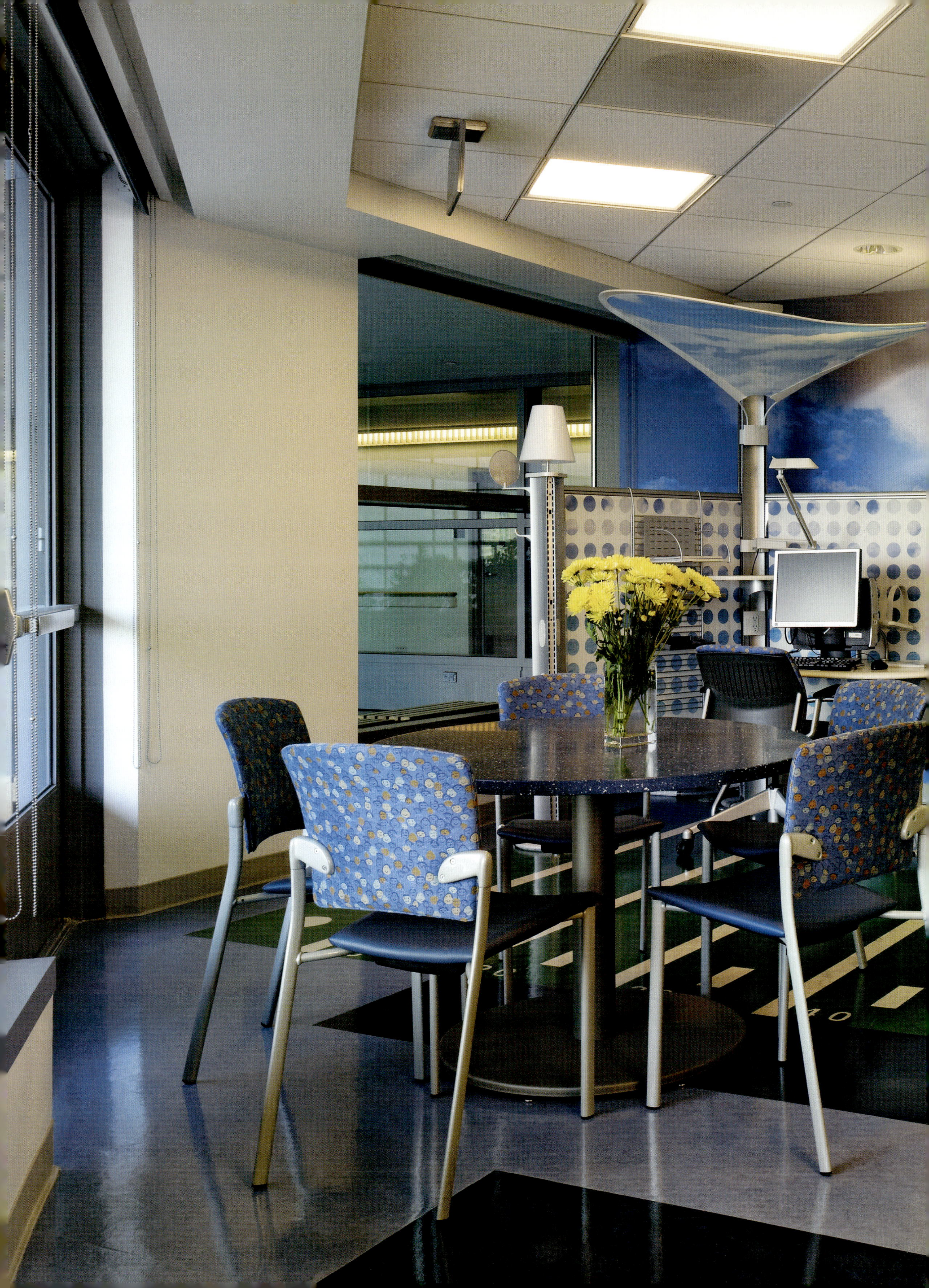

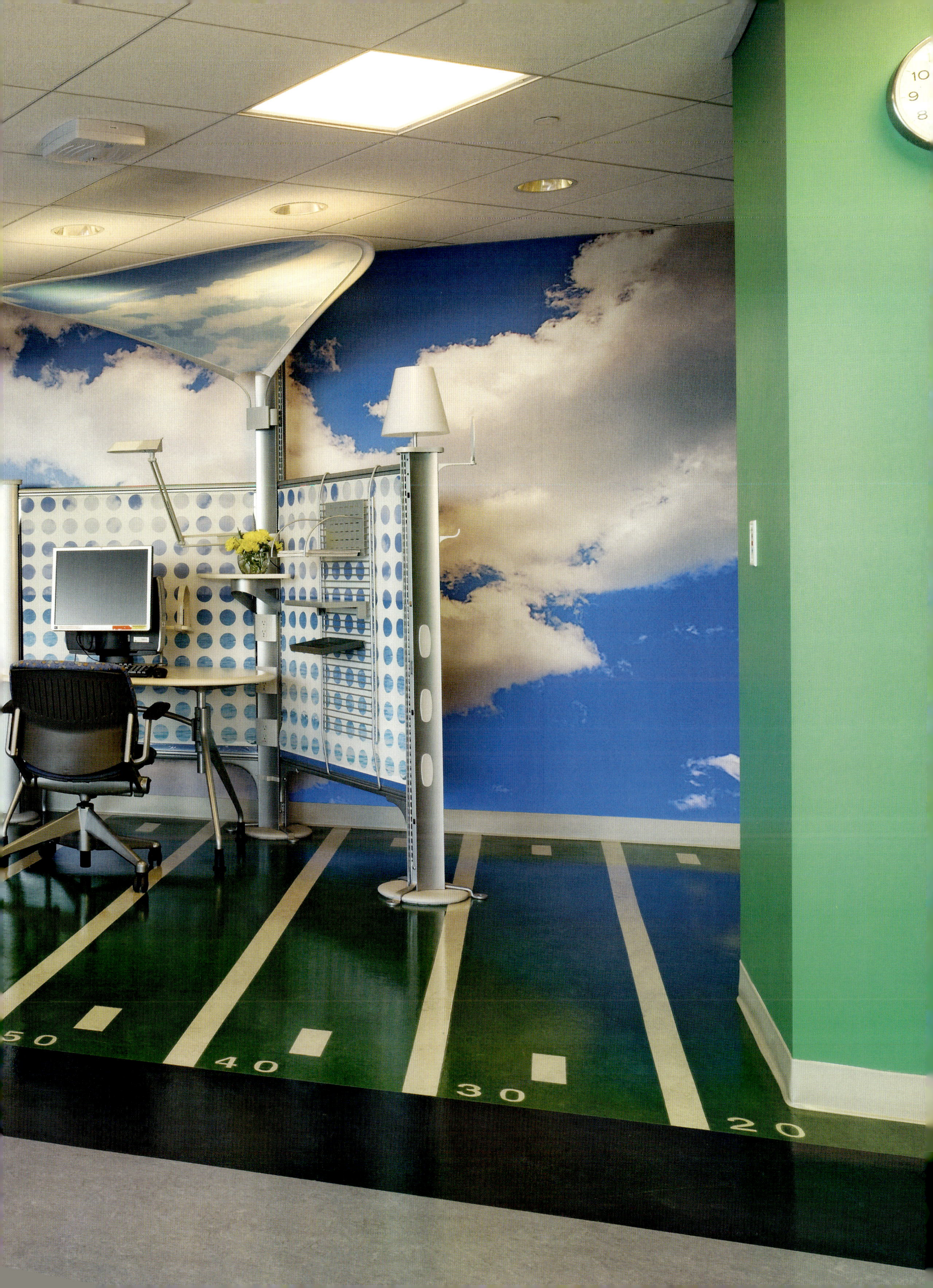
10
9
8
50
40
30
20

Previous pages: Mattel Children's Hospital UCLA, Los Angeles, CA
Photo: Benny Chan, fotoworks

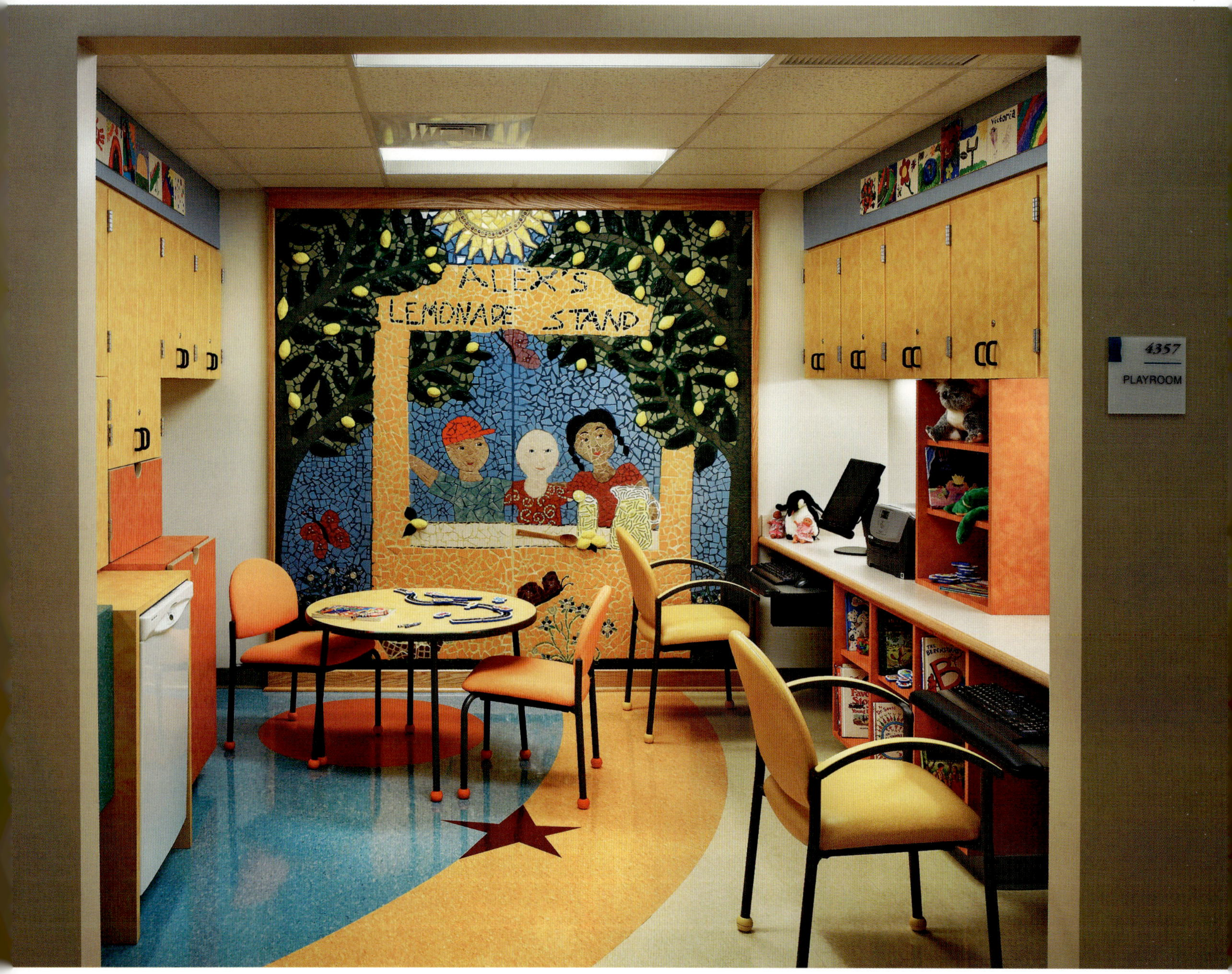

▲ Children's Hospital of Philadelphia, PA
Photo: Barry Halkin

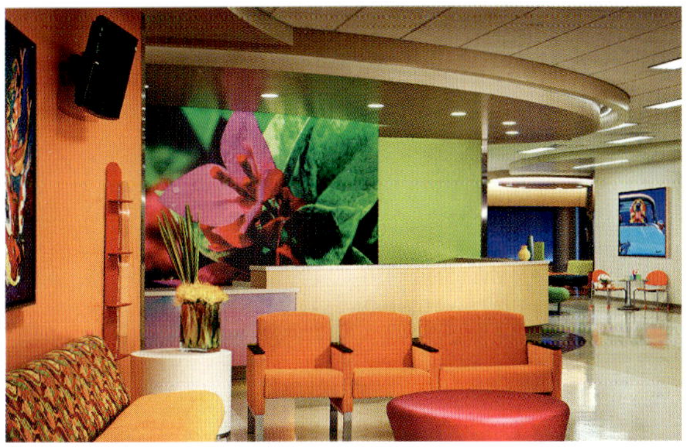

▲ Phoenix Children's Hospital, AZ
Photo: Blake Marvin

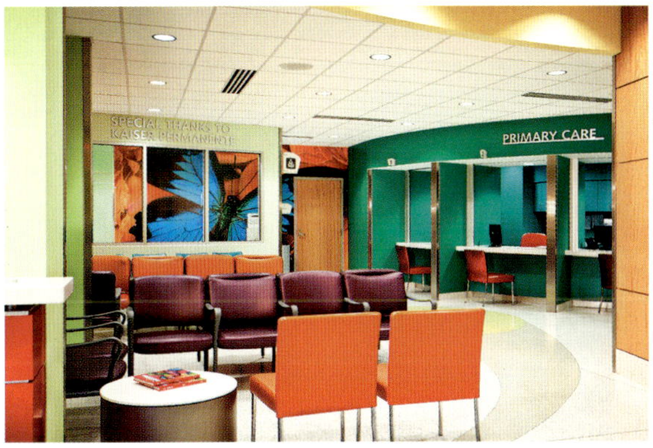

▲ Children's Healthcare of Atlanta, GA
Photo: Blake Marvin

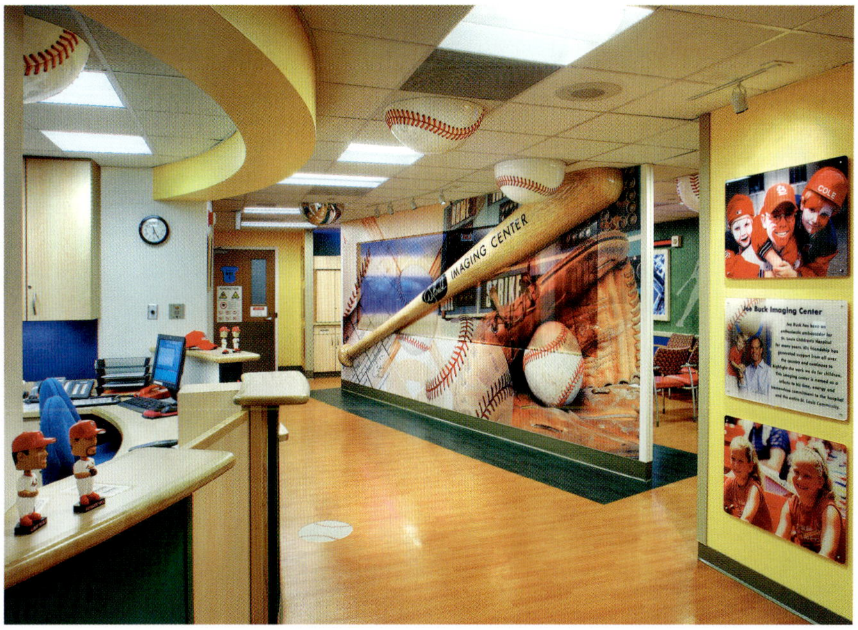

▲ St. Louis Children's Hospital, St, Louis, MI
▼ *Photos: Sam Fentress*

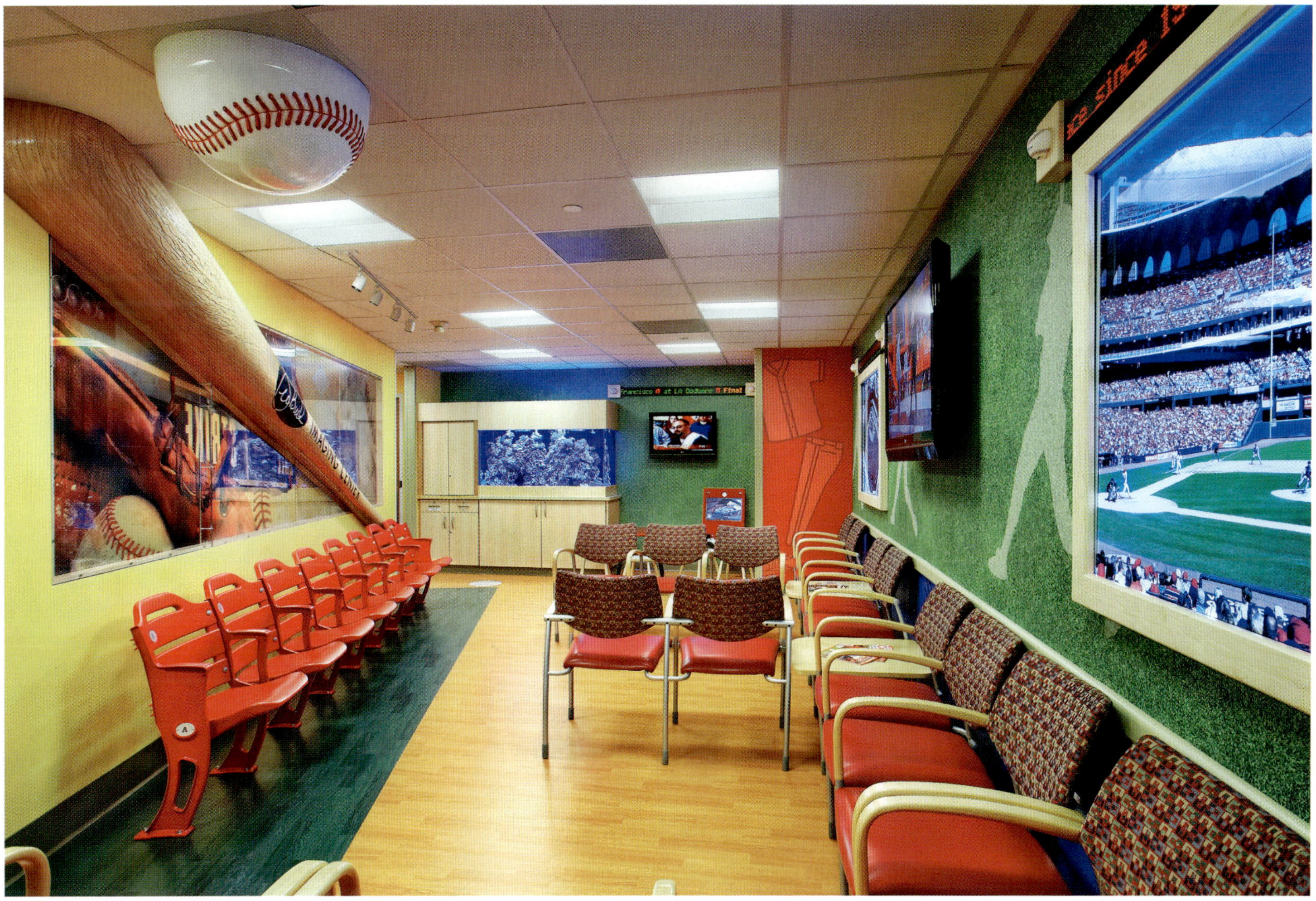

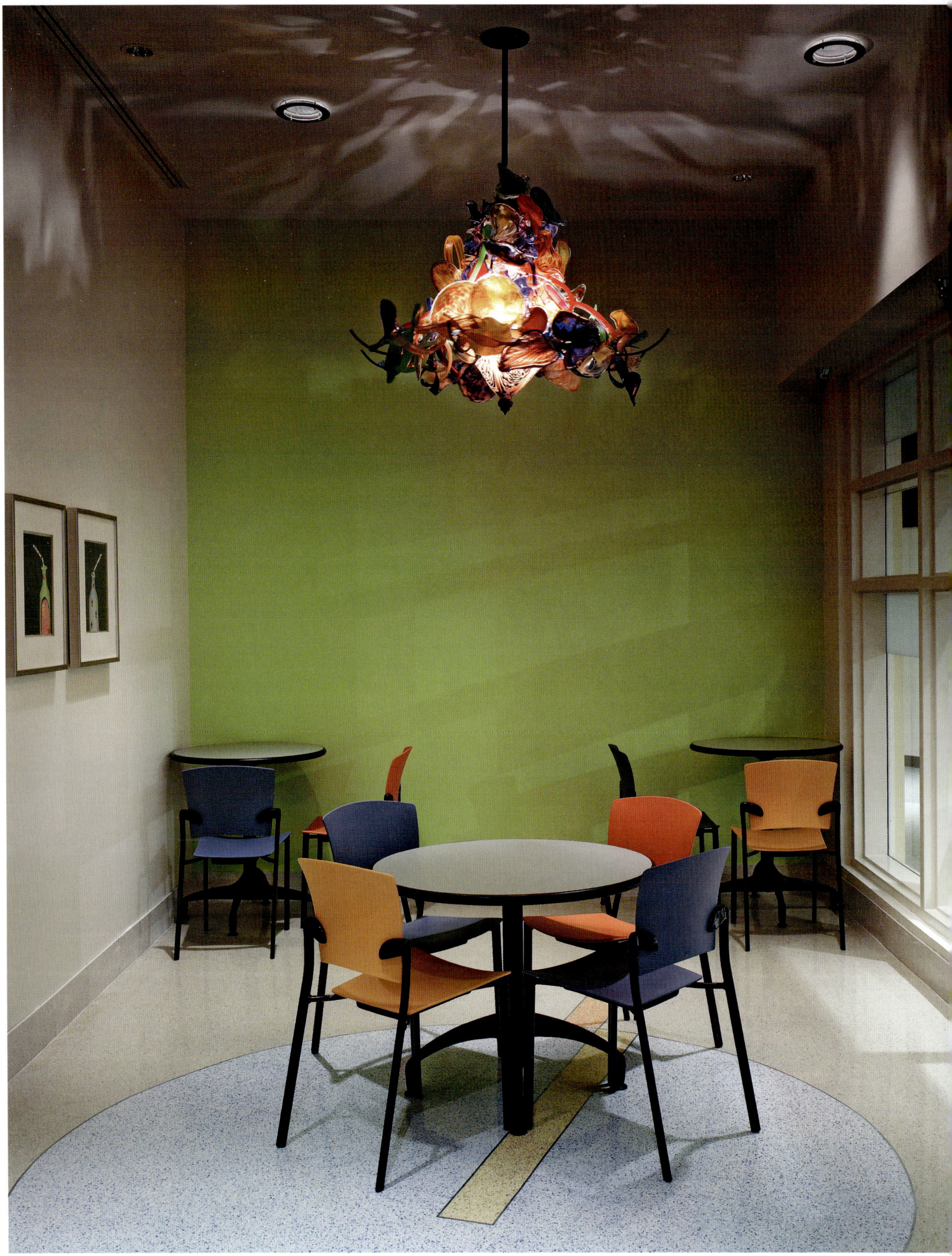

◀ Levine Children's Hospital, Charlotte, NC
Photo: Brad Feinknopf

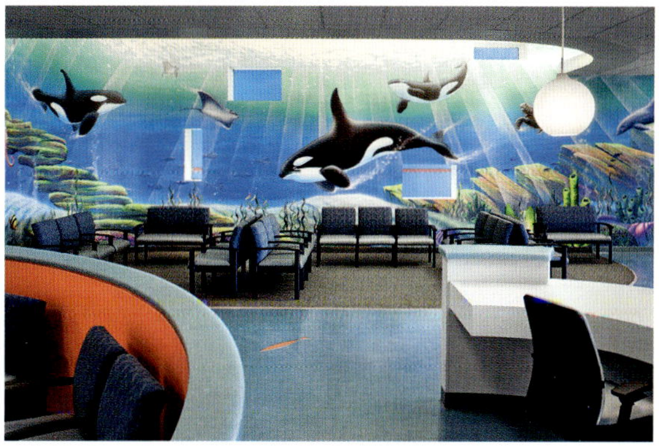

▲ Riverton Hospital Primary Children's Medical
▼ Center, Riverton, UT
Photos: Stantec © David Wakely Photography

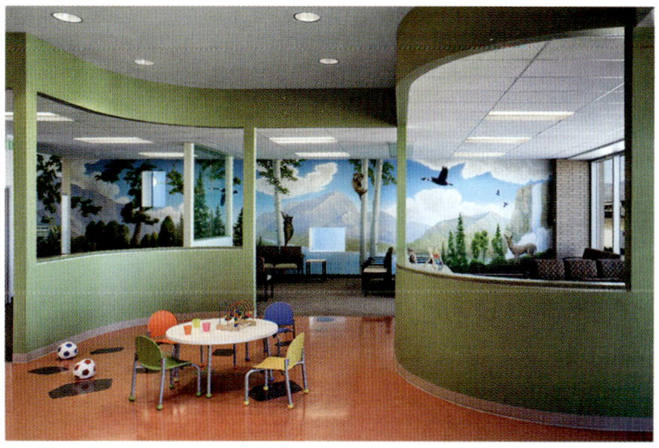

▼ Children's Hospital of Philadelphia, PA
Photo: Atlantic

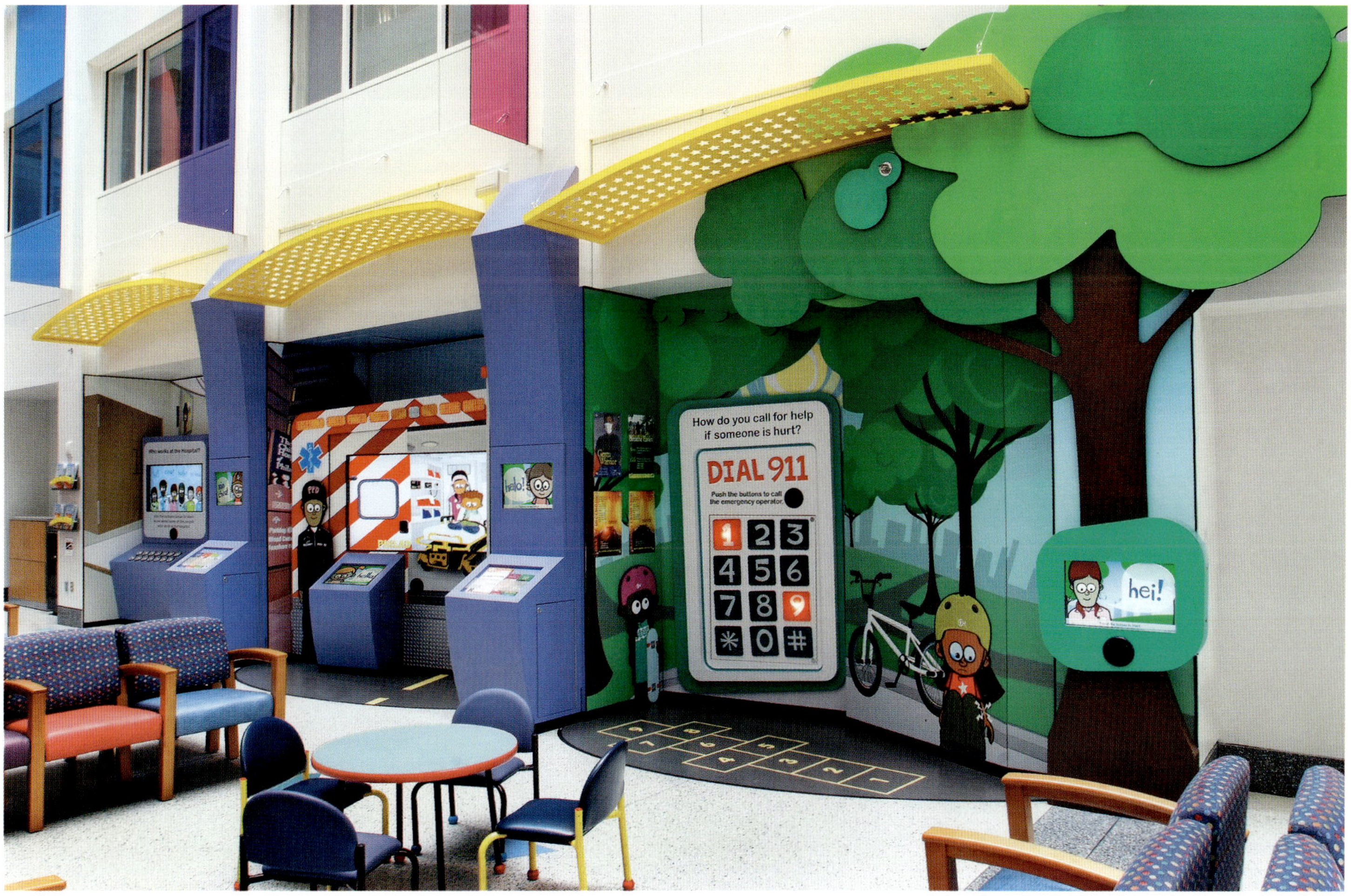
How do you call for help
if someone is hurt?
DIAL 911
Push the buttons to call
the emergency operator
1 2 3
4 5 6
7 8 9
* 0 #
hei!

▼ Maria Fareri Children's Hospital, Valhalla, NY
Photo: Westchester Medical Centre

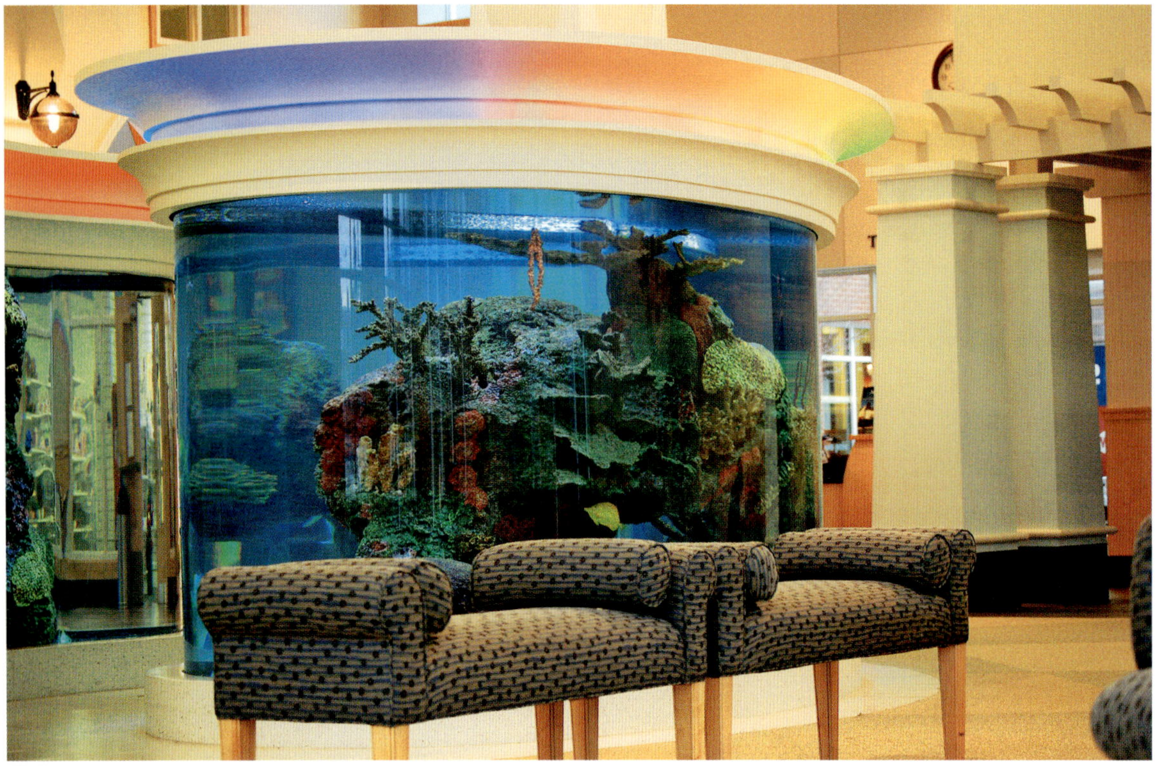

▼ Cardon Children's, Mesa, AZ
Photo: HDR Architecture, Inc.; © 2010 Mark Boisclair Photography Inc.

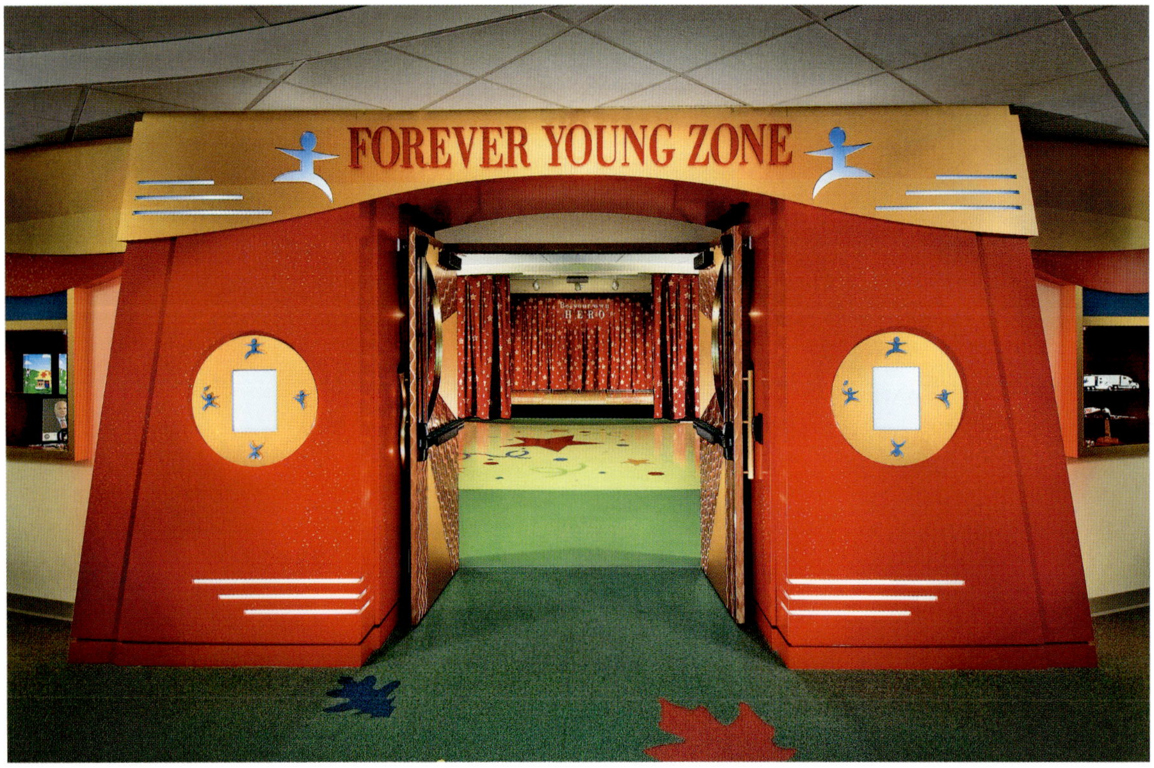

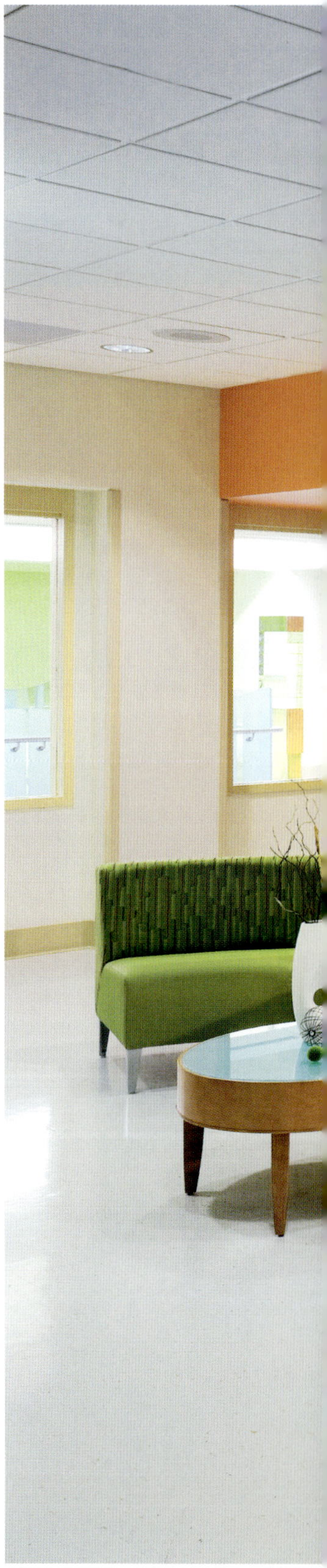

▼ Palmetto Health Children's Hospital, Columbia, SC

Following pages: The Children's Inn at NIH, Bethseda, MD

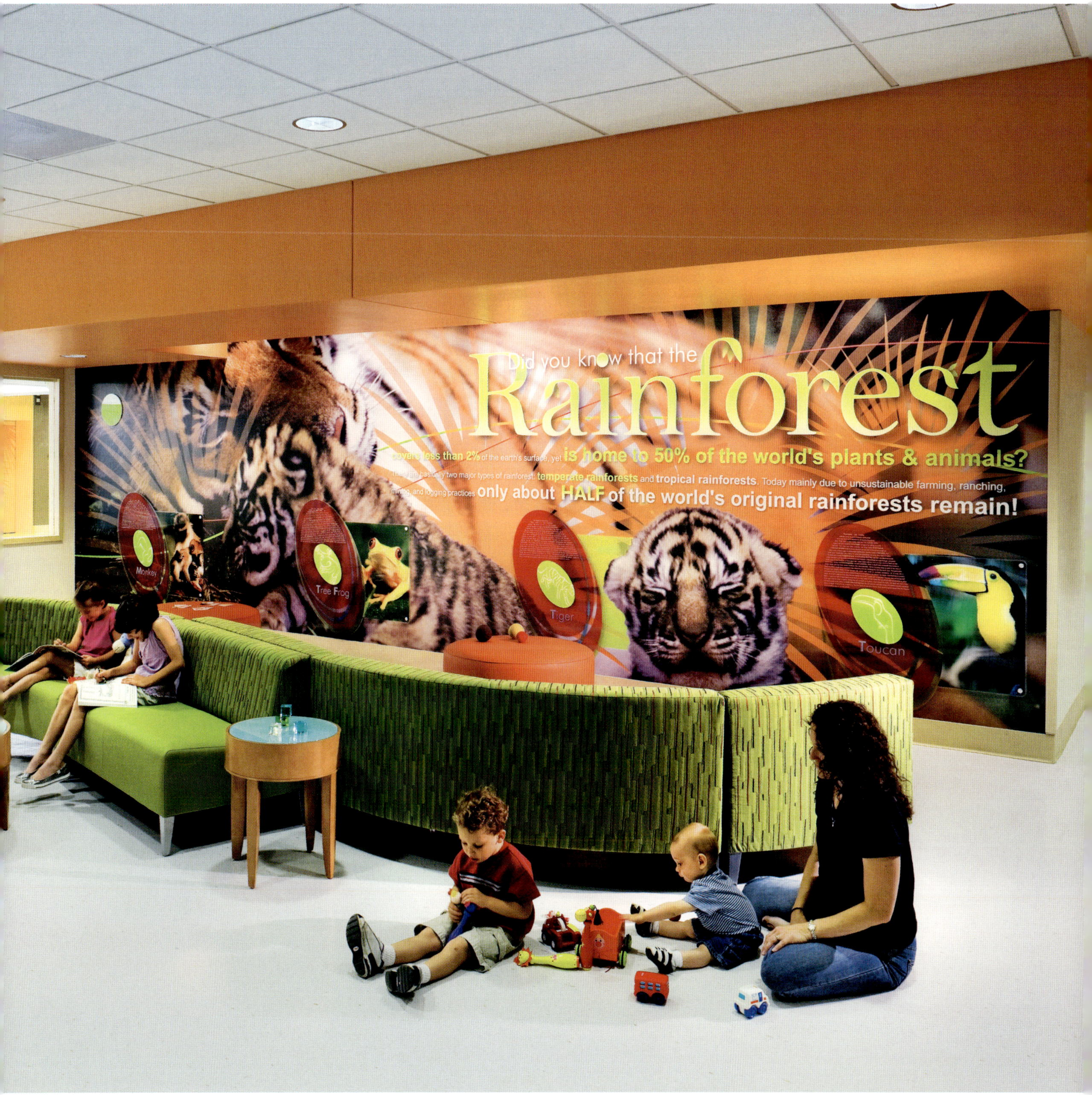
Did you know that the
Rainforest
covers less than 2% of the earth's surface, yet is home to 50% of the world's plants & animals?
There are basically two major types of rainforest: temperate rainforests and tropical rainforests. Today mainly due to unsustainable farming, ranching,
mining, and logging practices only about HALF of the world's original rainforests remain!
Monkey
Tree Frog
Tiger
Toucan

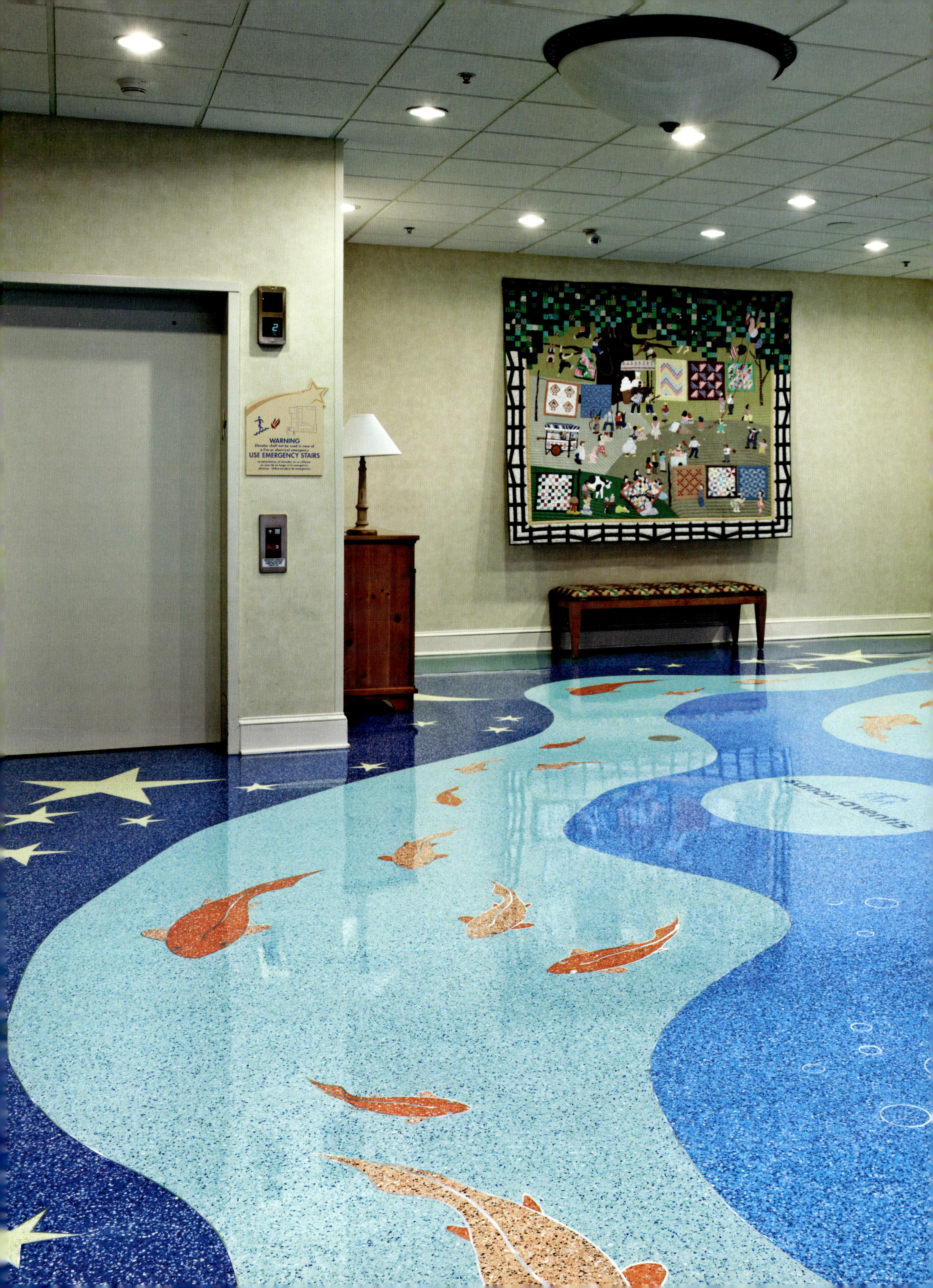
WARNING
Elevator shall not be used in case of
a fire or electrical emergency
USE EMERGENCY STAIRS
sanofi aventis

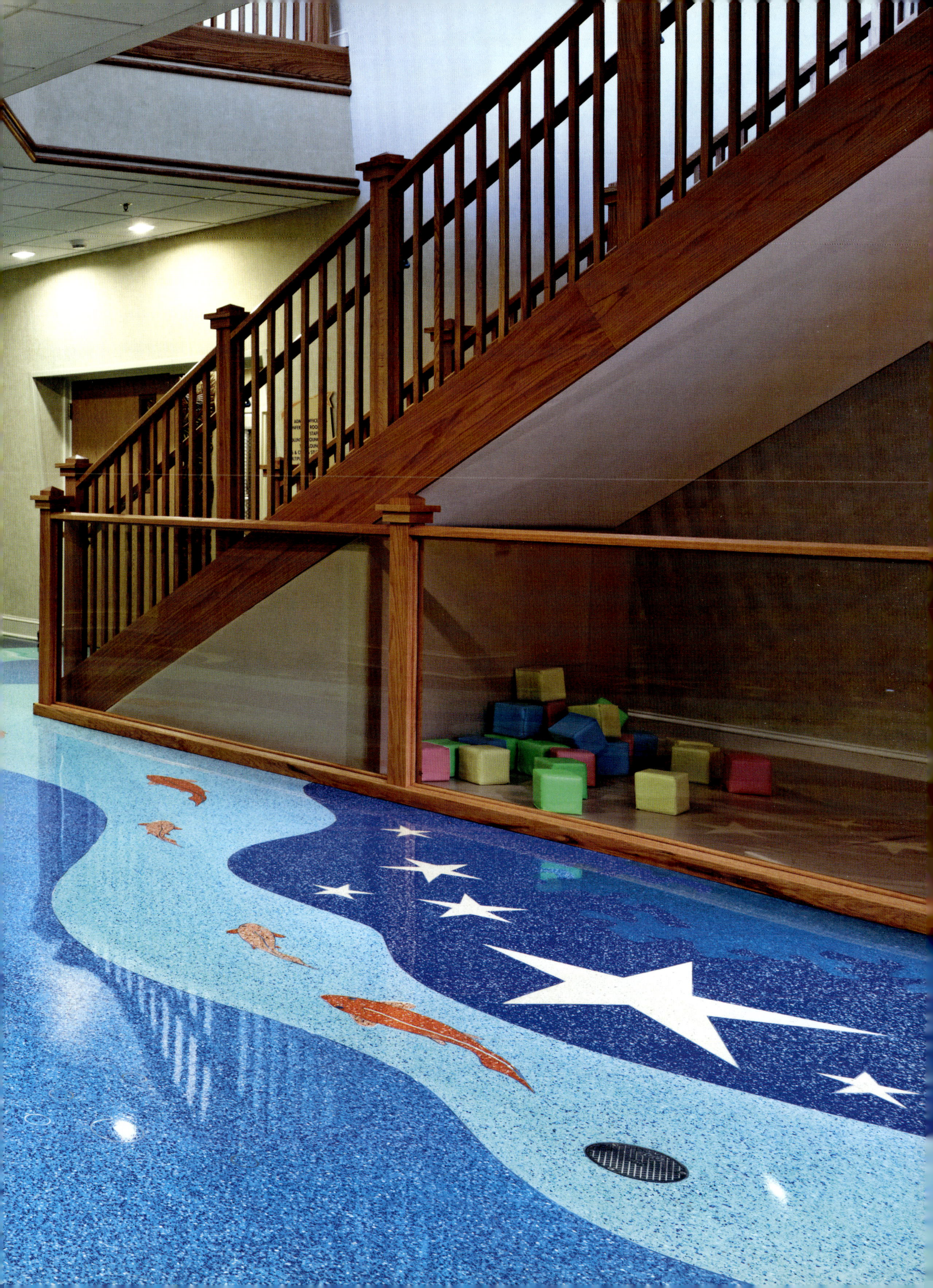

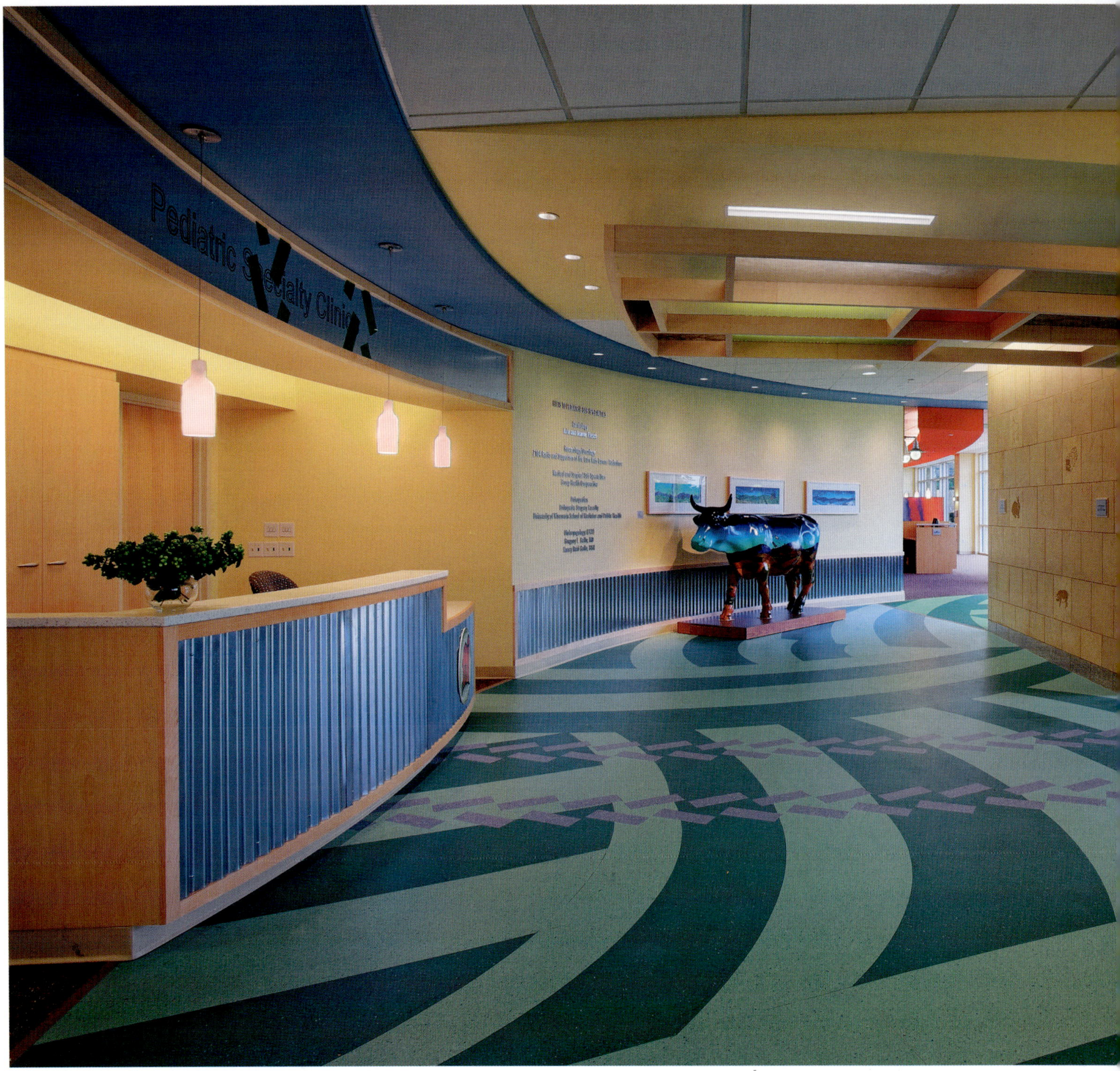

▲ American Family Children's Hospital, Madison, WI
Photo: HDR Architecture, Inc.; ©2007 Ballogg Photography Inc, Chicago

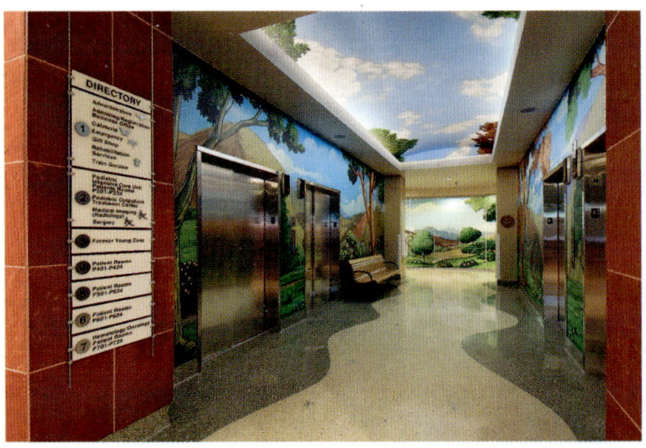

▲ Cardon Children's, Mesa, AZ
Photo: HDR Architecture, Inc.; © 2010 Mark Boisclair Photography Inc.

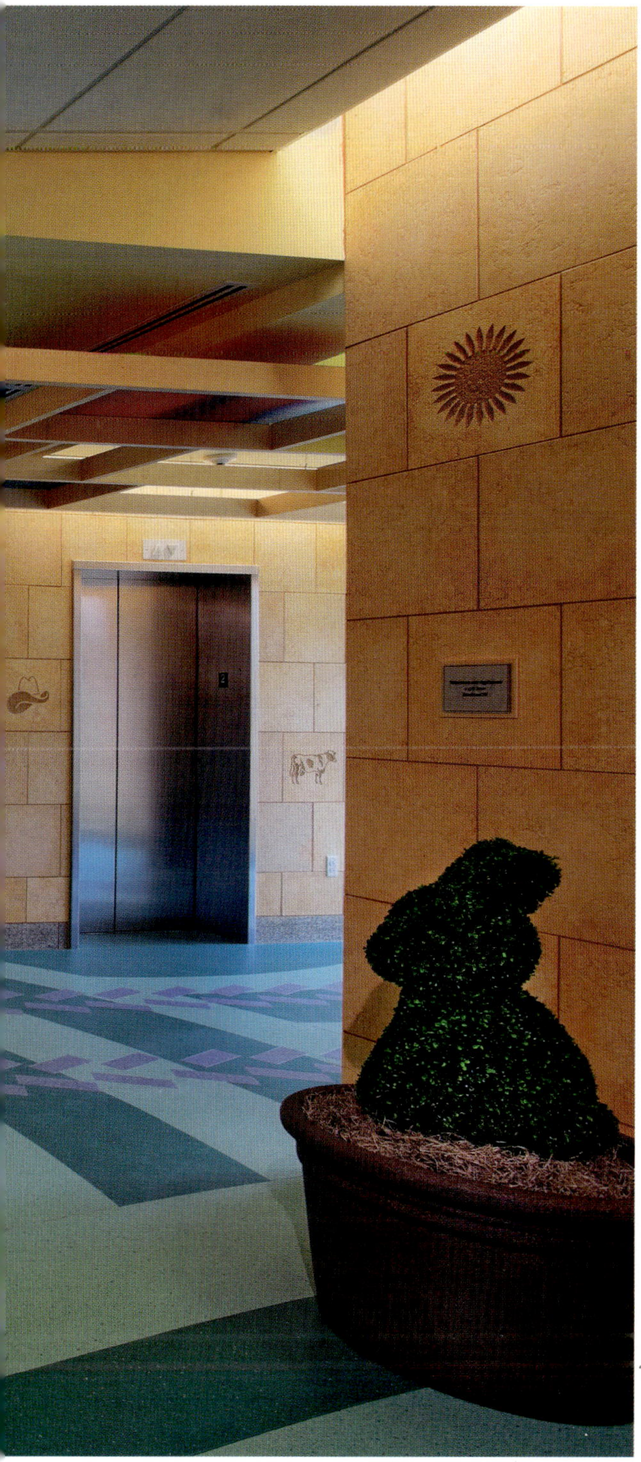

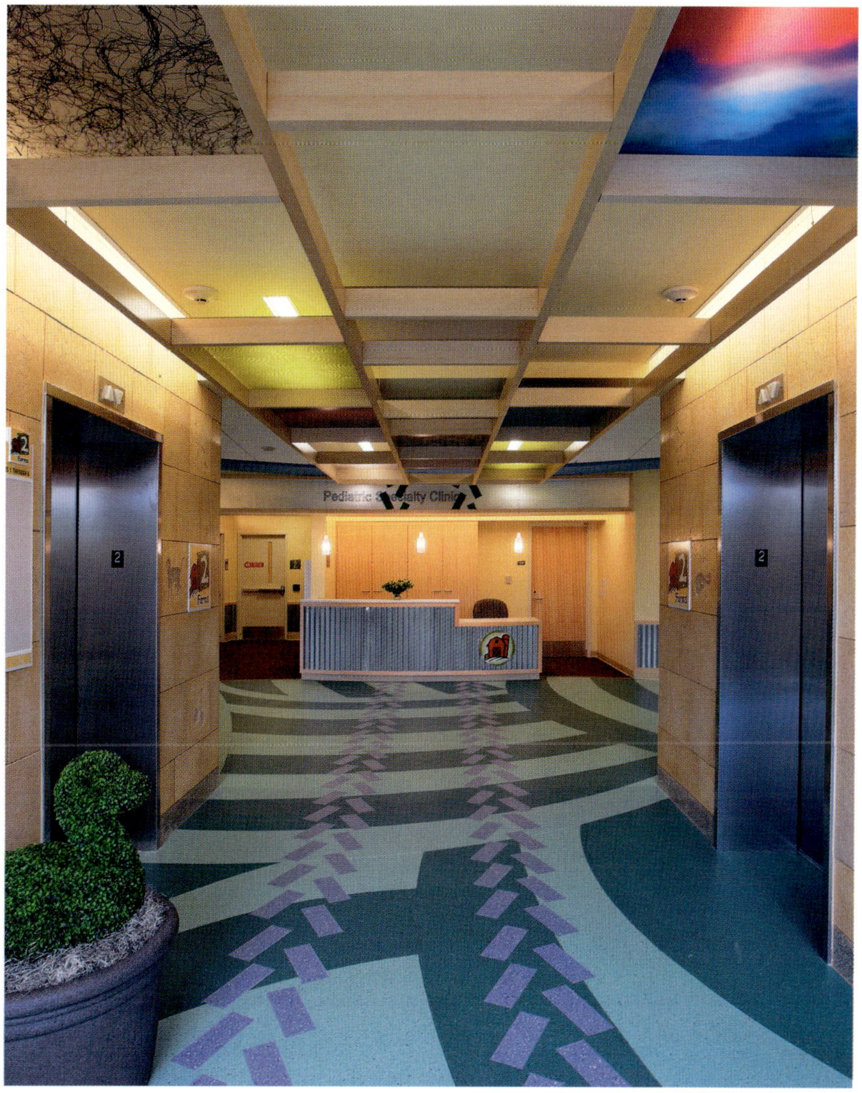

▲ American Family Children's Hospital, Madison, WI
Photo: HDR Architecture, Inc.; ©2007 Ballogg Photography Inc, Chicago

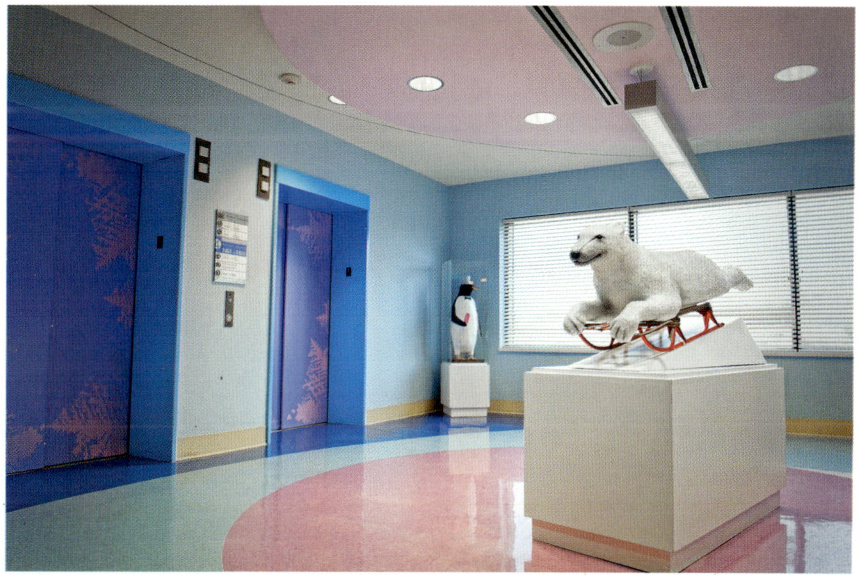

▲ Palmetto Health Children's Hospital, Columbia, SC

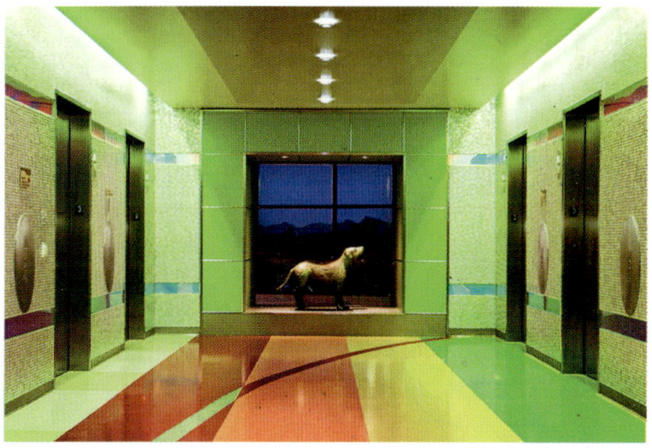

▲ Phoenix Children's Hospital, AZ
Photo: Blake Marvin, HKS

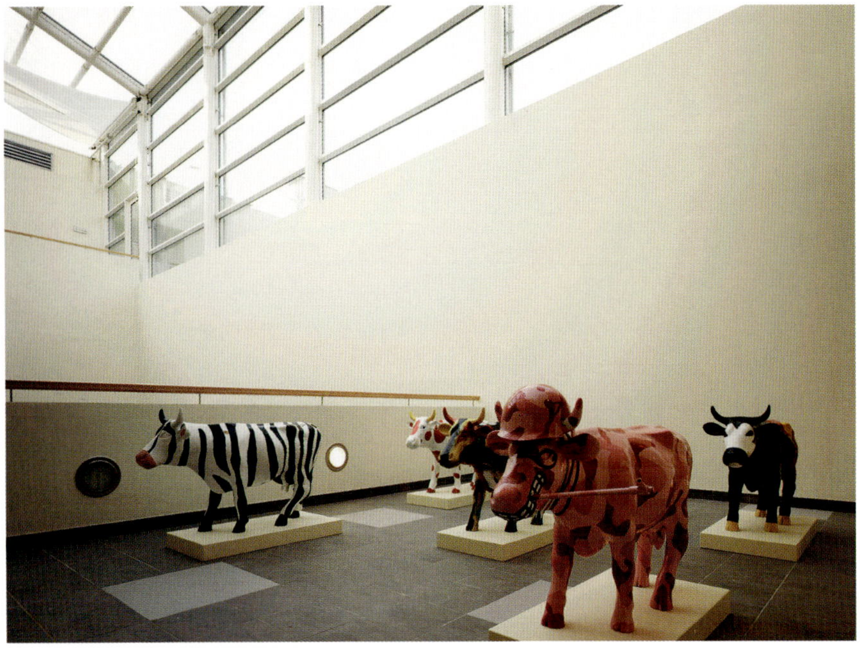

▲ Meyer Children's Hospital, Florence, Italy
Photo: Stantec © Alessandro Ciampi and Pietro Savorelli

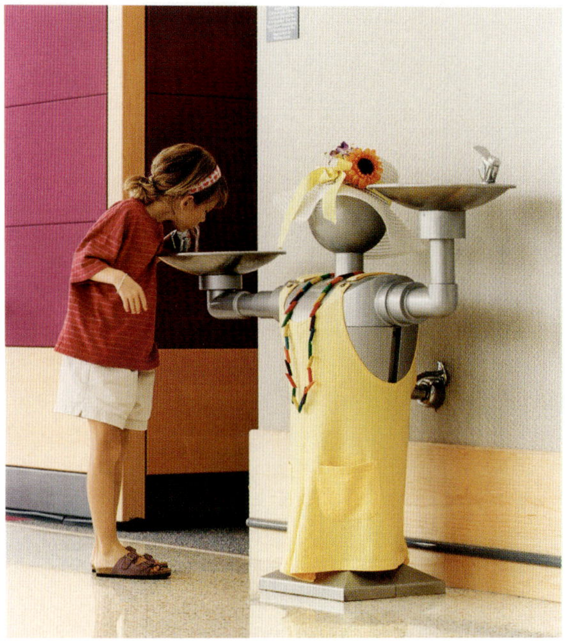

▲ Duke University Children's Hospital, Durham, NC
Photo: Jeff Goldberg/Esto Photography

▼ Ann & Robert H. Lurie Children's Hospital of Chicago, IL
Photo: Hedrich Blessing Photography, Nick Merrick

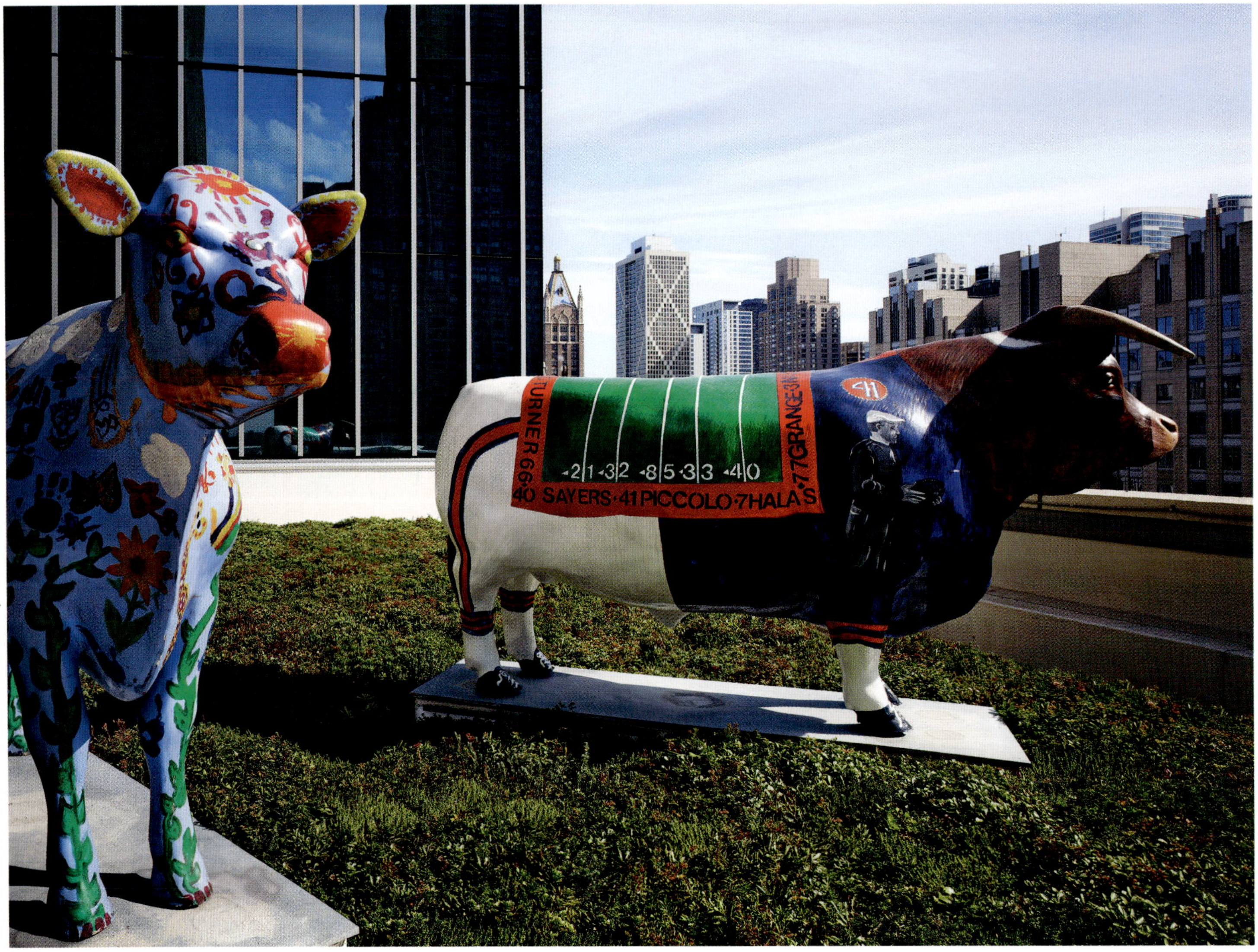

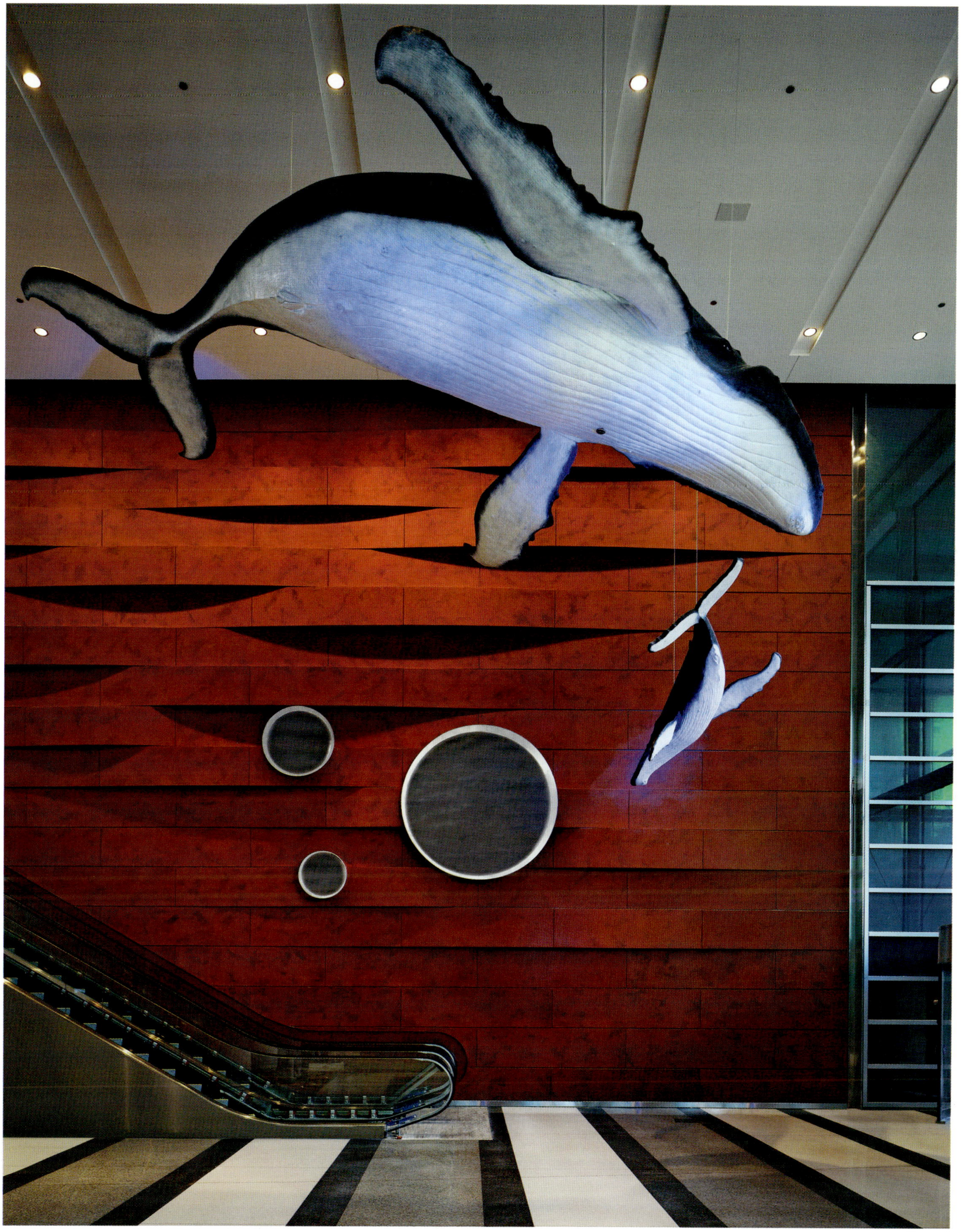

▲ Ann & Robert H. Lurie Children's Hospital of Chicago, IL
Photo: Hedrich Blessing Photography, Nick Merrick

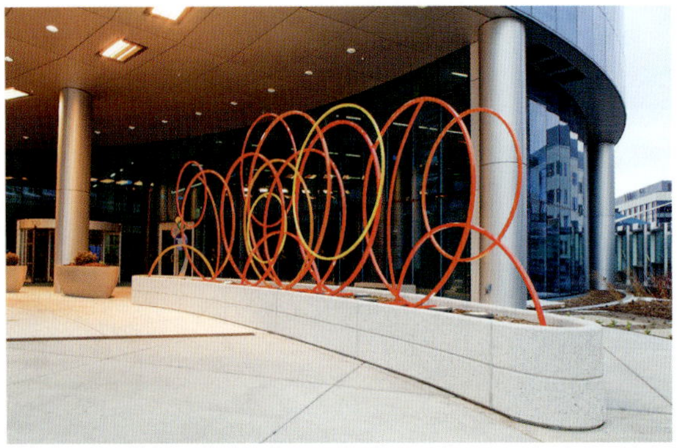

▲ Helen DeVos Children's Hospital, Grand Rapids, MI
Photo: Lucid Architecture, Eric DeWitt

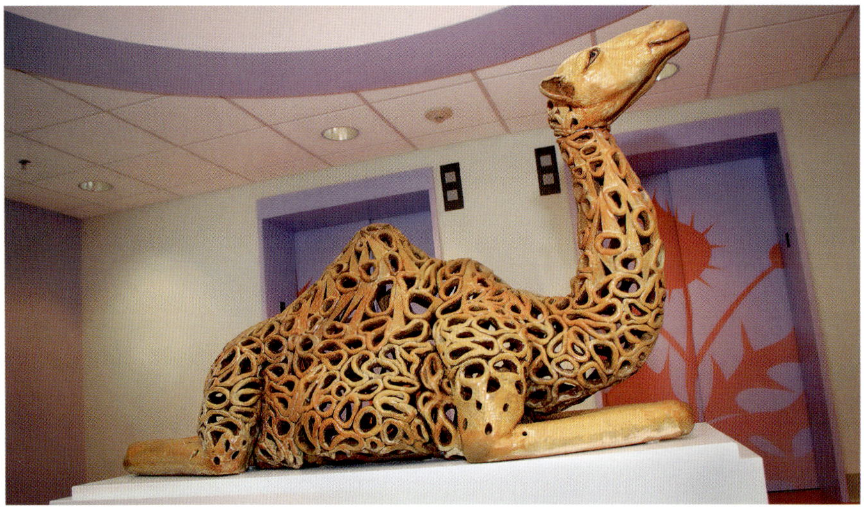

▲ Palmetto Health Children's Hospital, Columbia, SC

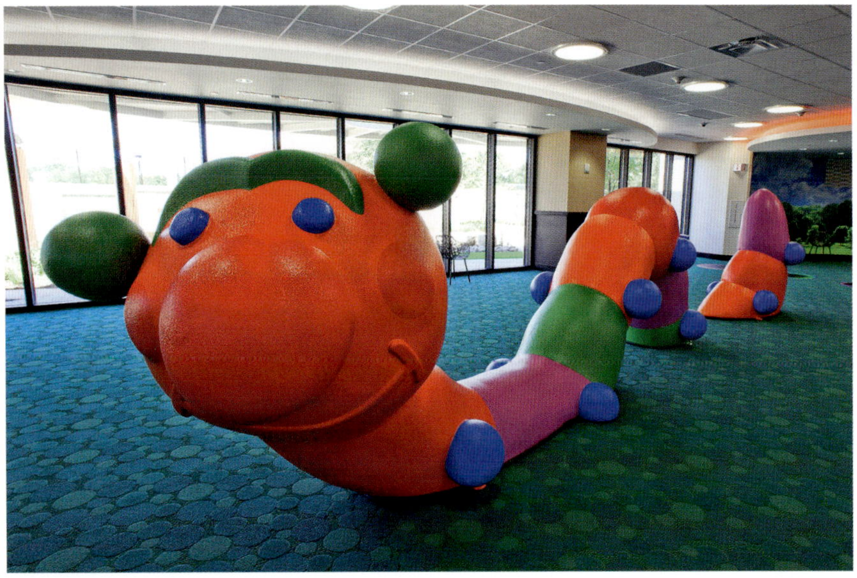

▲ Medical City Children's Hospital, Dallas, TX
▼ ***Photos: Terry Cockerham***

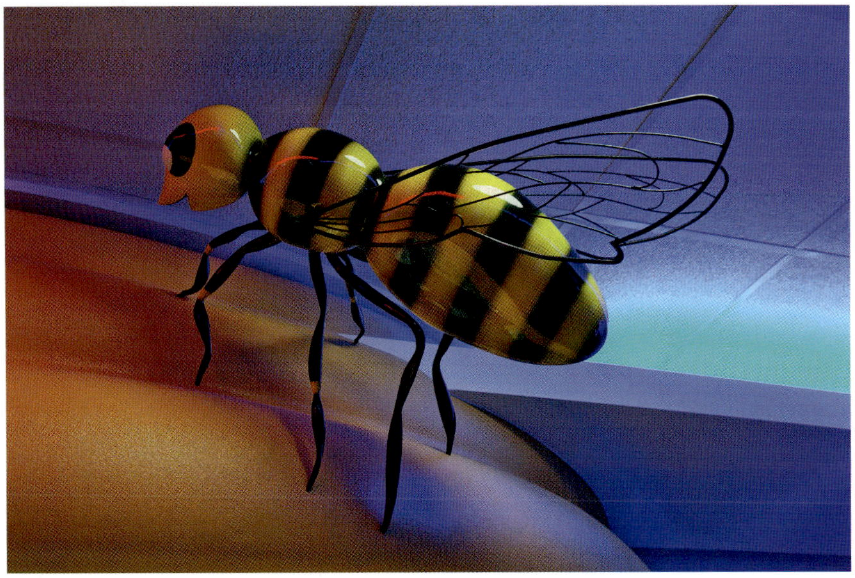

Upstate Golisano Children's Hospital, Syracuse, NY ▶
Photo: Susan Kahn

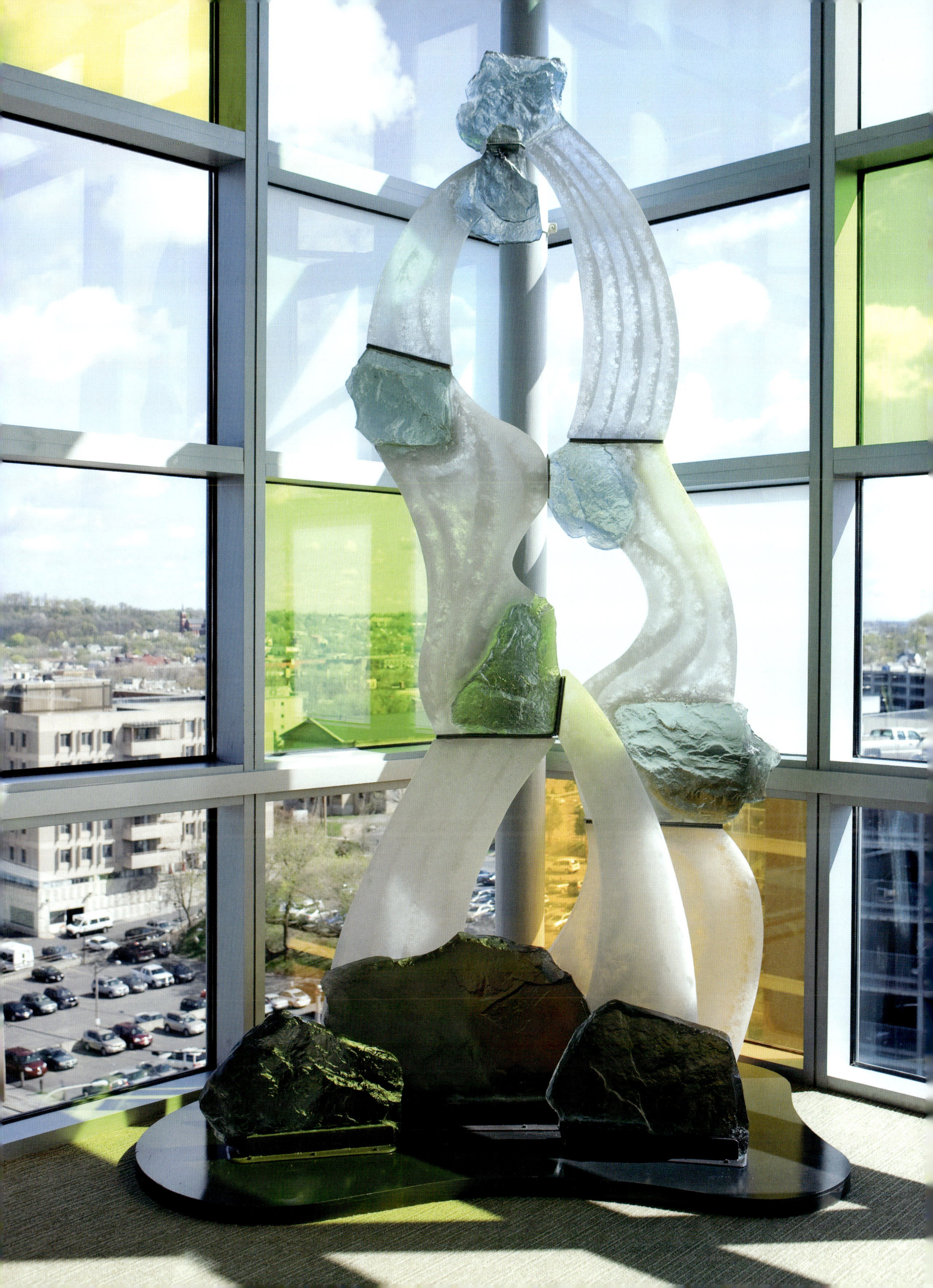

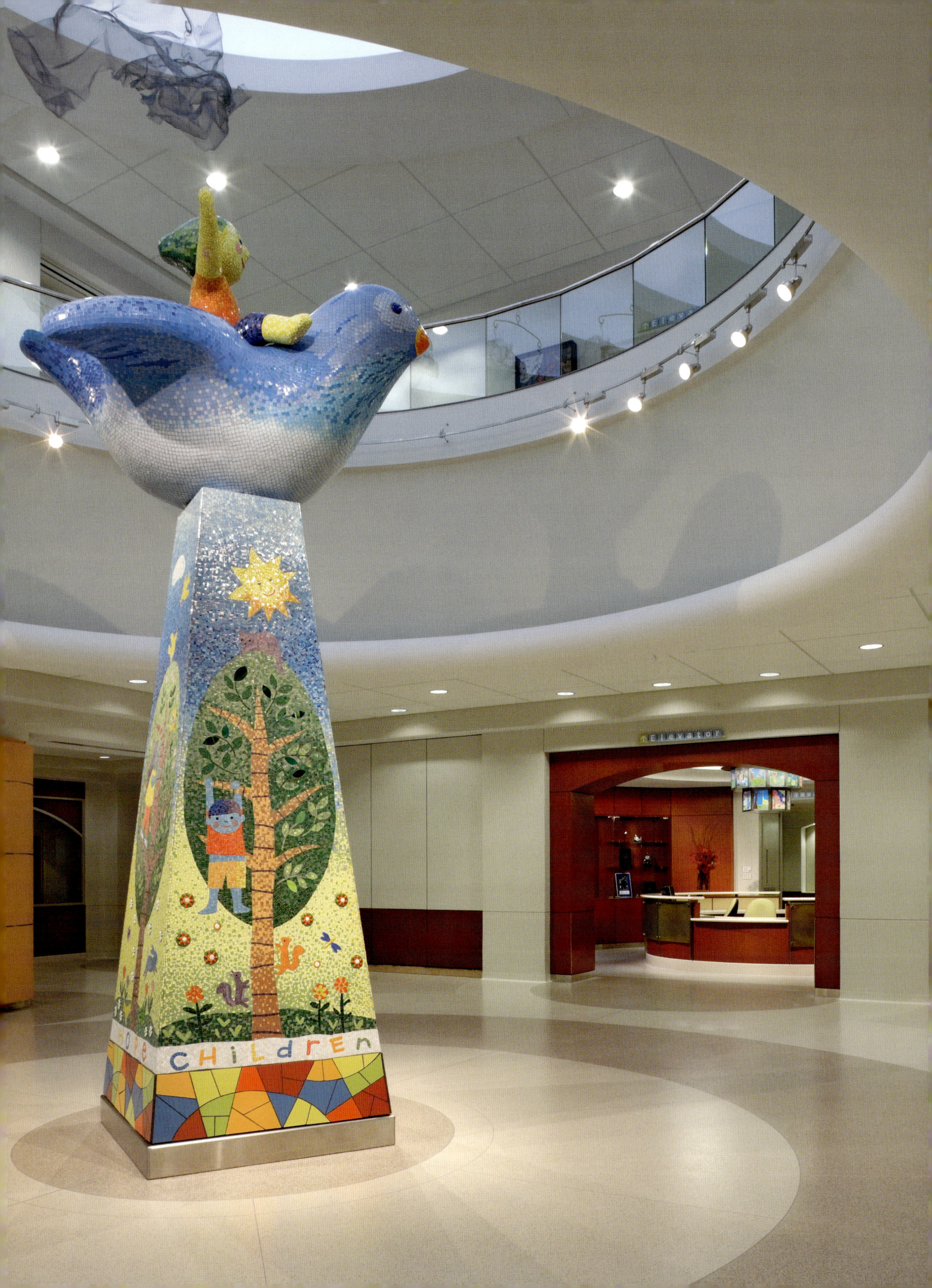
Elevator
Children

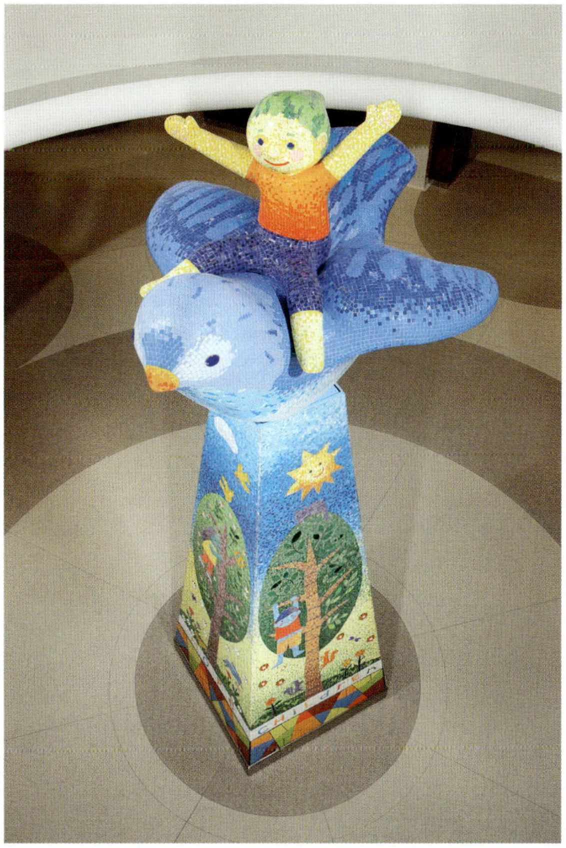

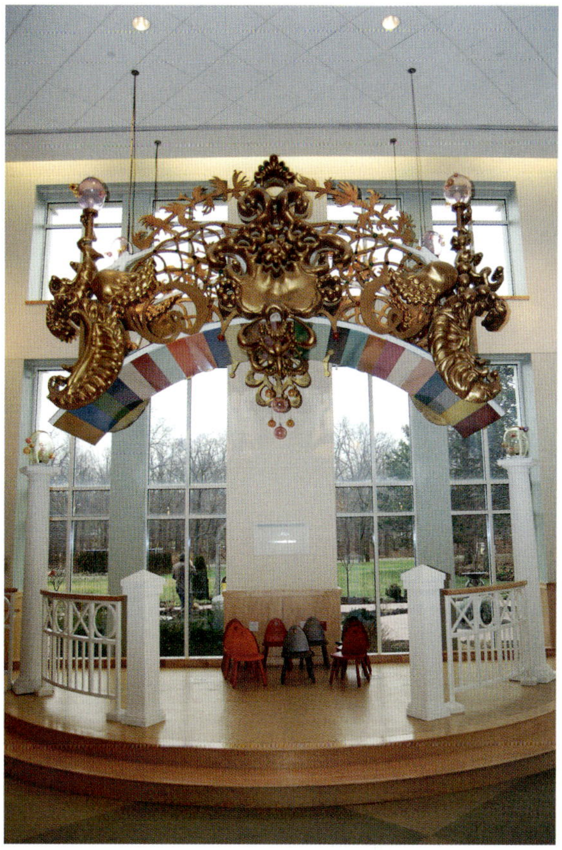

▲ Le Bonheur Children's Hospital, Memphis, TN
◀ ***Photos: Aker Imaging***
Sculpture: I Can Fly (by Jeanne Segal and Lee Holland)

▲ Maria Fareri Children's Hospital, Valhalla, NY
Photo: Westchester Medical Center

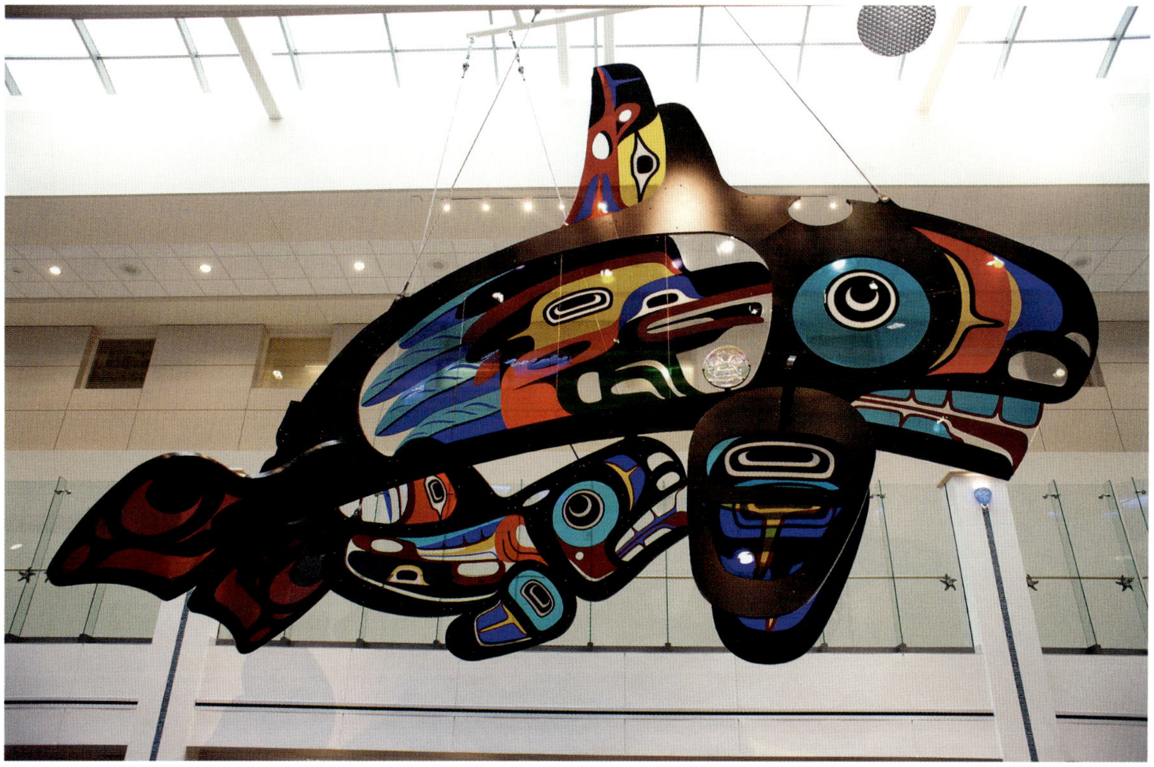

▲ Seattle Children's Hospital, WA
Photo: Nancy LeVine

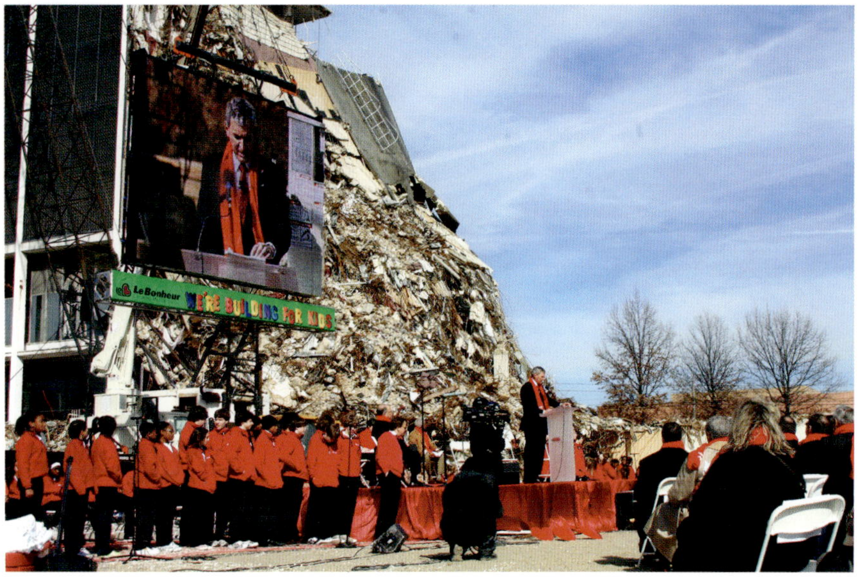

▲ Le Bonheur Children's Hospital, Memphis, TN
▶

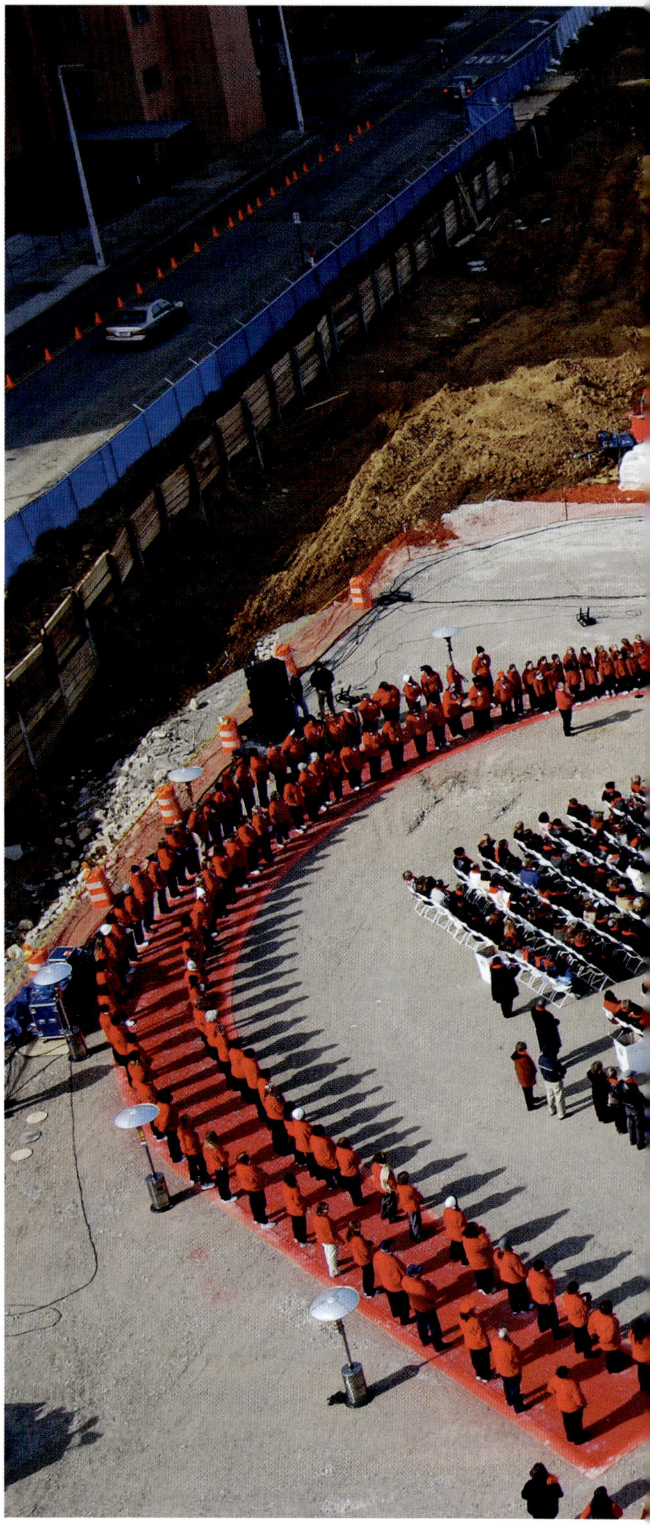

▼ Children's Hospital Los Angeles, CA
Photo: Eckert & Eckert

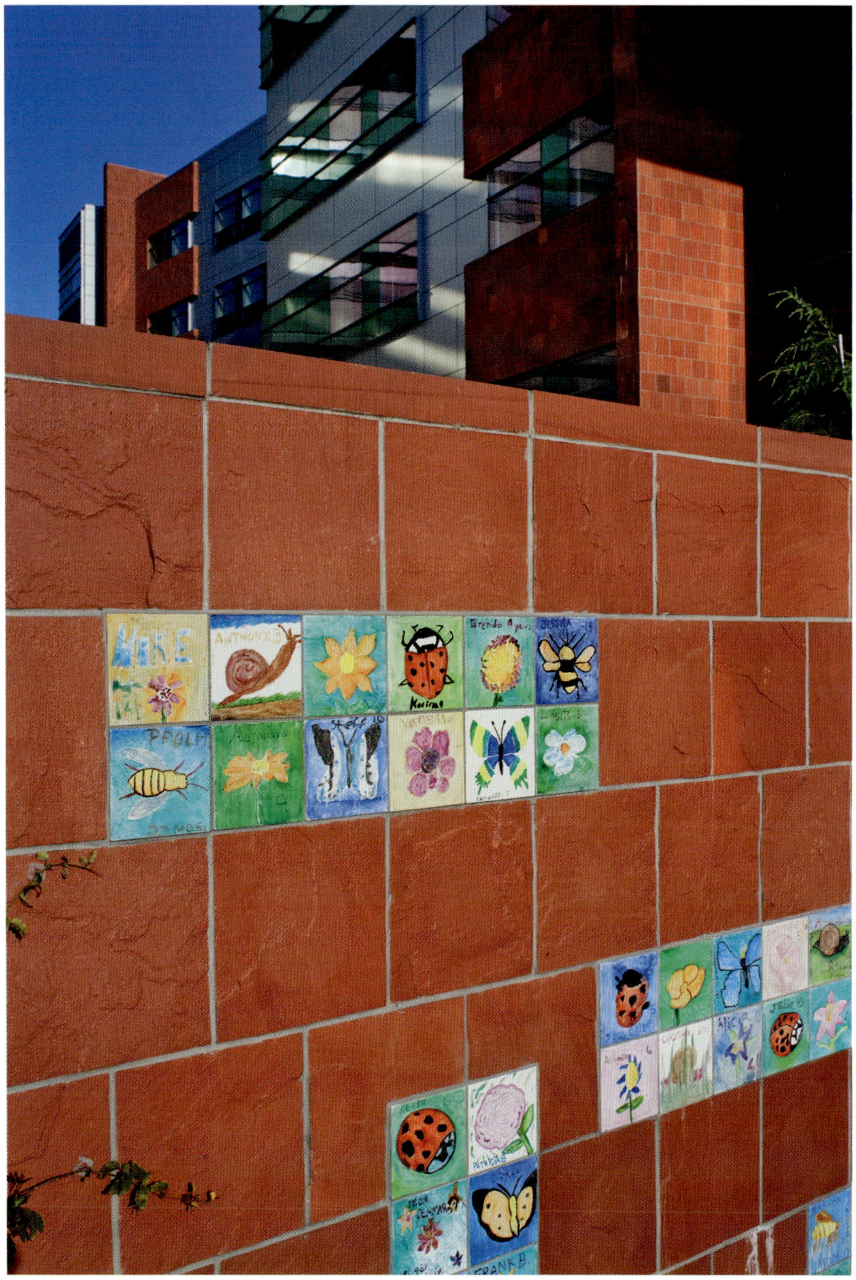

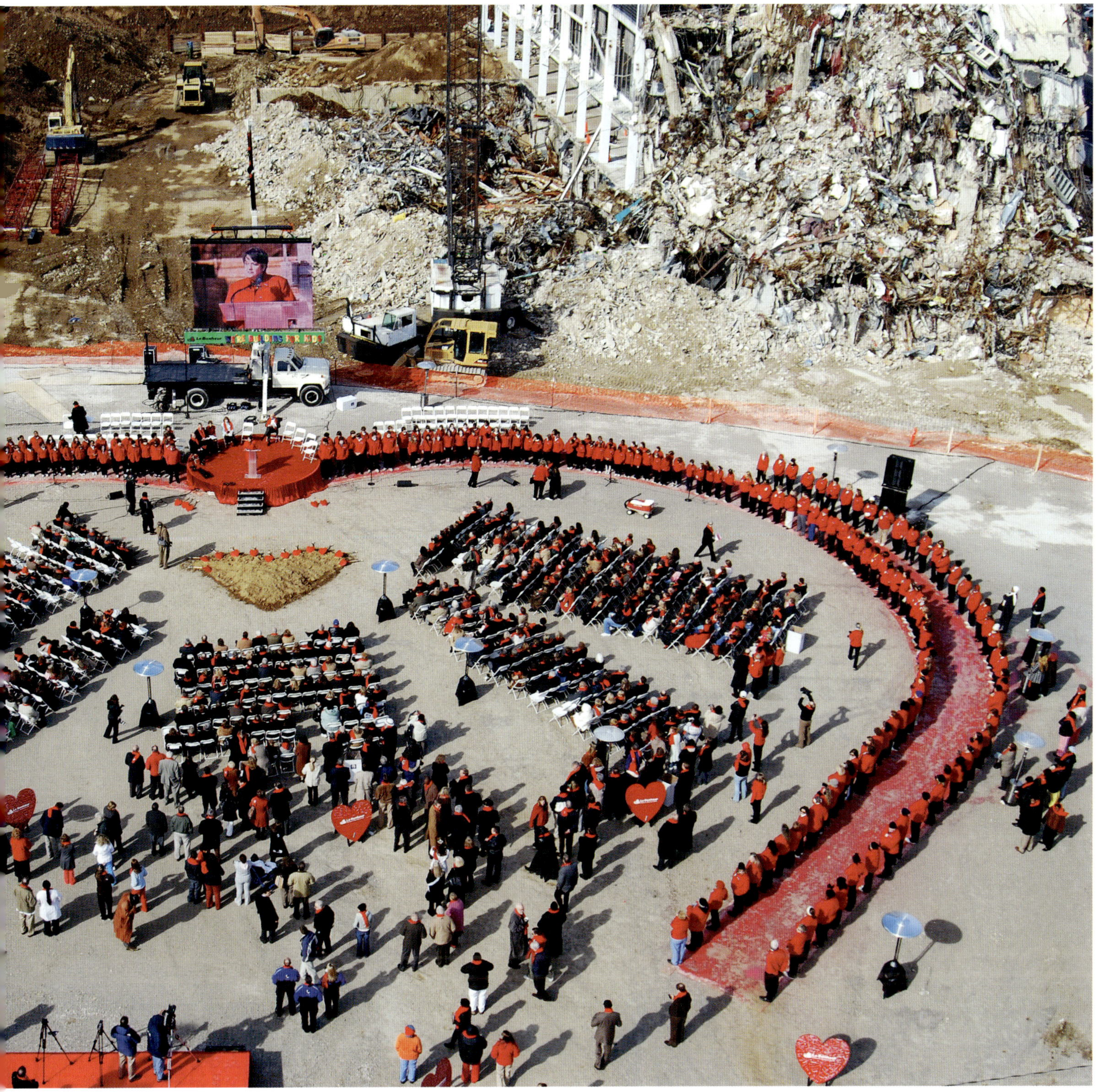

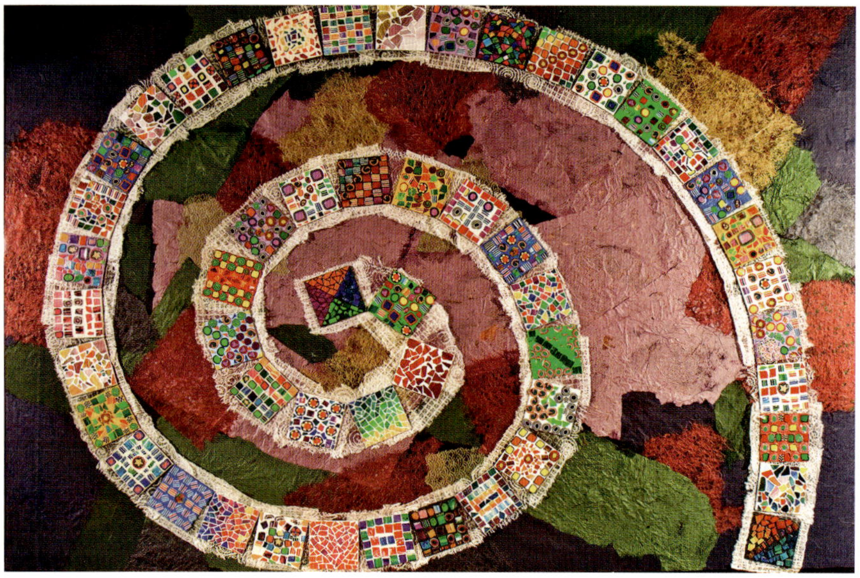

▲ Children's Hospital of Philadelphia, PA
Photo: Paul Crane

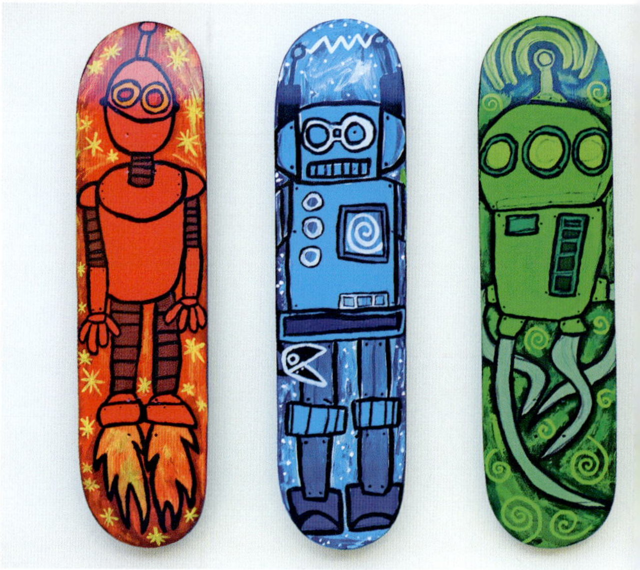

▲ Dayton Children's, Dayton, OH
▼ ***Photos: Ken Shory***

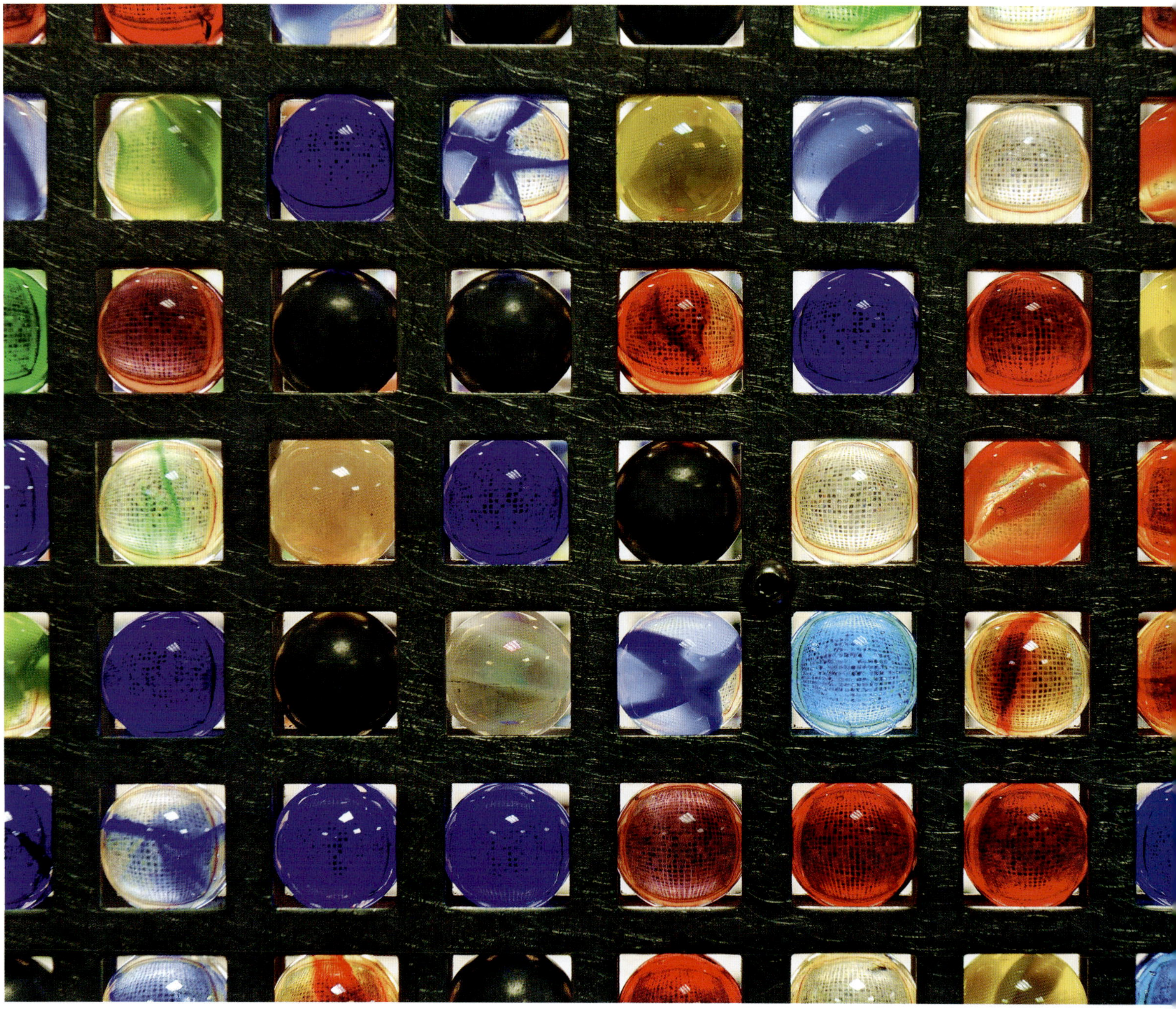

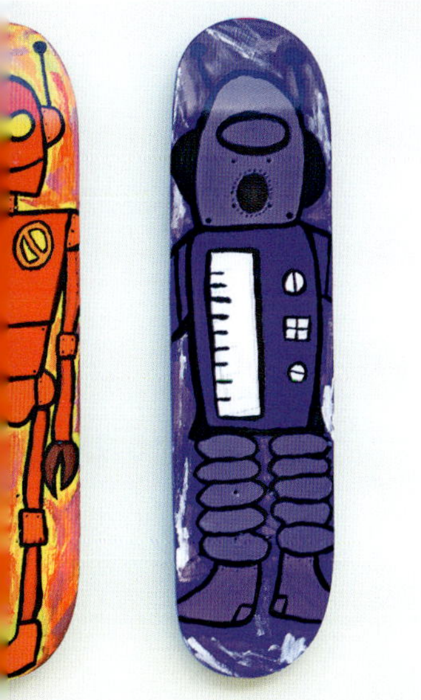

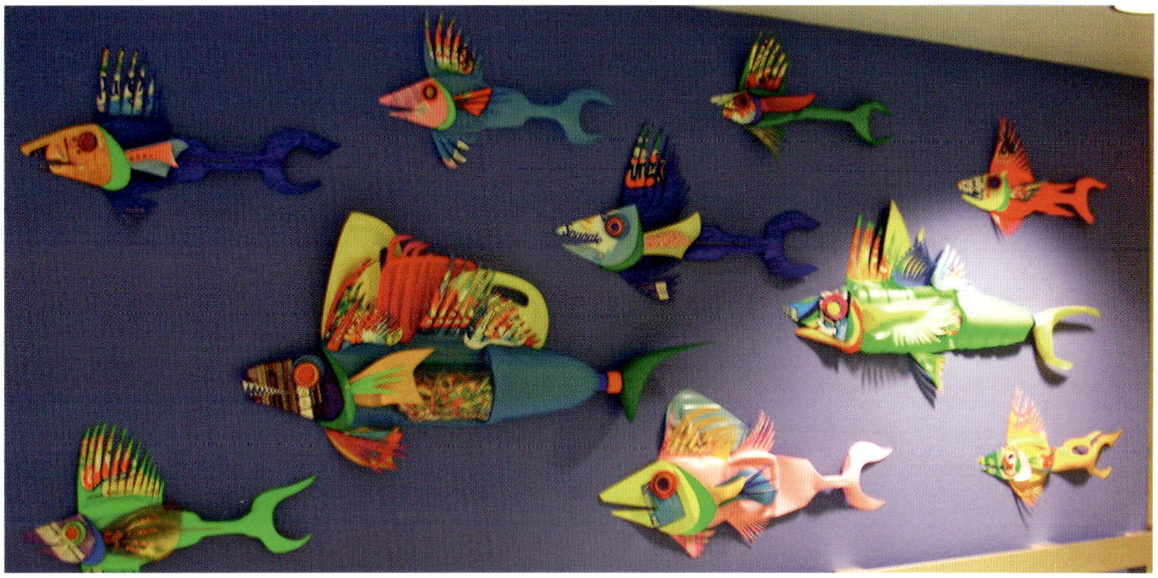

▲ Levine Children's Hospital, Charlotte, NC
Photo: Brad Feinknopf

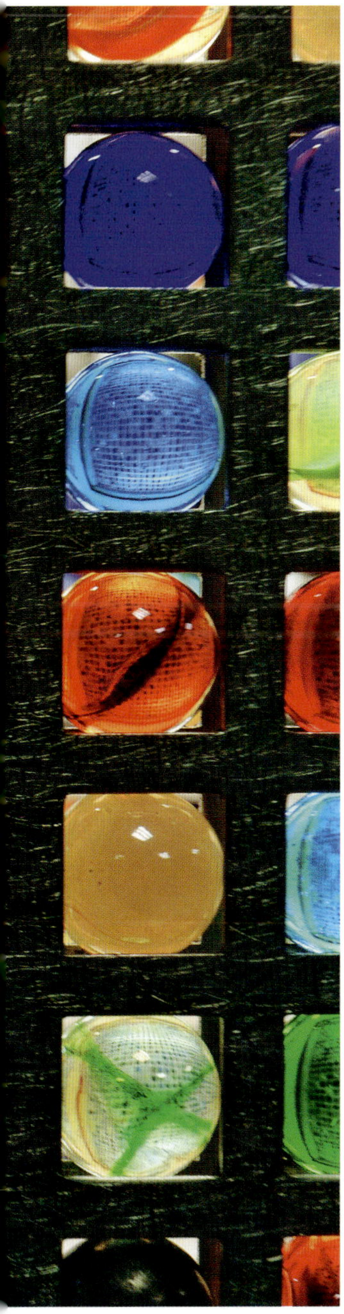

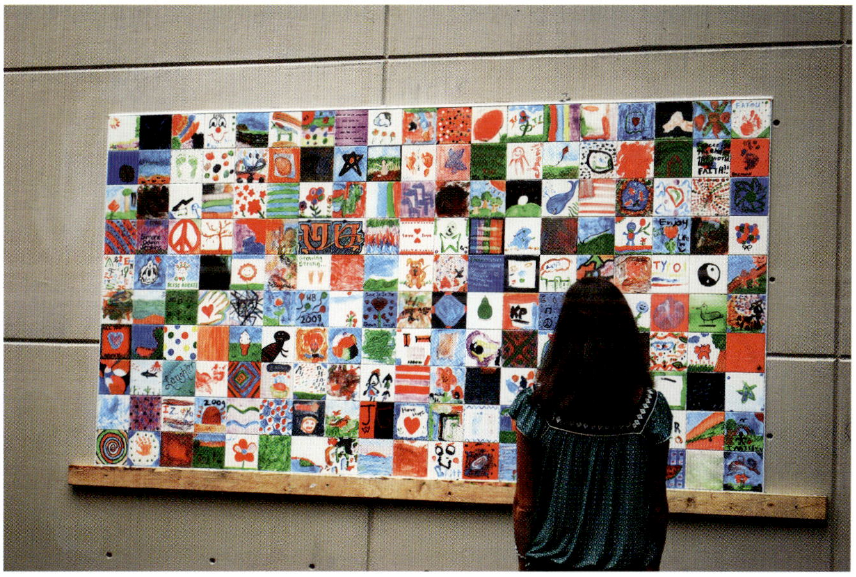

▲ Mt. Washington Pediatric Hospital, Baltimore, MD
Photo: Jeffrey Totaro Photographer

Following pages: Le Bonheur Children's Hospital, Memphis, TN
Photo: Aker Imaging
Mural: Enchilada, Caboodle, Shebang (by Mary Jo Karimnia)

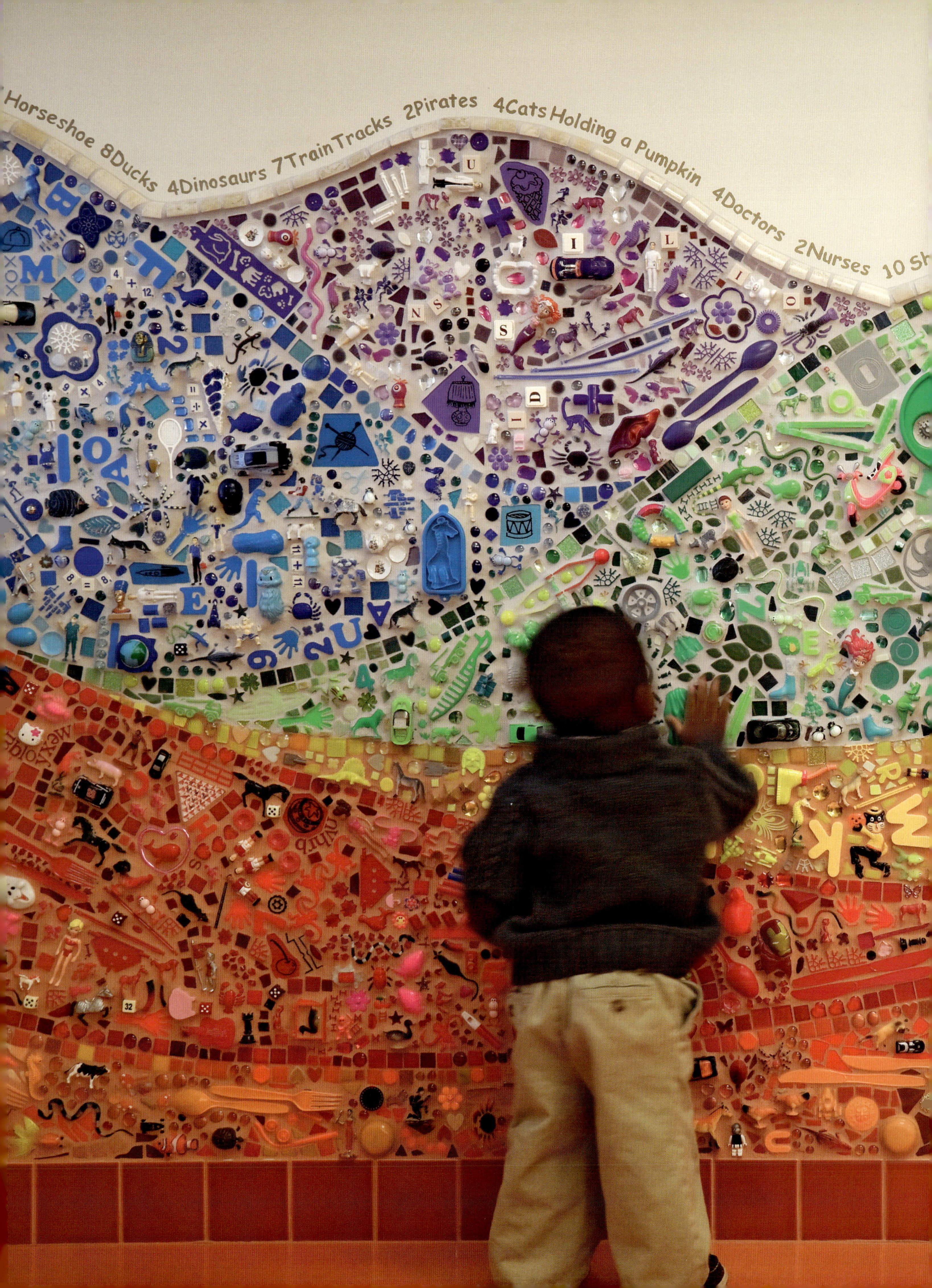
Horseshoe 8Ducks 4Dinosaurs 7Train Tracks 2Pirates 4Cats Holding a Pumpkin 4Doctors 2Nurses

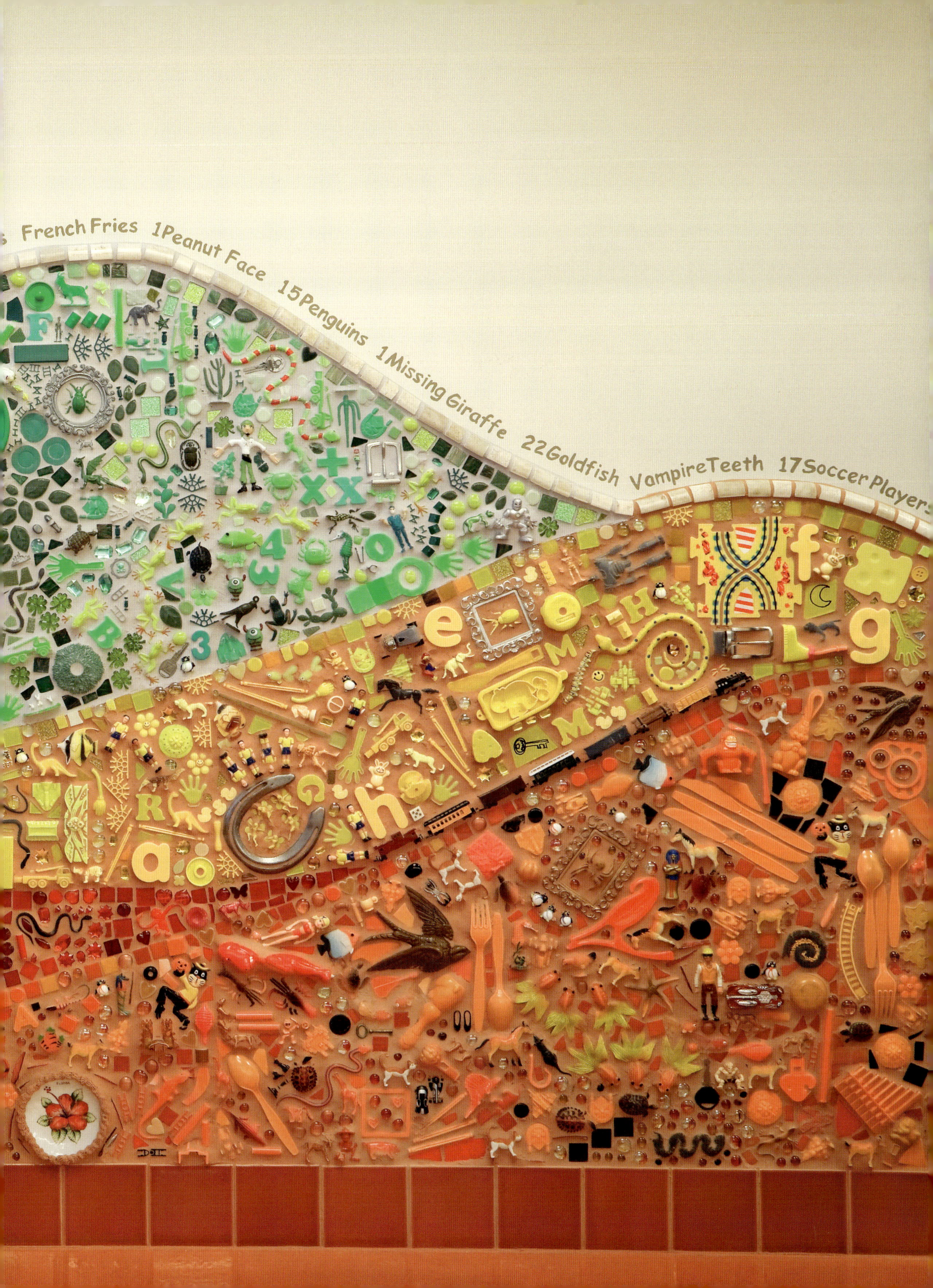
s French Fries 1 Peanut Face 15 Penguins 1 Missing Giraffe 22 Goldfish Vampire Teeth 17 Soccer Players

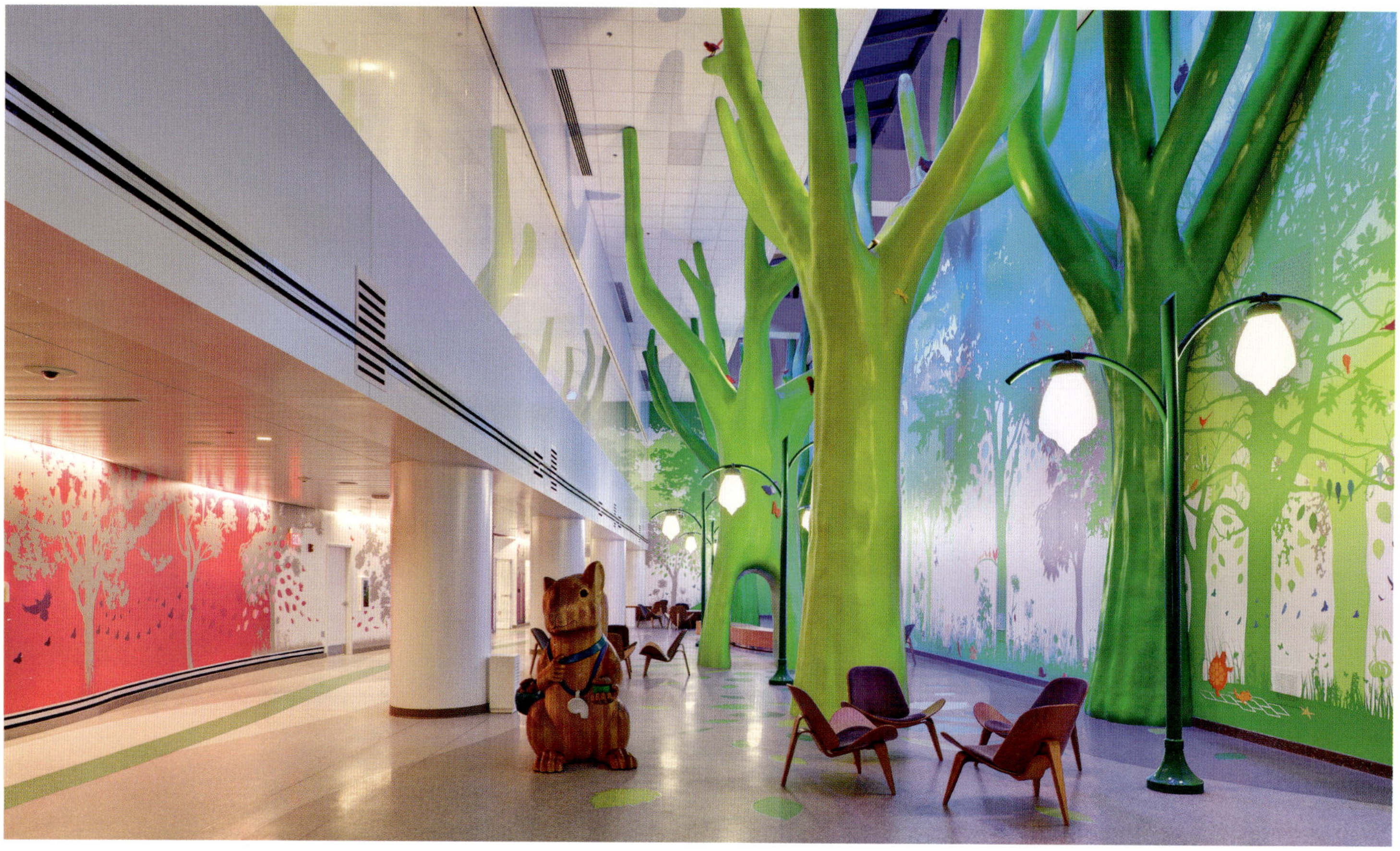

▲ Nationwide Children's Hospital, Columbus, OH
Photo: Brad Feinknopf

▼ Children's Hospital of Michigan, Detroit, MI

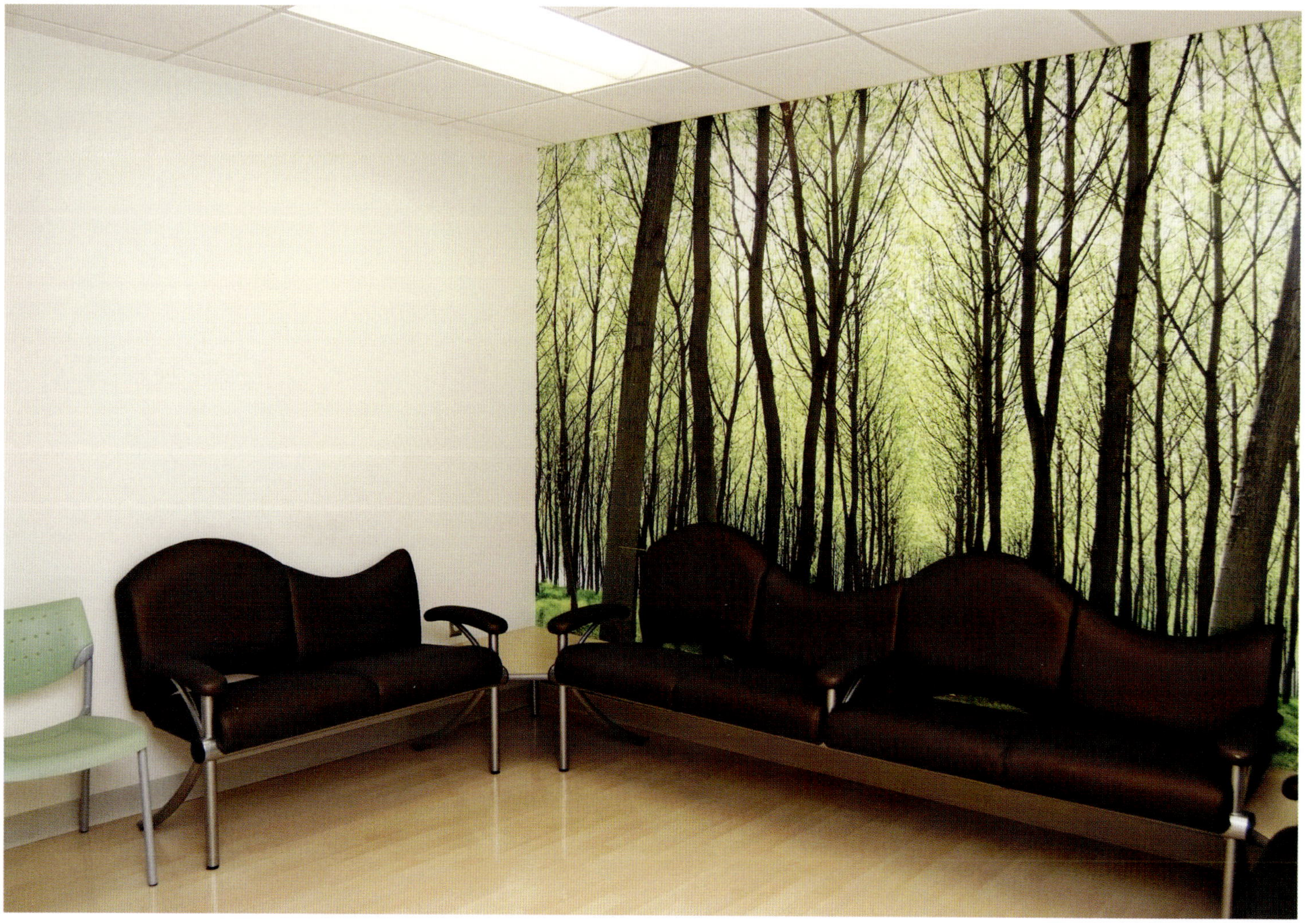

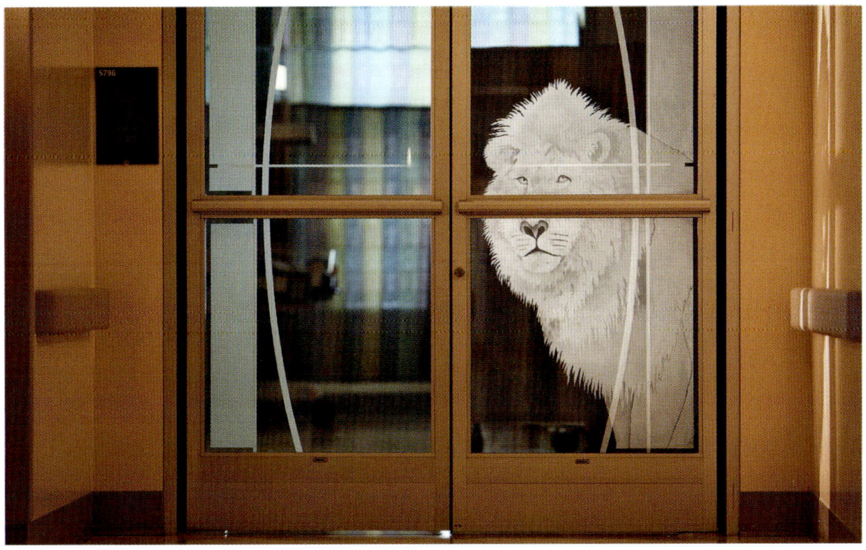

▲ UC Davis Children's Hospital, Sacramento, CA
Photo: University of California Regents

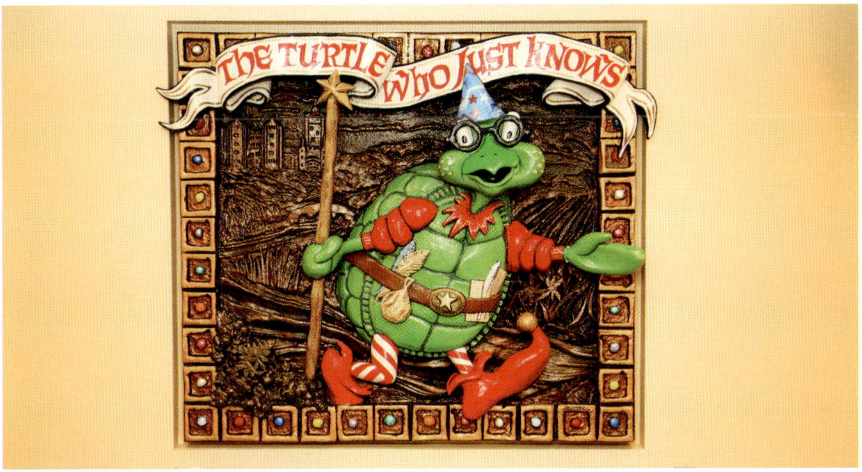

▲ Sanford Children's Hospital, Sioux Falls, SD

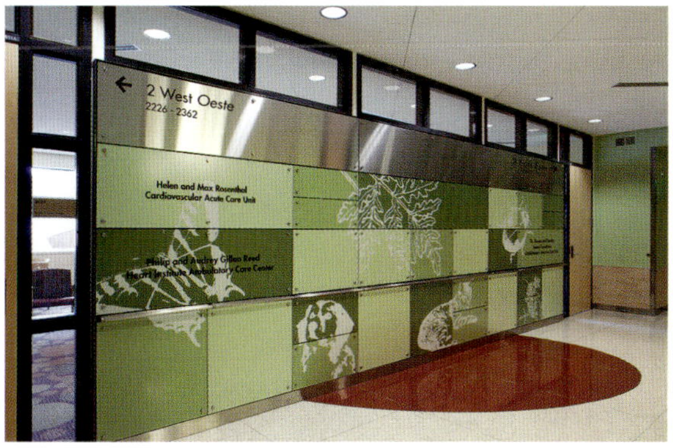

▲ Children's Hospital Los Angeles, CA
Photo: Pete Eckert

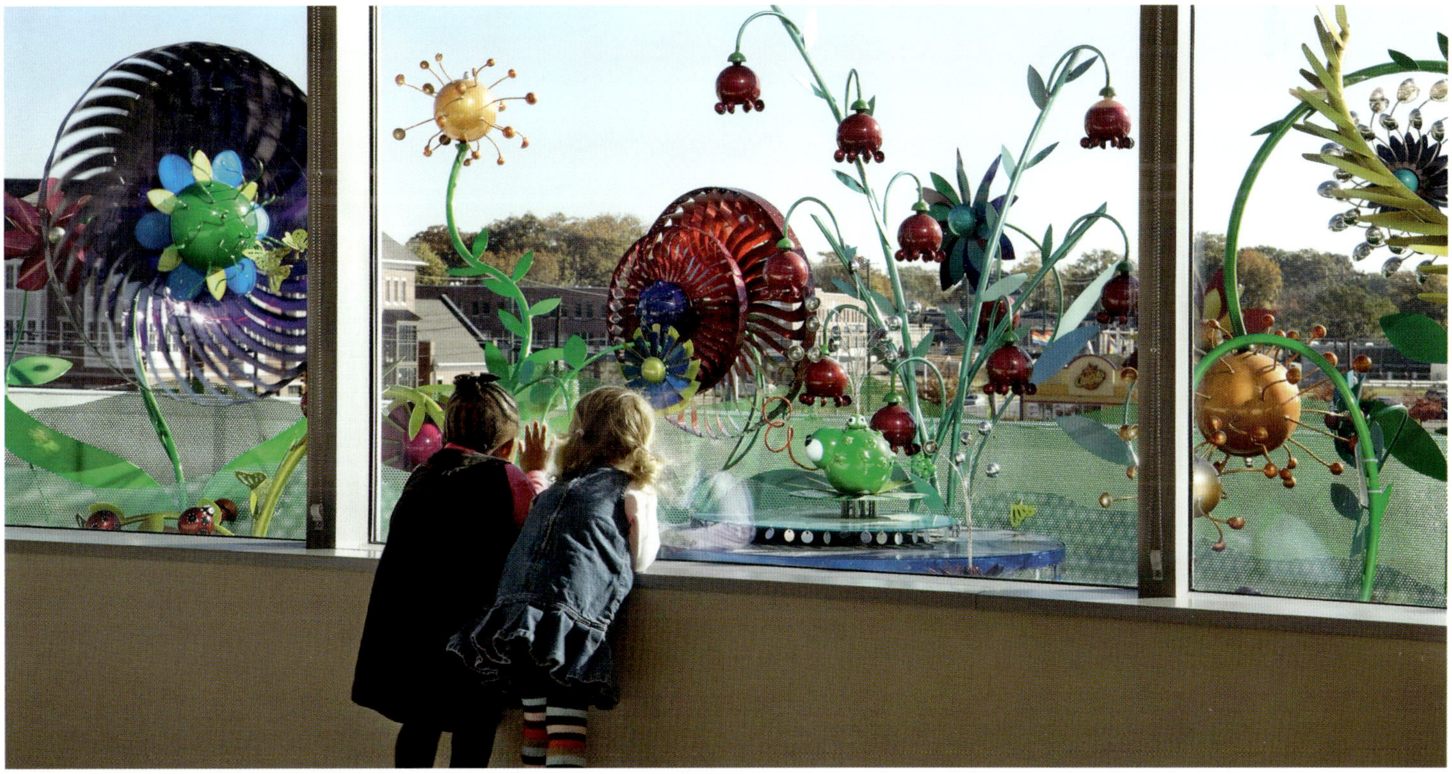

▲ Le Bonheur Children's Hospital, Memphis, TN
Photo: Aker Imaging
Sculpture: Where the Wind Plays (by Yvonne Bobo)

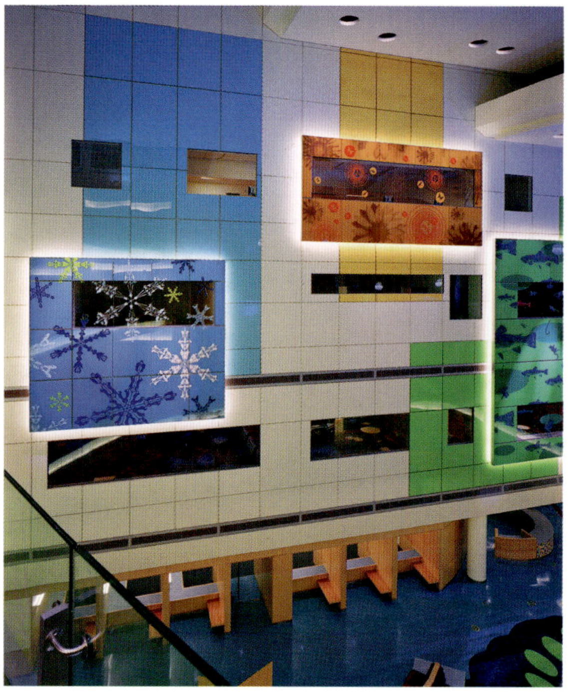

▲ Children's Hospital Colorado, Denver, CO
Photo: Eckert & Eckert

▼ Helen DeVos Children's Hospital, Grand Rapids, MI
Photo: Lucid Architecture, Eric DeWitt

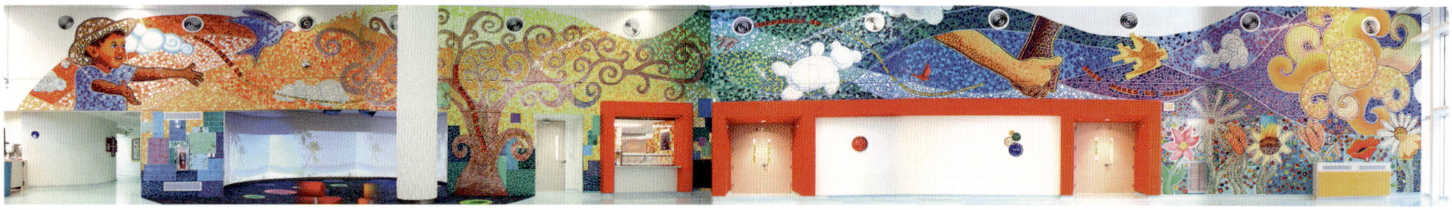

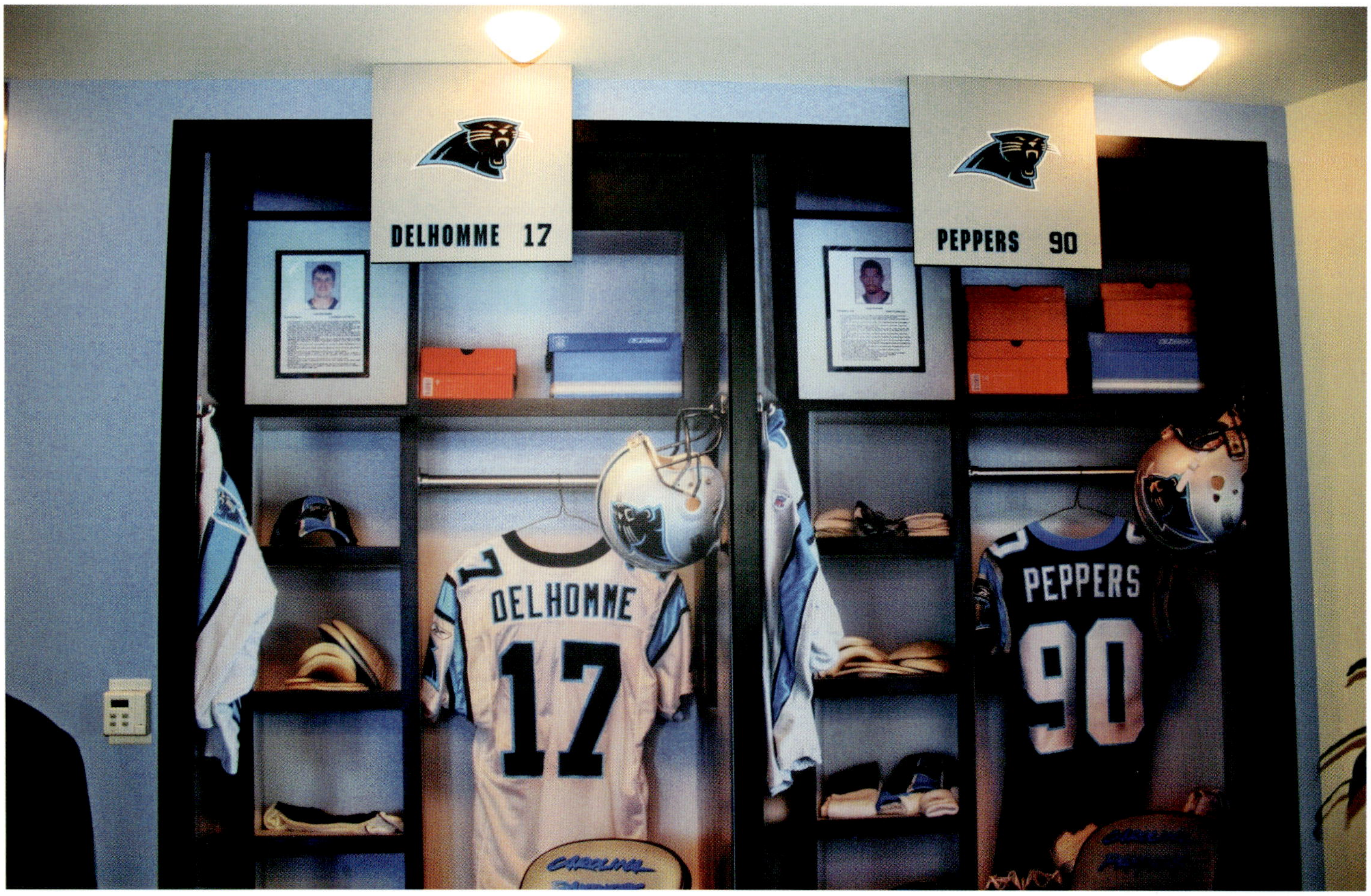

▲ Joseph M. Sanzari Children's Hospital at Hackensack University Medical Center, Hackensack, NJ
Photo: Basil Fargnoli

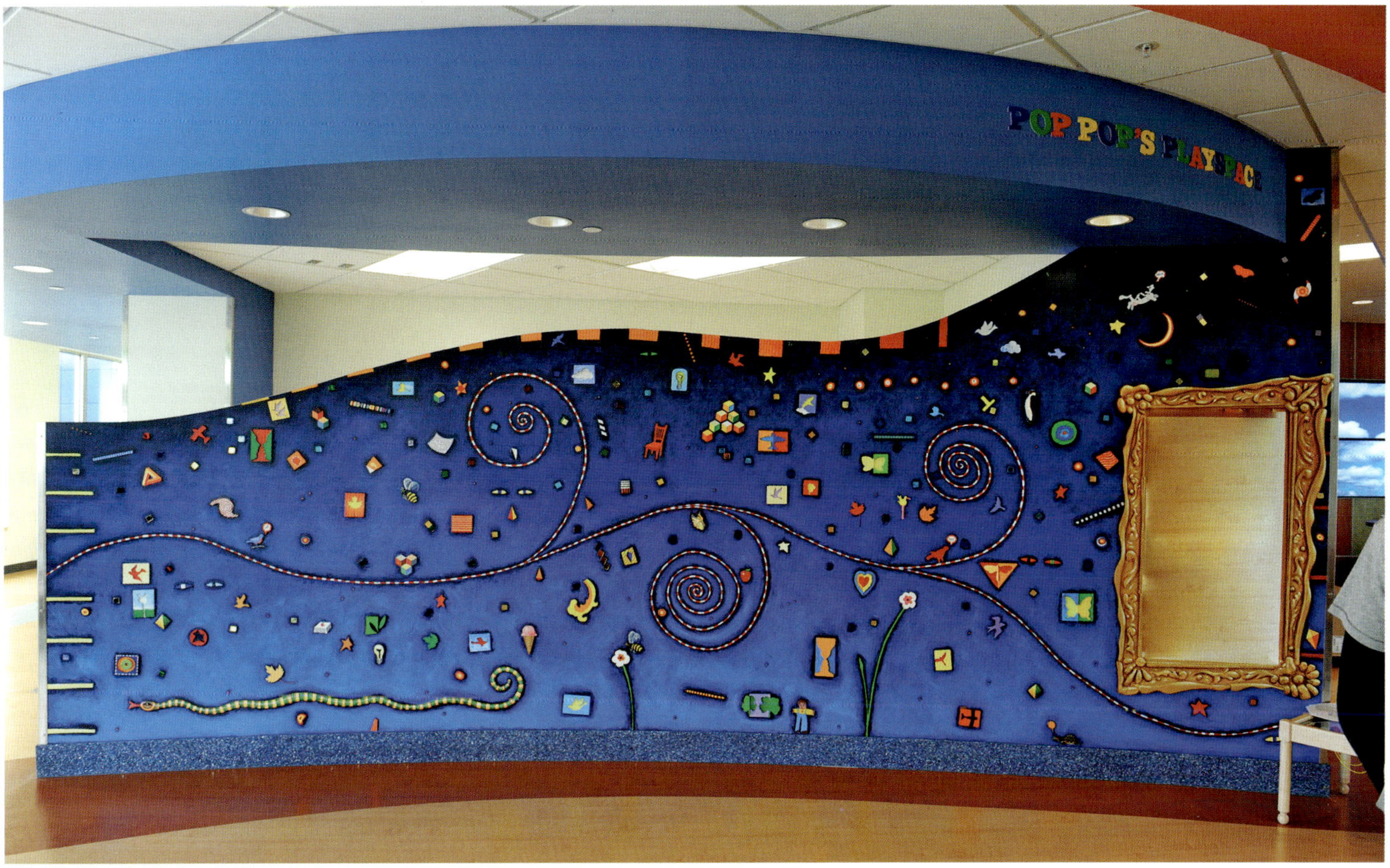

▲ Kosair Children's Hospital, Louisville, KY

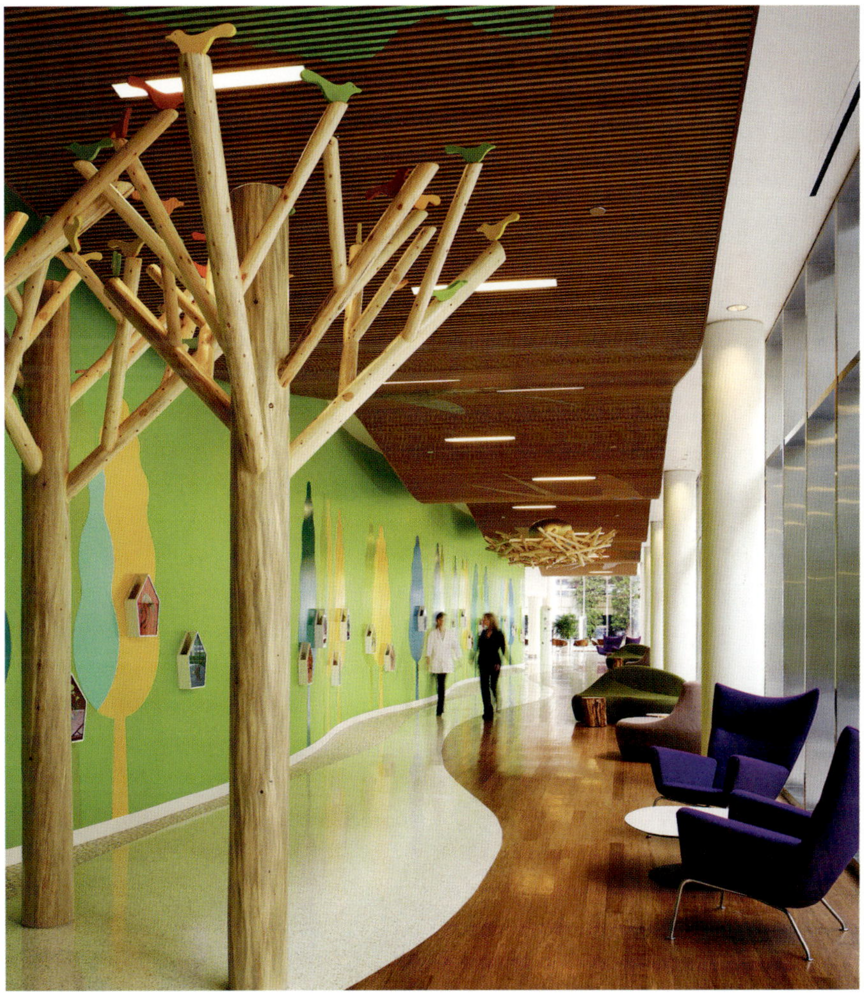

▲ Randall Children's Hospital at Legacy Emanuel, Portland, OR
Photo: Hedrich Blessing Photography, Nick Merrick

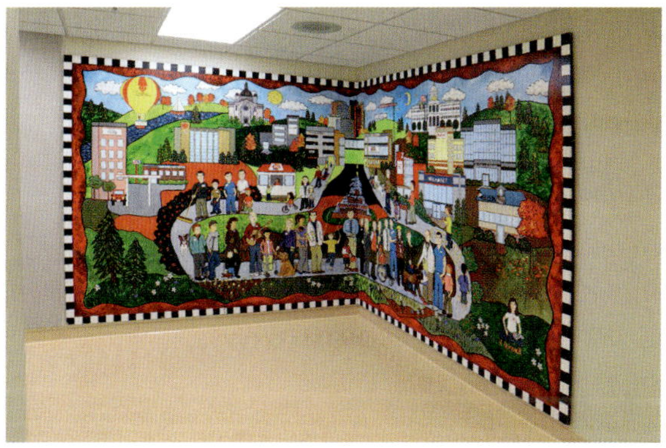

▲ Helen DeVos Children's Hospital, Grand Rapids, MI
Photo: Hedrich Blessing

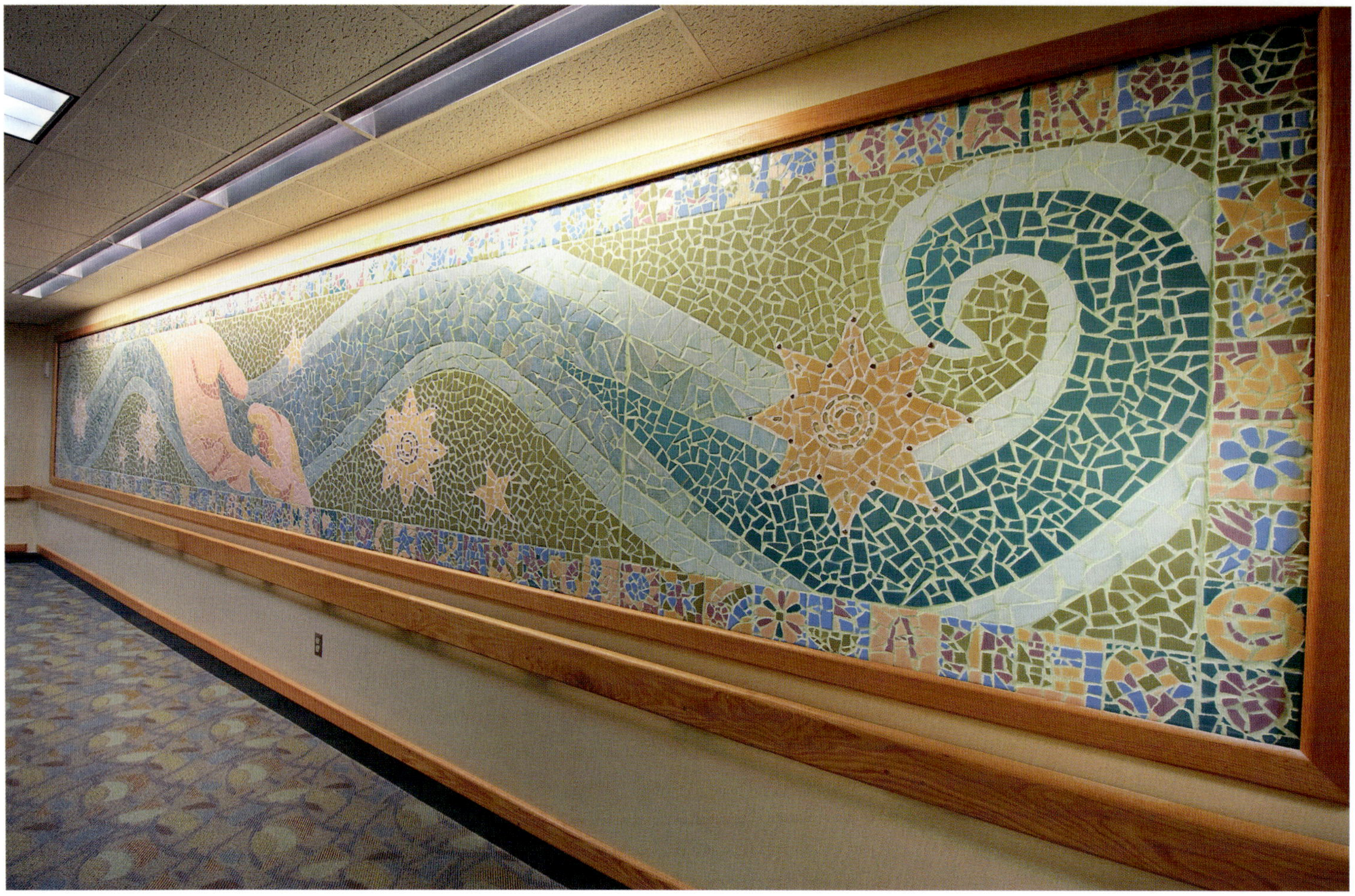

▲ Children's Hospital of Philadelphia, PA
Photo: Paul Crane

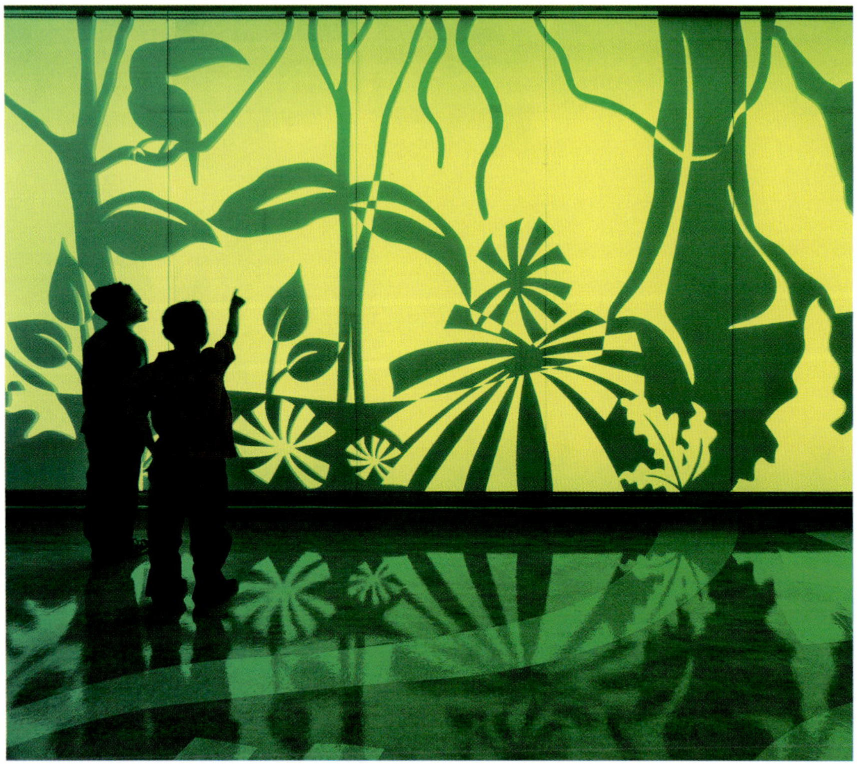

▲ University of Minnesota Amplatz Children's Hospital, Minneapolis, MN
Photo: Hedrich Blessing Photography, Nick Merrick

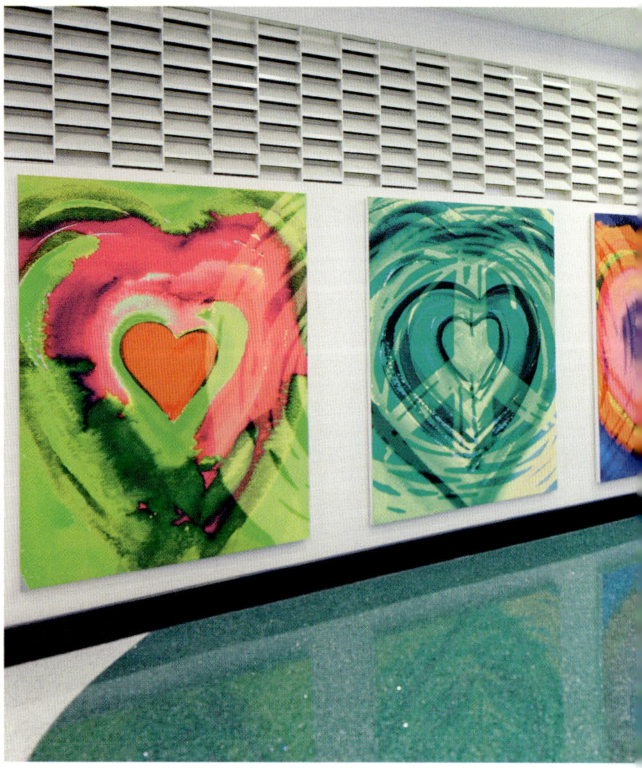

▲ Medical City Children's Hospital, Dallas, TX
Photo: Terry Cockerham

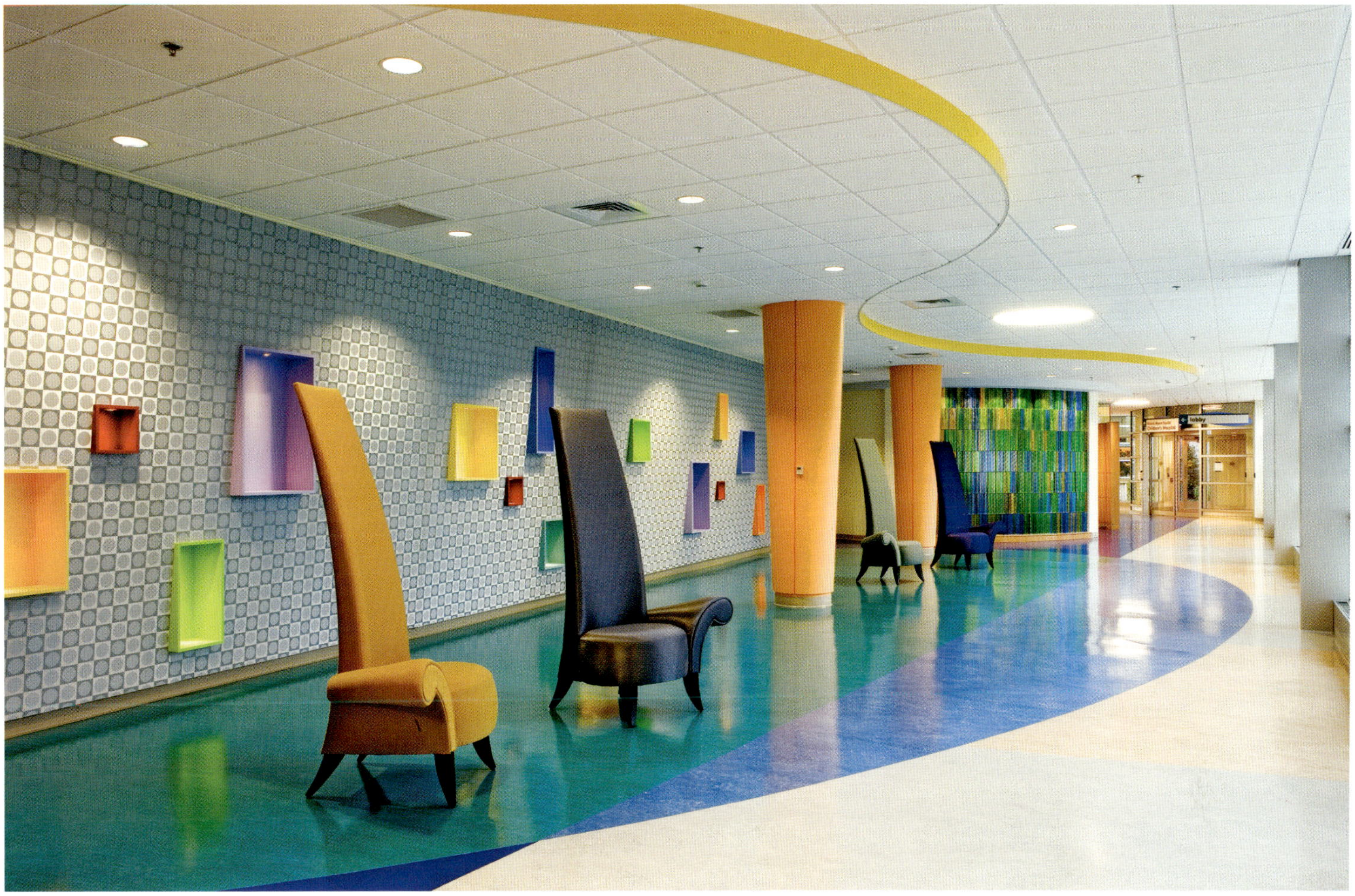

▲ PSE&G Children's Specialized Hospital, New Brunswick, NJ
Photo: Stantec © Tom Crane Photography, Inc.

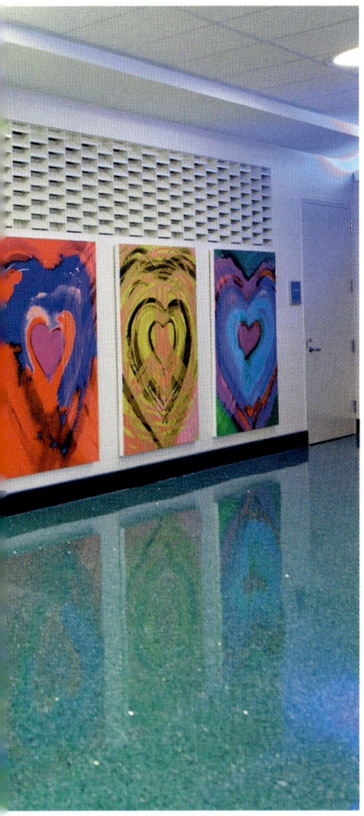

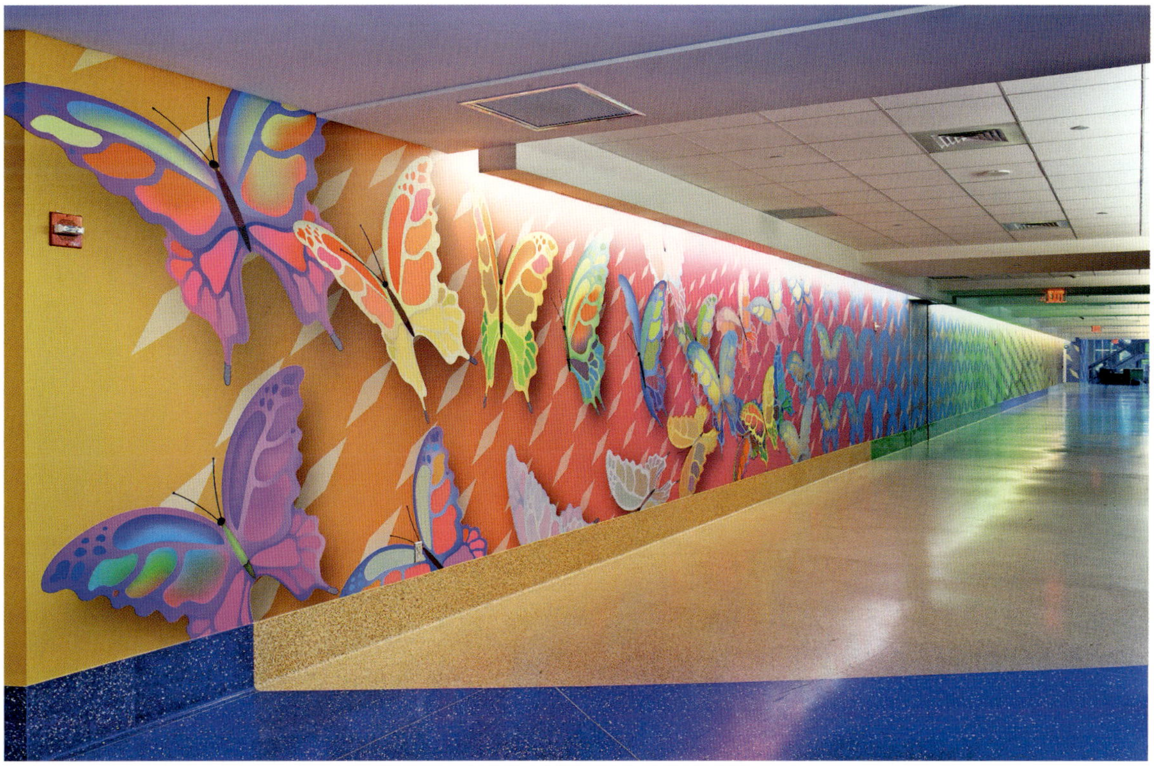

▲ Children's Hospital, Pittsburgh, PA
Photo: Alexander Denmars

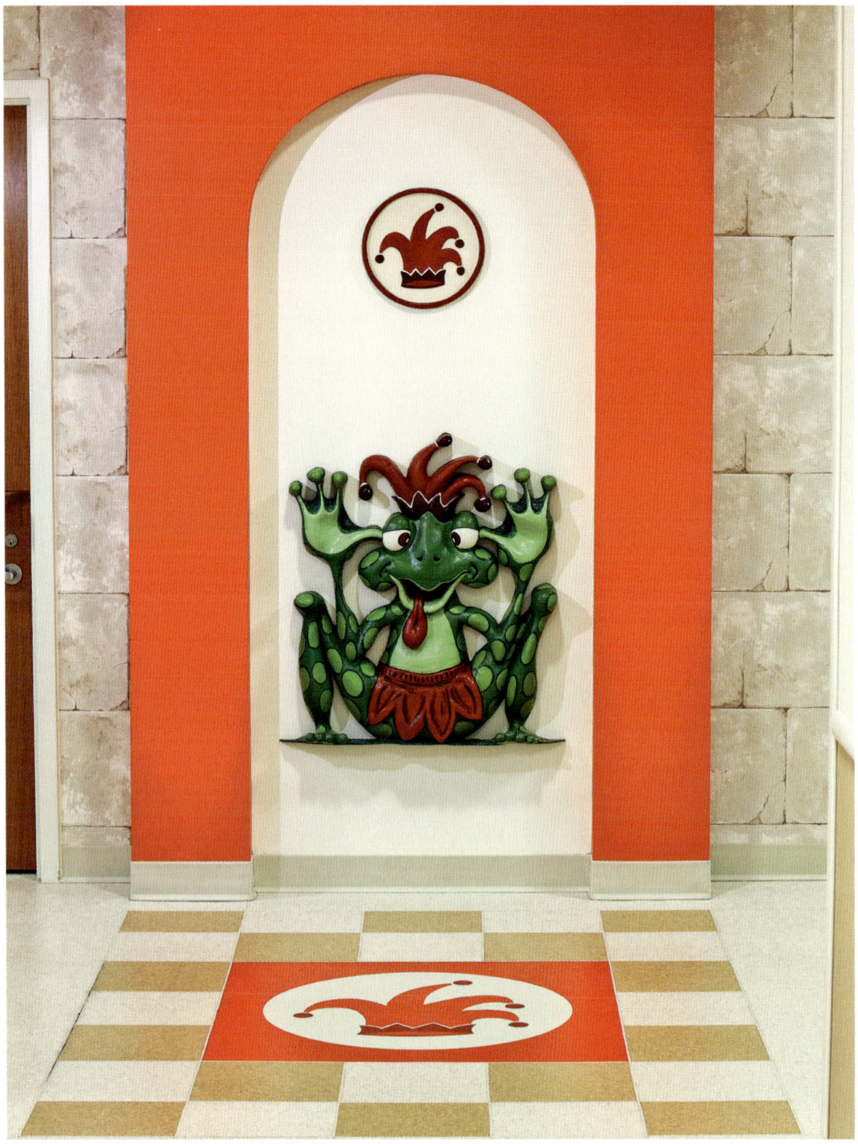

▲ Sanford Children's Hospital, Sioux Falls, SD

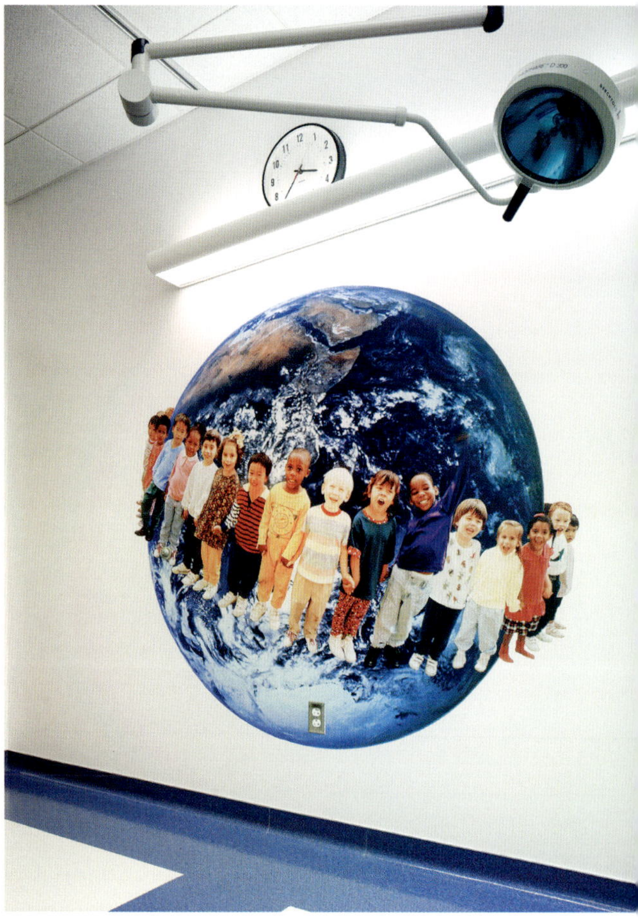

▲ Mattel Children's Hospital UCLA, Los Angeles, CA
Photo: Benny Chan, fotoworks

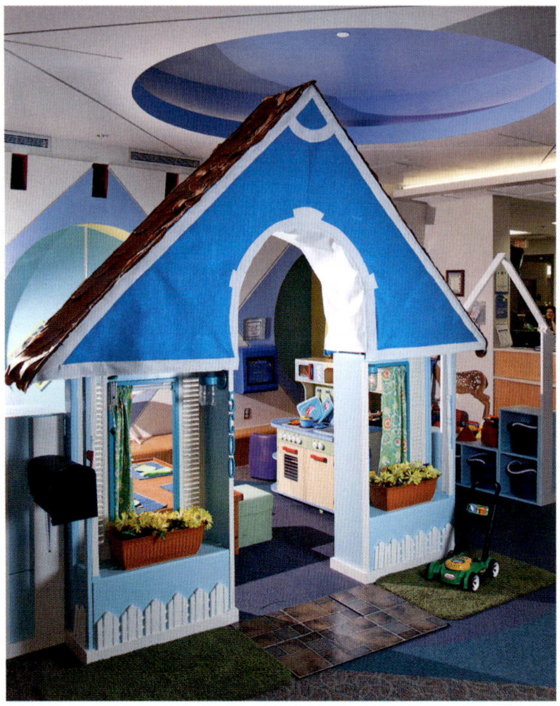

▲ UNC North Carolina Children's Hospital, Chapel Hill, NC
Photo: Brian Strickland

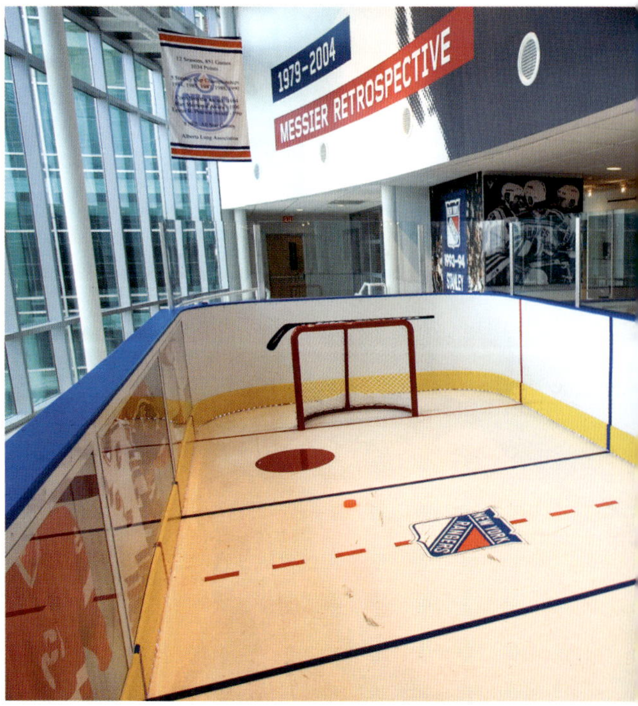

▲ Joseph M. Sanzari Children's Hospital at Hackensack University Medical Center, Hackensack, NJ
Photo: Steve Hockstein, Harvard Studio

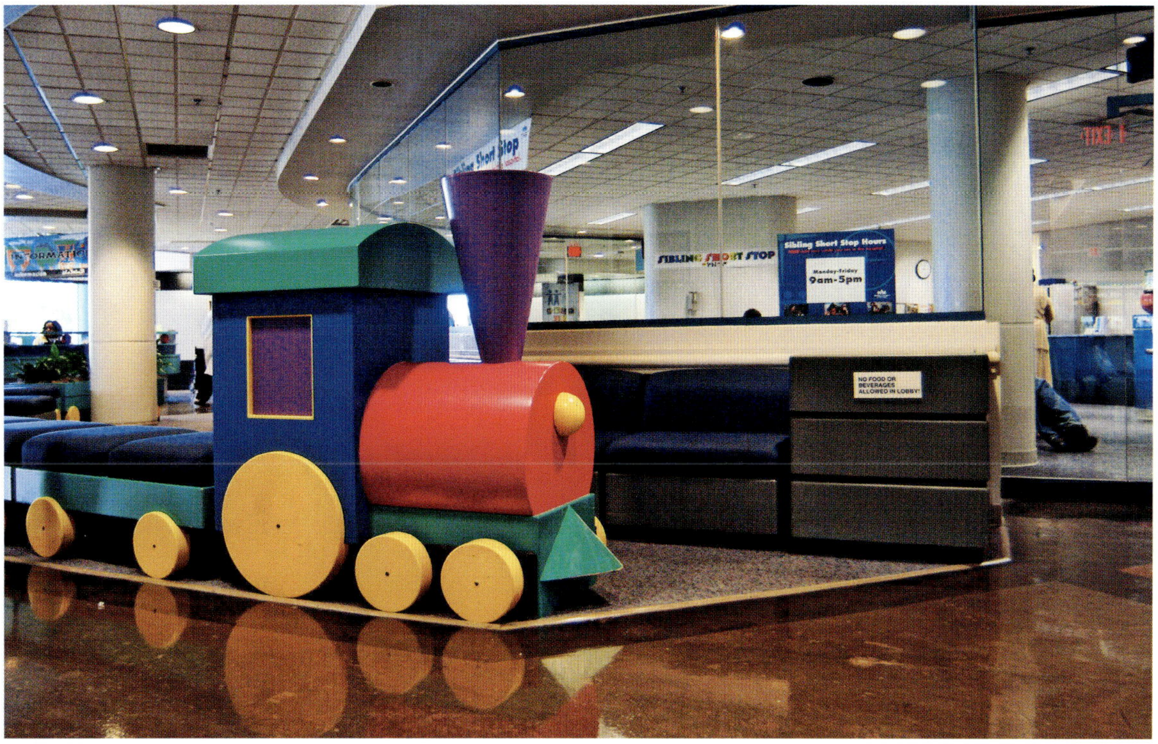

▲ Children's Hospital of Michigan, Detroit, MI
▼

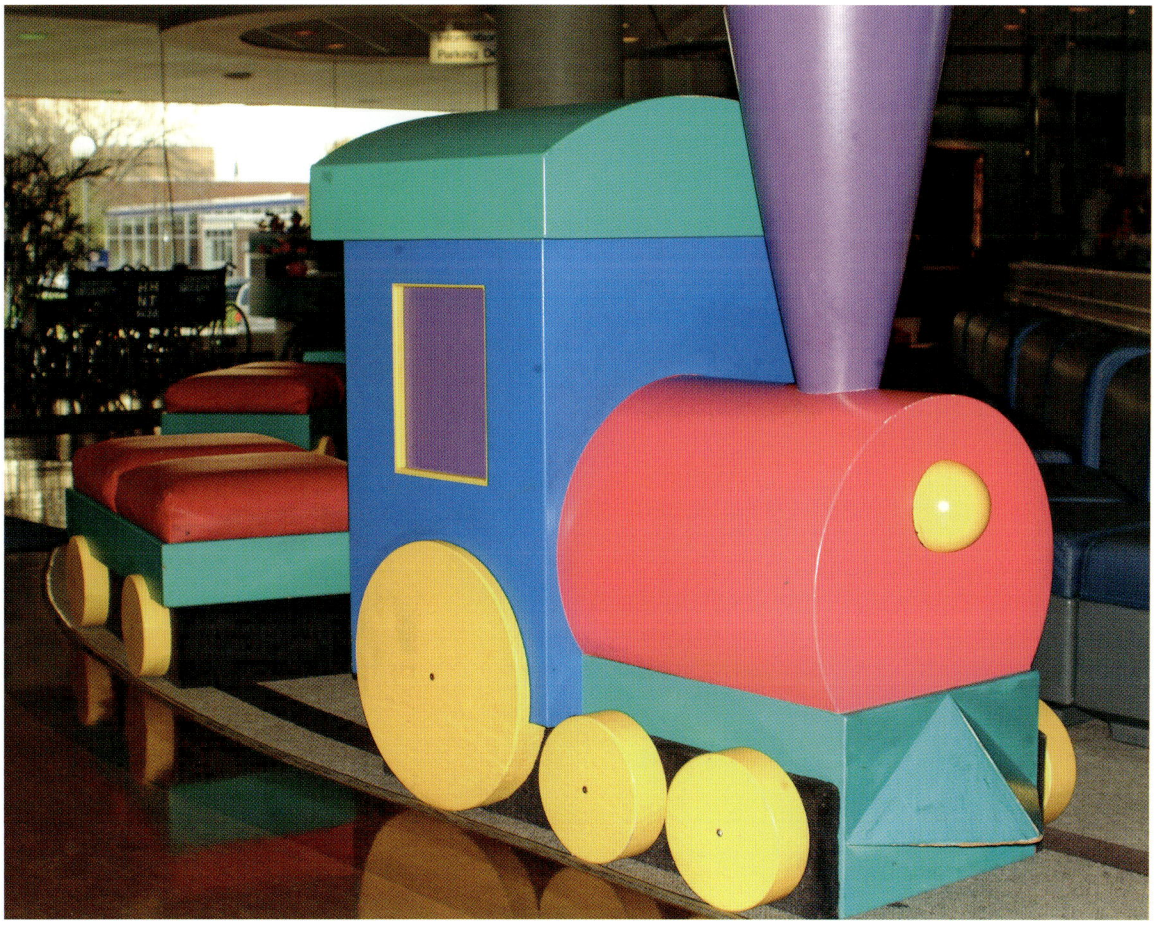

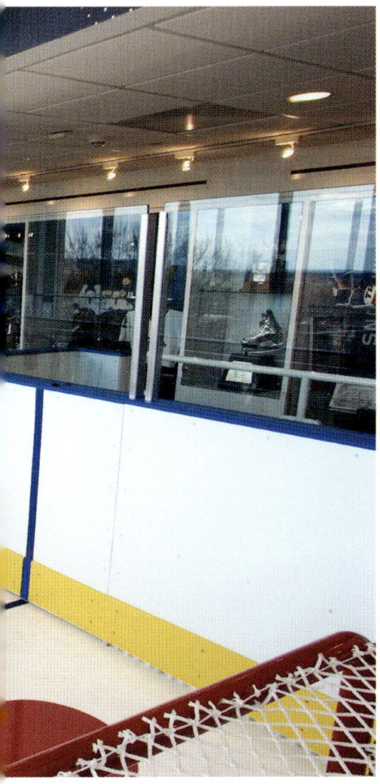

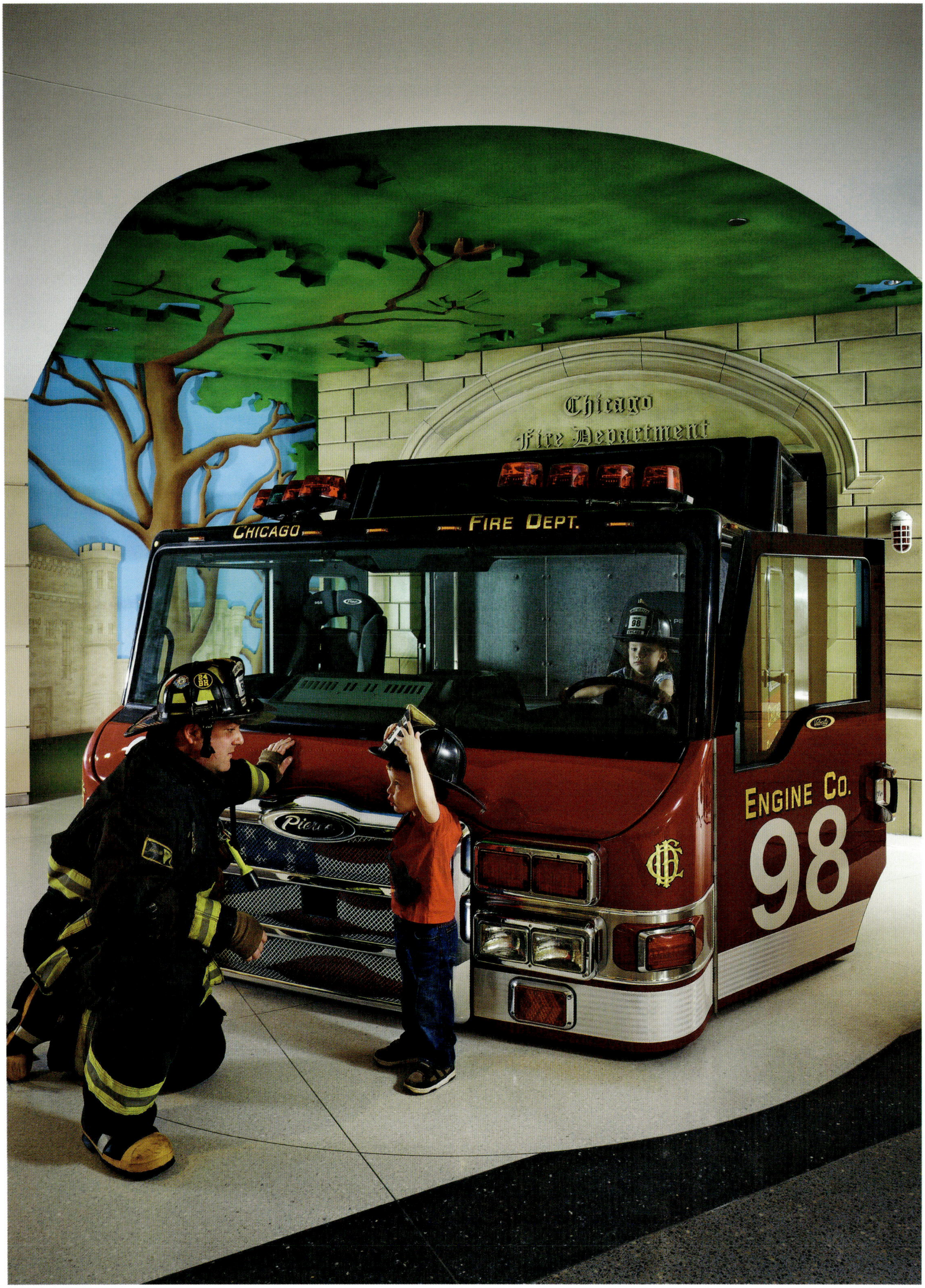
Chicago
Fire Department
CHICAGO
FIRE DEPT.
ENGINE CO.
98

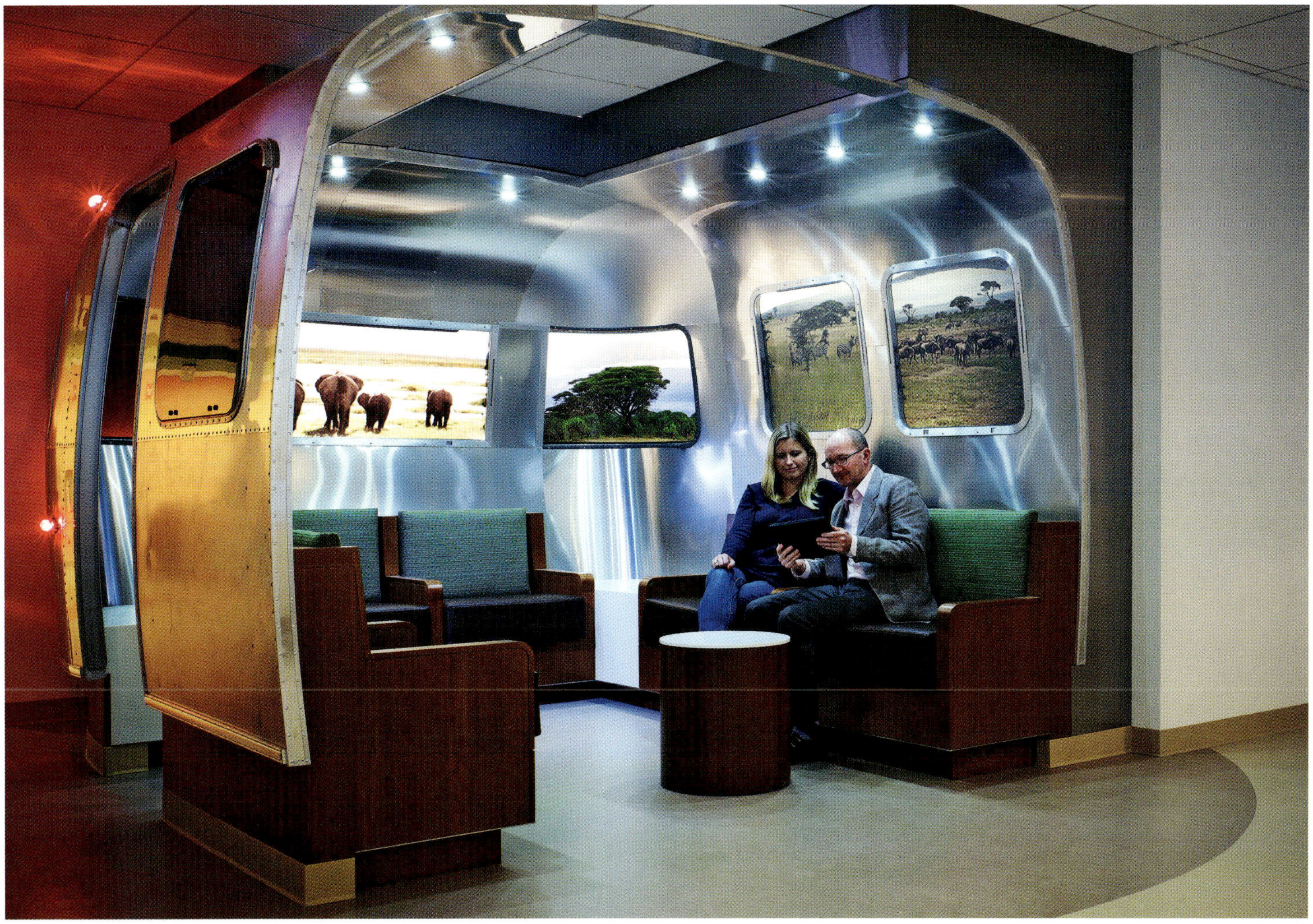

▲ Ann & Robert H. Lurie Children's Hospital of Chicago, IL

◀ ***Photos: Hedrich Blessing Photography, Nick Merrick***

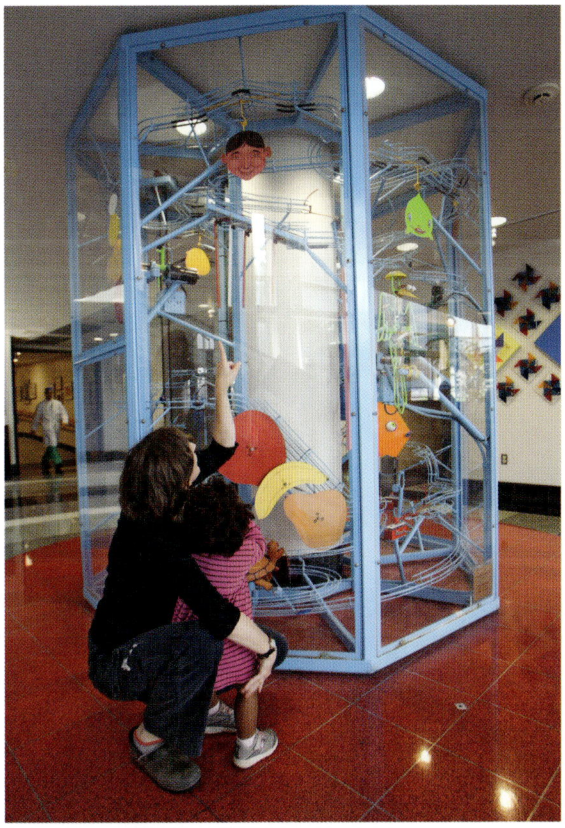

▲ UNC North Carolina Children's Hospital, Chapel Hill, NC

Photo: Brian Strickland

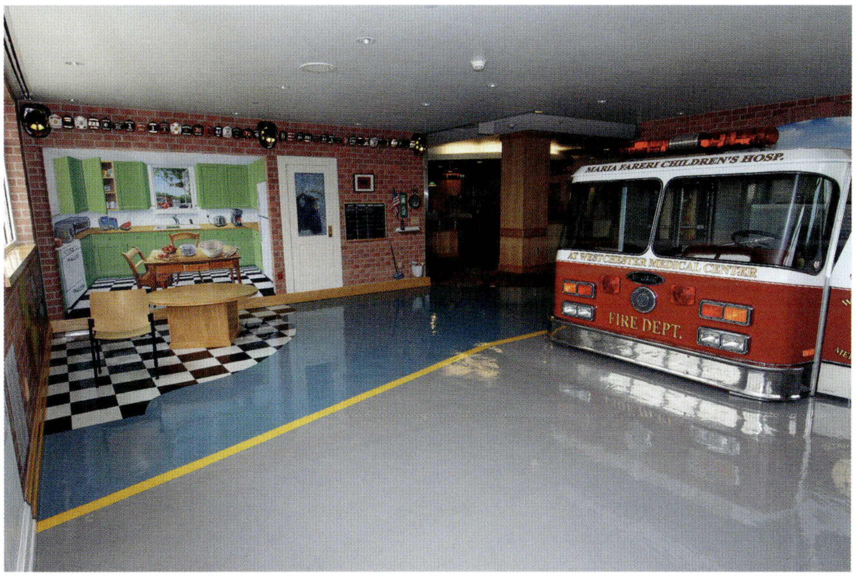

▲ Maria Fareri Children's Hospital, Valhalla, NY

Photo: Westchester Medical Center

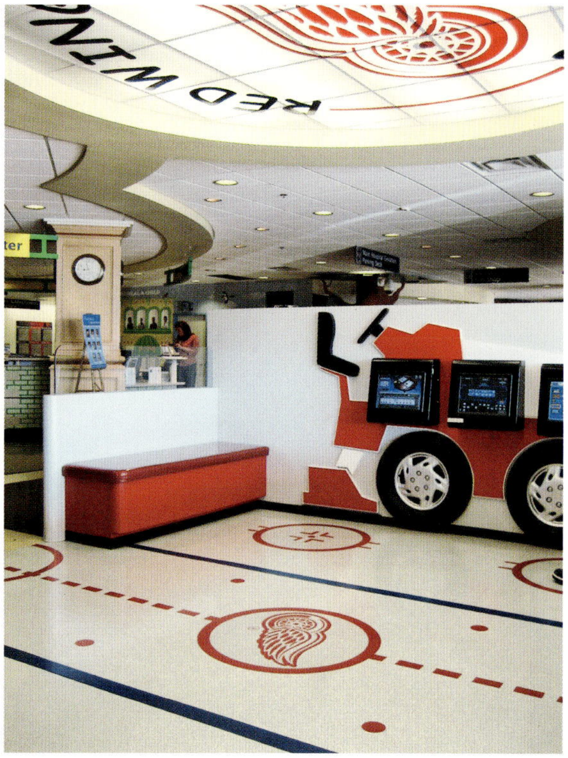

▲ Children's Hospital of Michigan, Detroit, MI

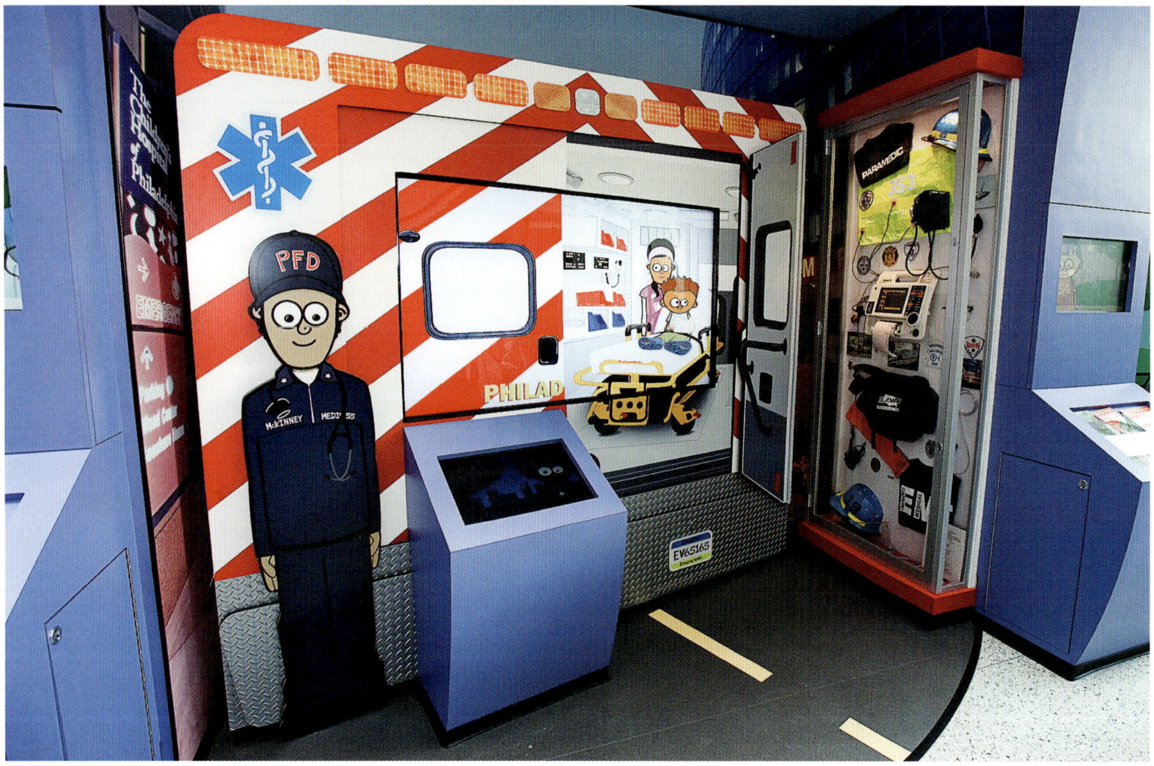

▲ Children's Hospital of Philadelphia, PA
Photo: Paul Crane

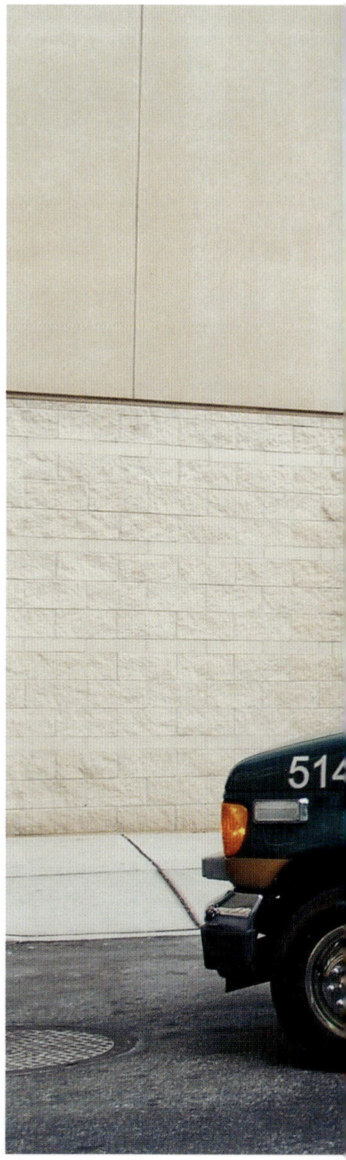

Joseph M. Sanzari Children's Hospital at Hackensack University Medical Center, Hackensack, NJ ▶
Photo: Basil Fargnoli

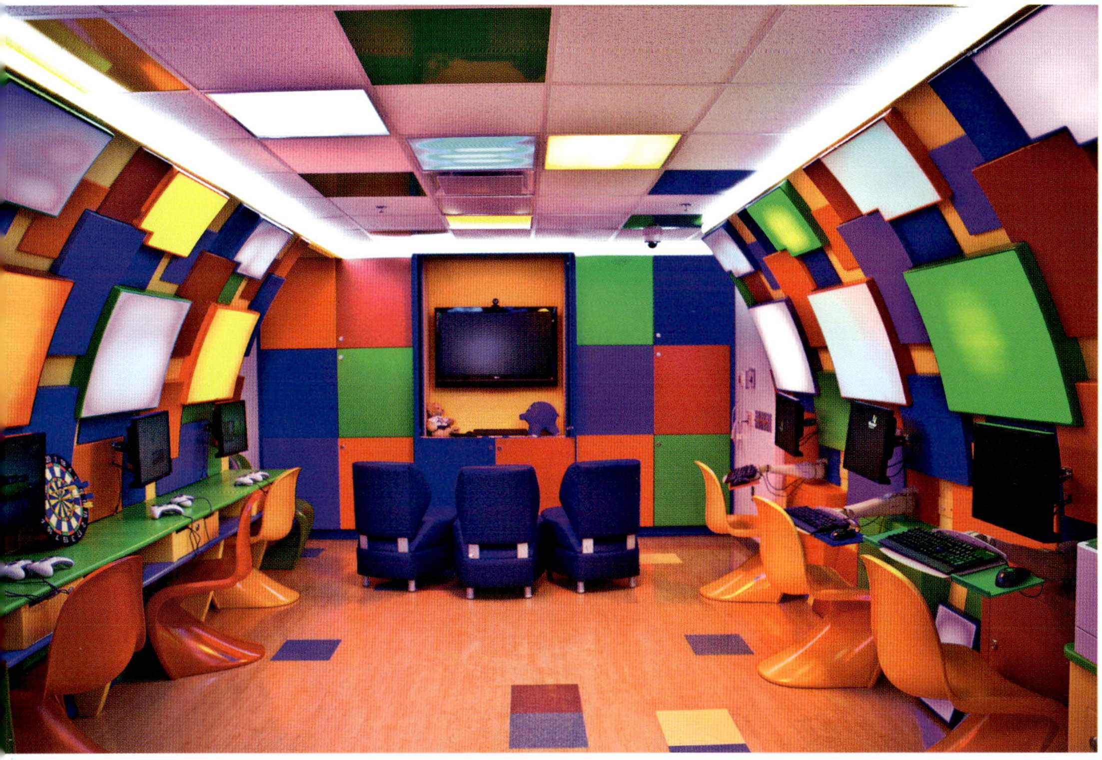

▲ Children's Hospital of Philadelphia, PA
Photo: Albert Chen

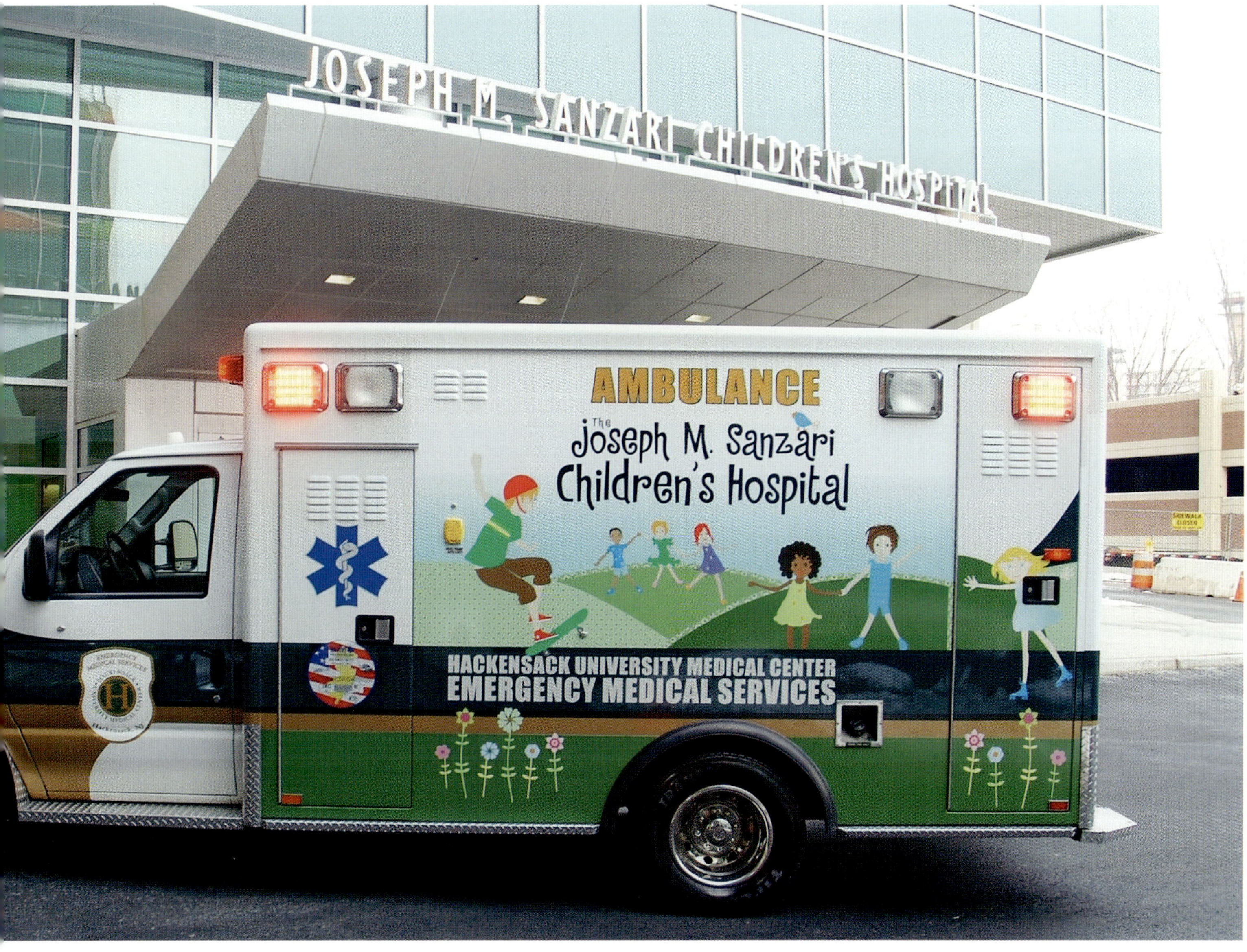

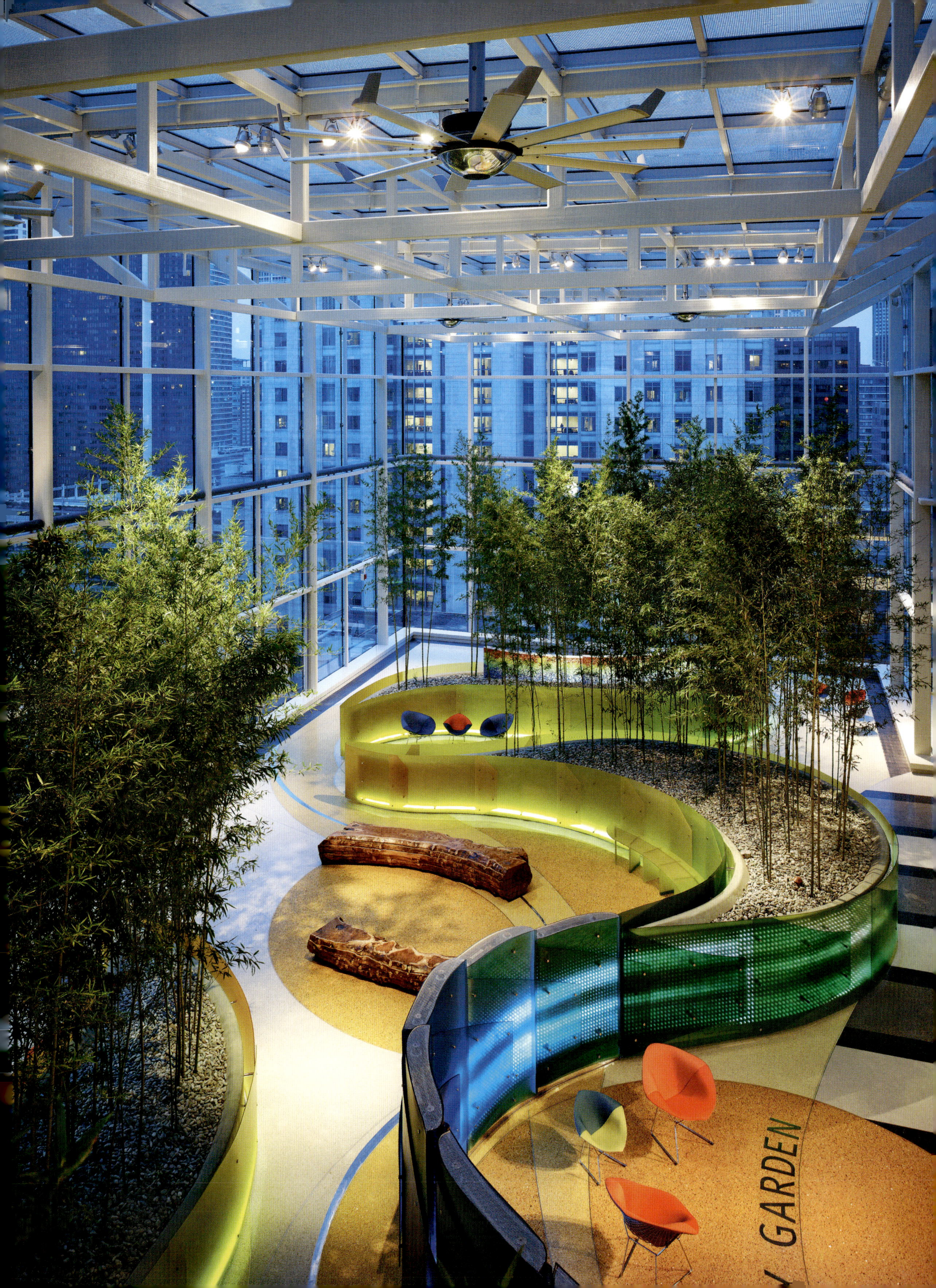
GARDEN

Healing Gardens

"Everybody needs beauty as well as bread, places to play in and pray in, where nature may heal and give strength to body and soul."
—John Muir

The renaissance of the garden as an integral part of the hospital environment is an extension of the long-held appreciation that humankind has for nature and its healing qualities. Studies have shown that exposure to nature, particularly in healthcare settings, has a restorative effect on patients, families, and staff.

The world of a hospital can be disorienting and confining, especially for children, with the focus on illness, protocols, and equipment. A garden can provide an important link to the outside world and reduce the sense of isolation. Whether viewed from the patient's room, or experienced as a place to retreat, socialize, or play, a garden space within the hospital setting has proven to reduce stress and promote healing.

From a beautifully landscaped suburban campus to an urban pocket garden, from blossoming terraces to an enclosed sky garden, from horticultural activity gardens to nature depicted in graphics, all can elicit pleasant memories and sensory experiences of time spent outdoors—providing stimulation and delight, a place for quiet contemplation, or an opportunity to regain optimism and composure.

In the following pages, you will see a range of gardens designed to enhance the human experience in the healthcare setting, inspired by and in support of all who are on their healing journey.

Sue Ann Barton, AIA
ZGF Architects LLP

◀ Ann & Robert H. Lurie Children's Hospital of Chicago, IL
Photo: Hedrich Blessing Photography, Nick Merrick

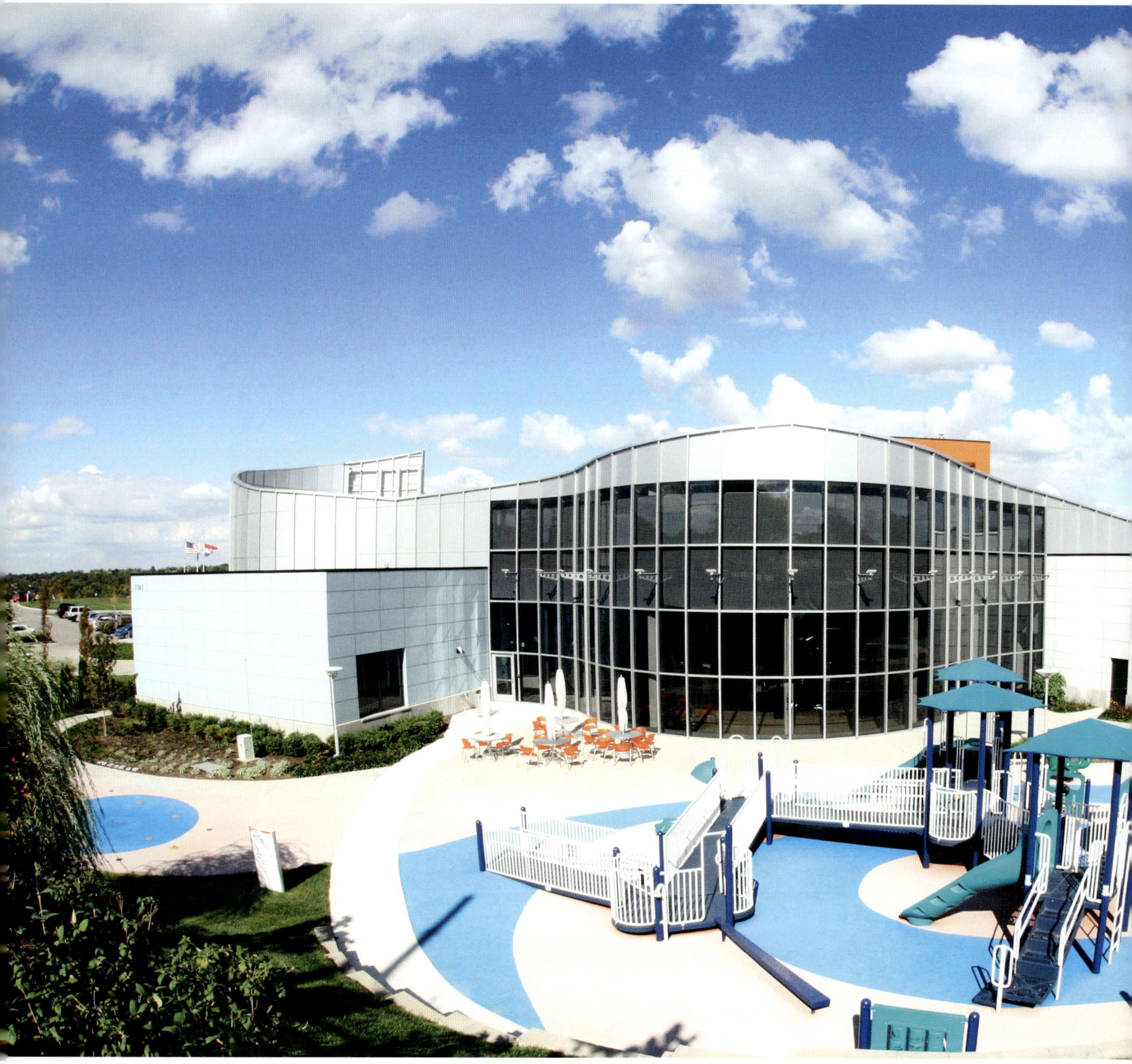

▲ Ranken Jordan - A Pediatric Specialty Hospital, Maryland Heights, MO
Photo: Brian Spurgeon

Following pages: Levine Children's Hospital, Charlotte, NC
Photos: Brad Feinknopf

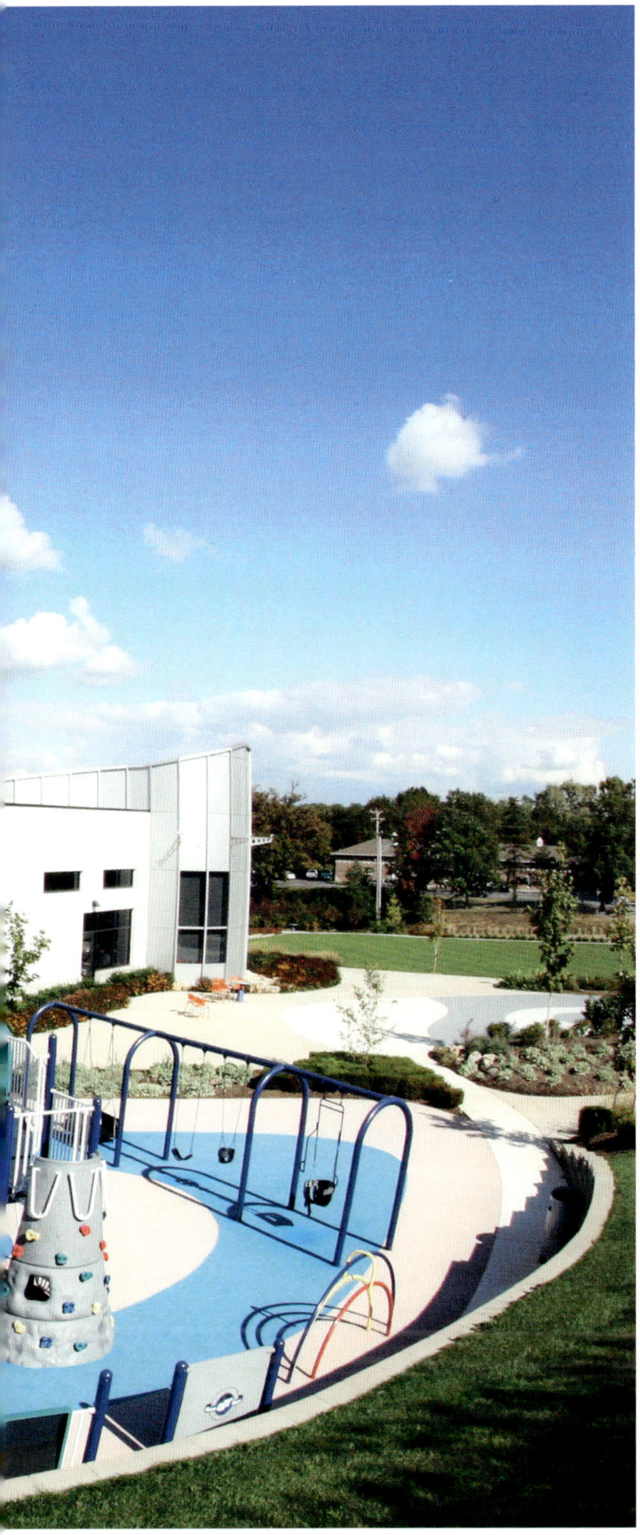

▼ Meyer Children's Hospital, Florence, Italy
Photo: Stantec © Alessandro Ciampi and Pietro Savorelli

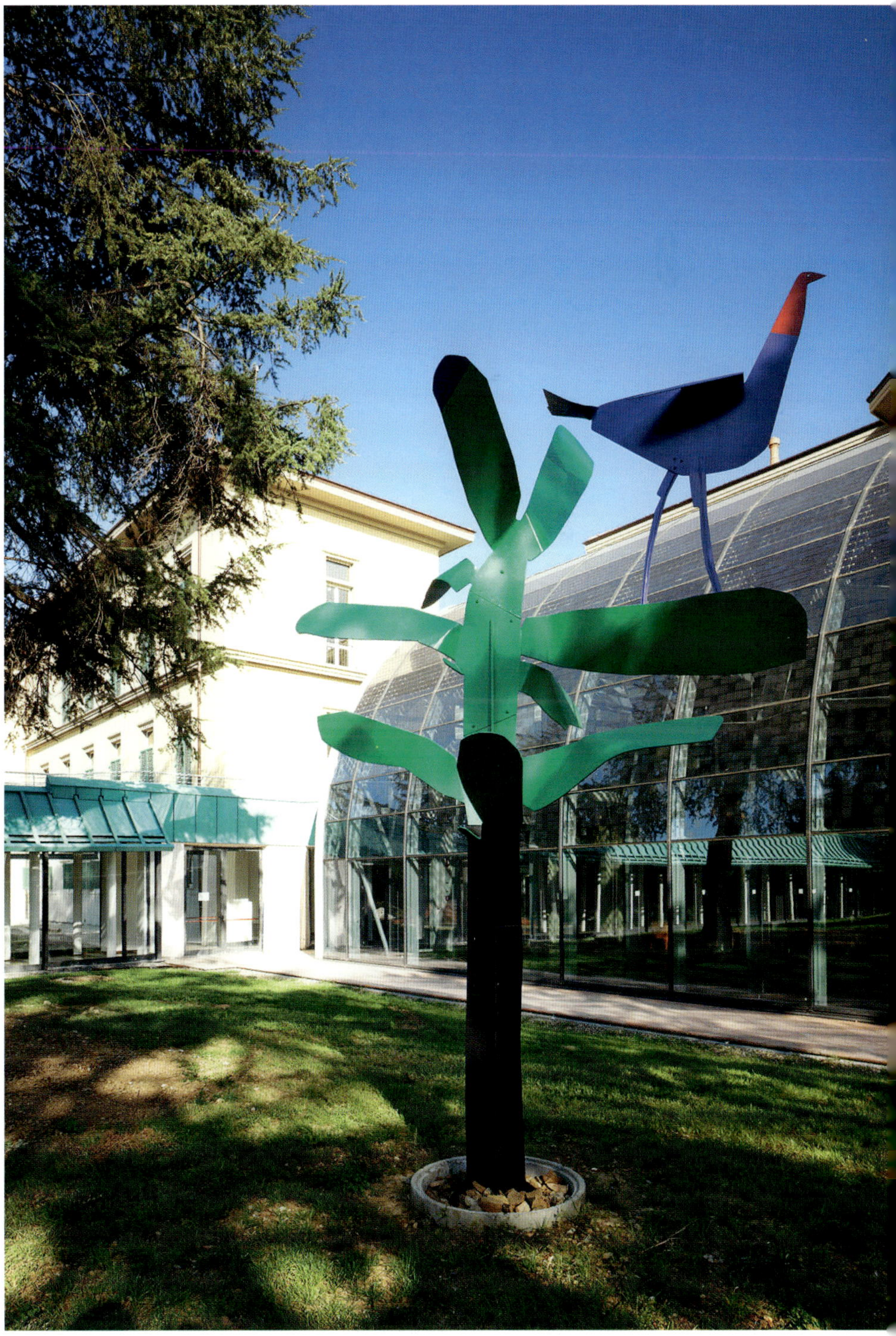

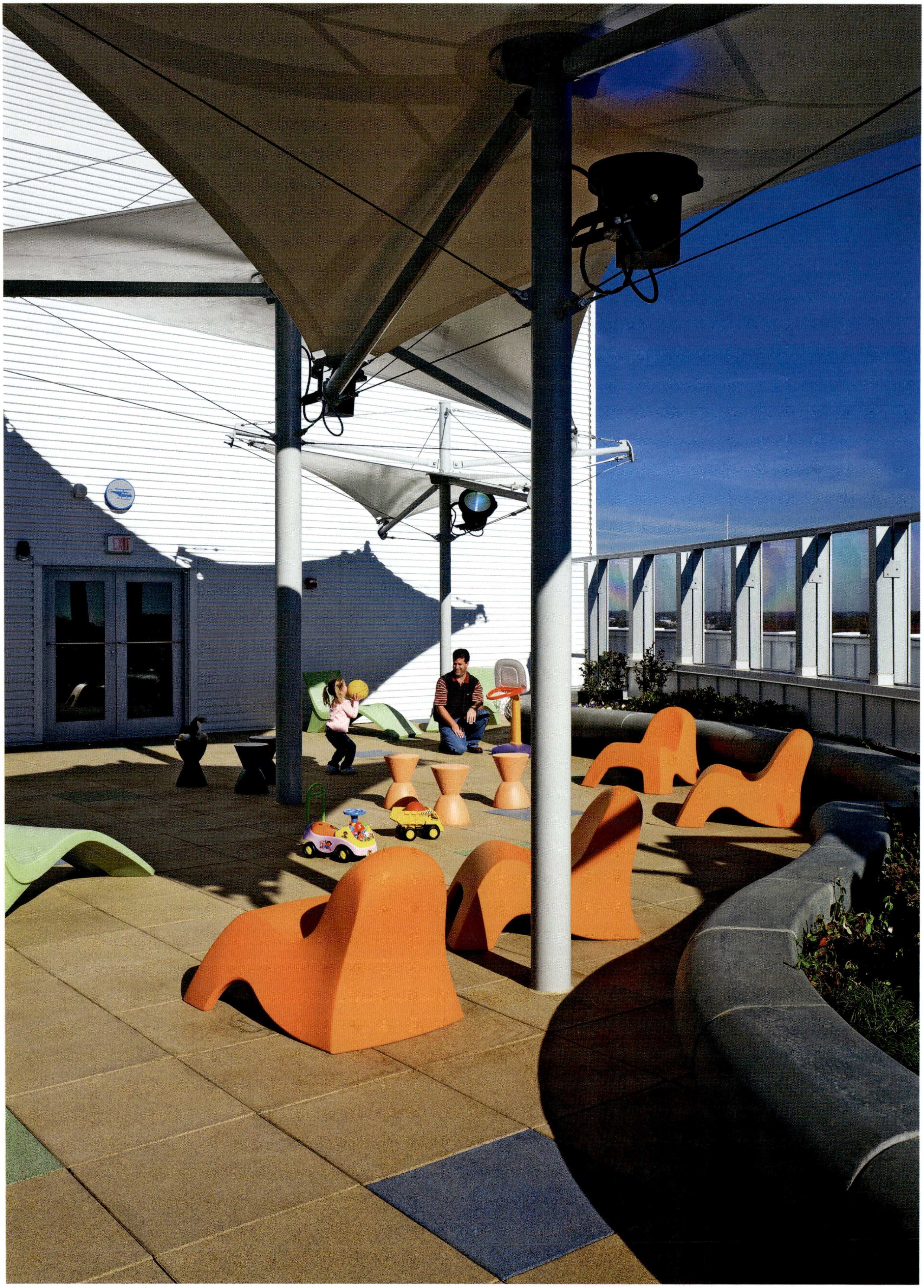
EXIT

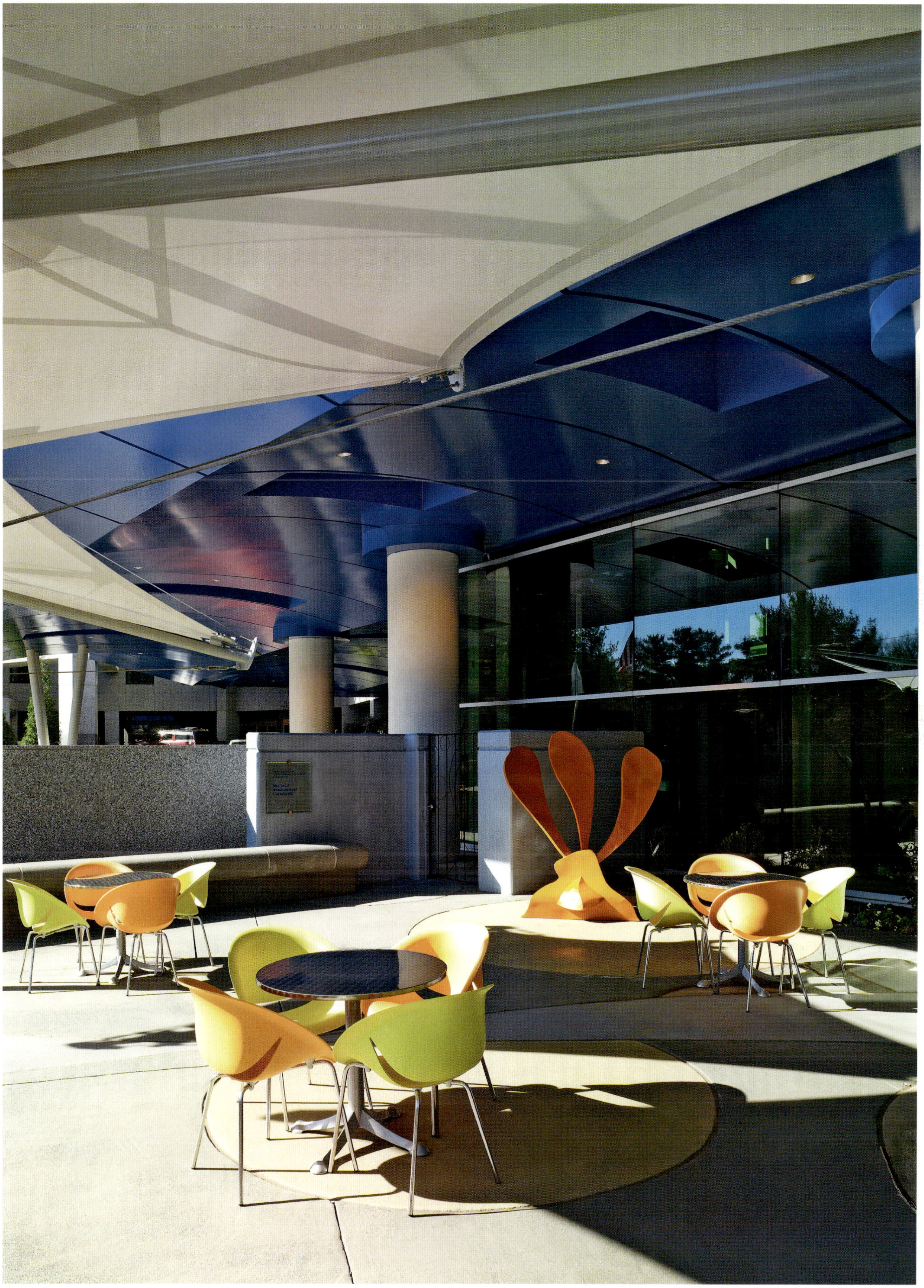

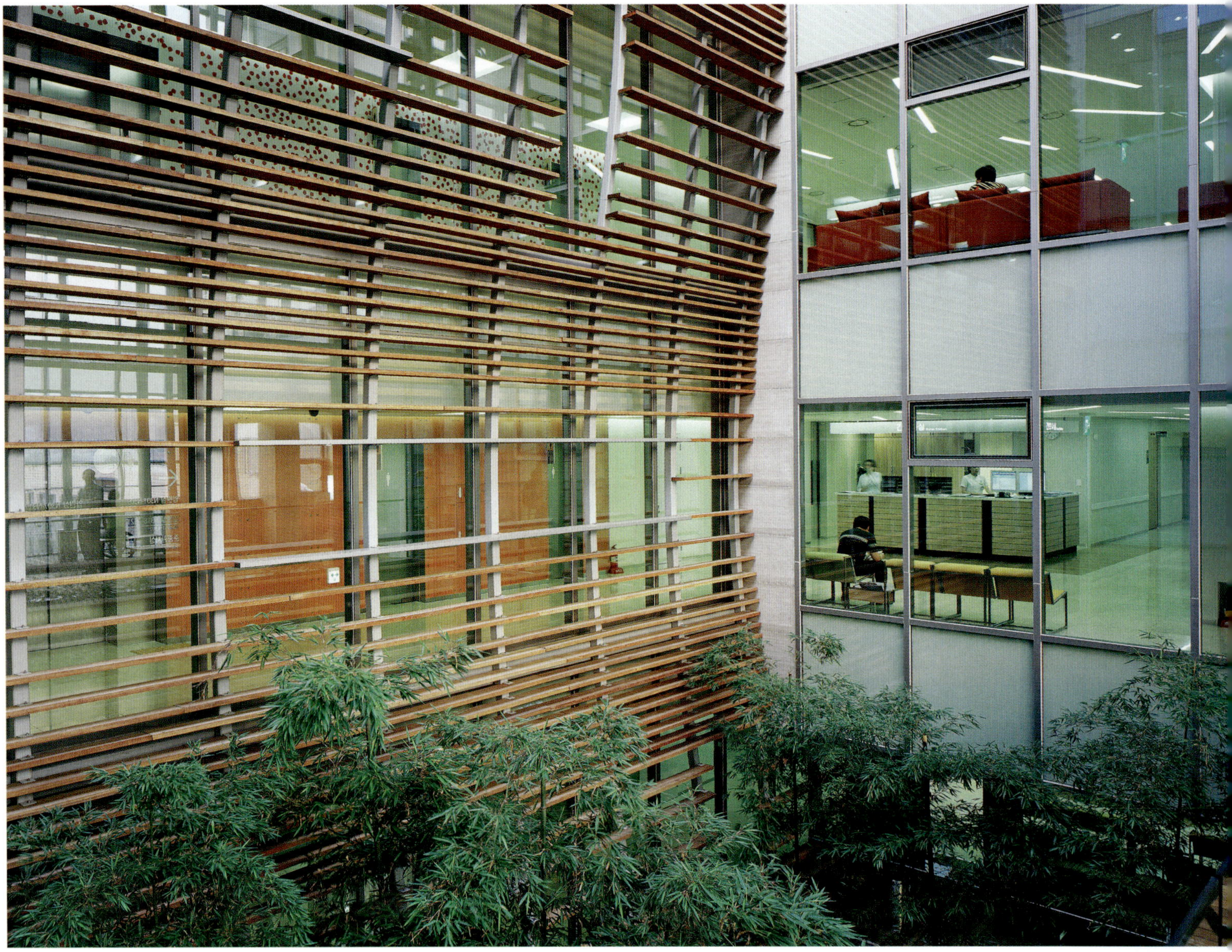

▲ Cha Women and Children's Hospital, Seongnam, South Korea
Photo: Jong O Kim

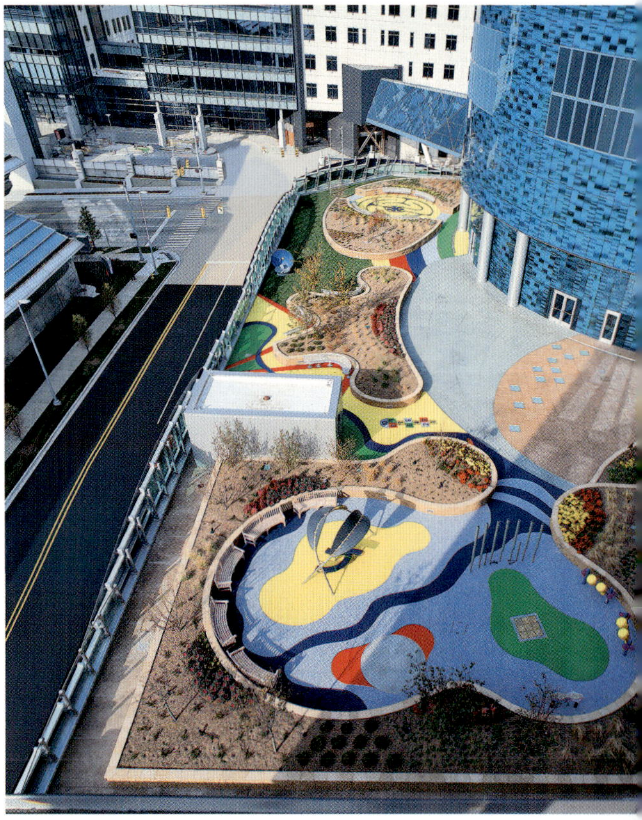

Helen DeVos Children's Hospital, Grand Rapids, MI ▶
Photo: Scott Wilson

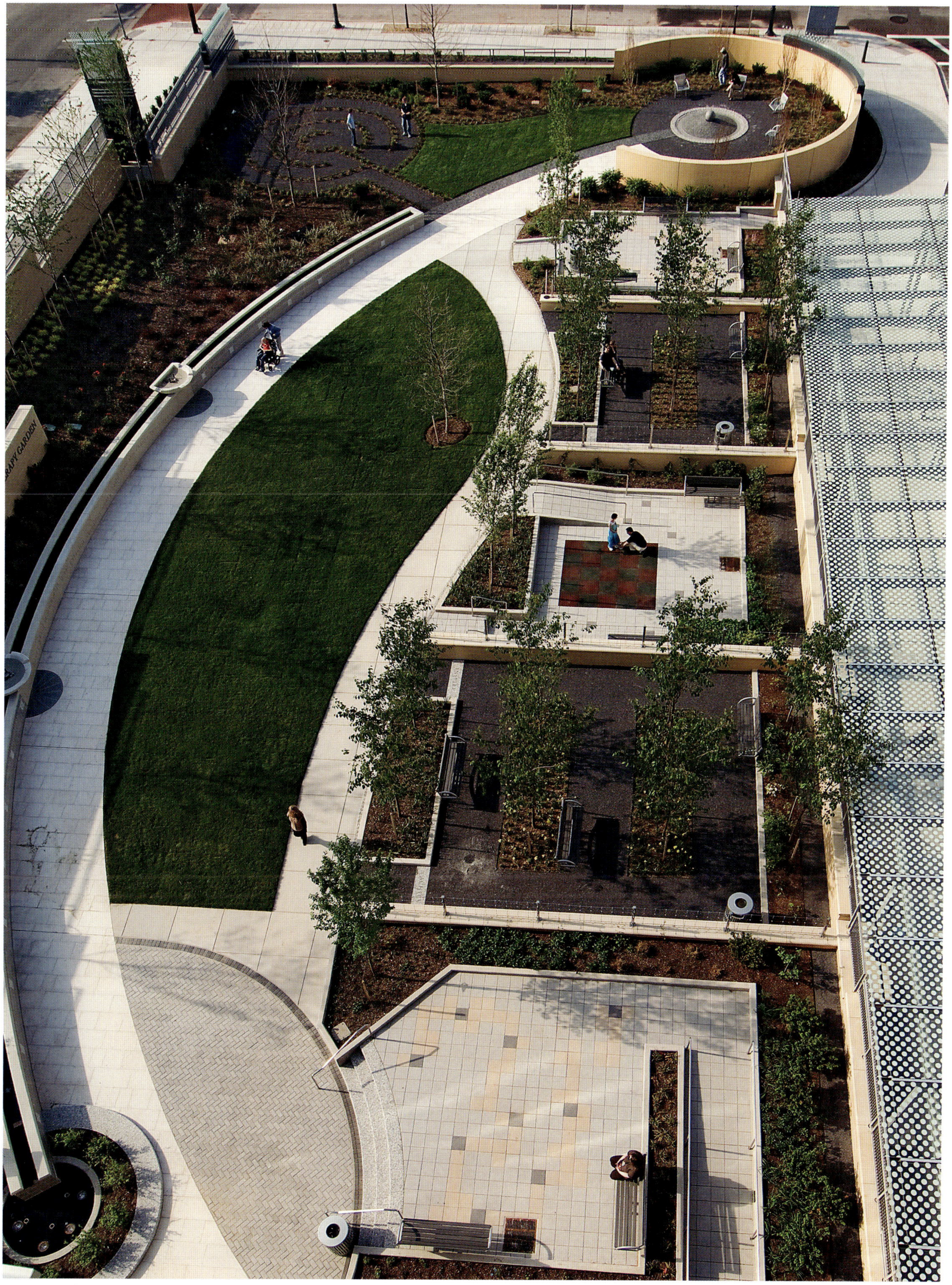

▲ Kennedy Krieger Institute, Kennedy Krieger Children's Hospital, Baltimore, MD
Photo: Jim Roof Creative

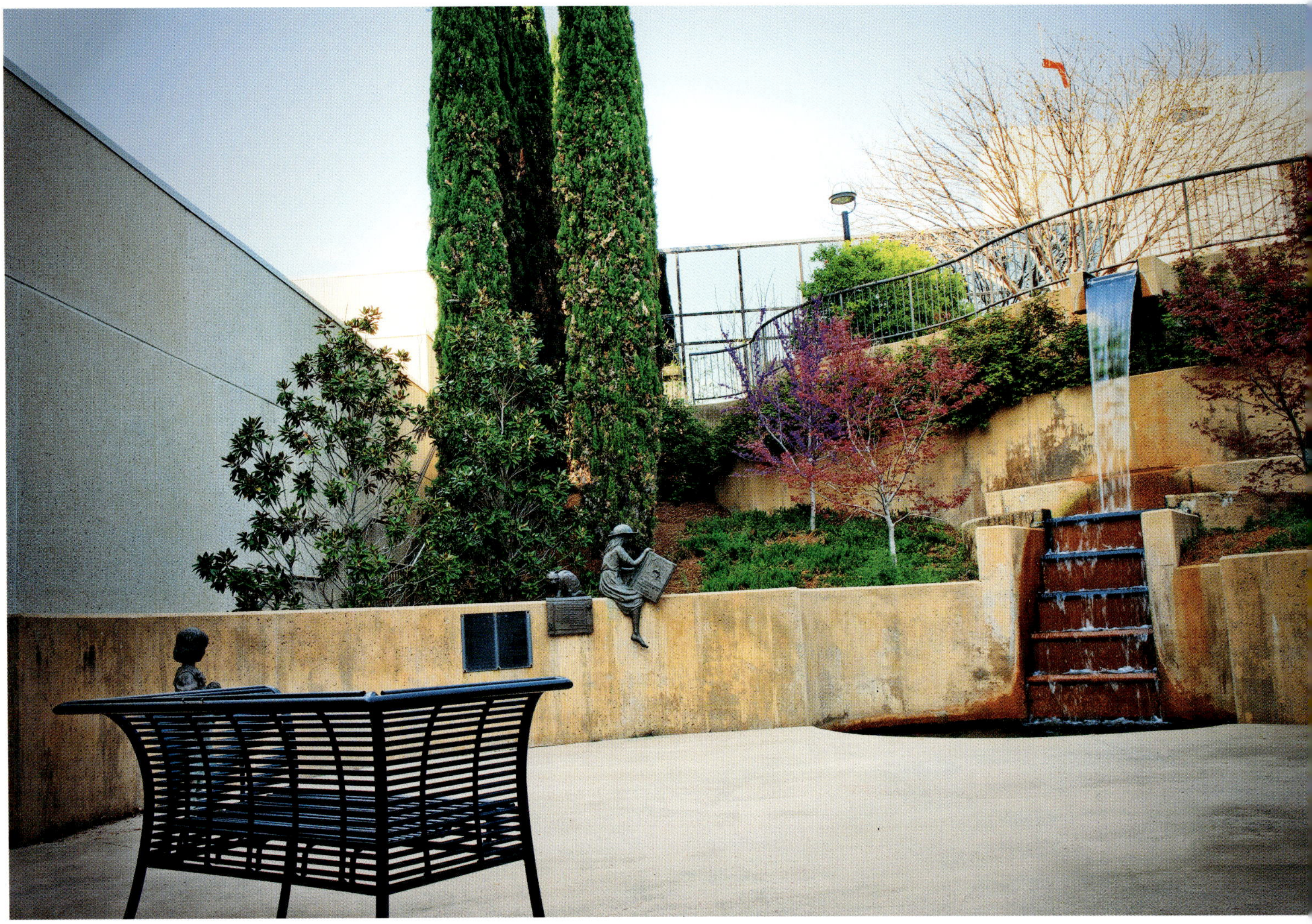

▲ Palmetto Health Children's Hospital, Columbia, SC

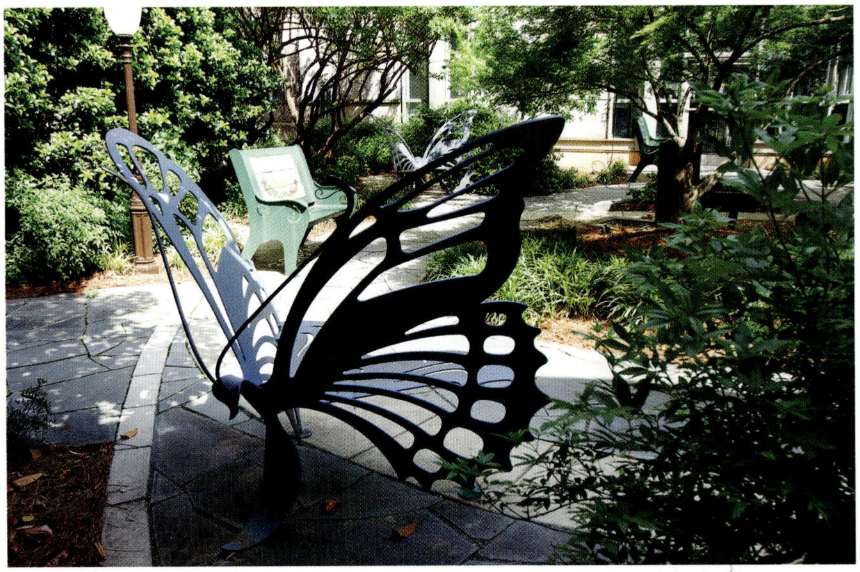

▲ UNC North Carolina Children's Hospital, Chapel Hill, NC
Photo: Brian Strickland

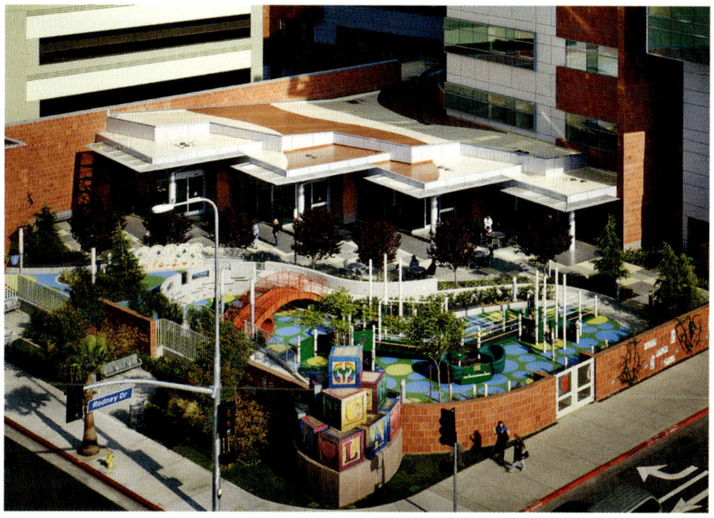

▲ Children's Hospital Los Angeles, CA
Photo: Hedrich Blessing Photography, Nick Merrick

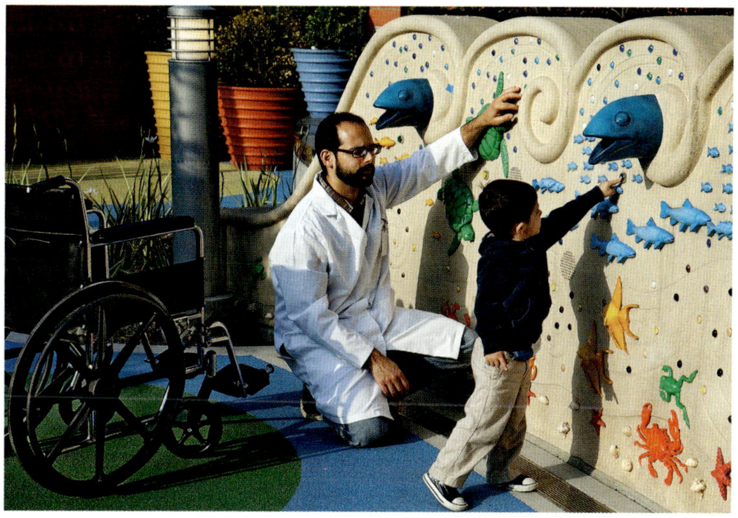

▲ Children's Hospital Los Angeles, CA
▼ ***Photos: Eckert & Eckert***

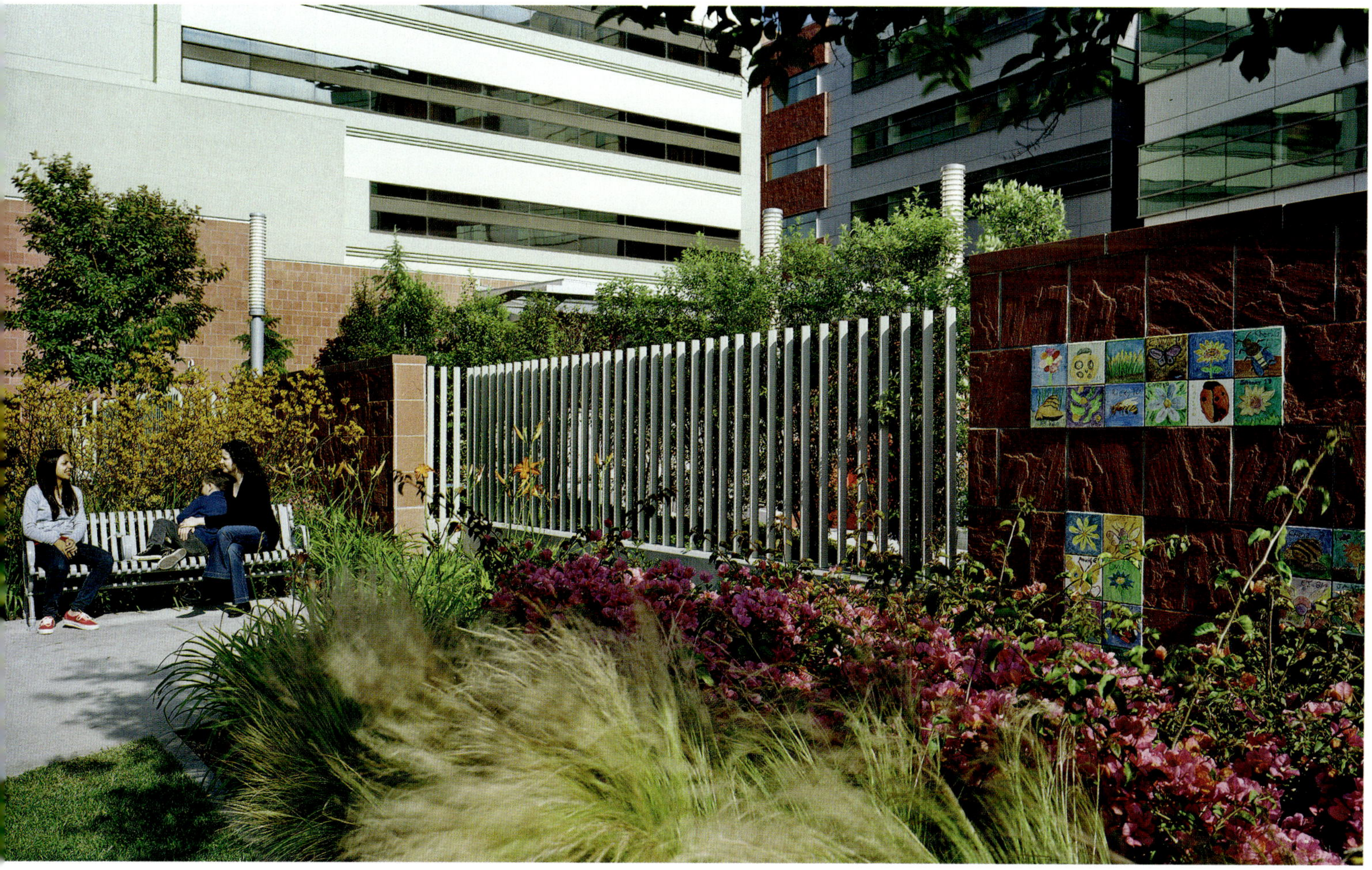

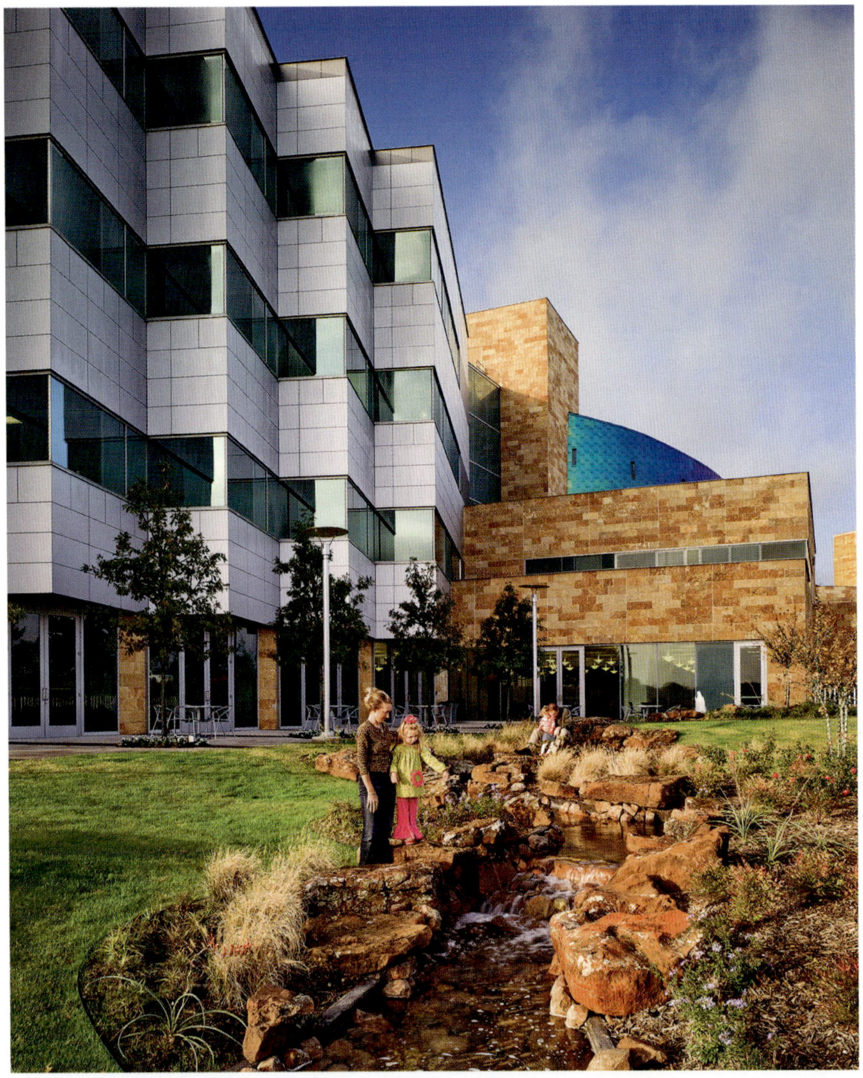

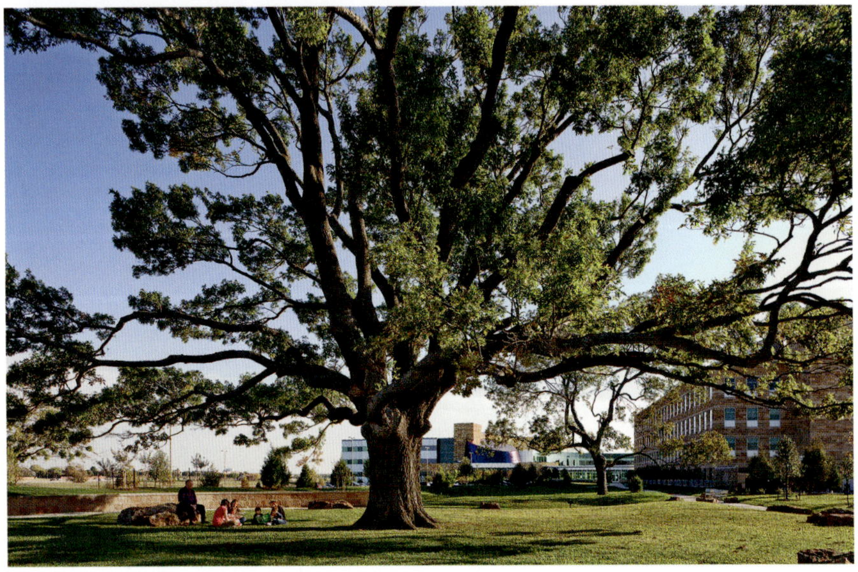

▲ Children's Medical Center at Legacy, Plano, TX
Photos: Robert Canfield

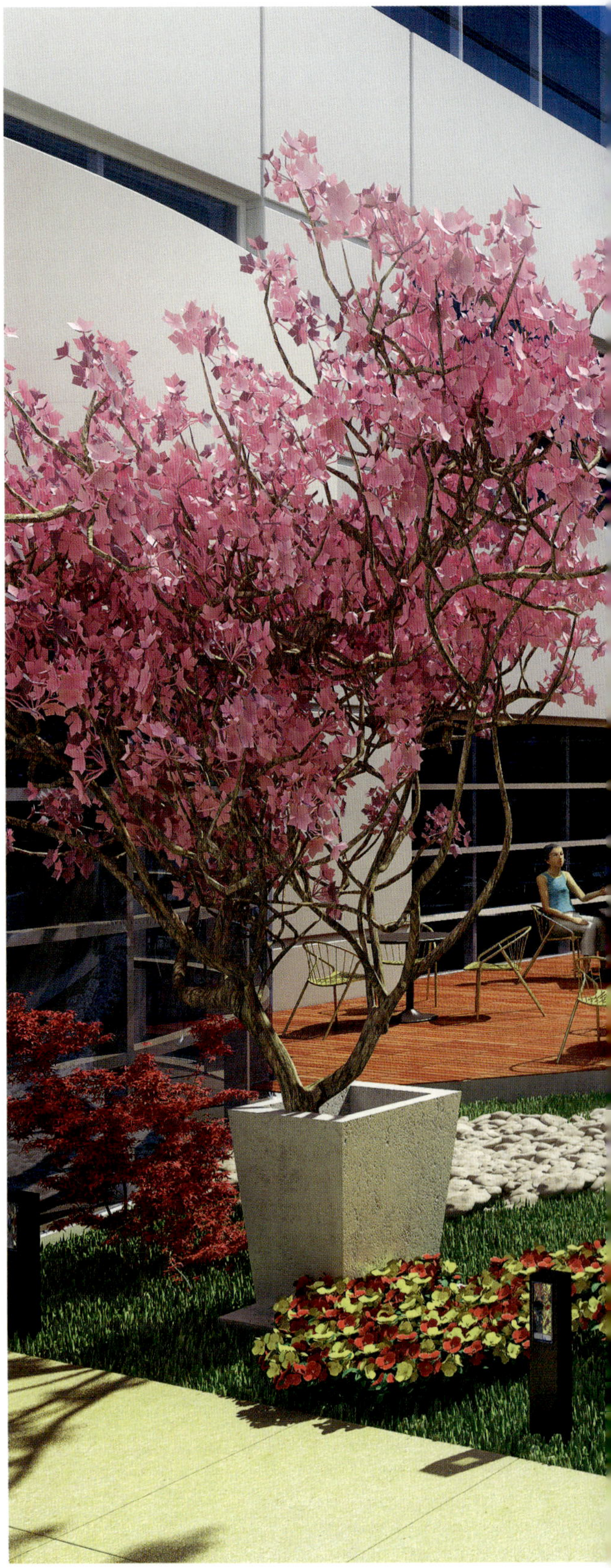

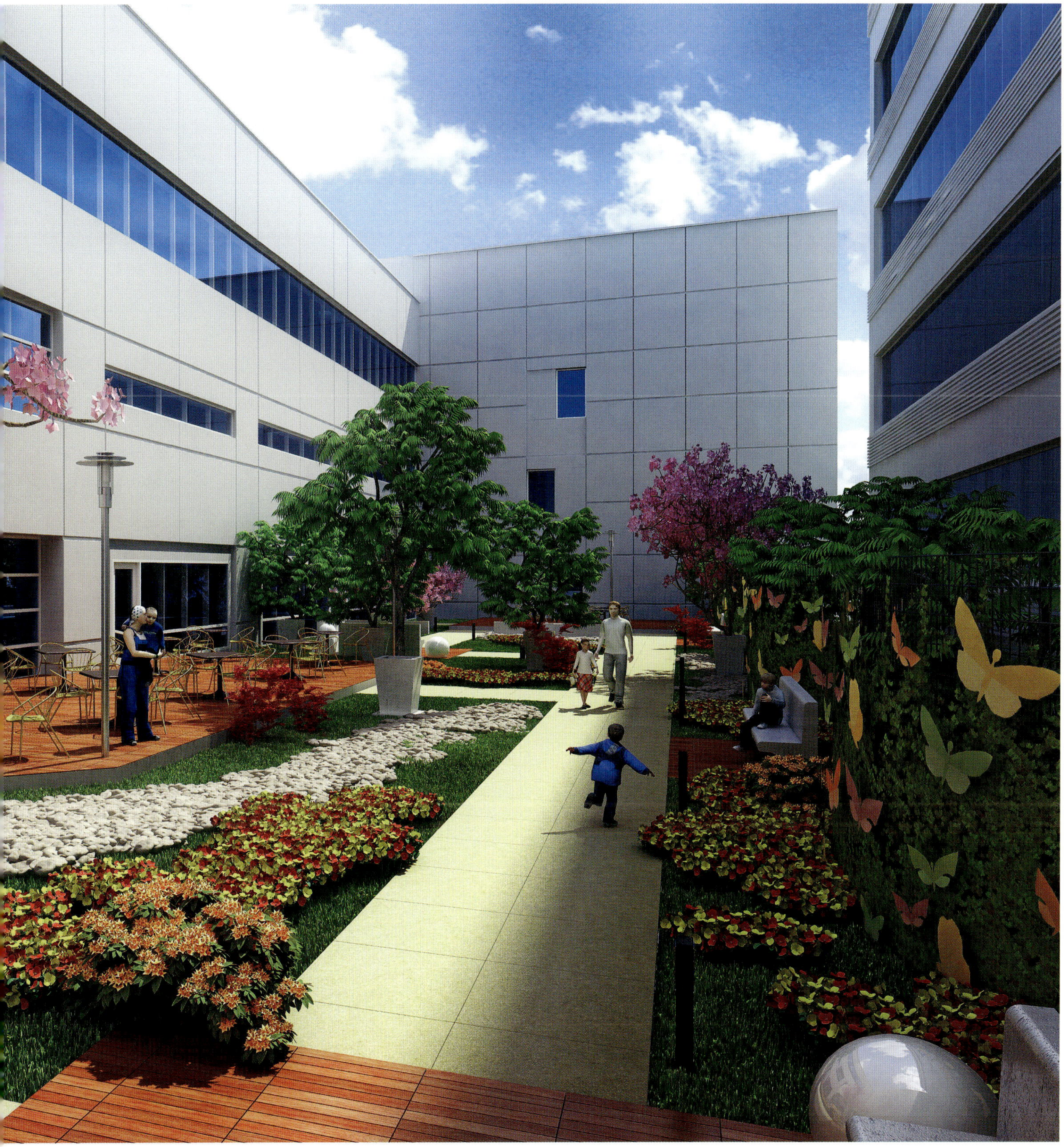

▲ CHOC Children's Hospital, Orange, CA
Photo: Provided by FKP Architects

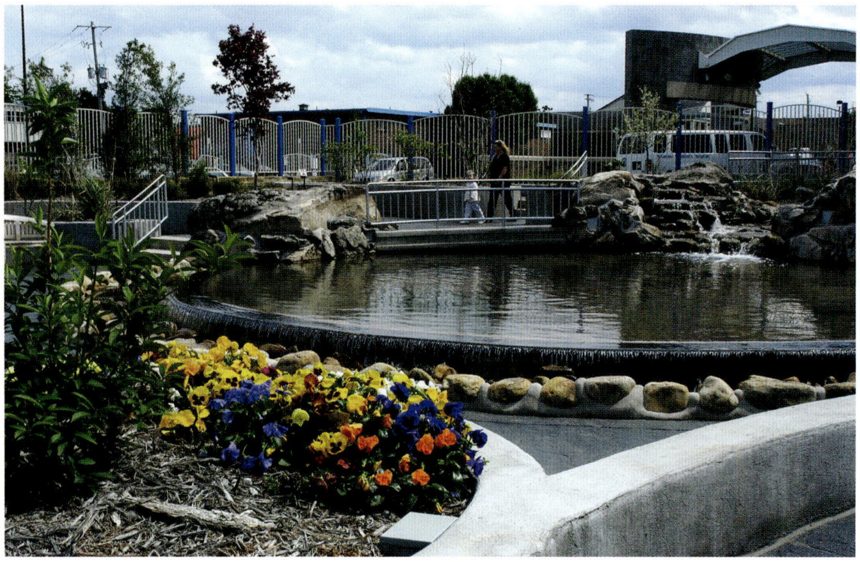

▲ Arkansas Children's Hospital, Little Rock, AR
Photo: Kelley Cooper

▼ Children's Medical Center, Dallas, TX
Photo: Scott Williams

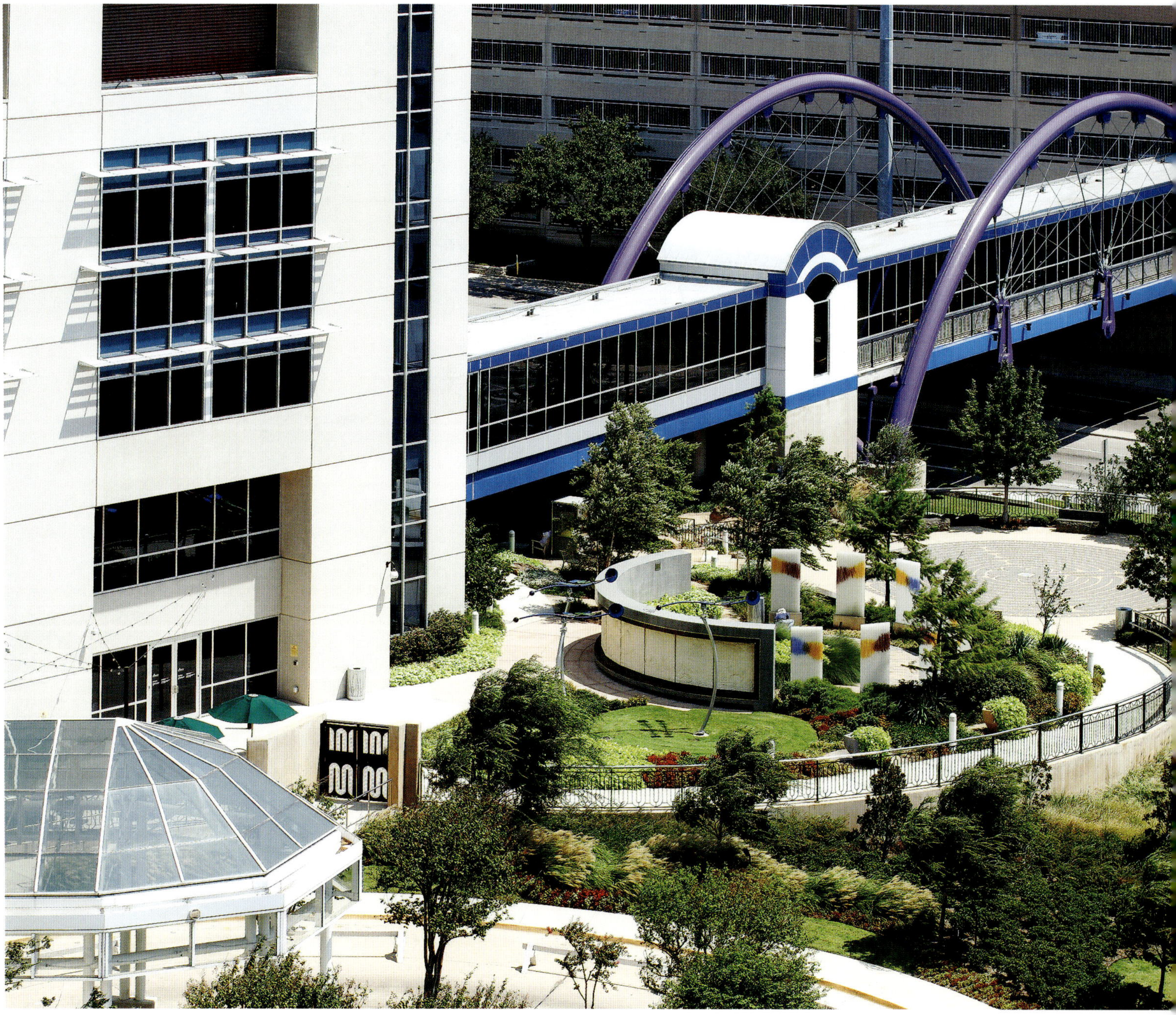

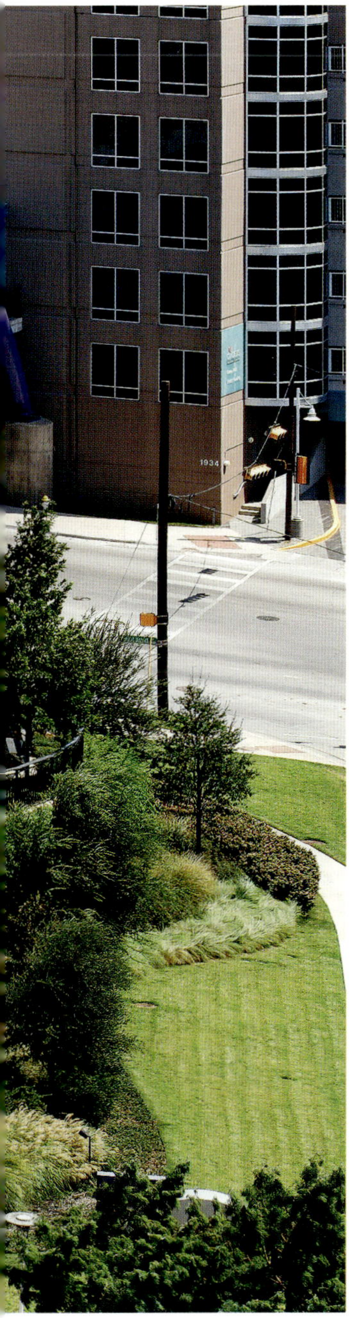

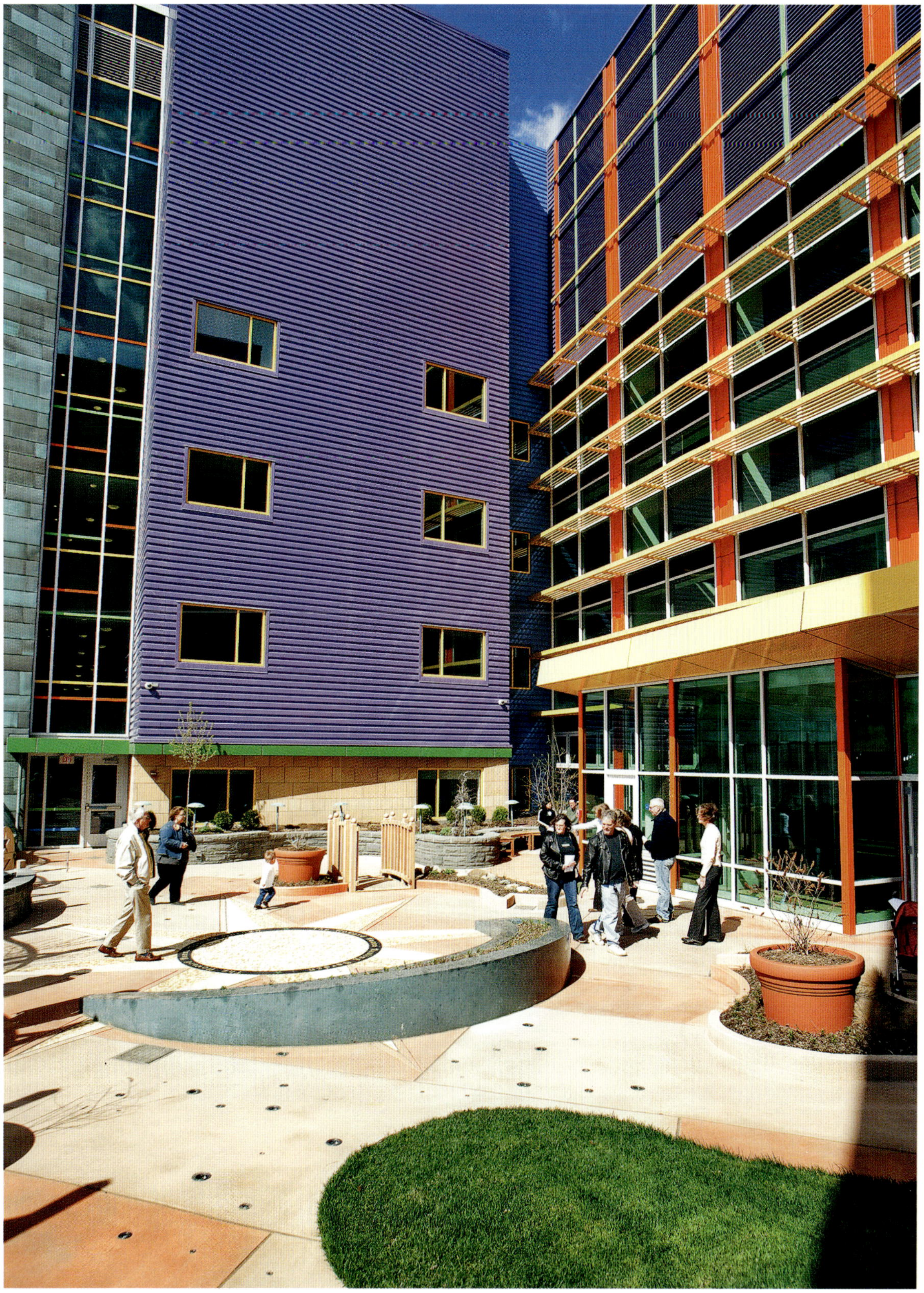

▲ Children's Hospital of Pittsburgh, PA

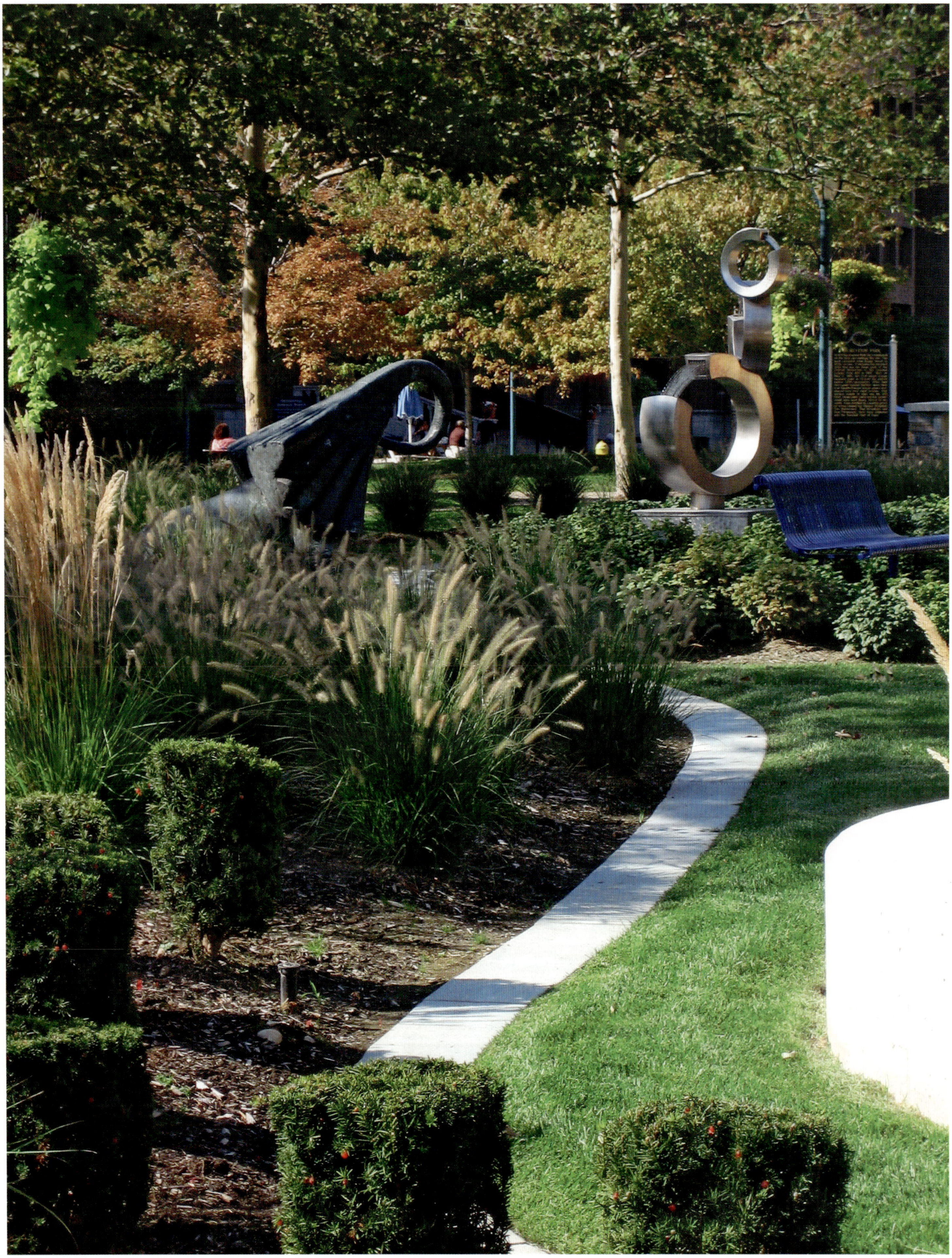

▲ Children's Hospital of Michigan, Detroit, MI

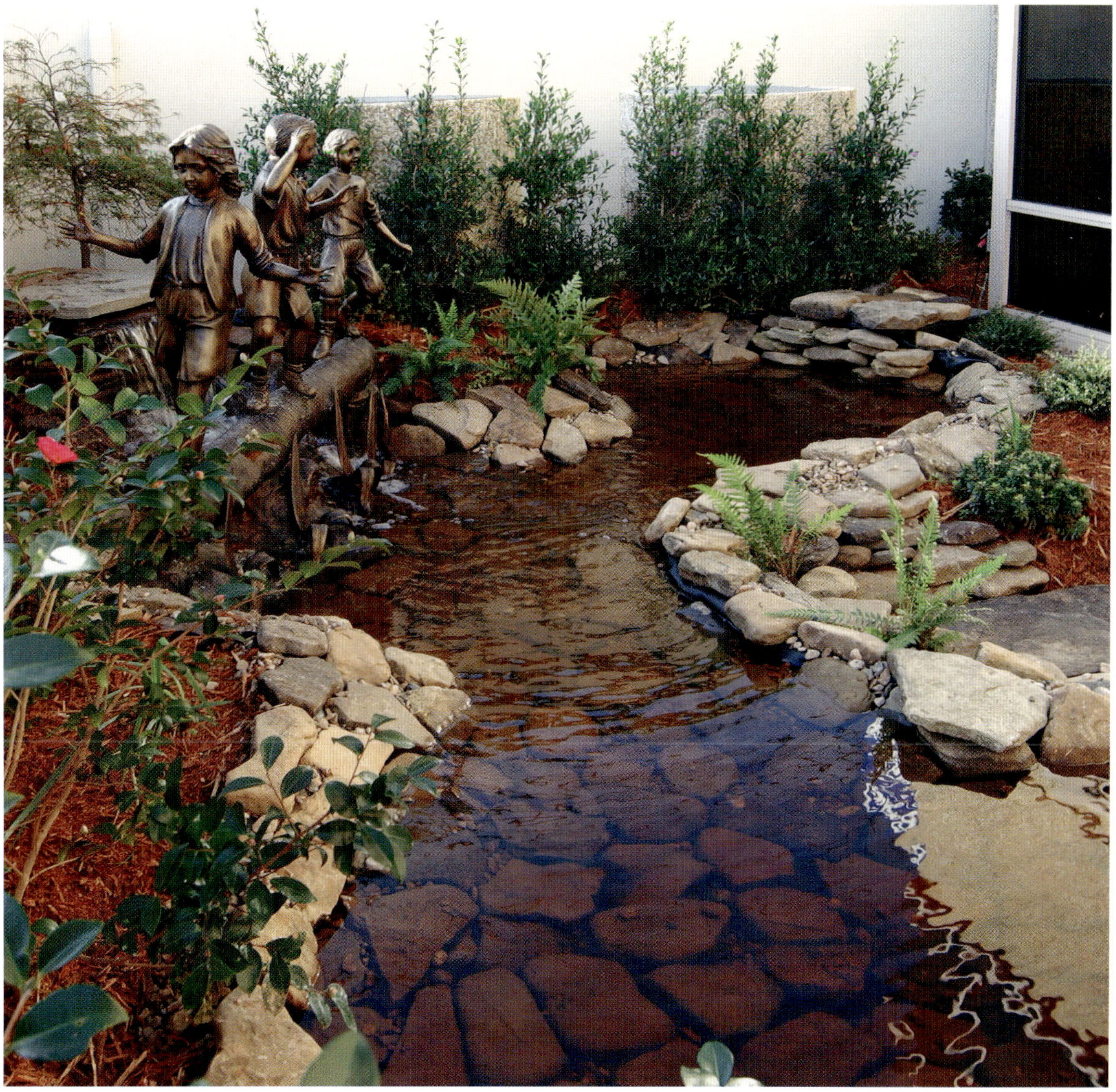

▲ Arkansas Children's Hospital, Little Rock, AR
Photo: Kelley Cooper

▼ Helen DeVos Children's Hospital, Grand Rapids, MI
Photo: Scott Wilson

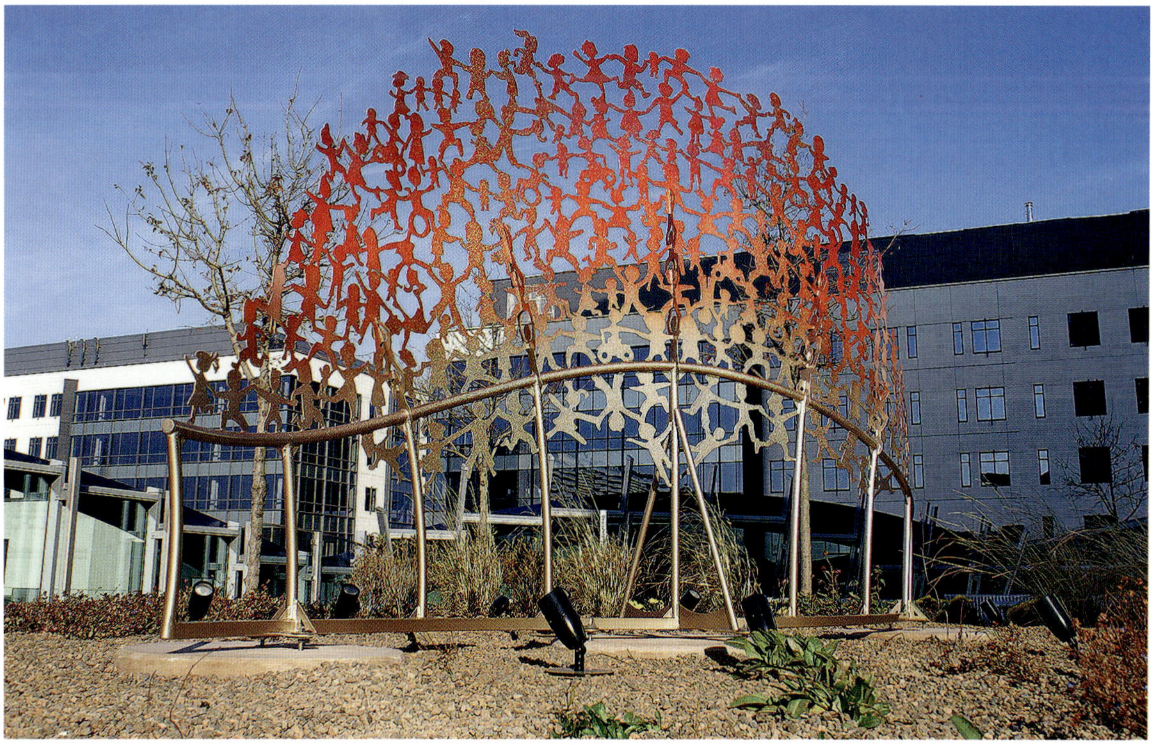

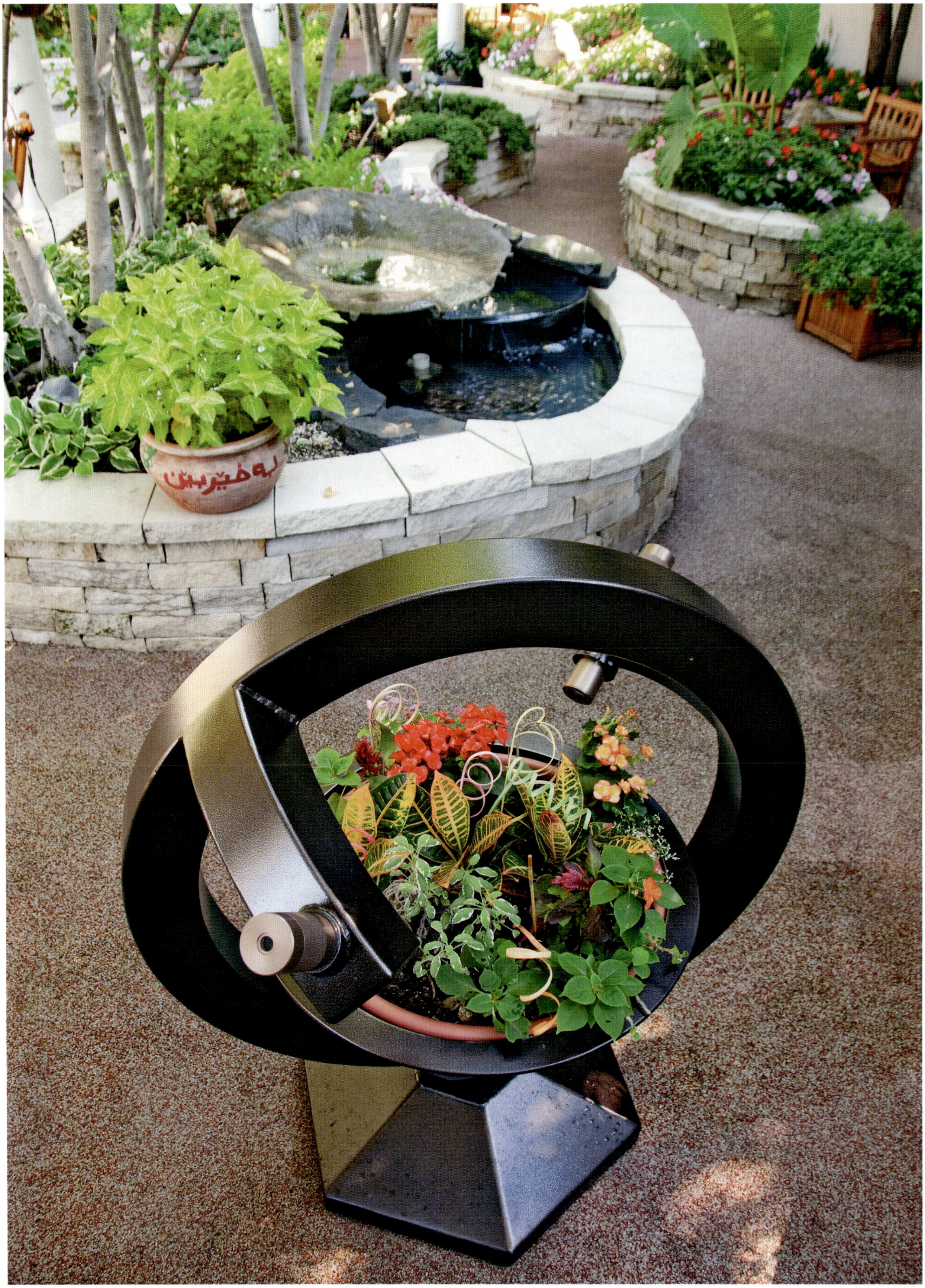

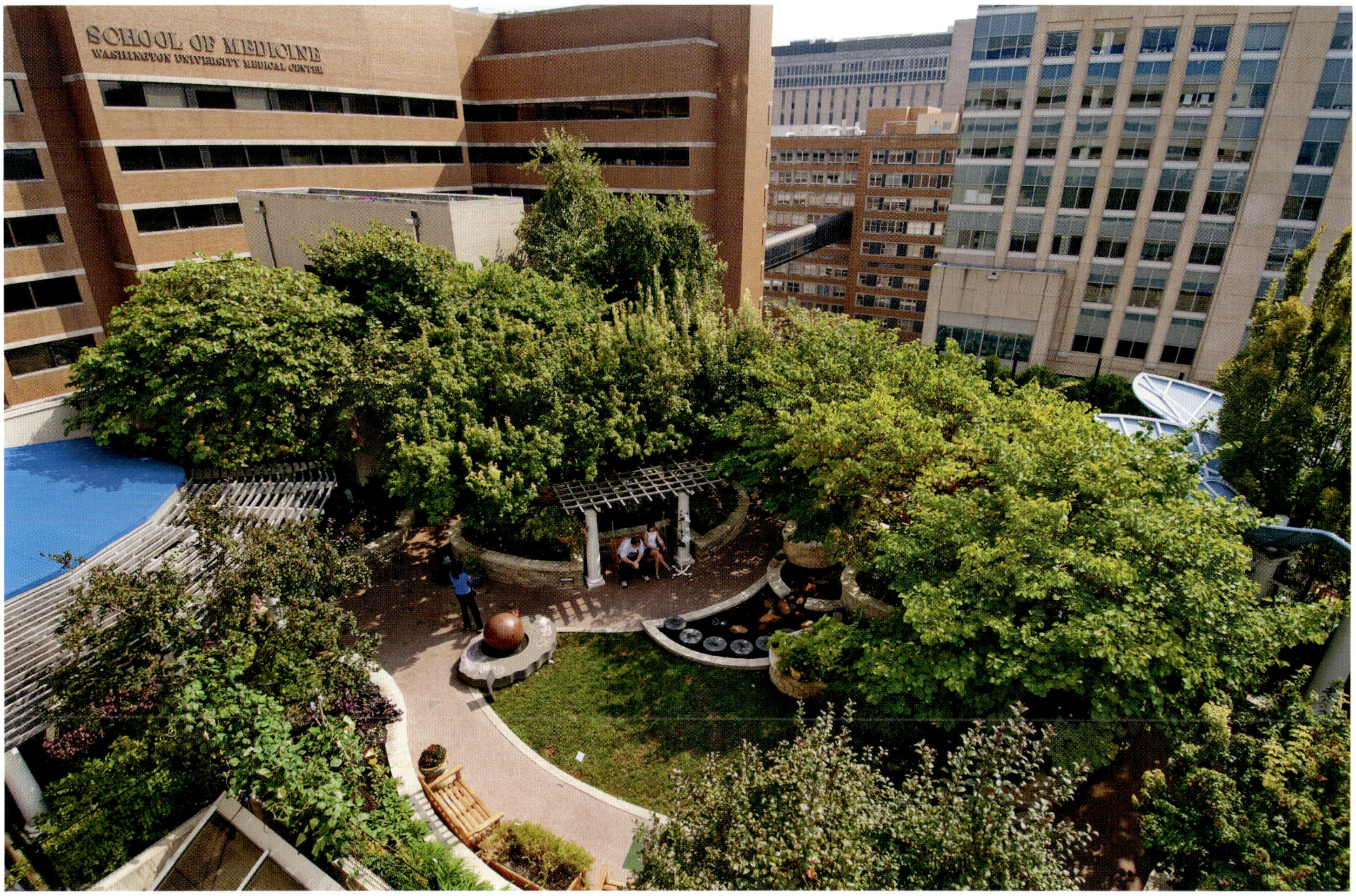

▲ St. Louis Children's Hospital, MO
◀ ***Photos: Bob Boston, Washington University***

▼ St. Louis Children's Hospital, MO
Photos: Bob Boston, Washington University

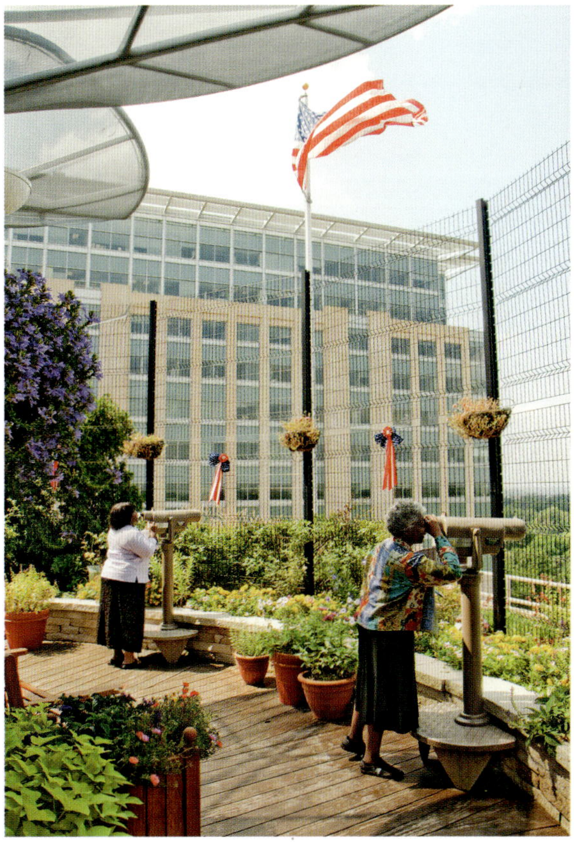

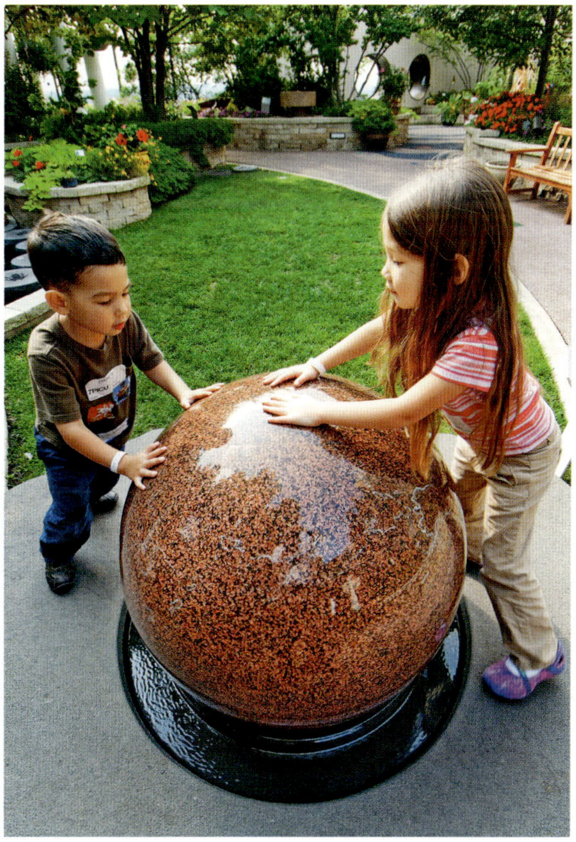

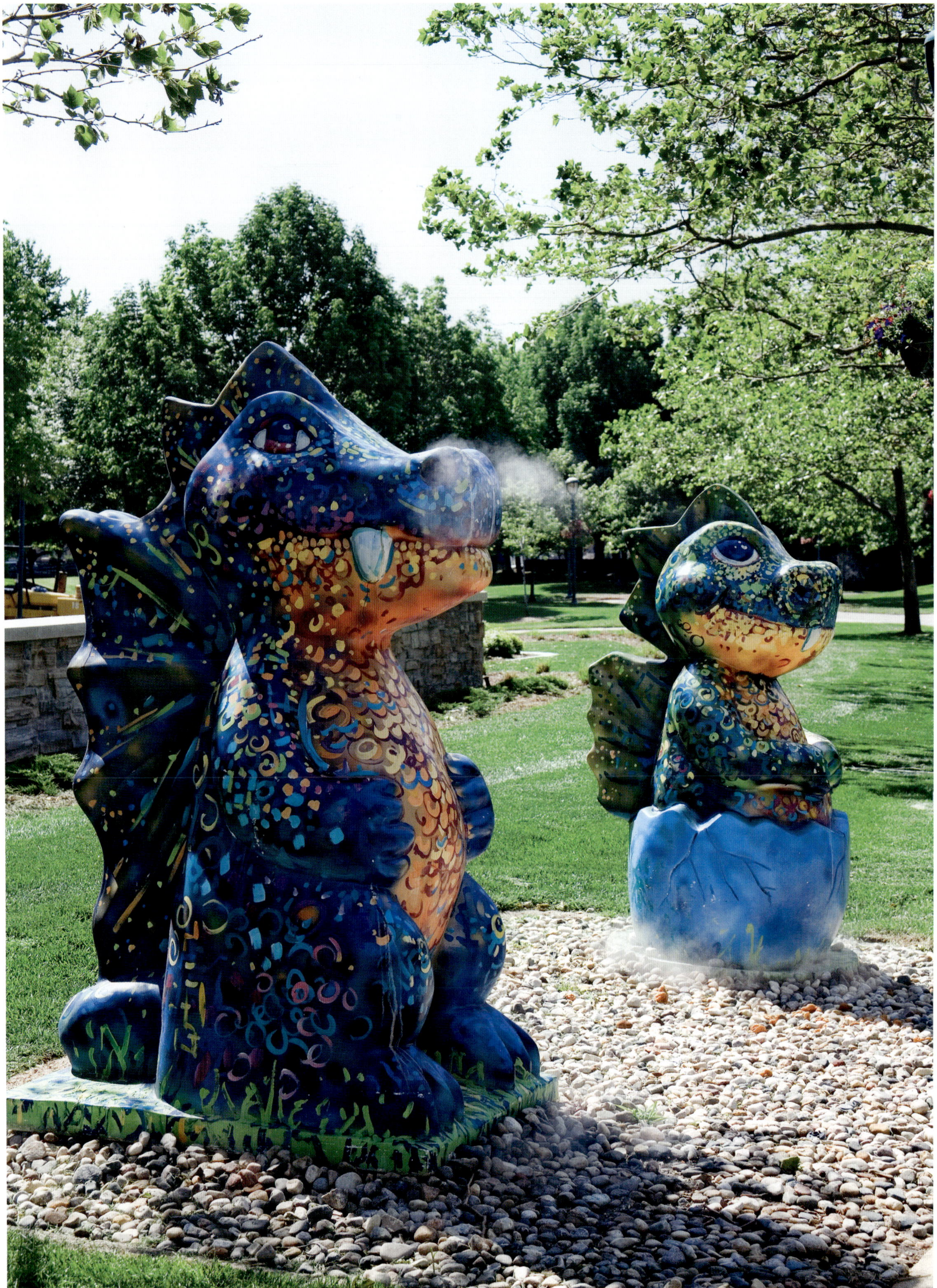

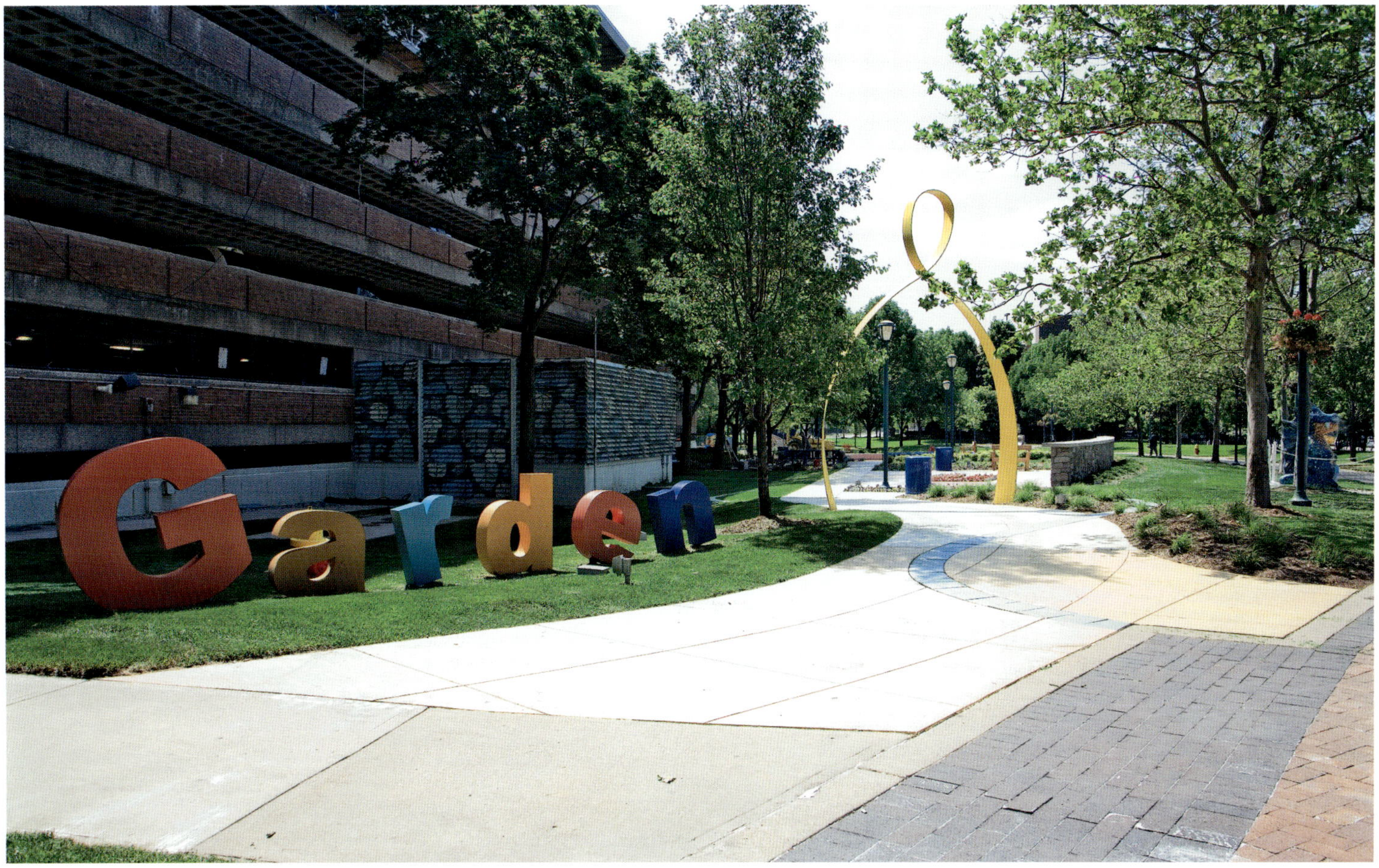

▲ Children's Hospital of Michigan, Detroit, MI
◀

▼ UNC North Carolina Children's Hospital, Chapel Hill, NC
Photo: Brian Strickland

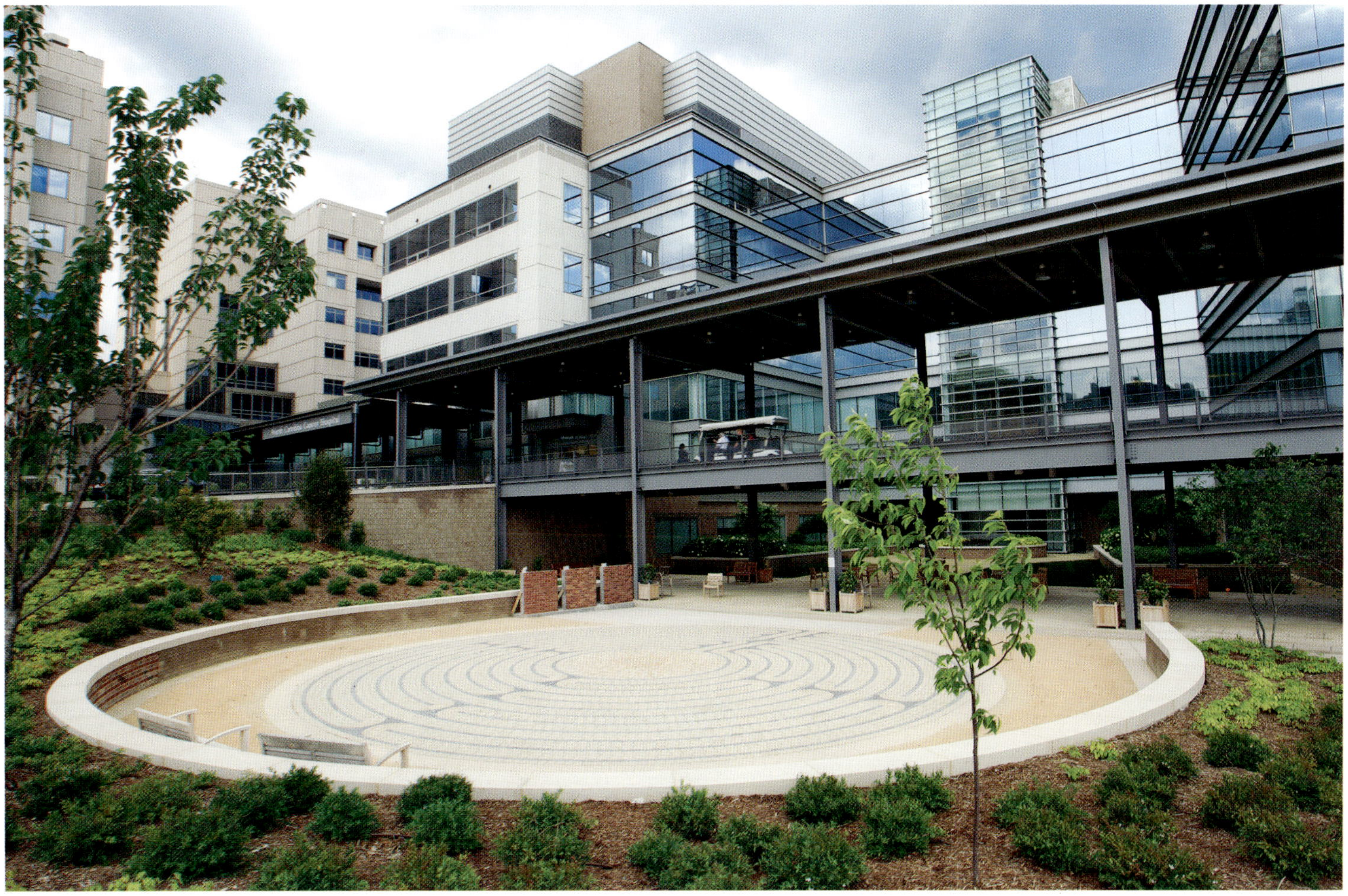

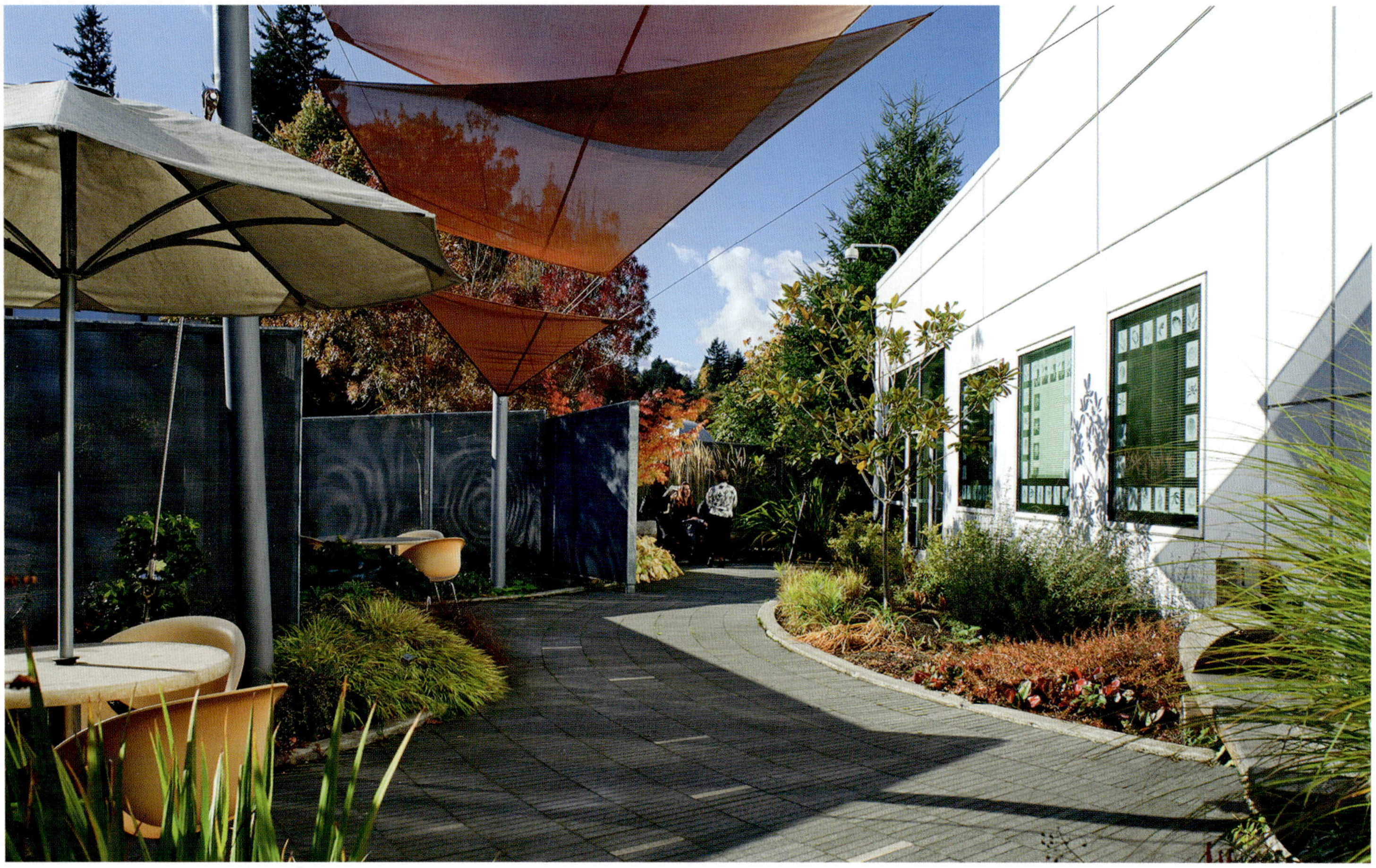

▲ Kenneth Ford Cancer Center, Doernbecher Children's Hospital, Portland, OR
▼ ***Photos: Eckert & Eckert***

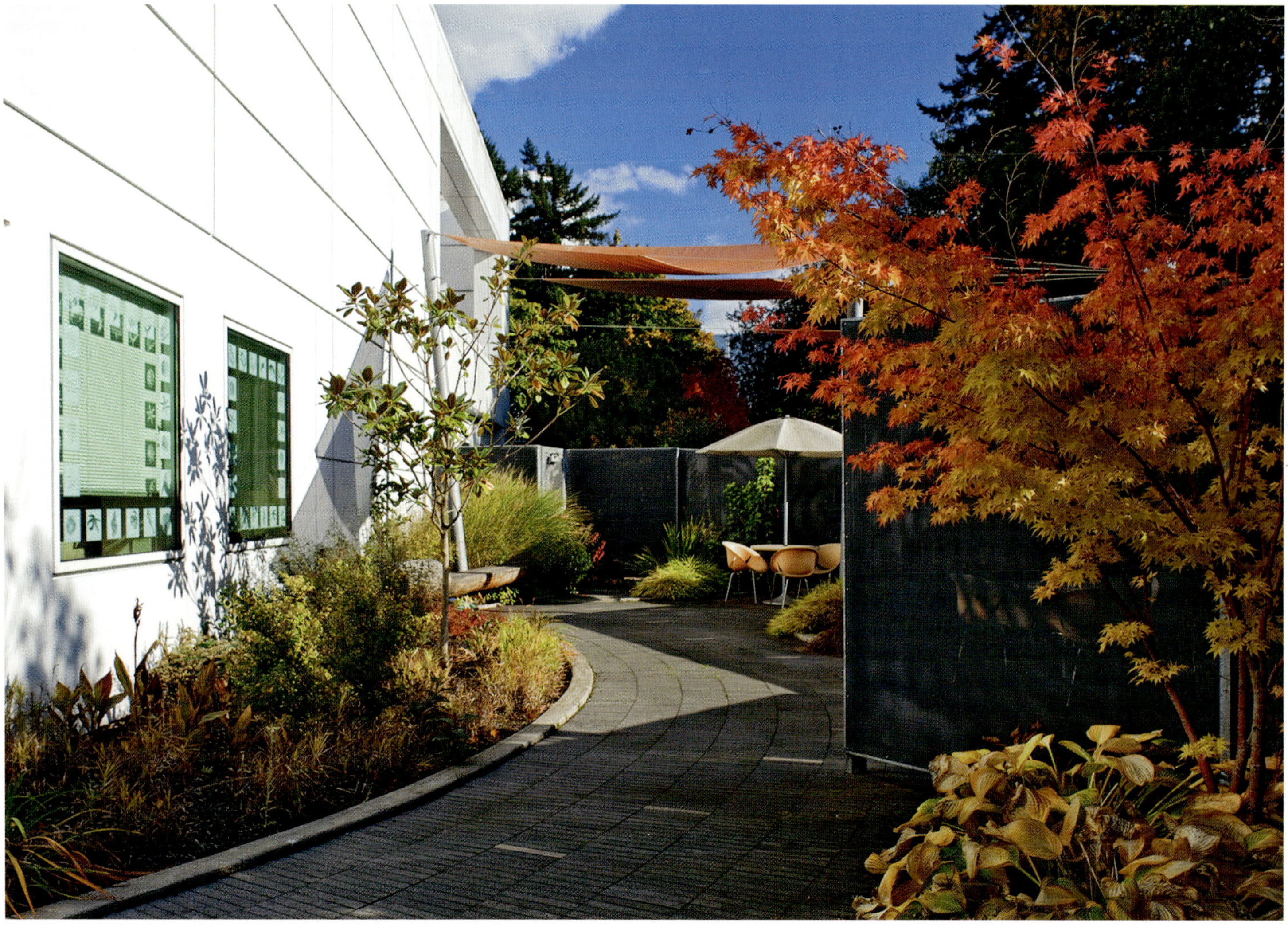

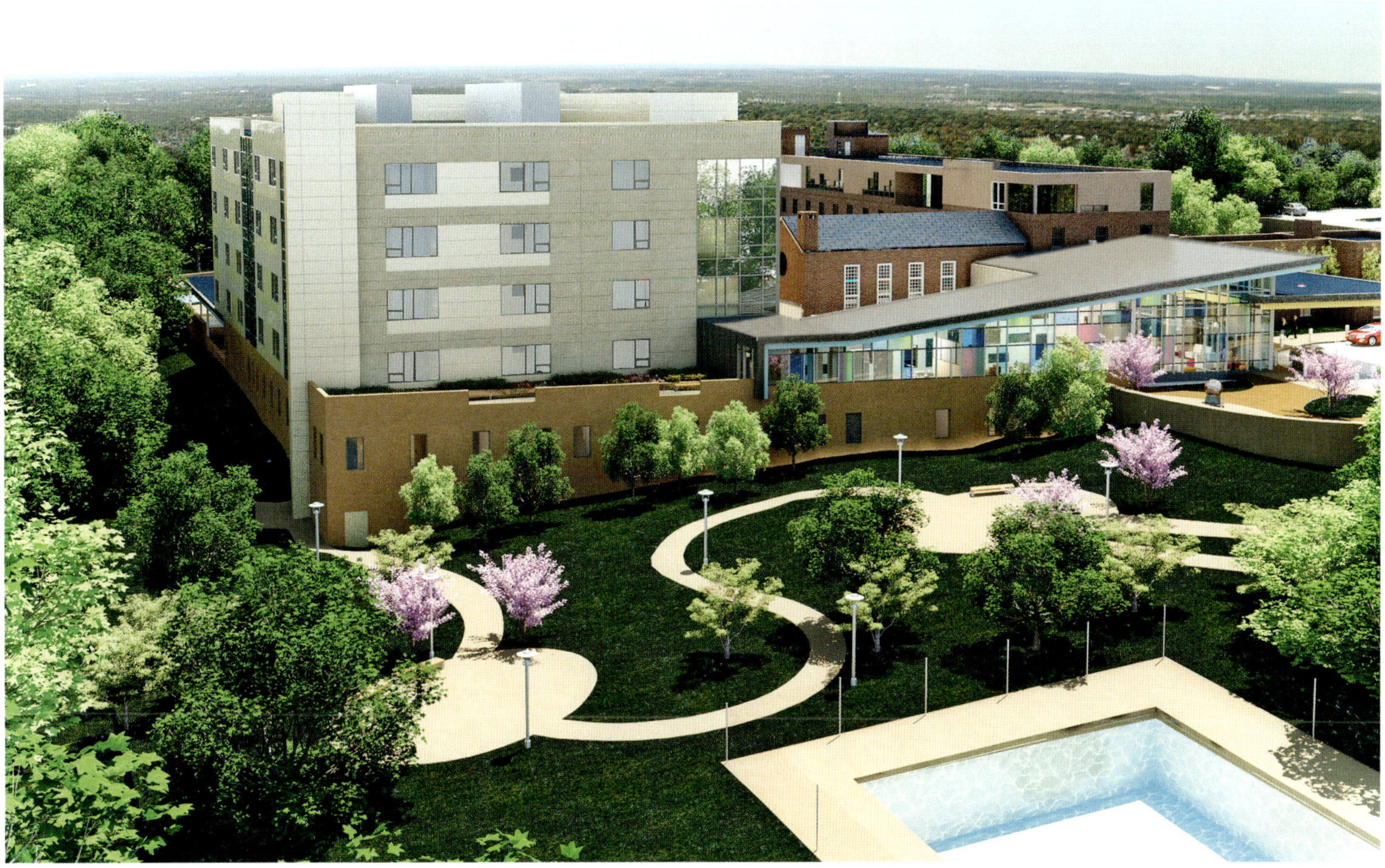

▲ St. Mary's Hospital for Children, Bayside, NY
▼ ***Photos: Stantec ©***

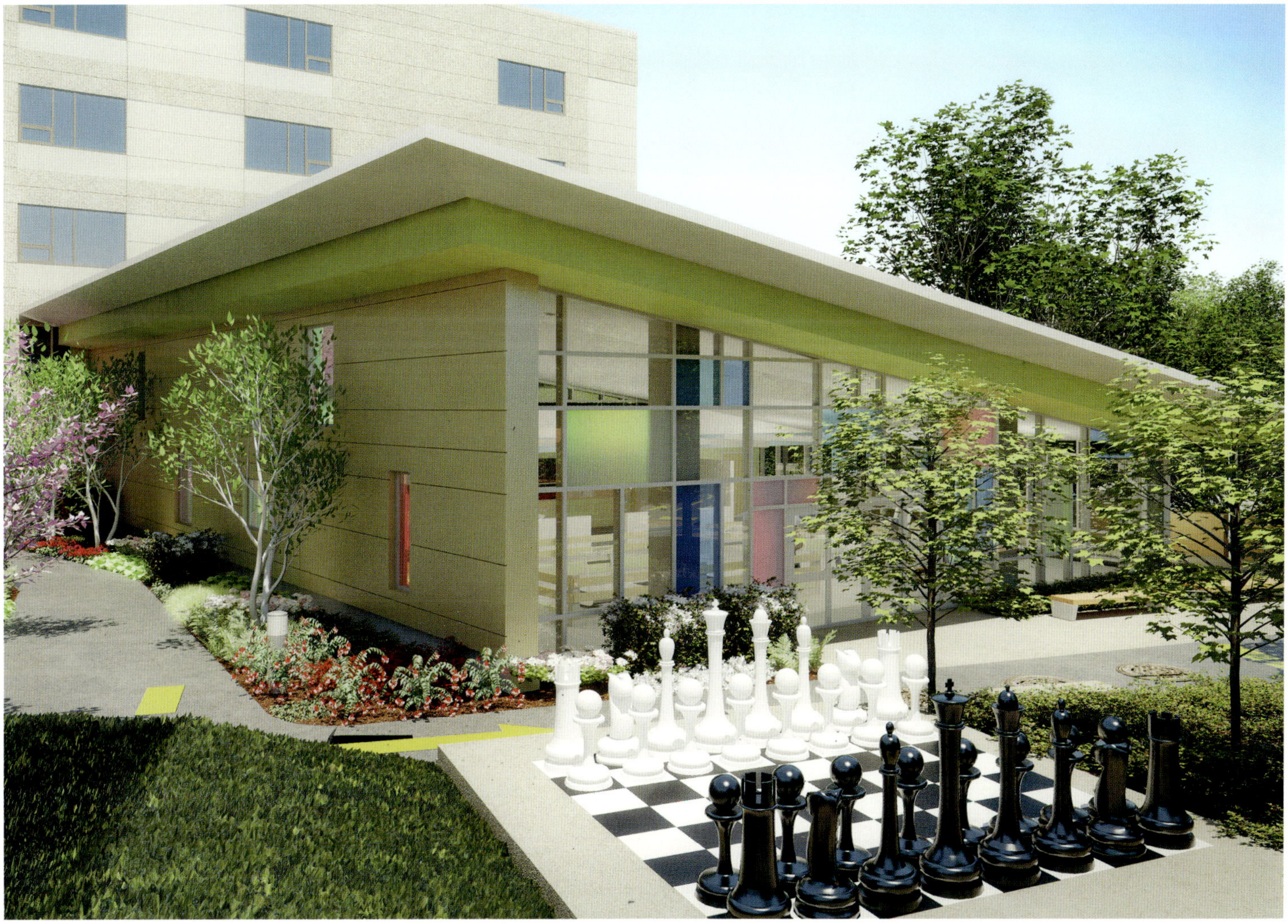

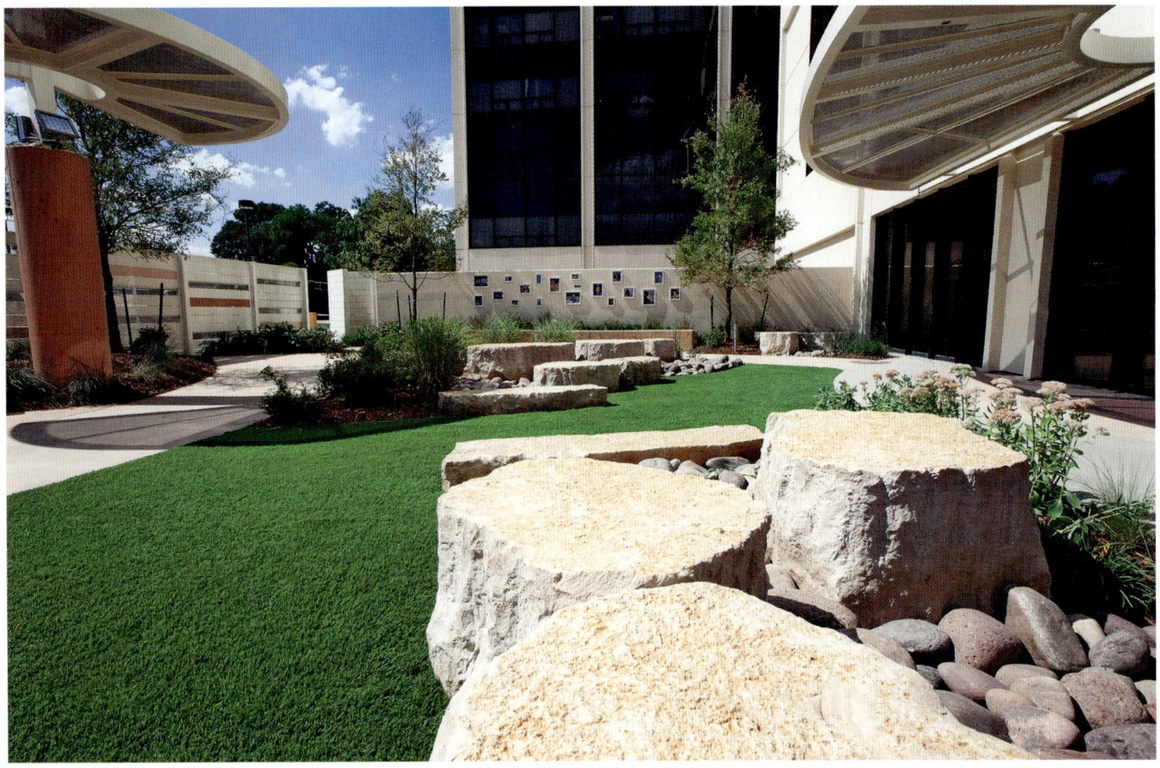

▲ Medical City Children's Hospital, Dallas, TX
Photo: Terry Cockerham

▼ Rady Children's Hospital, San Diego, CA
Photo: Stantec © RMA Photography

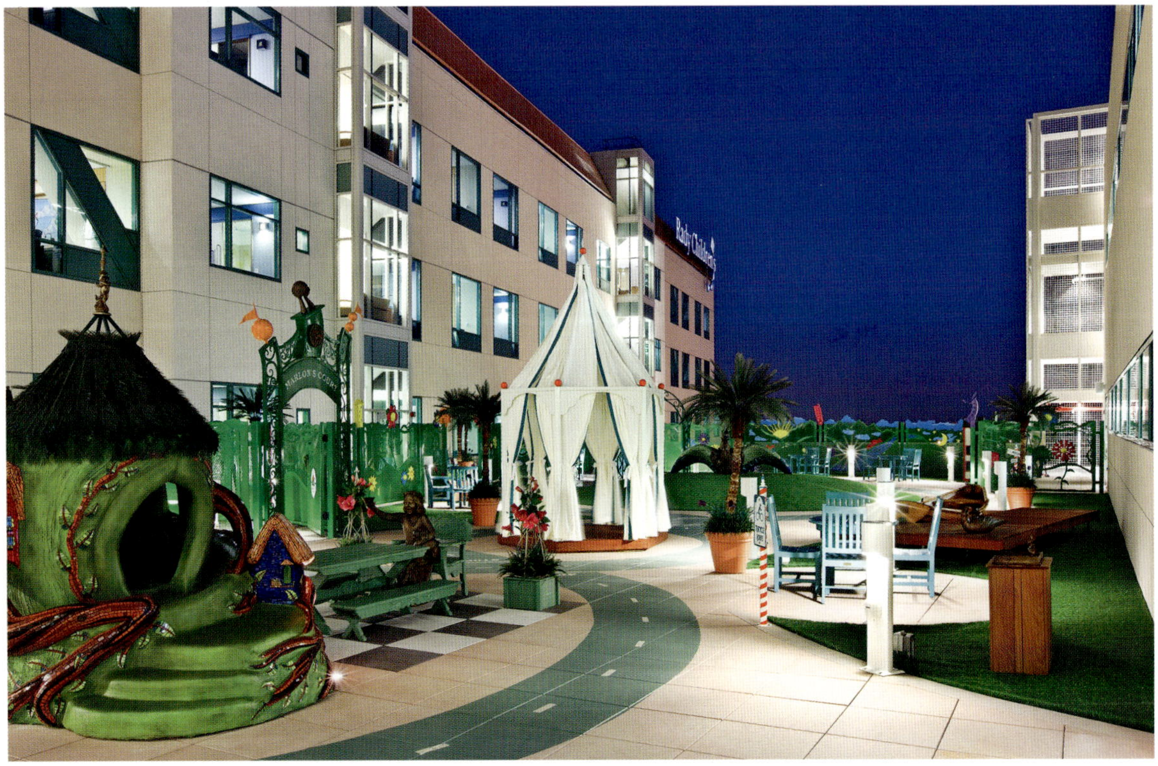

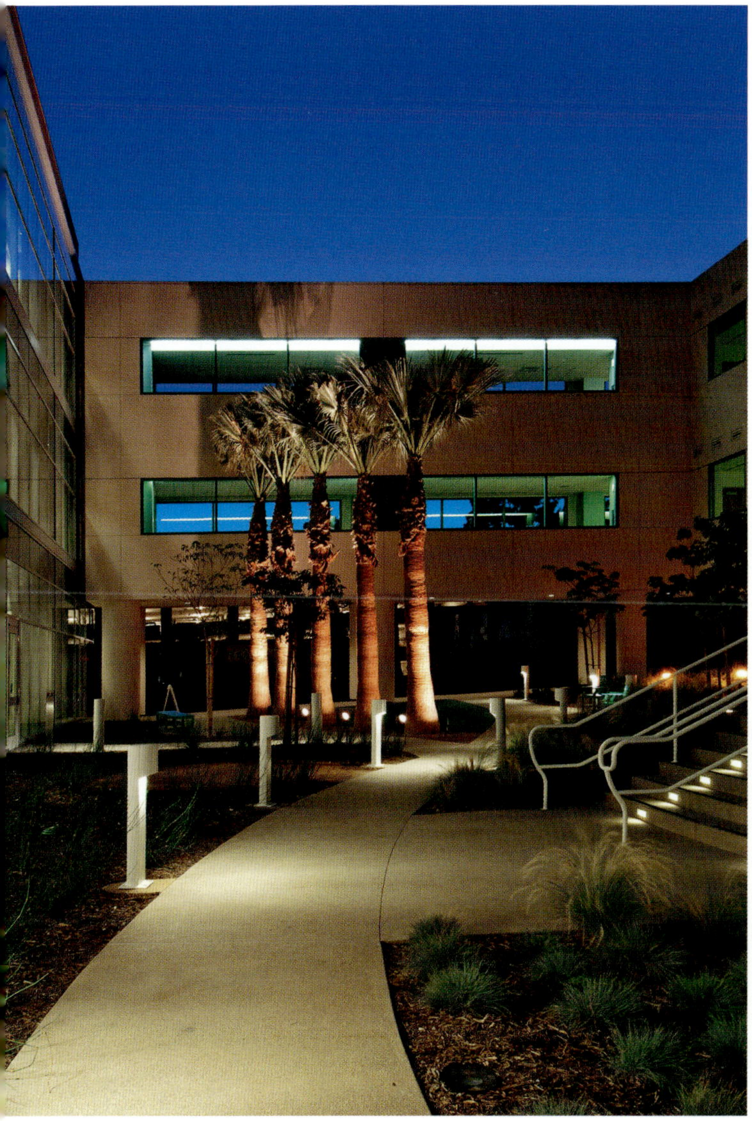

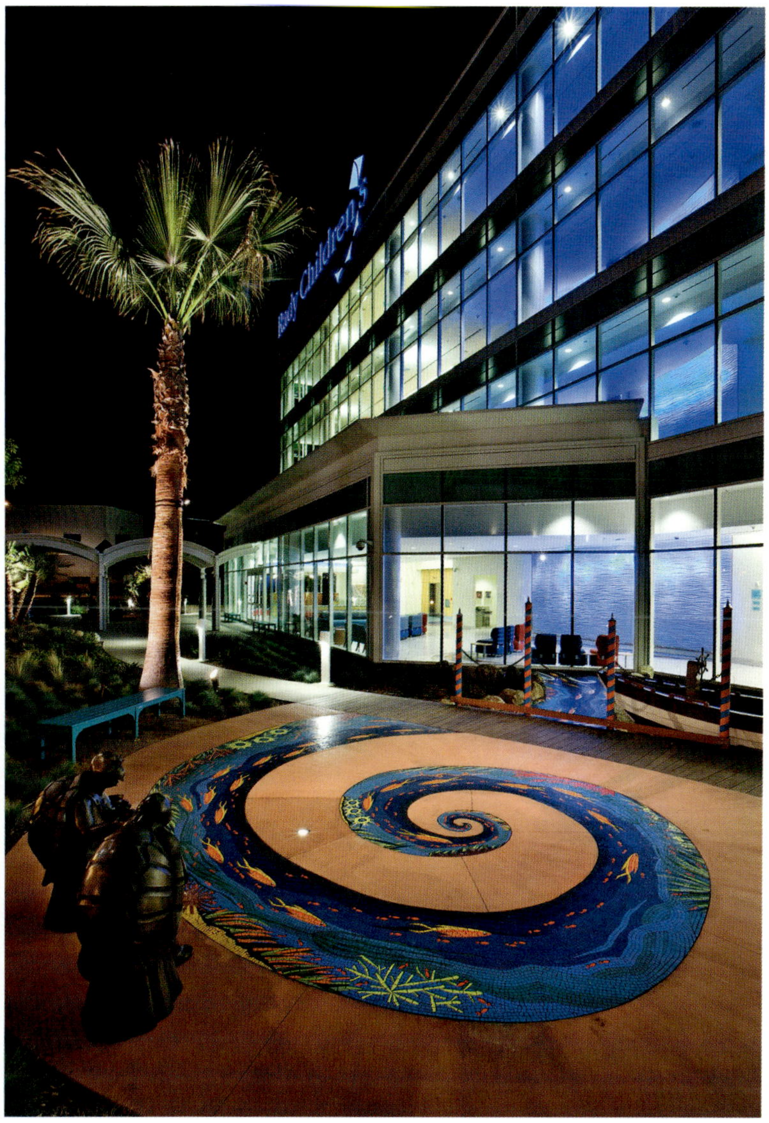

▲ Rady Children's Hospital, San Diego, CA
Photos: Stantec © RMA Photography

Following pages: Mattel Children's Hospital UCLA, Los Angeles, CA
Photo: Benny Chan, fotoworks

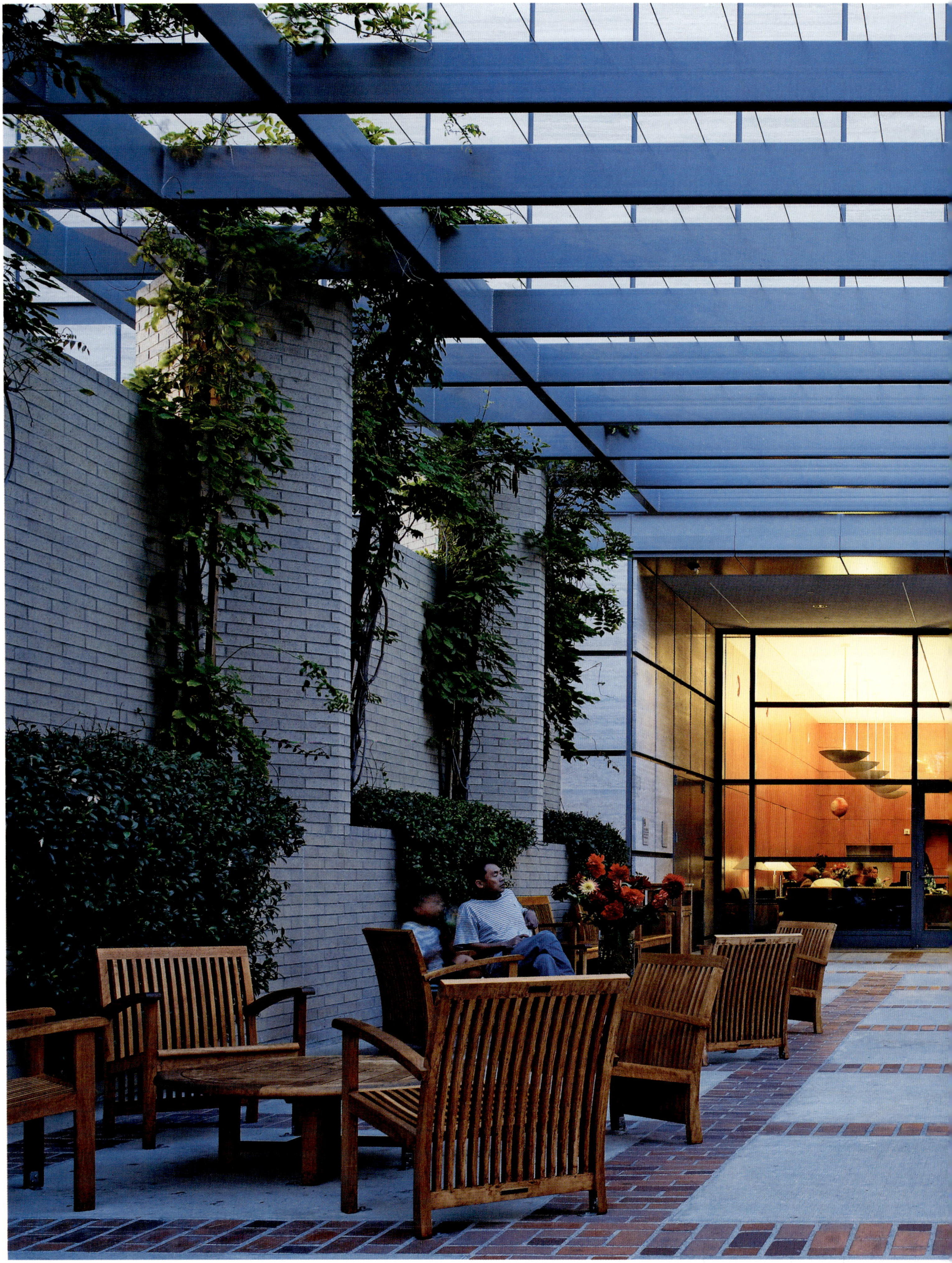

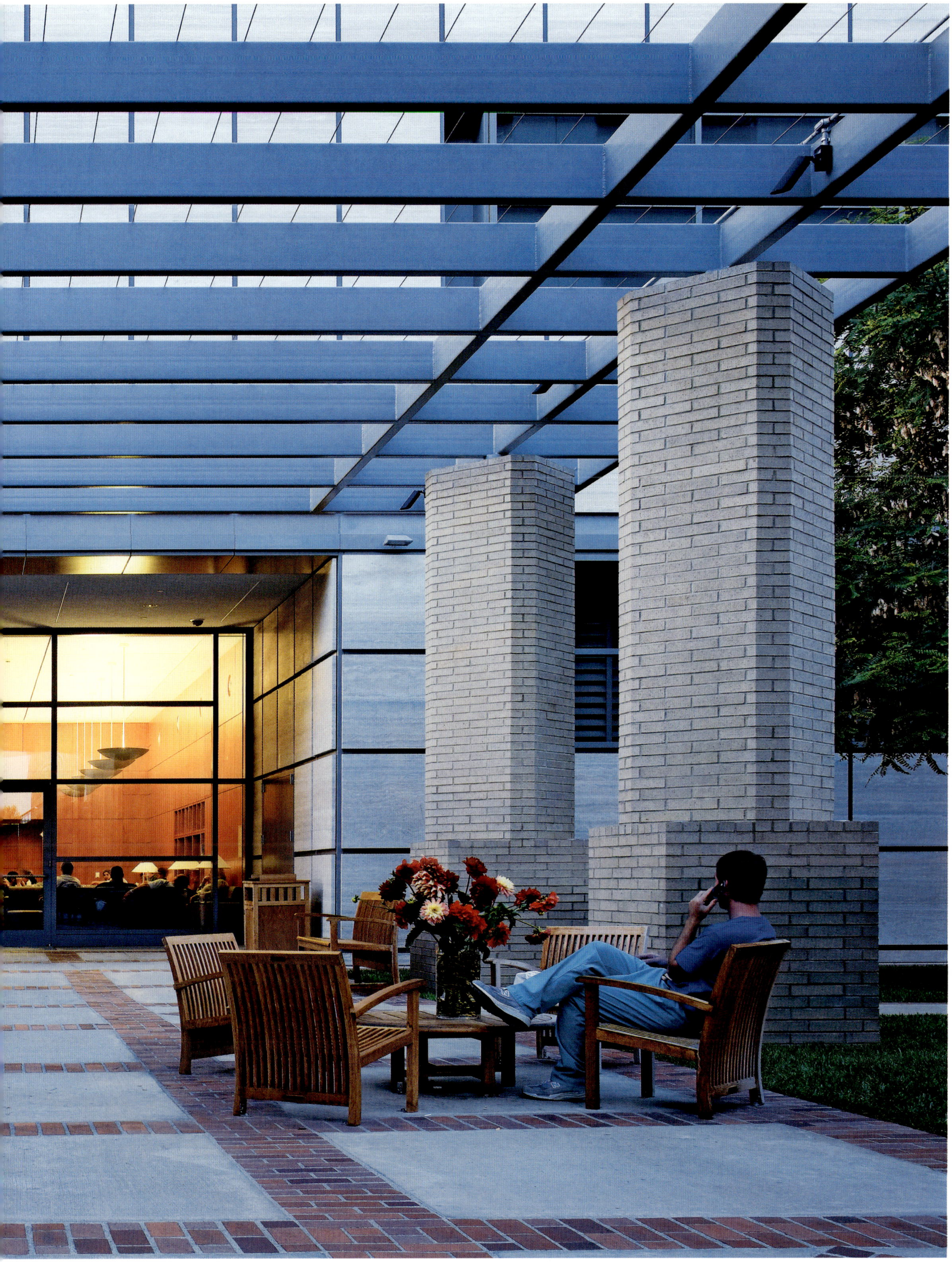

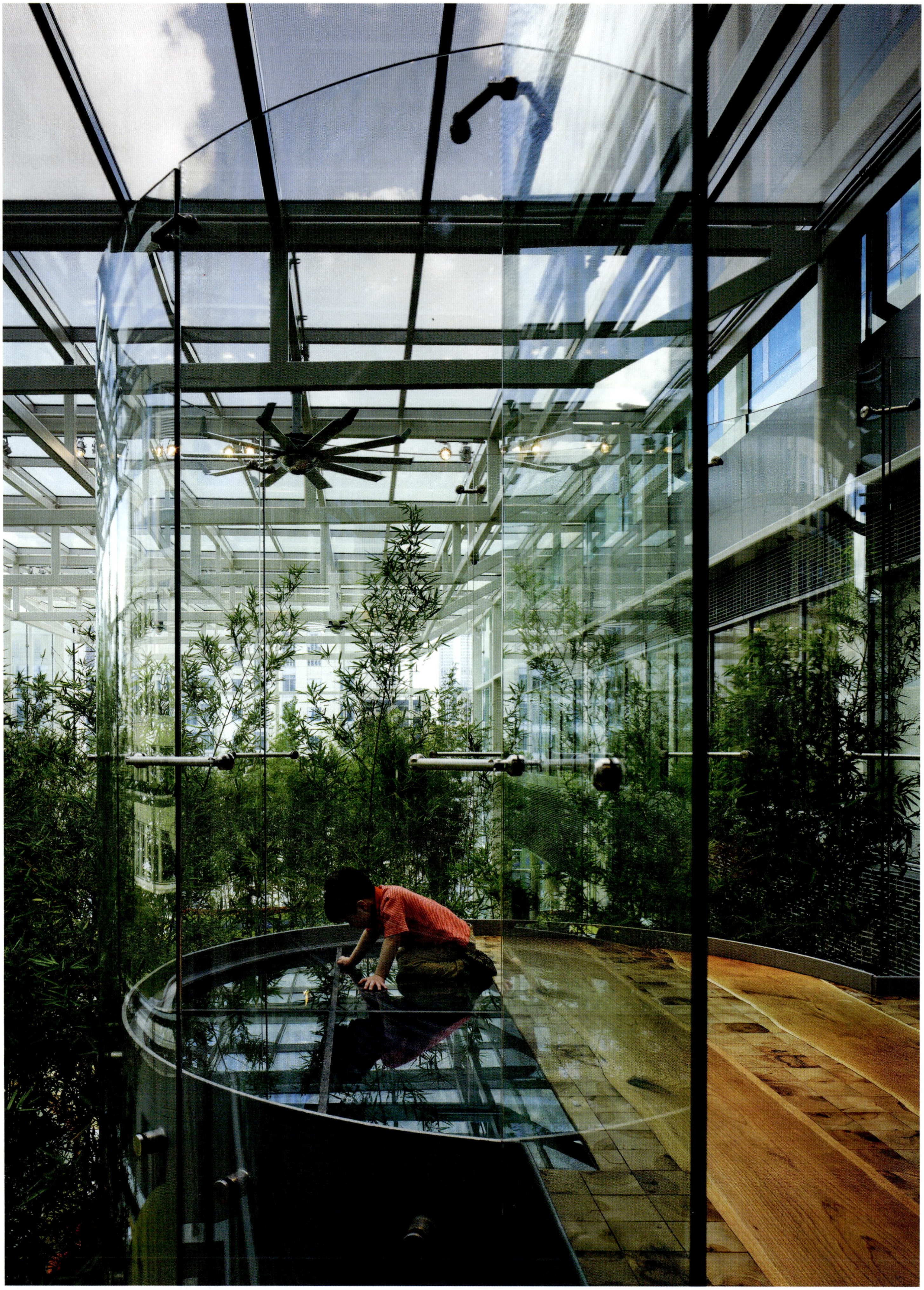

The Future

Pediatrics will be at the center of translational medicine research, with genetic and targeted therapies growing in volume rapidly. Since the infusion chair will be the "translational environment of the future," facility design today needs to consider flexibility of space and infrastructure to expand the genomics-based medicine environment and its required support in ambulatory care and clinical research areas. It is our responsibility as architects and clients to design clinic environments that can operate flexibly today, and be transformed with ease into family consultation and counseling, genetic intervention, and personalized medicine support areas tomorrow.

Other significant drivers of future design for children and families include the integration of obstetric and neonatal services (couplet care and maternal–fetal medicine); survival of very low birth weight and severely premature infants, which will require increasingly specialized environments and access to sophisticated technologies (MRI-compatible isolettes); the movement towards 'gentler imaging', which will result in increased use of non-ionizing radiation modalities (MRI, ultrasound, etc.); and the escalating rate of obesity in children, which suggests accommodation of increased services and staff for wellness, prevention, and community outreach. The role of the children's hospital in the future will be to both take care of the sickest children and to promote the Health of the next generation.

Annie Coull
Stantec Architecture

◀ Ann & Robert H. Lurie Children's Hospital of Chicago, IL
Photo: Hedrich Blessing Photography, Nick Merrick

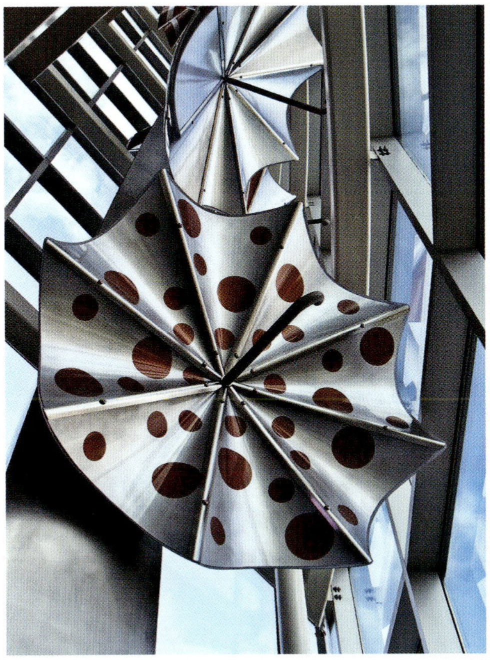

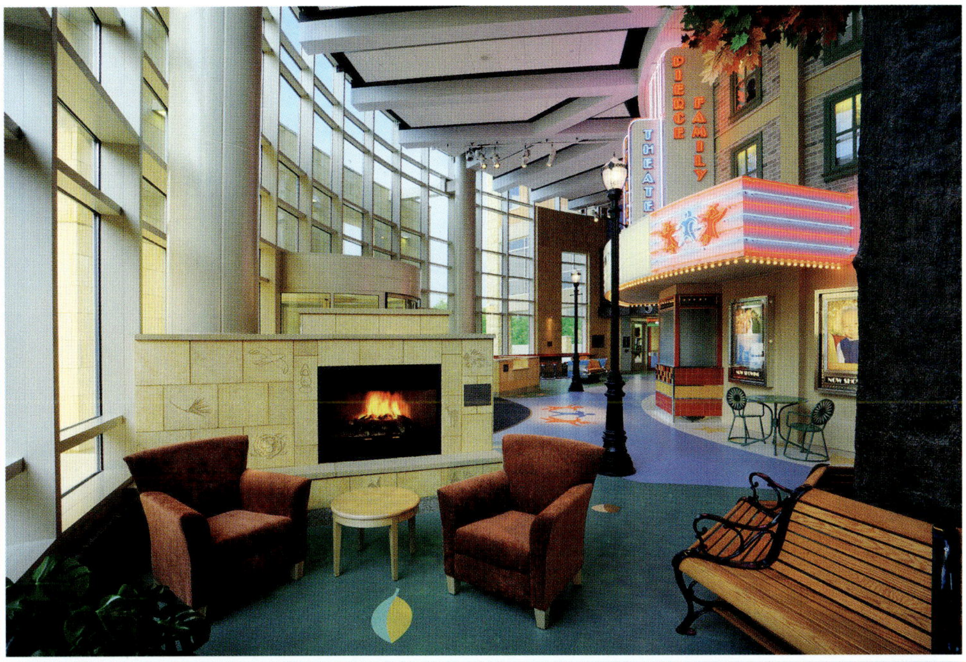

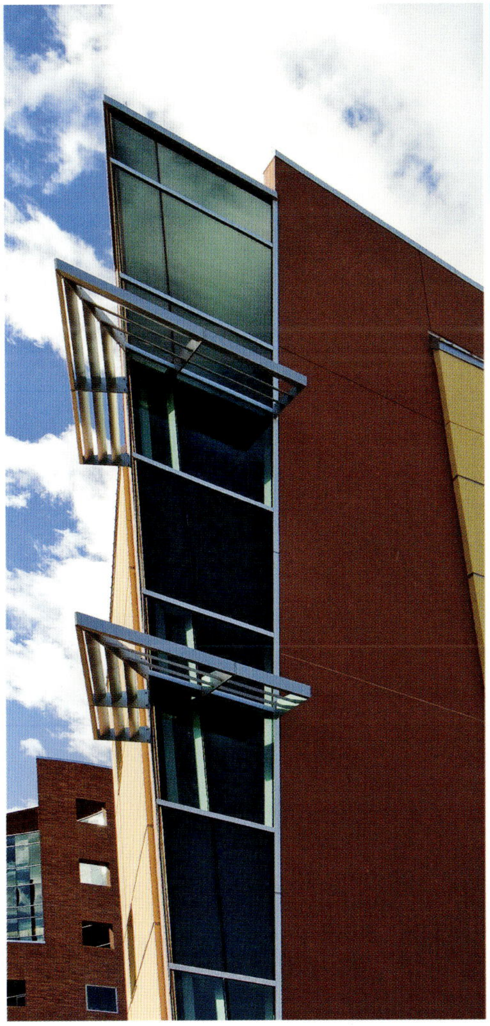

Healing Spaces for Little Faces

HDR Architecture is a global leader in integrated, multidisciplinary design. Our parent company was founded more than 90 years ago as a small Midwestern civil engineering firm; since the 1950s, our architecture practice has grown to nearly 1,700 employees, including architects, engineers, planners, consultants and designers located in more than 40 offices worldwide. HDR's talented team of designers is world-renowned for designing intelligent buildings that express our clients' missions and values.

Our design teams recognize the unique physical and emotional needs associated with creating healing and patient-centered spaces for children. We are dedicated to incorporating advanced evidence-based design concepts that contribute to the healing process of this very special patient population, and we understand the roles that a caregiver and family play in improving clinical outcomes. Our constant goal is the thoughtful design of innovative healthcare environments for every child.

HDR Architecture, Inc.
8404 Indian Hills Drive
Omaha, NE 68114
Phone: 800-366-4411
Fax: 402-399-1238
Email: info@hdrinc.com

Jim Hohenstein, AIA
Director of Pediatric Healthcare
Design & Planning
Jim.Hohenstein@hdrinc.com

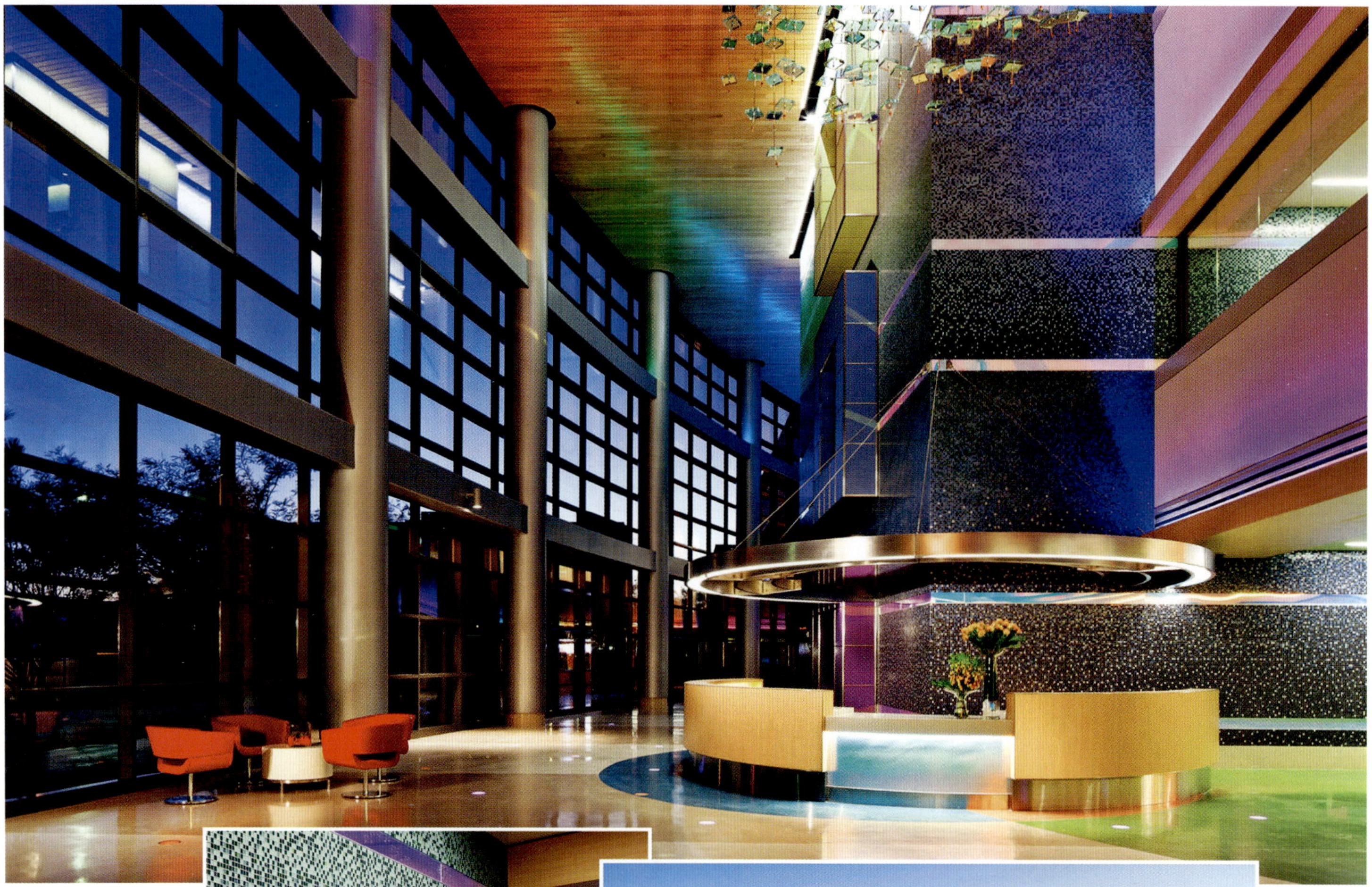

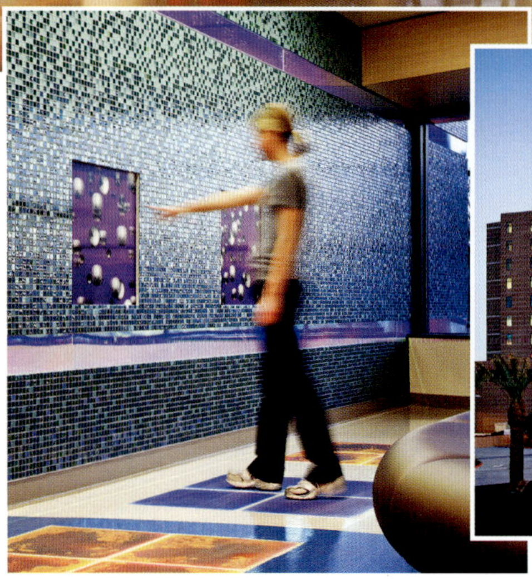

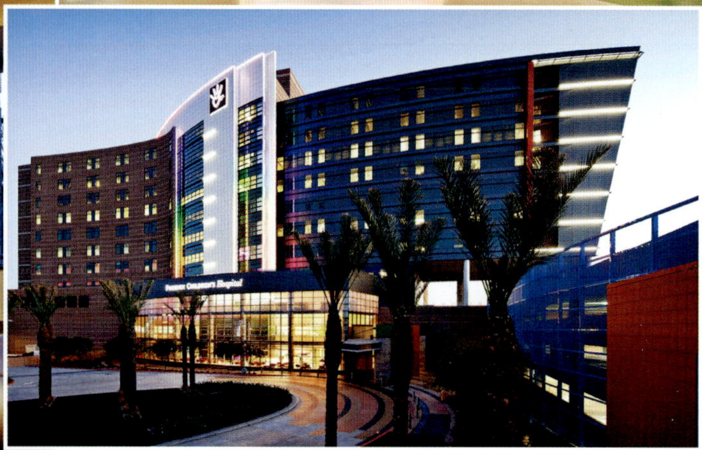

HKS

Enhancing the Human Experience

Today's children's medical facilities are transporting kids and their families into a world of healing, caring and learning. From the lobby to the patient room, the hospital's mission is clear – children of all ages and their families come first. Our designs are enhancing the human experience by addressing questions raised by parents including, "Is my child being cared for in the best, safest and most inspiring environment?" We infuse evidence-informed design principles, working with the client, family advisory groups and the community.

HKSINC.COM | 29 OFFICES WORLDWIDE
HKS, Inc. Jeffrey Stouffer, AIA Principal/Director of Pediatric Facilities jstouffer@hksinc.com

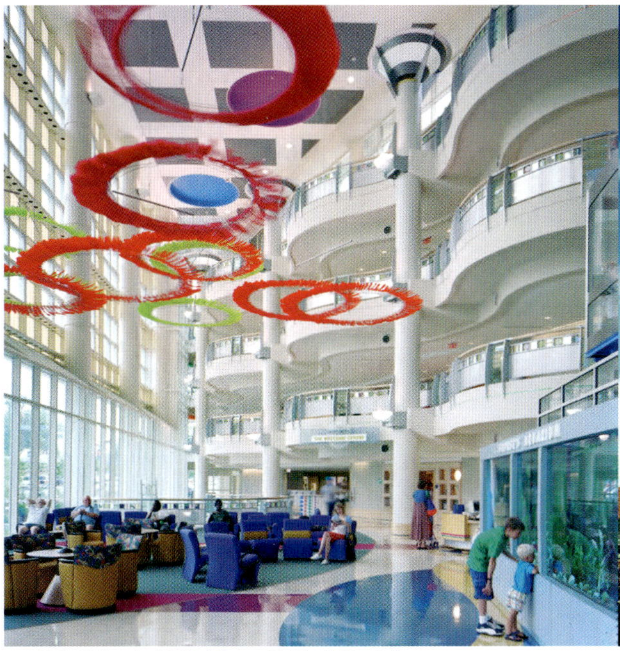

Duke University Medical Center Children's Hospital

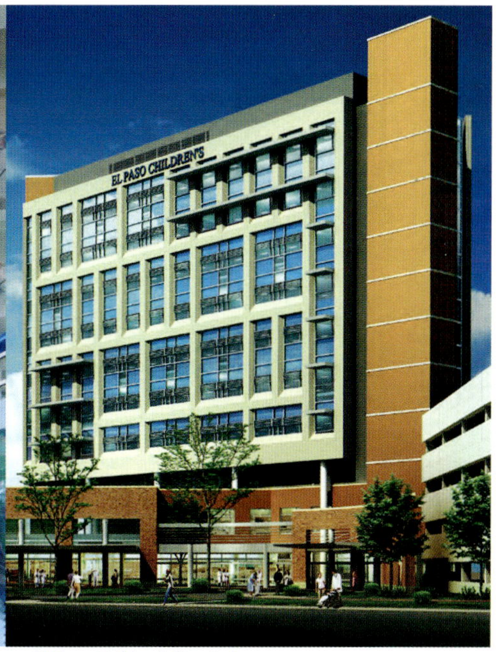

El Paso Children's Hospital

KMDARCHITECTS

san francisco • seattle • portland • los angeles • dallas • mexico city • dubai

www.kmdarchitects.com

Since 1963, KMD Architects has established itself as an international planning and design firm with practices in healthcare, mixed-use, corporate, retail, hospitality and academia.

The phased renovation and expansion of two entire floors of **Children's Medical Center Dallas** will create new homes for two centers of excellence for the Heart and Cancer programs. The designs of each Center will seamlessly join inpatient and outpatient care, procedures and diagnostics.

The **Children's Hospital** lobby at the **Duke University Medical Center** is a prime example of "placemaking." KMD created a fresh and captivating environment for children and families.

The new **El Paso Children's Hospital** is the culmination of a successful civic campaign and bond issue election to create a new, distinct hospital within the larger **University Medical Center**. Pediatric and women's services share a new eleven story tower and entrance lobby.

Children's Medical Center Dallas

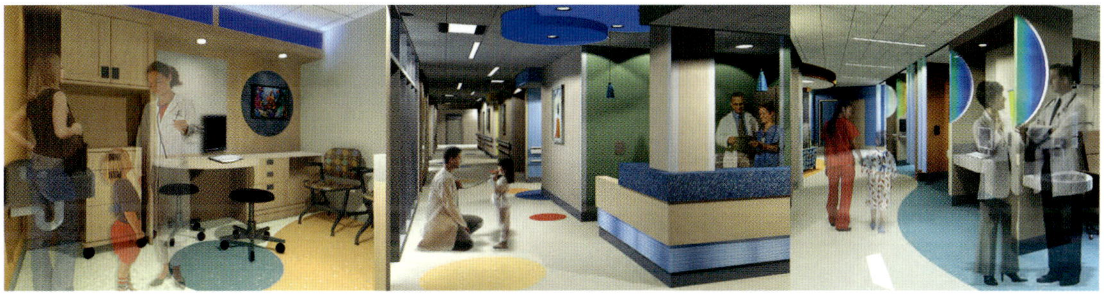

PUBLIC SPACES

Public space in a children's hospital is more than just a friendly entrance or a comforting waiting room. These popular environments provide a unique opportunity for design teams, hospital staff and patients to create an experience that speaks to each of the institutional stakeholders. More importantly, these common areas offer a way for children's hospitals to distinguish themselves appropriately from their adult counterparts.

Such spaces can be challenging to execute. Too often, the public realm in a children's hospital looks like it was born of a Saturday cartoon or a scene out of a movie. They need to be timeless, making sense to all hospitals users, whether staff, a mother of a PICU patient, or a teenager who has spent months, if not years, within its walls. What is more, public spaces must carefully balance a design vision with the medical culture of the hospital. They must be functional - from accommodating clinical needs to addressing a hospital's security regulations. To be truly successful they should create a sense of community, beckon interactivity, and inspire confidence in the patients, families and staff that use them daily.

Public space in a children's hospital can be a powerful and captivating experience.

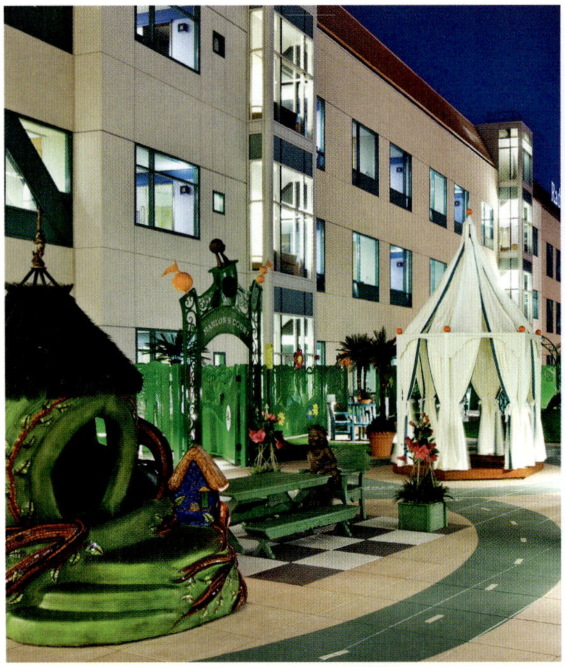

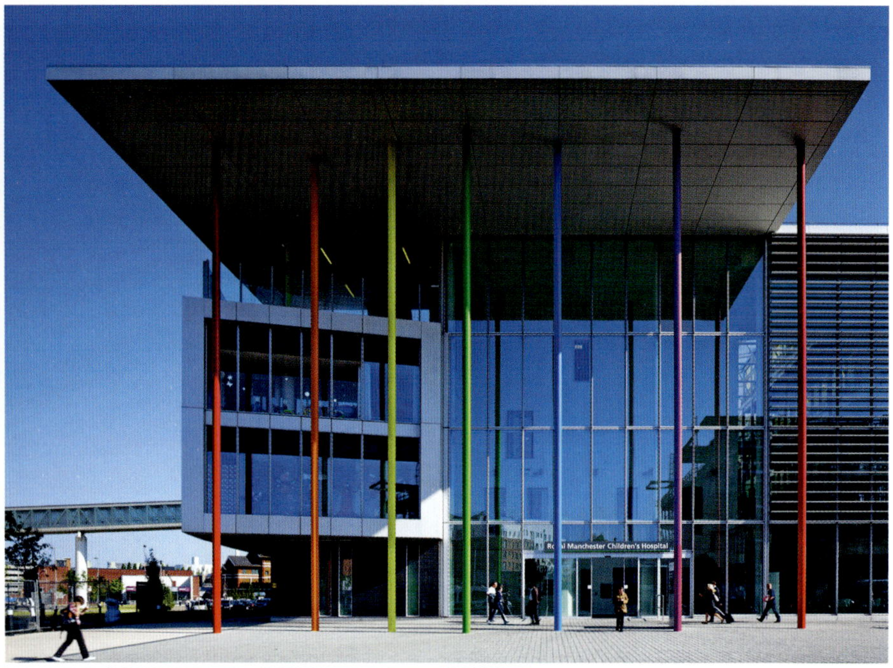

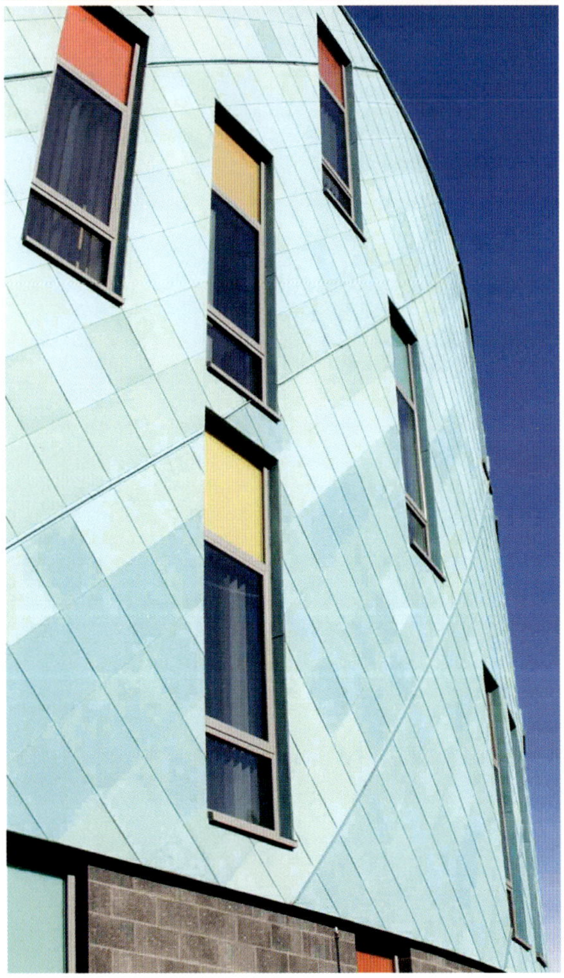

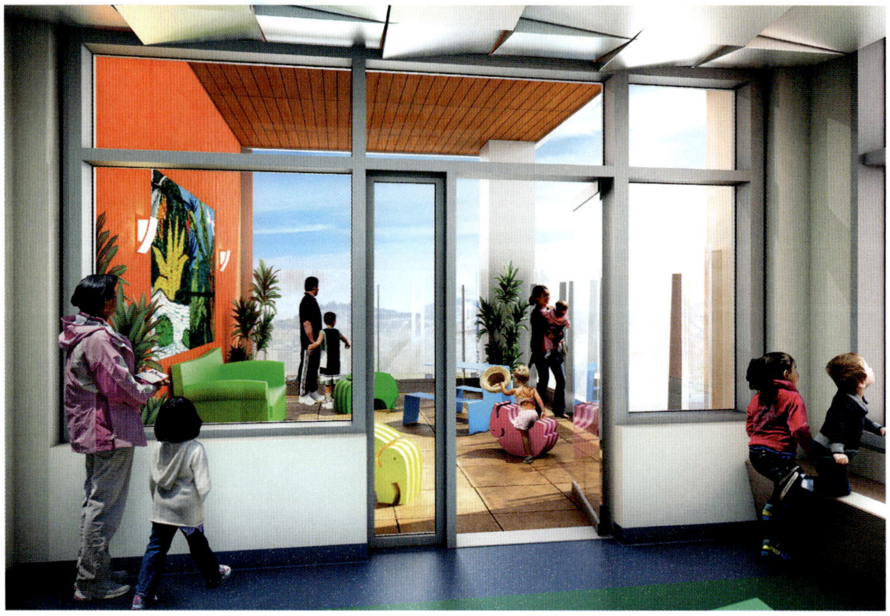

PORTLAND | SEATTLE | LOS ANGELES | WASHINGTON, DC | NEW YORK

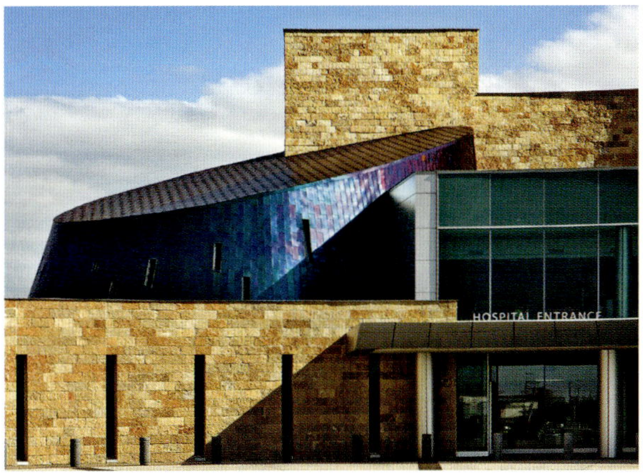

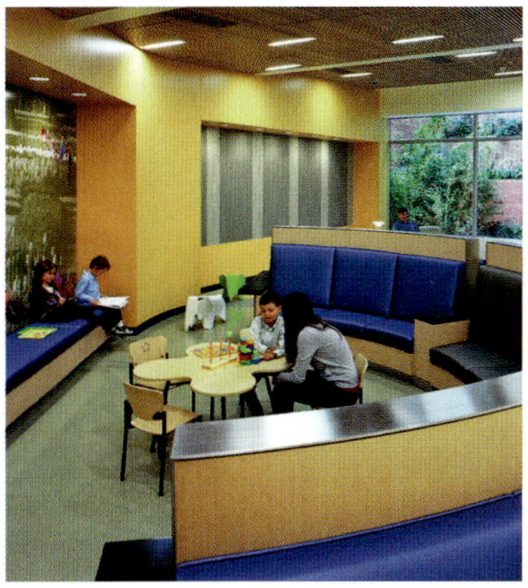

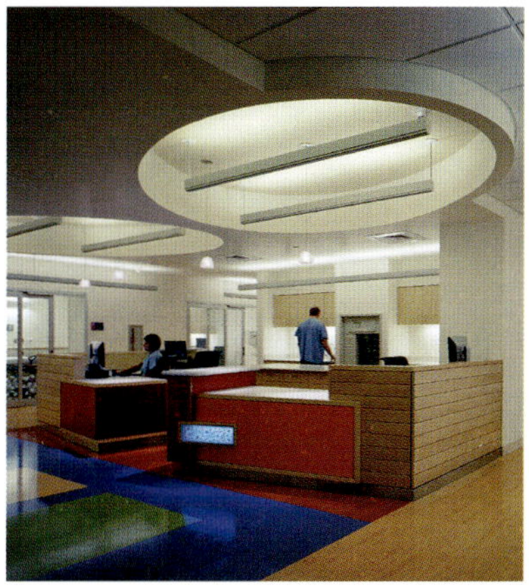

HEALTHCARE ENVIRONMENTS

FOR CHILDREN, THEIR FAMILIES, AND STAFF

ZGF creates healing environments that are influenced by the latest thinking in patient- and family-centered care. From public spaces to patient rooms, nursing units to corridors, our designers consider how patient care and safety issues can be enhanced by nature, daylight, and color, while positively affecting the experiences of patients, families, and staff. For more information visit www.zgf.com.

ZGF

ZIMMER GUNSUL FRASCA ARCHITECTS LLP

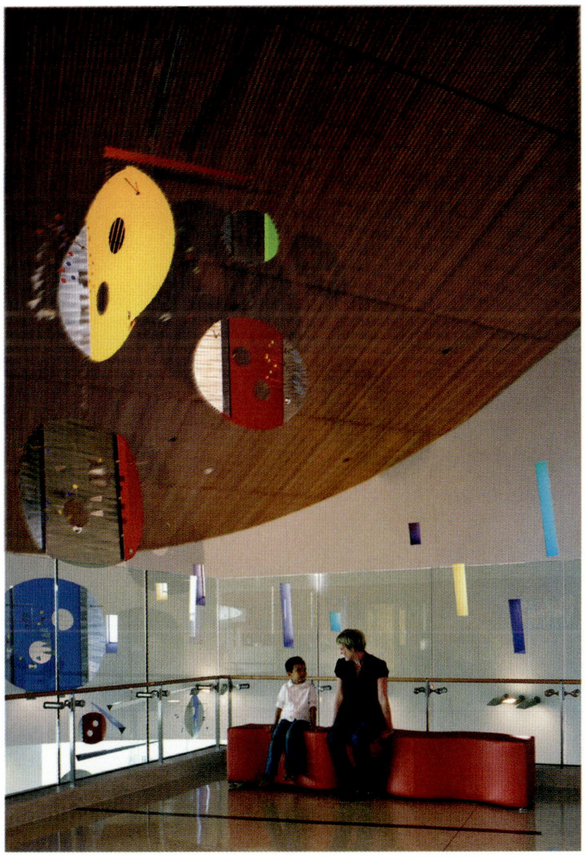

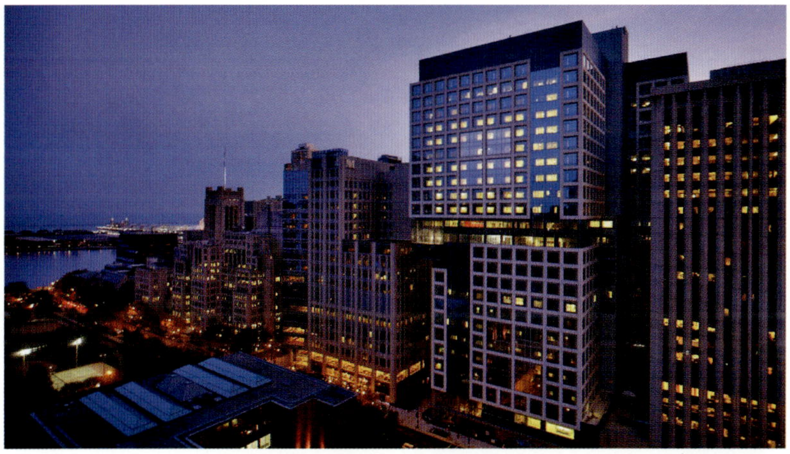

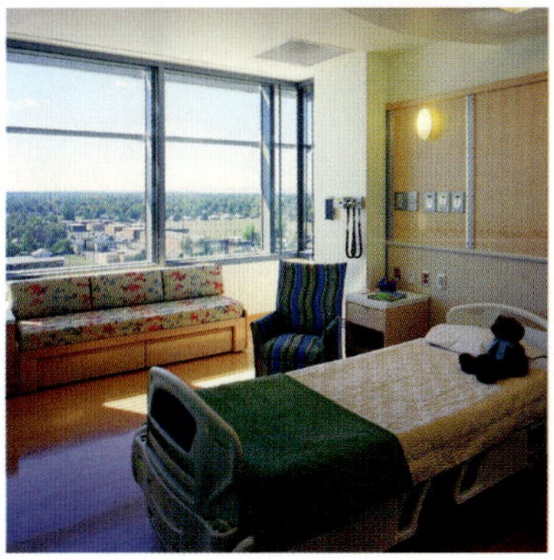

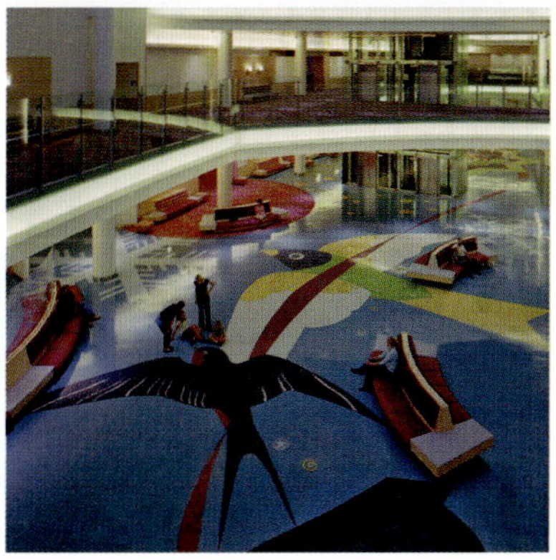

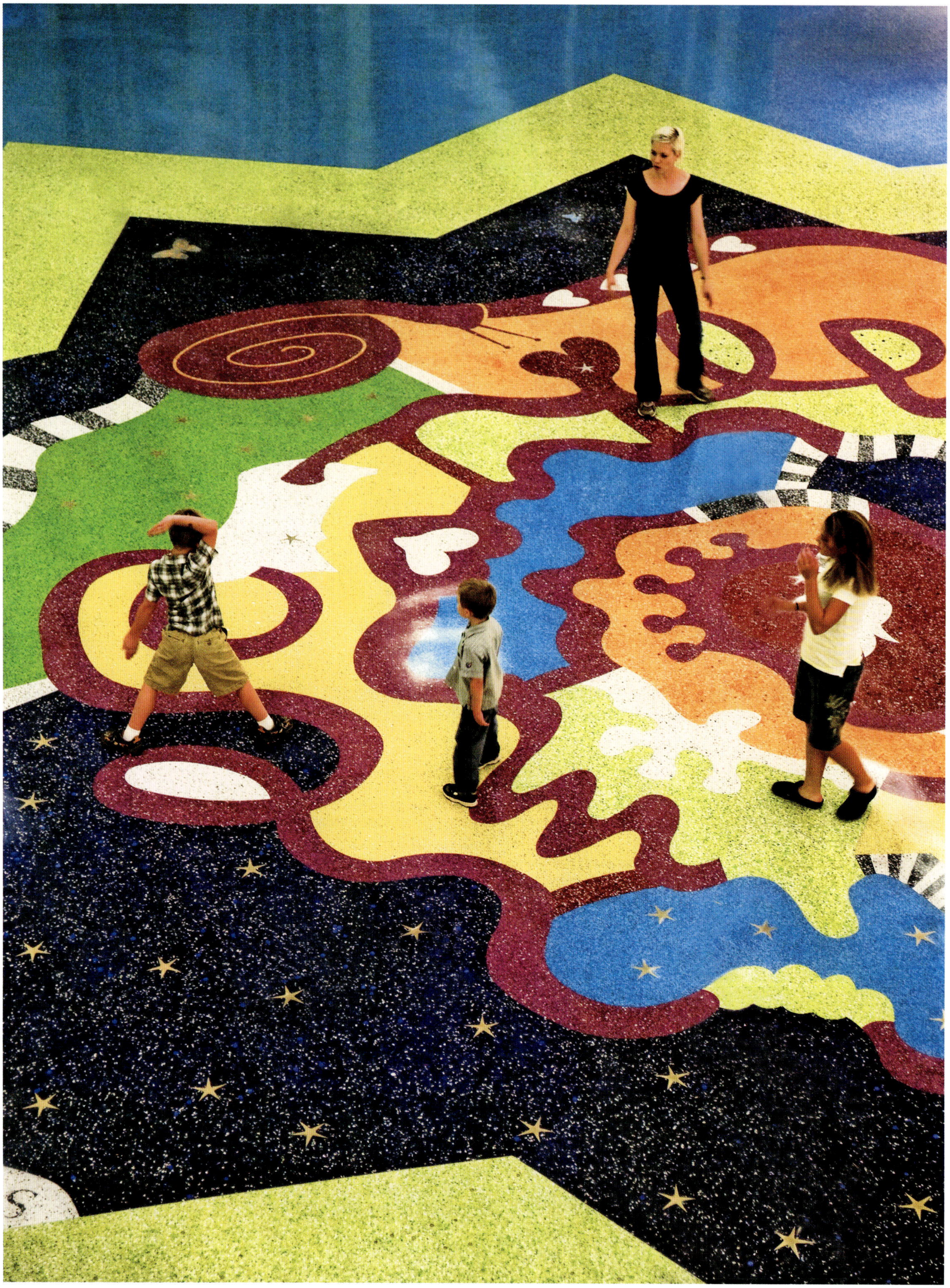

▲ Children's Hospital Colorado, Denver, CO
Photo: Eckert & Eckert

US State Abbreviations

Alabama	**AL**
Alaska	**AK**
Arizona	**AZ**
Arkansas	**AR**
California	**CA**
Colorado	**CO**
Connecticut	**CT**
Delaware	**DE**
District of Columbia	**DC**
Florida	**FL**
Georgia	**GA**
Hawaii	**HA**
Idaho	**ID**
Illinois	**IL**
Indiana	**IN**
Iowa	**IA**
Kansas	**KS**
Kentucky	**KY**
Louisiana	**LA**
Maine	**ME**
Maryland	**MD**
Massachusetts	**MA**
Michigan	**MI**
Minnesota	**MN**
Mississippi	**MS**
Missouri	**MO**
Montana	**MT**
Nebraska	**NE**
Nevada	**NV**
New Hampshire	**NH**
New Jersey	**NJ**
New Mexico	**NM**
New York	**NY**
North Carolina	**NC**
North Dakota	**ND**
Ohio	**OH**
Oklahoma	**OK**
Oregon	**OR**
Pennsylvania	**PA**
Rhode Island	**RI**
South Carolina	**SC**
South Dakota	**SD**
Tennessee	**TN**
Texas	**TX**
Utah	**UT**
Vermont	**VT**
Virginia	**VA**
Washington	**WA**
West Virginia	**WV**
Wisconsin	**WI**
Wyoming	**WY**

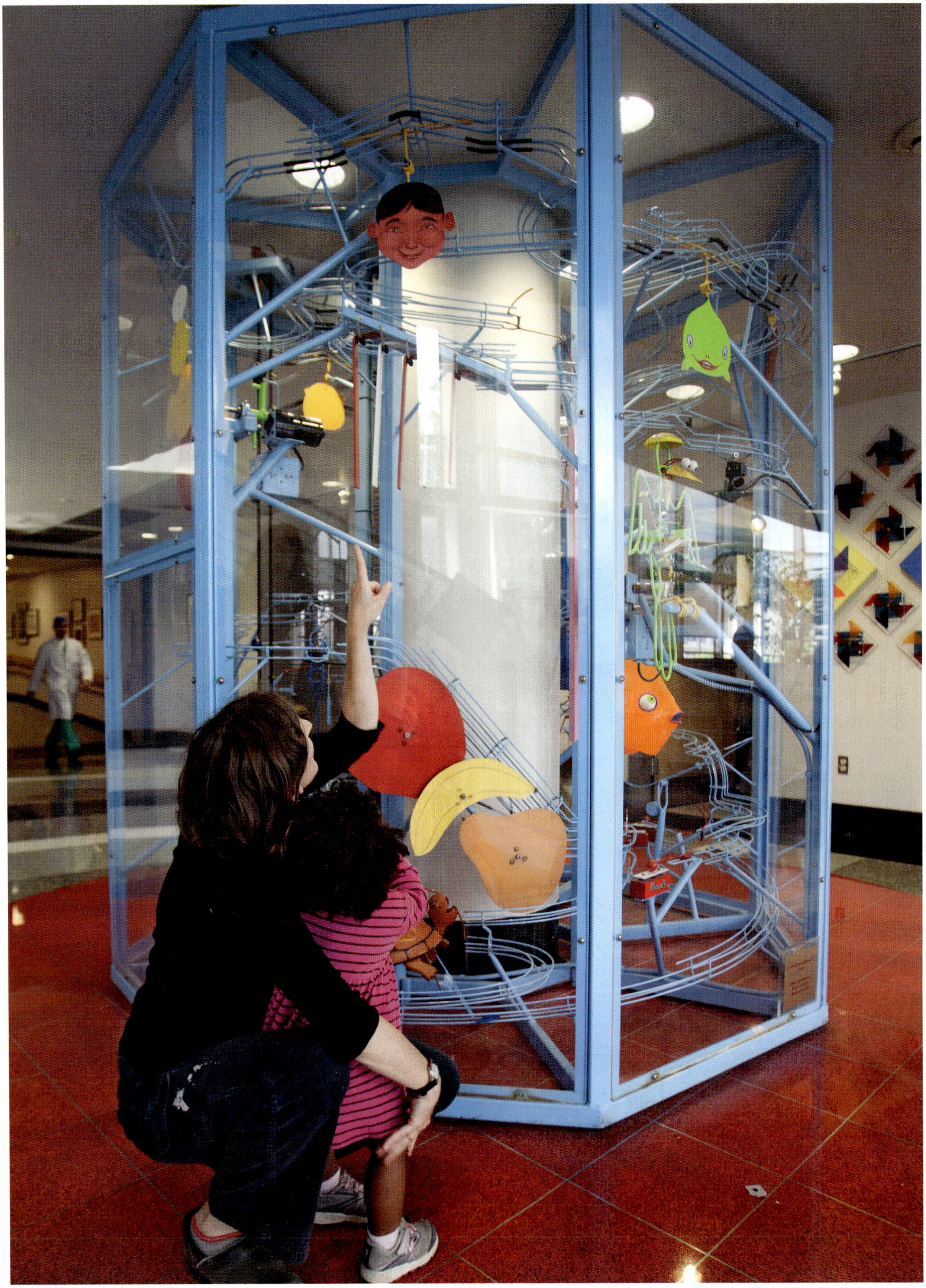

Acknowledgments

Special Thanks

- FKP, HDR, HKS, KMD, Stantec, ZGF—without their support there would be no book
- Larry McAndrews and the NACHRI staff for embracing the concept from the beginning
- All the NACHRI Hospitals and other organizations that have shared the photos of their facilities so that others will benefit
- Ken Labok for his tireless efforts in tracking, sorting, and compiling the 1,000s of images that were submitted, and Jim Gimple for his excellent editing skills
- Pat Magoon and the incredible staff at Children's Memorial Hospital for their continued inspiration

◀ UNC North Carolina Children's Hospital, Chapel Hill, NC
Photo: Brian Strickland